Inflammatory Bowel Disease
Basic Research, Clinical Implications and Trends in Therapy

Inflammatory Bowel Disease

Basic Research, Clinical Implications and Trends in Therapy

EDITED BY

L. R. Sutherland
Professor of Medicine, Head
Division of Gastroenterology
The University of Calgary
Alberta
Canada

S. M. Collins
Chief
Division of Gastroenterology
McMaster University
Faculty of Health Sciences
Hamilton, Ontario, Canada

F. Martin
Professor of Medicine
Chief
Division of Gastroenterology
St Luc Hospital
Montreal, Quebec, Canada

R. S. McLeod
Head of the Clinical Epidemiology
Program
Associate Professor
Department of Surgery
University of Toronto
Mount Sinai Hospital
Toronto, Ontario, Canada

S. R. Targan
Director
Inflammatory Bowel Disease Center
Cedars-Sinai Medical Center
Los Angeles
California, USA

J. L. Wallace
Professor of Medical Physiology and
Medicine
University of Calgary
Health Sciences Center
Calgary, Alberta, Canada

C. N. Williams
Professor and Head,
Division of Gastroenterology
Dalhousie University
Faculty of Medicine
Clinical Research Center
Halifax, Nova Scotia, Canada

The proceedings of two symposia held in Victoria, BC, Canada, in April 1994, co-sponsored by Axcan Pharma, Inc., The Crohn's and Colitis Foundation of Canada, and The Canadian Association of Gastroenterology.

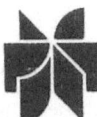

KLUWER ACADEMIC PUBLISHERS
DORDRECHT / BOSTON / LONDON

Distributors

for the United States and Canada: Kluwer Academic Publishers, PO Box 358, Accord Station, Hingham, MA 02018-0358, USA
for all other countries: Kluwer Academic Publishers Group, Distribution Center, PO Box 322, 3300 AH Dordrecht, The Netherlands

A catalogue record for this book is available from the British Library.

ISBN-13:978-94-010-6653-2

Library of Congress Cataloging in Publication Data

```
Inflammatory bowel disease : basic research, clinical implications,
  and trends in therapy / edited by L.R. Sutherland ... [et al.].
      p.   cm.
  "The proceedings of two symposia held in Victoria, BC, Canada, in
April 1994, co-sponsored by Axcan Pharma, Inc., the Crohn's and
Colitis Foundation of Canada, and the Canadian Association of
Gastroenterology."
  Includes bibliographical references and index.
  ISBN-13:978-94-010-6653-2       e-ISBN-13:978-94-009-0371-5
  DOI: 10.1007/978-94-009-0371-5


   1. Inflammatory bowel diseases--Congresses.   I. Sutherland, L.
II. Axcan Pharma, Inc.   III. Crohn's and Colitis Foundation of
Canada.   IV. Canadian Association of Gastroenterology.
  [DNLM: 1. Inflammatory Bowel Diseases--etiology--congresses.
2. Inflammatory Bowel Diseases--therapy--congresses.
3. Inflammatory Bowel Diseases--physiopathology--congresses.   WI
420 I423 1994]
RC862.I53I5233   1994
616.3'44--dc20
DNLM/DLC
for Library of Congress                                    94-38684
                                                               CIP
```

Copyright

Published in the United Kingdom by Kluwer Academic Publishers, PO Box 55, Lancaster, UK.

Kluwer Academic Publishers BV incorporates the publishing programmes of D. Reidel, Martinus Nijhoff, Dr W. Junk and MTP Press.

Typeset by Lasertext Ltd., Stretford, Manchester, UK

Contents

PART 2: TRENDS IN IBD THERAPY 1994

Section VI: CRITICAL APPRAISAL OF CLINICAL TRIALS

Section VII: BASIC SCIENCE: GENETICS, MARKERS AND MODELS

Section VIII: BASIC SCIENCE: PATHOGENESIS

CONTENTS

List of Principal Authors

RN Allan
Queen Elizabeth Hospital
Edgbaston
Birmingham B15 2TH
UK

KE Barrett
UCSD Medical Center, 8414
200 West Arbor Drive
San Diego, CA 92103-8414
USA

TM Bayless
Meyerhoff DD-IBD Centre
Johns Hopkins Hospital
600 North Wolfe Street
Baltimore, MD 21205
USA

IT Beck
Queen's University
Kingstown
Ontario
Canada

C Benoni
Department of Medicine
Helsingborg Hospital
S-251 87 Helsingborg
Sweden

I Bjarnason
Department of Clinical Biochemistry
King's College School of Medicine
Bessemer Road
London SE5 9PJ
UK

J Braun
Department of Pathology
UCLA School of Medicine
Los Angeles, CA 90024
USA

TC Chalmers
MetaWorks Inc.
32 Pinewood Village
West Lebanon, NH 03784
USA

Z Cohen
Department of Surgery
Mount Sinai Hospital
600 University Avenue Suite 451
Toronto
Ontario M5G 1X5
Canada

SM Collins
McMaster University Medical Centre
1200 Main Street West, Room 4W8
Hamilton
Ontario L8N 3Z5
Canada

K Croitoru
IDRP, Department of Medicine
McMaster University
1200 Main St West, Rm 4H17
Hamilton
Ontario L8N 3Z5
Canada

GS Eisenbarth
Barbara Davis Center for Child
 Diabetes
University of Colorado Health Science
 Center
4200 East 9th Ave, Box B140
Denver, CO 80262
USA

AM Ekbom
University Hospital
Cancer Epidemiology Unit
S-751 85 Uppsala
Sweden

CO Elson
Division of Gastroenterology
UAB Station
Birmingham, AL 35294–8493
USA

RG Farmer
Georgetown University Medical
  Center
Georgetown
USA

C Fiocchi
Division of Gastroenterology
Case Western Reserve University
School of Medicine
Cleveland, OH 44195-5014
USA

MB Grisham
Department of Physiology
LSU Medical Center
1501 Kings Highway
Shreveport, LA 71130
USA

SB Hanauer
University of Chicago
Medical Centre
5841 Maryland Avenue
Chicago, IL 60637
USA

TL Hull
Department of Colon and Rectal
  Surgery
Cleveland Clinic Foundation
Cleveland
OH 44195
USA

EJ Irvine
Division of Gastroenterology
McMaster University
1200 Main Street West, Rm 4W8-HSC
Hamilton
Ontario L8N 3Z5
Canada

KN Jeejeebhóy
Department of Medicine
Division of Gastroenterology
University of Toronto
St Michael's Hospital
30 Bond Street 3F-372
Toronto
Ontario M5B 1W8
Canada

D Johnston
Academic Unit of Surgery
The General Infirmary
Leeds LS1 3EX
UK

EH Leiter
Senior Staff Scientist
The Jackson Laboratory
Bar Harbour, ME 04609
USA

RS McLeod
Department of Surgery, Suite 451
Mt Sinai Hospital
600 University Ave
Toronto
Ontario M5G 1X5
Canada

F Martin
Division of Gastroenteroly
St Luc Hospital
Montreal
Quebec
Canada

RJ Nicholls
Consultant Surgeon
St Mark's Hospital
City Road
London EC1V 2PS
UK

SR Nordgren
Department of Surgery
Göteborg University
Göteborg
Sweden

MH Perdue
McMaster University, HSC-3N5C
1200 Main Street West
Hamilton
Ontario L8N 3Z5
Canada

RB Sartor
Division of Digestive Diseases and
  Nutrition
University of North Carolina School of
  Medicine
CB #7080, Room 326, Burnett-Womack
  Bldg
Chapel Hill, NC 27599-7080
USA

LIST OF PRINCIPAL AUTHORS

F Shanahan
Department of Medicine
Cork Regional Hospital
Cork
Eire

KA Sharkey
Department of Medical Physiology
The University of Calgary
3330 Hospital Drive NW
Calgary
Alberta T2N 4N1
Canada

LR Sutherland
Division of Gastroenterology
The University of Calgary
3330 Hospital Drive NW
Calgary
Alberta T2N 4N1
Canada

SR Targan
IBD Center, Cedars-Sinai Medical
 Center
8700 Beverly Blvd, Suite D4063
Los Angeles, CA 90048
USA

ABR Thomson
University of Alberta
Department of Medicine
519 Newton Research Bldg
Edmonton
Alberta T6G 2C2
Canada

AJ Wakefield
University Department of Medicine
Royal Free Hospital School of
 Medicine
Rowland Hill St
London NW3 2PF
UK

JL Wallace
Gastrointestinal Research Group
University of Calgary
Calgary
Alberta T2N 4N1
Canada

CH Warden
Department of Medicine
Division of Cardiology
UCLA
Los Angeles, CA 90024-167917
USA

HP Weingarten
Department of Psychology and IDRP
McMaster University
Hamilton
Ontario L8S 4K1
Canada

CN Williams
Division of Gastroenterology
Department of Medicine
Dalhousie University
Halifax
Nova Scotia B3H 4H7
Canada

NA Wright
Department of Histopathology
RPMS, Hammersmith Hospital
DuCane Road
London
UK

H Yang
Division of Medical Genetics and IBD
 Center
Departments of Medicine and
 Pediatrics
Cedars-Sinai Medical Center
8700 W Beverly Blvd
Los Angeles, CA 90048
USA

Preface

The inflammatory bowel diseases, of unknown etiology and for which there are no cures, continue to attract the attention and interest of gastroenterologists, internists and surgeons. International symposia are common and it is safe to say that there is at least one major symposium held somewhere in the world each year.

This book encompasses the proceedings of two recent symposia held in Victoria, British Columbia, Canada. The symposia were the fifth and sixth international meetings focused on inflammatory bowel disease in Canada in the last eight years. Once again they were sponsored by Axcan Pharma, Inc. (formerly Interfalk Canada, Inc.) and endorsed by the Canadian Association of Gastroenterology. As has become traditional at such meetings the faculty was drawn from an international roster of leaders in the field of inflammatory bowel disease and gastroenterology.

The chapters of the proceedings provide a timely, up-to-date review of the major issues, including those within the realm of basic science and others dealing with clinical problems. The first symposium, 'Basic Research and Clinical Implications', was co-ordinated by John Wallace in association with Stephen Collins and Stephan Targan. The themes of this section were organized under the general topics of predisposing factors (genetics, animal models, infection, permeability, and immune deficits) and the pathophysiology of intestinal inflammation.

The second symposium, 'Trends in Therapy' was organized by Lloyd Sutherland along with François Martin, Robin McLeod and Noel Williams. The range of topics included the methodology of clinical trials, a review of basic science issues for the clinician, surgical controversies, lifestyle and its influence on inflammatory bowel disease, and therapeutics. The symposium concluded with two special 'State of the Art' lectures': Therapy of IBD in 1994: A gastroenterologist's perspective and a surgeon's perspective.

All members of the two organizing committees participated in the editing of the proceedings. We wish to express our appreciation to Léon and Diane Gosselin at Axcan Pharma for their dedicated, ongoing support of educational events related to gastrointestinal disease. The next Canadian symposium on inflammatory bowel disease will be held in Ottawa, June 1996.

Lloyd R. Sutherland

PART 1:
BASIC RESEARCH AND
CLINICAL IMPLICATIONS IN
IBD

Section I
Predisposing factors in the etiology of IBD: what we can learn from animal models

1
Subclinical markers of human IBD

H. YANG and J. I. ROTTER

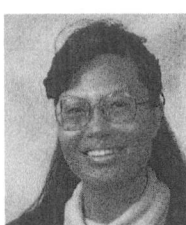

H. YANG

INTRODUCTION

Genetic studies utilizing clinical techniques and clinical disease definition alone have their limits, since clinically unaffected individuals with the variant genotype will not be recognized. Such studies can be greatly aided by the use of subclinical markers that are closer to the basic defect and thus likely to detect more individuals with the abnormal genotype[1]. Subclinical markers are parameters used to detect the abnormal genotype in the absence of the full phenotype; e.g. abnormal glucose tolerance and islet cell antibodies in diabetes or serum cholesterol in coronary artery disease. These markers represent abnormalities having a direct role in the pathogenesis of the disease. They are useful in genetic studies, because in many disorders not all individuals with the mutant genotype may manifest the disorder (reduced penetrance), the variability of the phenotype may be so great that the clinical features are too mild to be readily apparent (variable expressivity), or there may be a delayed age of onset of the disease such that the younger genetically predisposed individuals would be clinically normal[1]. Thus, subclinical markers maximize the number of affected individuals that can be detected.

In addition, the detection of subclinical abnormalities in unaffected family members similar to those found in the probands can distinguish between a primary defect indicating the presence of disease pathophysiology and a secondary abnormality due to the disease process. Therefore finding such abnormalities in clinically unaffected family members helps establish an etiological role for a certain abnormality in a disease. Such an abnormality may either indicate the genetic abnormality predisposing to a disease, or identify those in whom an earlier, subclinical phase of the disease process is

Table 1 Subclinical marker studies in IBD

Marker		Observation	Reference
↑ Antibodies to colonic epithelial cells	UC, CD	Relative	2
↑ Antibodies to crude colonic and *E. coli*	UC	Female relative	3
↓ Mucin species IV	UC	Twin	4
↑ Mucosal cellular IgG1	UC	Twin	5
↑ IgA titres against gliadin	UC	Twin	6
↑ Antineutrophil cytoplasmic antibodies	UC	Relative	7
↑ Lymphocytotoxic antibody	CD	Relative	8
↑ Complement dysfunction	CD	Relative	9
↑ Intestinal permeability	CD	Relative	10
↑ Obligate anaerobic faecal flora (Gram-positive coccoid rods, Gram-negative rods)	CD	Children	11

Table 2 ANCAs in UC and other associated diseases

Location	Percentage of positive pANCA					Reference
	UC	CD	PSC	Control	Other	
USA	68	12	–	0	–	12
USA, Canada	61	6	–	0	< 2	14
USA	68	–	65	–	0	17
USA, Canada	68	–	–	3	–	7
Norway	27	0	63	0	–	18
Germany	83	25	40 (88 PSC + UC)	–	–	13
France	50	–	–	0	–	19
Sweden	50	8	50	–	–	16
Netherlands	79	13	–	9	–	20
Greece	30	–	–	–	–	21
UK	–	–	80	0 (all in children)	–	22
UK	54	10	–	0	–	15
Hong Kong	32	–	–	0	–	23

occurring that may or may not eventuate in clinical disease. Although several abnormalities have been described in IBD, only a few have yet been extended beyond the patients to include family members (Table 1). The important characteristics of a subclinical marker for genetic studies include high specificity, constancy, and familiality. Antineutrophil cytoplasmic antibodies (ANCAs) have all of these characteristics.

ANTINEUTROPHIL CYTOPLASMIC ANTIBODIES

Specificity

A distinct subset of antineutrophil cytoplasmic antibodies was recently discovered to be highly specific for UC by Targan and co-workers[12]. Approximately 70% of UC patients are ANCA-positive compared with other forms of colitis, which include CD (as low as 6%)[12-16]. ANCA is rare in normal controls. Table 2 summarizes all of the available ANCA studies in IBD and related diseases. Although there are differences in the frequency of

ANCAs between studies from different countries, it is consistent that the prevalence of ANCAs is significantly increased in UC compared with CD. ANCAs observed in UC patients have higher titers, with a perinuclear immunofluorescence binding pattern (pANCA), whereas in CD, ANCAs have lower titers, with cytoplasmic pattern (cANCA)[12,14]. A high specificity indicates that this marker is disease-specific, and therefore more likely to be involved in the pathogenesis of the disease.

The prevalence of ANCAs is also significantly increased in patients with primary sclerosing cholangitis (PSC), which is clinically associated with UC. The shared increase in ANCAs in both UC and PSC may indicate that there is a common antigenic target for immune-mediated attack on both colonic and biliary epithelial cells. Further support of this concept is that a 40 000 molecular weight colonic epithelial protein has been identified with a unique epitope or epitopes that is shared by the skin and biliary tract epithelial cells[24].

Constancy

To date the presence of ANCAs appears to be independent of disease activity, duration of illness, localization, extent of disease, previous bowel operations or medical treatment[12,15,20,21]. ANCAs are also found in UC patients who are 5 or more years postcolectomy. ANCAs are not only persistent, but also may have clinical implications. For example, ANCAs have been reported to occur with increased frequency in those postcolectomy UC patients who experience the subsequent inflammation termed pouchitis, as compared with those who did not develop pouchitis[25,26]. The presence of ANCA is not only an indicator of the risk for UC, but also an indicator of the high risk for complications of postcolectomy in UC patients. The presence of ANCAs is thus not simply an epiphenomenon related to active colonic inflammation, but may reflect a fundamental disturbance of immune regulation.

Familiality

Since the relatives of IBD patients have a higher risk than the general population of developing IBD, the prevalence of a subclinical marker is expected to be increased among relatives compared with the general population, an observation termed increased familial aggregation, or simply familiality. Family or twin studies can be used to demonstrate familiality.

In a family study of ANCAs the authors have demonstrated that the clinically healthy relatives of UC patients have an increased frequency of positive ANCAs (16%) compared with environmental controls (3%)[7]. We also observed that second-degree relatives who are not sharing the same household with the probands have an increased prevalence of ANCAs, and that the household controls are not at an increased risk for ANCA[7]. These important epidemiologic observations suggest that the familial aggregation of ANCAs is due to shared genetic factors among the family members, and

Table 3 Characteristics of UC-associated antineutrophil cytoplasmic antibodies (ANCAs)

A subset of ANCAs associated with UC (50–86% UC)
Specific for UC compared with other forms of colitis
Independent of clinical features
Present in healthy relatives of UC cases
Familial distribution in the presence of ANCAs (ANCA (+) and ANCA (−) UC families)
Differential association of HLA class II alleles as a function of ANCA status

not due to shared environmental factors.

A second important finding in this published family study was the significant difference in the frequency of ANCAs in the relatives of probands whose sera were ANCA(+) compared with the relatives of probands whose sera were ANCA(−)[7]. This concordant familial distribution indicates heterogeneity within UC.

Genetic marker studies with ANCAs

Although epidemiological observations have suggested the important genetic contributions to the development of ANCAs, genetic marker studies provide definitive evidence for the genetic determination of ANCAs in IBD.

HLA class II genes

It has been shown that UC is associated with the HLA DR2 allele[27,28]. When we subdivided UC into ANCA(+) and ANCA(−) groups, ANCA-positive UC patients had a significantly increased frequency of DR2 compared with ANCA-negative controls (44% vs 22%). In contrast, the frequency of DR2 in ANCA-negative UC cases (21%) was virtually identical to that in controls (22%)[29]. In addition, the ANCA-negative UC patients had an increase in the DR4 allele compared with ANCA-positive UC. Therefore, the heterogeneity within UC indicated by ANCAs has a genetic basis. This genetic marker study further supports the epidemiologic observations – genetic susceptibility is an essential factor for the development of ANCAs.

At the present time, by the combination of family and gene marker studies, ANCAs are the most established subclinical marker for any form of IBD (Table 3).

PERMEABILITY STUDIES

Since the initial family study of permeability in CD[10], there have been several additional studies (Table 4). On first inspection, the results appear somewhat inconsistent. It seems that a number of related factors may affect the results of an intestinal permeability study. These may include the type of probes; the method of administration of the probe, e.g. fasting/non-fasting; with meals/without meals[38]; day urine collection/overnight urine collection; length of urine collection; and use of aspirin as a challenge[39]. It is important for this area of investigation to identify a sensitive and reproducible protocol

Table 4 Permeability studies in relatives of patients with Crohn's disease

	Probes					
	PEG		Lactulose		$[^{51}Cr]EDTA$	
Reference	Mean↑	10%↑	Mean↑	10%↑	Mean↑	10%↑
10	+	+				
30			−	+		
31					−	−
32	−	+				
33			±	+		+
34			−	+		
35*			+	+		
36			±	+		

10%↑ indicates that at least 10% of relatives have a significantly increased permeability compared with controls (estimated in Hollander's review, ref. 37)
+, Significant increase compared with controls
±, Increase in relatives, but not statistically significant
−, No difference between relatives and controls
*Used prior aspirin to augment permeability test

for permeability testing that reliably separates Crohn's patients (or a subgroup of CD) from controls. In addition, it has been proposed that some of the statistical methods used to illustrate the increased permeability in the relatives of patients with CD may give misleading results[37]. Rather than comparing the means of permeability between the two groups – relatives and controls – one can examine the proportion of the asymptomatic relatives of patients with CD who have permeability values above the upper limits of the range of values in normal controls. The logic of this latter approach is that presumably only a proportion of CD relatives are genetically susceptible. This was recently done, and the investigators found that approximately 10% of these relatives had a significant increase in intestinal permeability[36]. When re-examining the published studies by this same approach (i.e. defining an increased level as greater than two standard deviations above the mean in controls), Hollander found that the majority of such studies showed a significant increase in intestinal permeability in a fraction of the asymptomatic relatives of patients with CD[37] (Table 4). The possibility of abnormal permeability in relatives remains an attractive hypothesis either as a genetic abnormality or as a marker of early inflammation[40]. But this field needs additional studies and methodological standardization. Possibly the most interesting approach was presented by Pironi et al.[35]. In their study, both healthy relatives of CD patients and healthy controls were given the lactulose/mannitol (L/M) test before and after the administration of aspirin. These investigators concluded that the relatives of CD patients were more sensitive to nonsteroidal anti-inflammatory drugs than healthy controls, i.e. the mean percentage increase of above baseline L/M values observed after aspirin was greater in relatives than in controls. Thus, these results suggest that an enhanced small bowel mucosal sensitivity to factors increasing permeability can play a primary role in the pathogenesis of the disease. However, more subjects need to be studied to confirm their findings.

OTHER POTENTIAL SUBCLINICAL MARKERS

Both UC and CD

Antibodies to colonic epithelial cells

Antibodies to colonic epithelial cells have been reported in both CD and UC patients[28]. One study assessed the immune reactivity to gut epithelial cell antigens in healthy members of families of patients with IBD[2]. Specific lysis against epithelial cell-associated component antigens (colon-derived) (ECAC-C) among patients with IBD and among their unaffected first-degree family members was significantly higher than in control groups (70% in IBD patients, 56% in relatives, and 8% in controls). The possibility has been raised that these antibodies might reflect environmental in addition to genetic factors, because of their high prevalence in nonrelated family members[41].

In UC

Antibodies to crude colonic and Escherichia coli

Elevated titers of antibodies to crude colonic and *Escherichia coli* 0:14 antigens have been found not only in patients with UC but also in their healthy female relatives[3].

Mucosal production of IgG subclasses

The importance of immunoglobulin (IgG)-mediated immunopathological processes in IBD has been suggested by the increased IgG cell fraction[42] and the elevated secretion of IgG[43] in the affected tissues. It has also been shown that there is a significant difference between UC and CD in terms of IgG subclass production in the mucosal lesion: the proportion of IgG1 immunocytes has been found to be higher in UC than in CD, while the reverse was true for the IgG2 cell fraction[44]. A recent twin study revealed an interesting result: there was no difference in the cellular IgG subclass pattern between healthy and affected UC twins (i.e. where the index twin had UC), and the proportion of IgG1 in these healthy and diseased twins was significantly correlated[5]. In UC the aberrant mucosal production of IgG1 and IgG2 did not depend on active disease, and the raised IgG1 proportion appeared to be disease-specific[5]. These findings suggest that genetic mechanisms appear to be involved in the regulation of the IgG subclass response.

Antibodies to gliadin

In a twin study examining antibody (IgG, IgA and IgM) to baker's yeast, yeast mannan, gliadin, ovalbumin and beta-lactoglobulin, high IgA titers against gliadin were found in healthy and diseased UC monozygotic twins[6]. This could indicate a subclinical and/or genetically determined gluten intolerance.

Mucin abnormalities

The gastrointestinal tract is lined with a mucus layer that forms a barrier against exotoxins and microorganisms. One etiological hypothesis is that inborn abnormalities in colonic mucin species may be related to the pathogenesis of UC[45-47].

The content of the chromatographically defined component of colonic mucin designated HCM species IV has been reported to be reduced in both patients with ulcerative colitis and their apparently healthy twins[4]. Composition of the mucins in CD patients and their unaffected twins was not significantly different from that in controls. These observations suggest that altered profiles of mucin glycoprotein may be present before the onset of UC and therefore may be genetically defined.

In CD

Lymphocytotoxic antibodies

Autoantibodies to lymphocyte surface membrane antigens (lymphocytotoxic antibodies) have been found in increased frequency in patients with CD and their relatives, but these have been found in increased frequency in their spouses as well[8]. In addition, these antibodies are not specific to IBD and have been found in a variety of other diseases such as systemic lupus erythematosus, rheumatoid arthritis, malaria and others, all involving active immune responses[48].

Complement dysfunction

In a study of CD patients and their clinically unaffected first-degree relatives, 38% of cases and 18% of relatives showed subnormal generation of chemotactic activity and decreased utilization of C3 by the alternative complement pathway[9]. All of the relatives with C3 abnormalities were confined to families of probands with similar abnormalities, suggesting that: (a) the abnormalities are not simply secondary to the CD; (b) the abnormalities are familial; (c) since these occurred only in some families and not others, these abnormalities predispose in only a subset of Crohn's disease.

Obligate anaerobic fecal flora

The obligate anaerobic fecal flora of patients with CD has been shown to be different from that of healthy controls (CD flora has more Gram-positive coccoid rods and Gram-negative rods than the flora of healthy subjects)[49-51]. To investigate whether the abnormal fecal flora is a genetically determined condition that predisposes an individual to the development of CD[52], a family study was conducted[11]. The investigators observed that 35% (9/26) of clinically healthy children of CD patients had abnormal anaerobic flora, similar to the frequency in CD patients. In 5–7 years of follow-up, three of the nine children with abnormal flora developed symptoms suggestive of CD, and one was diagnosed as having CD, while none of the 17 children with a normal flora showed symptoms consistent with CD. Thus, the abnormal flora may be indigenous to subjects predisposed to CD. It appears this may be limited to the early-onset patient population, since the siblings and parents of the CD patients did not show an abnormal flora. If the basic observation is confirmed, then it needs to be determined whether the relationship between the abnormal fecal flora and CD is direct (products or cell wall fragments consisting of peptidoglycan and/or lipopolysaccharides could initiate the inflammatory reaction)[53] or indirect (the abnormal flora were less resistant to colonization of the bowel by pathogenic bacteria).

In summary, IBD is a genetically heterogeneous group of disorders. We are still at the beginning stage of using subclinical markers to understand the genetics of IBD. In future genetic studies these subclinical markers (currently, at the minimum ANCAs) should be taken into consideration for classification of the patients and families to obtain etiologically homogeneous groups. Natural history studies are needed to understand the role of ANCAs and eventually other subclinical markers in the development of clinical IBD.

Acknowledgements

This work was supported in part by grants from the Crohn's and Colitis Foundation of America, NIH Program Project grant DK46763, the Stuart Foundations, and the Cedars-Sinai Board of Governors' Chair in Medical Genetics (J.I.R.).

References

1. King RA, Rotter JI, Motulsky AG, editors. The genetic basis of common diseases. New York: Oxford University Press; 1992.
2. Fiocchi C, Roche JK, Michener WM. High prevalence of antibodies to intestinal epithelial antigens in patients with inflammatory bowel disease and their relatives. Ann Intern Med. 1989;110:786–94.
3. Lagercrantz R, Perlmann P, Hammerstrom S. Immunological studies in ulcerative colitis. V. Family studies. Gastroenterology. 1971;60:381–9.
4. Tysk C, Riedesel H, Lindberg E, Panzini B, Podolsky D, Jarnerot G. Colonic glycoproteins in monozygotic twins with inflammatory bowel disease. Gastroenterology. 1991;100:419–23.
5. Helgeland L, Tysk C, Jarnerot G et al. IgG subclass distribution in serum and rectal mucosa of monozygotic twins with or without inflammatory bowel disease. Gut. 1992;33:1358–64.
6. Lindberg E, Magnusson K-E, Tysk C, Jarnerot G. Antibody (IgG, IgA and IgM) to baker's yeast (Saccharomyces cerevisiae), yeast mannan, gliadin, ovalbumin and betalactoglobulin in monozygotic twins with inflammatory bowel disease. Gut. 1992;33:909–13.
7. Shanahan F, Duerr RH, Rotter JI et al. Neutrophil autoantibodies in ulcerative colitis: familial aggregation and genetic heterogeneity. Gastroenterology. 1992;103:456–61.
8. Korsmeyer SJ, Williams RC Jr, Wilson ID, Strickland RG. Lymphocytotoxic antibody in inflammatory bowel disease – a family study. N Engl J Med. 1974;293:1117–20.
9. Elmgreen J, Both H, Binder V. Familial occurrence of complement dysfunction in Crohn's disease: correlation with intestinal symptoms and hypercatabolism of complement. Gut. 1985;26:151–7.
10. Hollander D, Vadheim CM, Brettholtz E, Petersen GM, Delahunty T, Rotter JI. Increased intestinal permeability in Crohn's patients and their relatives: an etiological factor? Ann Intern Med. 1986;105:883–95.

11. Van de Merwe JP, Schroder AM, Wensinck F, Hazenberg MP. The obligate anaerobic faecal flora of patients with Crohn's disease and their first-degree relatives. Scand J Gastroenterol. 1988;23:1125–31.
12. Saxon A, Shanahan F, Landers C, Ganz T, Targan S. A subset of antineutrophil anticytoplasmic antibodies is associated with inflammatory bowel disease. J Allergy Clin Immunol. 1990;86:202–10.
13. Seibold F, Weber P, Klein R, Berg PA, Wiedmann KH. Clinical significance of antibodies against neutrophils in patients with inflammatory bowel disease and primary sclerosing cholangitis. Gut. 1992;33:657–62.
14. Duerr RH, Targan SR, Landers CJ, Sutherland LR, Shanahan F. Anti-neutrophil cytoplasmic antibodies in ulcerative colitis. Comparison with other colitides/diarrheal illnesses. Gastroenterology. 1991;100:1590–6.
15. Cambridge G, Rampton DS, Stevens TRJ, McCarthy DA, Kamm M, Leaker B. Anti-neutrophil antibodies in inflammatory bowel disease: prevalence and diagnostic role. Gut. 1992;33:668–74.
16. Peen E, Almer S, Bodemar G, Ryden BO, Sjolin C, Tejle K, Skogh T. Anti-lactoferrin antibodies and other types of ANCA in ulcerative colitis, primary sclerosing cholangitis, and Crohn's disease. Gut. 1993;34:56–62.
17. Duerr RH, Targan SR, Landers CJ et al. Neutrophil cytoplasmic antibodies: a link between primary sclerosing cholangitis and ulcerative colitis. Gastroenterology. 1991;100:1385–91.
18. Zauli D, Baffoni L, Cassani F et al. Antineutrophil cytoplasmic antibodies in primary sclerosing cholangitis, ulcerative colitis, and autoimmune diseases. Gastroenterology. 1992;102:1088–95.
19. Reumaux D, Delecourt L, Colombel JF, Noël LH, Duthilleul P, Cartot A. Anti-neutrophil cytoplasmic autoantibodies in relatives of patients with ulcerative colitis. Gastroenterology. 1992;103:1706.
20. Oudkerk-Pool M, Ellerbroek PM, Ridwan BU et al. Serum antineutrophil cytoplasmic autoantibodies in inflammatory bowel disease are mainly associated with ulcerative colitis. A correlation study between perinuclear antineutrophil cytoplasmic autoantibodies and clinical parameters, medical, and surgical treatment. Gut. 1993;34:46–50.
21. Dalekos GN, Manoussakis MN, Goussia AC, Tsianos EV, Moutsopoulos HM. Soluble interleukin-2 receptors, antineutrophil cytoplasmic antibodies, and other autoantibodies in patients with ulcerative colitis. Gut. 1993;34:658–64.
22. Lo SK, Chapman RWG, Cheeseman P et al. Antineutrophil antibody: a test for autoimmune primary sclerosing cholangitis in childhood? Gut. 1993;34:199–202.
23. Sung JY, Chan KL, Hsu R, Liew CT, Lawton JW. Ulcerative colitis and antineutrophil cytoplasmic antibodies in Hong Kong Chinese. Am J Gastroenterol. 1993;88:864–9.
24. Das KM, Vecchi M, Sakamaki S. A shared and unique epitope(s) on human colon, skin, and biliary epithelium detected by a monoclonal antibody. Gastroenterology. 1990;98:464–9.
25. Sandborn WJ, Landers CJ, Tremaine WJ, Targan SR. The presence of antineutrophil cytoplasmic antibody correlates with pouchitis after ileal pouch–anal anastomosis for ulcerative colitis. Gastroenterology. 1993;104:A774.
26. Vecchi M, Giochetti P, Bianchi MB et al. p-ANCA reactivity in ulcerative colitis patients with and without pouchitis after proctocolectomy. Gastroenterology. 1993;104:A796.
27. Toyoda H, Wang S-J, Yang H et al. Distinct association of HLA class II genes with inflammatory bowel disease. Gastroenterology. 1993;104:741–8.
28. Yang H, Rotter JI. The genetics of inflammatory bowel disease: genetic predispositions, disease markers, and genetic heterogeneity. In: Targan SR, Shanahan F, editors. Inflammatory bowel disease: from bench to bedside. Baltimore: Williams & Wilkins; 1994:32–64.
29. Yang H, Rotter JI, Toyoda H et al. Ulcerative colitis: a genetic heterogeneous group defined with genetic (DR2) and subclinical markers (anti-neutrophil cytoplasmic antibodies). J Clin Invest. 1993;92:1080–4.
30. Katz KD, Hollander D, Vadheim CM et al. Intestinal permeability in Crohn's disease patients and their healthy relatives. Gastroenterology. 1989;97:927–31.
31. Ainsworth M, Eriksen J, Rasmussen JW, Schaffalitzky de Muckadell OB. Intestinal permeability of ^{51}Cr-labelled ethylenediaminetetraacetic acid in patients with Crohn's disease and their healthy relatives. Scand J Gastroenterol. 1989;24:993–8.

32. Ruttenberg D, Young GO, Wright JP, Isaacs S. PEG-400 excretion in patients with Crohn's disease, their first-degree relatives, and healthy volunteers. Dig Dis Sci. 1992;37:705–8.
33. Teahon K, Smethurst P, Levi AJ, Menzies IS, Bjarnason I. Intestinal permeability in patients with Crohn's disease and their first degree relatives. Gut. 1992;33:320–3.
34. Valpiani D, Ornigotti L, Ricca Rosellini S et al. Intestinal permeability in patients with Crohn's disease and in first grade relatives. Gastroenterology. 1992;102:A708.
35. Pironi L, Miglioli M, Ruggeri E et al. Effect of non-steroidal anti-inflammatory drugs (NSAID) on intestinal permeability in first degree relatives of patients with Crohn's disease. Gastroenterology. 1992;102:A679.
36. May GR, Sutherland LR, Meddings JB. Is small intestinal permeability really increased in relatives of patients with Crohn's disease? Gastroenterology. 1993;104:1627–32.
37. Hollander D. Permeability in Crohn's disease: altered barrier functions in healthy relatives? Gastroneterology. 1993;104:1848–51.
38. Bjarnason I, Smethurst P, Macpherson A et al. Glucose and citrate reduce the permeability changes caused by indomethacin in humans. Gastroenterology. 1992;102:1546–50.
39. Bjarnason I, Smethurst P, Levi AJ, Menzies IS, Peters TJ. The effect of polyacrylic acid polymers on small-intestinal function and permeability changes caused by indomethacin. Scand J Gastroenterol. 1991;26:685–8.
40. Hollander D. The intestinal permeability barrier. Scand J Gastroenterol. 1992;27:721–6.
41. Seiden MV. Environmental or genetic effects in inflammatory bowel disease. Ann Intern Med. 1989;111:445–6.
42. Baklien K, Brandtzaeg P. Comparative mapping of the local distribution of immunoglobulin-containing cells in ulcerative colitis and Crohn's disease of the colon. Clin Exp Immunol. 1975;22:197–209.
43. Scott MG, Nahm MH, Macke K, Nash GS, Bertovich MJ, MacDermott RP. Spontaneous secretion of IgG subclasses by intestinal mononuclear cells: differences between ulcerative colitis, Crohn's disease, and controls. Clin Exp Immunol. 1986;66:209–15.
44. Kett K, Rognum TO, Brandtzaeg P. Mucosal subclass distribution of immunoglobulin G-producing cells is different in ulcerative colitis and Crohn's disease of the colon. Gastroenterology. 1987;93:919–24.
45. Cope GF, Heatley RV, Kelleher J, Axon ATR. In vitro mucus glycoprote in production by colonic tissue from patients with ulcerative colitis. Gut. 1988;29:229–34.
46. Podolsky DK, Isselbacher KJ. Comparison of human colonic mucin. Selective alteration in inflammatory bowel disease. J Clin Invest. 1983;72:142–53.
47. Podolsky DK, Isselbacher KJ. Glycoprotein composition of colonic mucosa. Specific alterations in ulcerative colitis. Gastroenterology. 1984;87:991–8.
48. Elson CO. The immunology of inflammatory bowel disease. In: Kirsner JB, Shorter RG, editors. Inflammatory bowel disease, 3rd edn. Philadelphia: Lea & Febiger; 1988:97–164.
49. Wensinck F. Proceedings: The faecal flora of patients with Crohn's disease. Antonie Van Leeuwenhoek. 1975;41:214–15.
50. Wensinck F, Custers-Van Lieshout LMC, Poppelaars-Kustermans PAJ, Schroder AM. The faecal flora of patients with Crohn's disease. J Hyg. 1981;87:1–12.
51. Ruseler-Van Embden JGH, Both-Patoir HC. Anaerobic gram-negative faecal flora in patients with Crohn's disease and healthy subjects. Antonie Van Leeuwenhoek. 1983;49:125–32.
52. Van de Merwe JP, Stegeman JH, Hazenberg MP. The resident faecal flora is determined by genetic characteristics of the host. Implications for Crohn's disease? Antonie Van Leeuwenhoek. 1983;49:119–24.
53. Sartor RB, Cromartie WJ, Powell DW, Schwab JH. Granulomatous enterocolitis induced in rats by purified bacterial cell wall fragments. Gastroenterology. 1985;89:587–95.

2
Genetic factors in animal models of intestinal inflammation

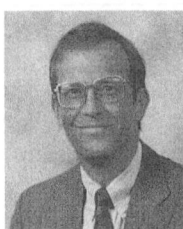

R. B. SARTOR

INTRODUCTION

Clinical investigators have compellingly documented a genetic component in ulcerative colitis and Crohn's disease[1]. There is an increased incidence of inflammatory bowel disease (IBD) in family members, a predilection for these disorders in certain genetically defined ethnic groups, higher concordance of disease in monozygotic versus dizygotic twins, and familial patterns of clinical phenotypes. However, human genetic research has not yet provided clinically useful disease susceptibility markers, or an understanding of the immuno-pathogenesis of IBD.

The critical importance of host genetic susceptibility in determining chronicity, aggressiveness and complications of intestinal inflammation is clearly demonstrated by studies in inbred rodents, transgenic rats, gene knockout mice and spontaneous mutants (Table 1). This chapter will summarize evidence of genetic control of intestinal and extraintestinal inflammation in these models, briefly outline possible immunologic mechanisms of enhanced genetic susceptibility and discuss the relevance of these observations to the pathogenesis of human IBD.

SPONTANEOUS INFLAMMATORY MODELS

The cottontop tamarin and the recently developed C_3H/HeJ Bir substrain mouse develop chronic, spontaneously relapsing colitis. The mechanisms of

Table 1 Genetic influence on animal models of intestinal inflammation

A. *Spontaneous mutations (presumed)*
Cottontop tamarin
C_3H/HeJ Bir mouse
B. *Genetically engineered models*
HLA-B27/β2 microglobulin transgenic rats
IL-2, IL-10 TGFβ, $\alpha\beta$ TCR knockout mice
C. *Differential susceptibility of inbred rodent strains to induced inflammation*
Peptidoglycan-polysaccharide enterocolitis
Indomethacin enterocolitis
Small bowel bacterial overgrowth-induced hepatobiliary inflammation
TNBS/ethanol colitis
$\alpha\beta$ TCR-deleted colitis
Citrobacter freundii colitis

intestinal inflammation in these animals are unknown, but presumably are the result of a spontaneous genetic mutation, since closely related strains do not develop colitis and aggressive searches have not identified environmental microbial pathogens.

At least 11 different species and hybrids of tamarins, a group of New World monkeys, spontaneously develop mild chronic colitis with mucosal atrophy[2]. Cottontop tamarins are unique in that they exhibit acute relapsing colitis complicated by adenocarcinoma of the colon[2-4]. Captive cottontop tamarins frequently develop a wasting syndrome characterized by weight loss, anorexia and diarrhea. An age-related chronic colitis is almost universally present by 2 years of age. Underlying chronic colitis is relatively mild, characterized by a thickened mucosa with hyperplastic, elongated crypts, pseudopolyps and mild mononucler cell infiltration of the lamina propria. Approximately one-half to two-thirds of marmosets at any given time will have histologic evidence of acute colonic inflammation, with neutrophilic infiltration, crypt abscesses and goblet cell depletion but rare ulceration. The adenocarcinoma which complicates chronic colitis is not preceded by epithelial cell dysplasia or adenomatous polyps. Some tamarins develop chronic periportal inflammation with fibrosis.

The mechanism(s) of intestinal inflammation in cottontop tamarins remain unclear. The inflammatory mediator profile of increased interleukin 1 (IL-1) and eicosanoids is characteristic of intestinal inflammation and the colitis responds to sulfasalazine and a 5-lipoxygenase inhibitor[4,5]. These marmosets share several biochemical and immunologic alterations with ulcerative colitis patients. They have a selective reduction in mucus glycoprotein fraction IV which does not correlate with inflammatory activity[6]. In addition their serum contains antineutrophil cytoplasmic autoantibodies (ANCA) which react with human but not marmoset neutrophils[7], and slightly increased concentrations of serum antibodies which stimulate cell-mediated cytotoxicity to colonic epithelial cell-associated components[8]. However, the precise genetic alteration which predisposes these marmosets to chronic, relapsing colitis with associated adenocarcinoma remains uncharacterized.

C₃H/HeJ Bir SUBSTRAIN MOUSE COLITIS

Birkenmeier and colleagues[9] have recently described a heritable form of murine colitis. It had become apparent that sporadic diarrhea and perianal ulceration was frequent in individual members of the Jackson Laboratory C_3H/HeJ mouse breeding colony, but that no microbial pathogens were demonstrable. Selective breeding of mice which developed diarrhea resulted in a pedigree of mice in which there is a 50% incidence of spontaneous colitis. Colitis is more frequent in males (67% incidence) than females (31% incidence), and exhibits a seasonal variation (winter > summer). Inflammation follows a biphasic time-course with onset around the time of weaning (3–5 weeks of age), spontaneous resolution in most mice and a less predictable chronic phase. Clinical manifestations include occasional diarrhea, fecal blood (not grossly apparent) and perianal ulceration. Inflammation is most frequently found near the ileocecal valve, but can involve the entire colon. Histologic findings include focal linear ulcers and a mixed mononuclear and neutrophilic infiltration. Extraintestinal manifestations have not been described.

Attempts to identify the presumed spontaneous genetic mutation are in progress. Like the parent C_3H/HeJ strain, monocytes from mice with spontaneous colitis are unresponsive to lipopolysaccharide (endotoxin)[10]. Comparison of *in-vitro* reactivity of T lymphocytes derived from parent strain and substrain mice and colonic cytokine profiles have not been reported. In preliminary studies, serum antibodies from 50% of C_3H/HeJ Bir mice react with luminal bacterial extracts compared with no detectable antibacterial antibodies from serum of C_3H/HeJ mice[11].

GENETICALLY ENGINEERED MODELS

Molecular engineering techniques permit selected genes to be overexpressed (transgenic) or deleted (embryonic stem cell recombination) in rodents. These methods have been powerful tools in determining the *in-vivo* functionof a targeted gene, and at times have provided unanticipated results. Deletion of several immunoregulatory cytokines, including IL-2, IL-10, and transforming growth factor $\beta1$ (TGF-$\beta1$) and α or β T cell receptor (TCR) chains induces spontaneous colitis[12-15]. These studies show that a single mutation of a key immunoregulatory cytokine or T lymphocyte protein can lead to spontaneous intestinal inflammation, and that the colon is particularly susceptible to injury in immunodeficient hosts.

Overexpression of human HLA-B27/$\beta2$-microglobulin ($\beta2\mu$) in transgenic rats induces a systemic inflammatory syndrome in which the first manifestation is diarrhea, followed by arthritis, dermatitis, hair loss, psoriatic nail changes, epididymitis and a wasting syndrome[16,17]. Histologic patterns of inflammation include focal chronic gastritis and duodenitis and diffuse infiltration of the colonic lamina propria by mononuclear cells. Severely inflamed rats exhibit focal mucosal ulcerations and crypt abscesses in the colon. Cell transfer experiments demonstrate that HLA-B27/$\beta2\mu$ expressing

Table 2 Differential susceptibility of inbred rats to experimental enterocolitis and systemic inflammation

High responder	Intermediate responders	Low responders
Lewis	Sprague-Dawley	Fischer F344
	Wistar	Buffalo

bone marrow cells mediate the disease, and that B27/$\beta2\mu$ protein expression by nonimmune cells is neither necessary nor sufficient to cause disease[18]. The absence of colitis and arthritis in germ-free B27/$\beta2\mu$ transgenic rats and attenuated inflammation in specific pathogen-free rats clearly demonstrate the importance of luminal bacteria in initiation and perpetuation of intestinal inflammation and associated extraintestinal disease[19] (RB Sartor, unpublished observations). The incidence and onset of colitis and systemic inflammation are dependent on high copy numbers of HLA-B27/$\beta2\mu$[17]. In contrast to induced rat models of enterocolitis (see below), the incidence of intestinal inflammation in Lewis and Fischer rats expressing equivalent copy numbers of the HLA-B27/$\beta2\mu$ transgene is similar, although extraintestinal inflammation is somewhat more frequent and rapid in onset in Lewis than Fischer rats[17].

INDUCED INFLAMMATION IN INBRED RODENT STRAINS

Differential susceptibility of inbred rodents to intestinal and systemic inflammation powerfully illustrates the key role of genetic regulation of chronic inflammation and its complications, including fibrosis.

Inbred rat strains

We have used three experimental models to demonstrate that with identical stimuli inbred Lewis rats develop chronic relapsing enterocolitis with extraintestinal inflammation and fibrosis, whereas inbred Buffalo and Fischer F344 (MHC matched with Lewis) rats develop only transient inflammation and no systemic manifestations (Table 2). Lewis rats injected subserosally with the bacterial cell wall polymer, peptidoglycan-polysaccharide (PG-PS), develop chronic, spontaneously relapsing, granulomatous enterocolitis with fibrosis and associated polyarthritis, granulomatous hepatitis, leukocytosis, and anemia which persists at least 16 weeks[5,20]. With identical exposure to PG-PS, Buffalo or Fischer rats exhibit only transient local inflammation, which resolves by 14 days with residual damage and no chronic enterocolitis or extraintestinal manifestations. Outbred Sprague-Dawley rats develop chronic granulomatous enterocolitis, but the chronic intestinal inflammation is less pronounced, and there is no extraintestinal disease[21]. In a second model, Lewis rats injected subcutaneously with indomethacin (7.5 mg/kg a day for 2 days) develop chronic mid-small bowel longitudinal ulcers with fibrosis and associated hepatobiliary inflammation, anemia and leukocytosis which persist for at least 77 days, whereas Fischer rats have no residual inflammation 14 days after indomethacin[22]. Similarly, Lewis rats, but not Buffalo or Fischer rats, develop chronic, fibrotic hepatobiliary inflammation in response to experimental small intestinal overgrowth of anaerobic bacteria following surgical creation of jejunal self-filling blind loops (SFBL)[23]. In this model, Lewis rats develop clinical (hepatomegaly), biochemical (increased plasma AST), histologic and cholangiographic evidence of hepatobiliary inflammation 2–4 weeks after creation of the SFBL. Wistar rats develop similar lesions by 8 and 12 weeks, but Fischer and Buffalo rats fail to develop hepatobiliary injury despite very similar luminal bacterial concentrations in all rat strains. Thus, with identical stimuli, Lewis rats develop chronic, spontaneously relapsing inflammation with extraintestinal inflammation, but Buffalo and Fischer rats develop transient, self-limited inflammation with no local or systemic complications.

Lewis rats are high responders in a number of inflammatory models, including autoimmune encephalitis, uveitis, and arthritis (adjuvant, collagen and PG-PS-induced)[24,25]. Experimental data support two theories to explain mechanisms of enhanced susceptibility to inflammation in Lewis rats: (a) defective acute hypothalamic/pituitary/adrenal responses to IL-1 and PG-PS[26] and (b) disordered regulation of the immune response. In support of the latter theory, Lewis rats have an increased ratio of cecal IL-1/IL-1ra mRNA during the chronic phase of PG-PS-induced inflammation relative to resistant Buffalo and Fischer rats[20]. Moreover, noninflamed intestinal tissues from Lewis but not Fischer and Buffalo rats constitutively express mRNA for TNF and an IL-8-like molecule[27], suggesting that the mucosal immune system of the Lewis rat is in a 'primed' state. We have also demonstrated that T lymphocytes regulate the chronic, relapsing granulomat-ous phase of PG-PS-induced enterocolitis and systemic inflammation, based on observations that Lewis athymic (nude) rats fail to develop enterocolitis and arthritis, and cyclosporin A prevents and treats chronic intestinal and systemic inflammation[28]. These results complement observations by Bristol et al.[29] that PG-PS-stimulated peritoneal macrophages from Lewis rats have an increased IL-1/IL-1ra ratio relative to Buffalo rats and our observations in IBD patients. Patients with active Crohn's disease and ulcerative colitis have significantly increased tissue IL-1/IL-1ra and mRNA protein ratios compared with normal controls[30,31].

Inbred mouse strains (Table 3)

Beagley et al.[32] have reported that Balb/C and C3H/HeN mice develop a chronic colitis upon repeated weekly administration of trinitrobenzene sulfonic acid/ethanol enemas, but DBA/2 and C57/BL mice were resistant to chronic inflammation. Similarly, C3H/HeJ mice develop more extensive colonic inflammation and ulcerations than DBA/2J mice following experi-mental infection with Citrobacter freundii, although the two strains develop similar degrees of epithelial hyperplasia[33]. However, inbred mouse strain susceptibility is not entirely consistent, since Mombaerts et al.[15] found that

Table 3 Differential host susceptibility of inbred mice to experimental colitis

Model	High responders	Low responders
TNB-SA/ethanol	Balb/C, C$_3$H/HeN	DBA/2, C57/BL
Citrobacter freundii	C$_3$H/HeJ	DBA/2J
αTCR knockout	C$_3$H/He	Balb/C, C57BL/6

TCRα chain-deficient mice on the 129/SV background and 129/SV × C3H/He crosses develop severe intestinal inflammation more rapidly (4–6 months of age) and with a higher incidence than those 129/SV mice crossed with C57BL/6 or Balb/C strain, which develop a less severe disease with a slower onset. The only mouse strain which displayed consistent high susceptibility in these models is the C3H/He background (C3H/HeN or C3H/JHeJ), which is the parent strain for the C3H/HeJ Bir mice that spontaneously develop colitis[9].

SUMMARY AND CONCLUSIONS

The studies discussed above clearly demonstrate that the chronicity, aggressiveness and complications of induced intestinal inflammation are dependent on host genetic susceptibility. Furthermore, spontaneous mutation or altered expression of a single gene can produce spontaneous colitis. Genetically engineered models demonstrate that alteration of any of a number of key immunoregulatory cytokine or T lymphocyte gene products can lead to phenotypically similar intestinal inflammatory conditions. Furthermore, inbred rodent strains susceptible to induced intestinal inflammation exhibit immunoregulatory defects (Lewis rats increased IL-1/IL-1ra ratio and C3H/HeJ LPS-unresponsiveness). These observations in animal models suggest that human IBD could arise from a number of mutations of immunoregulatory molecules, supporting the concept of genetic heterogeneity for ulcerative colitis and Crohn's disease.

We suggest that genetically determined defects in immunoregulation or perhaps mucosal barrier integrity could alter the delicate balance between phlogistic luminal bacterial constituents, dietary antigens and mucosal protective forces[34]. We propose that the genetic susceptibility of high-responding hosts (Lewis rats and perhaps IBD patients) is due to an inability to appropriately down-regulate the inflammatory response to ubiquitous luminal antigens, probably of bacterial origin. This theory predicts that events initiating inflammation may be nonspecific (self-limited infection, nonsteroidal anti-inflammatory drugs, toxins), and produce acute inflammation of similar degree in all hosts (Fig. 1). The normal, genetically resistant host appropriately down-regulates inflammation, which heals with no residual damage. However, the genetically susceptible host (Lewis rat, IBD patient) due to defective immunosuppression, amplifies the inflammatory response to develop aggressive tissue injury, fibrosis, and extraintestinal inflammation. Better understanding of genetically determined defects in immunoregulation

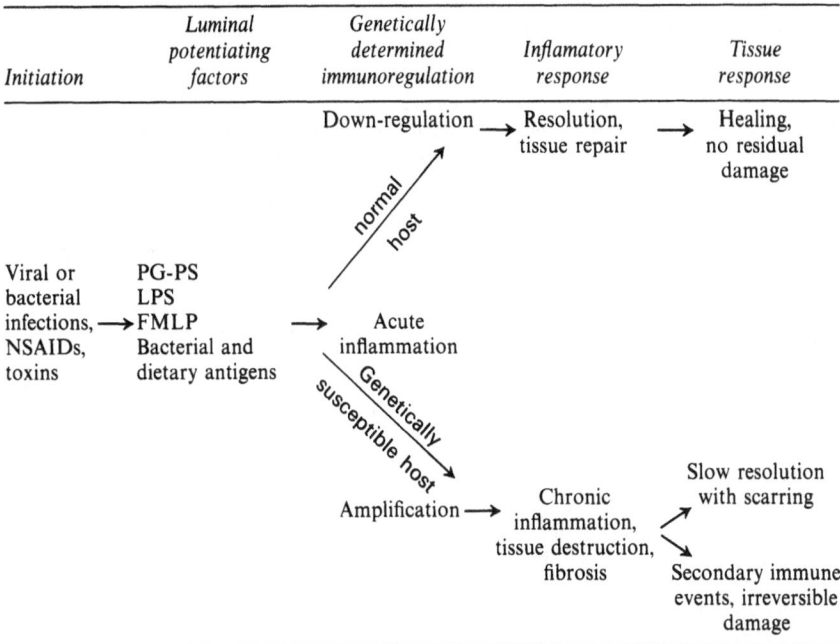

Fig. 1 Influence of genetic susceptibility on chronicity of inflammation. Episodic enteric infections, environment toxins and enhanced mucosal uptake of ubiquitous bacterial constituents induce transient injury in all hosts. The normal response is appropriate suppression of inflammation with no residual damage (upper arm). However, genetically susceptible hosts amplify the inflammatory response, which leads to chronic tissue damage. NSAIDs, non-steroidal anti-inflammatory drugs; PG-PS, peptidoglycan-polysaccharide; LPS, lipopolysaccharide, endotoxin; FMLP, n-formyl-methionyl-leucyl phenylalanine. (Reprinted with permission from Sartor RB, Microbial factors in the pathogenesis of Crohn's disease, ulcerative colitis and experimental intestinal inflammation. In: Kirsner JB, Shorter RG, editors. Inflammatory bowel disease, 4th edn. Baltimore: Williams & Wilkins, 1994: in press)

of the Lewis rat, C3H/HeJ and C3H/HeN mice and identification of the spontaneous genetic mutation(s) of the C3H/HeJ Bir mouse should lead to valuable insights into the genetic regulation of experimental chronic intestinal and extraintestinal inflammation which can be rapidly tested in IBD patients.

Acknowledgements

This work was supported by USPHS grants DK 40249, DK 47700 and DK 34987 and the Crohn's and Colitis Foundation of America. The authors gratefully acknowledge the expert secretarial assistance of Robert Tuttle and Shirley Willard.

References

1. Yang H, Rotter JI. Subclinical markers of human IBD. In Sutherland LR, Collins SM, Martin F, et al, editors. Inflammatory bowel disease: basic research, clinical implications

and trends in therapy. Lancaster: Kluwer Academic Publishers; 1994: chap 1.

2. Lushbaugh C, Humason G, Clapp N. Histology of colitis: *Saguinus oedipus* and other marmosets. Dig Dis Sci. 1985;30:45–51S.

3. Chalifoux IV, Brieland JK, King KW. Evolution and natural history of colonic disease in cotton-top tamarins (*Saguinus oedipus*). Dig Dis Sci. 1985;30:54–8S.

4. Madara JL, Podolsky DK, King NW, Sehgal PK, Moore R, Winter HS. Characterization of spontaneous colitis in cotton-top tamarins (*Saguinus oedipus*) and its response to sulfasalazine. Gastroenterology. 1985;88:13–19.

5. Sartor RB. Animal models of intestinal inflammation: relevance to IBD. In: MacDermott RP, Stenson W, editors. Inflammatory bowel disease. New York: Elsevier; 1991:337–54.

6. Podolsky DK, Madara JL, King N et al. Colonic mucin composition in primates. Gastroenterology. 1985;88:20–5.

7. Targan SR, Landers CJ, King NW, Podolsky DJ, Shanahan F. Ulcerative colitis-linked antineutrophil cytoplasmic antibody in the cotton-top tamarin model of colitis. Gastroenterology. 1992;102:1493–8.

8. Winter HS, Crum PM Jr, King NW, Sehgal PK, Roche JK. Expression of immune sensitization to epithelial cell-associated components in the cotton-top tamarin: a model of chronic ulcerative colitis. Gastroenterology. 1989;97:1075–82.

9. Birkenmeier EH, Sundberg JP, Elson CO. A heritable form of colitis in mice. Gastroenterology. 1991;102:A596.

10. McCabe RP, Mills T, Ridwan B et al. Immunologic reactivity in C3H/HeJ mice with spontaneous colitis. Gastroenterology. 1993;104:A739.

11. Brandwein SL, McCabe RP, Dadrat A et al. Immunologic reactivity of colitic C3H/HeJ Bir mice to enteric bacteria. Gastroenterology. 1994;106:A656.

12. Sadlack B, Merg H, Schorle H et al. Ulcerative colitis-like disease in mice with a disrupted interleukin-2 gene. Cell. 1993;75:253–61.

13. Kuhn R, Lohler J, Rennick D, Rajowsky K, Muller W. Interleukin-1-deficient mice develop chronic enterocolitis. Cell. 1993;75:263–79.

14. Kulkarni AB, Huh CG, Becker D et al. Transforming growth factor $\beta1$ null mutation in mice causes excessive inflammatory response and early death. Proc Natl Acad Sci. 1993;90:770–4.

15. Mombaerts P, Mizoguchi E, Grusby M et al. Spontaneous development of inflammatory bowel disease in T cell receptor mutant mice. Cell. 1993;75:275–82.

16. Hammer RE, Maika SD, Richardson JA, Tang J, Taurog JD. Spontaneous inflammatory disease in transgenic rats expressing HLA-B27 and human β_2m: an animal model of HLA-B27-associated human disorders. Cell. 1990;63:1099–112.

17. Taurog JD, Maika SD, Simmons WA, Breban M, Hammer RE. Susceptibility to inflammatory disease in HLA-B27 transgenic rat lines correlates with the level of B27 expression. J Immunol. 1993;150:4186.

18. Breban M, Hammer RE, Richardson JA, Taurog JD. Transfer of the inflammatory disease of HLA-B27 transgenic rats by bone marrow engraftment. J Exp Med. 1993;178:1607–16.

19. Taurog JD, Hammer RE, Balish E et al. Effect of the germfree state on the inflammatory disease of HLA-B27 transgenic rats: a split result. Arthritis Rheum. 1993;36:S46.

20. McCall RD, Haskill S, Zimmerman E et al. Tissue IL-1 and IL-1 receptor antagonist expression in enterocolitis in resistant and susceptible rats. Gastroenterology. 1994;106: 960–72.

21. Sartor RB, Cromartie WH, Powell DW et al. Granulomatous enterocolitis induced in rats by purified bacterial cell wall fragments. Gastroenterology. 1985;89:587–95.

22. Sartor RB, Bender DE, Holt LC. Susceptibility of inbred rat strains to intestinal and extraintestinal inflammation induced by indomethacin. Gastroenterology. 1992;102:A690.

23. Lichtman SN, Sartor RB, Schwab JH, Keku J. Hepatic inflammation in rats with experimental small bowel bacterial overgrowth. Gastroenterology. 1990;98:414–23.

24. Moore MJ, Singer DE, William RM. Linkage of severity of experimental allergic encephalomyelitis to the rat major histocompatibility locus. J Immunol. 1980;124:1815–20.

25. Schwab JH. Phlogistic properties of peptidoglycan-polysaccharide polymers from cell walls of pathogenic and normal-flora bacteria which colonize humans. Infect Immun. 1993;61:4535–9.

26. Sternberg EM, Hill JM, Chrousos GP et al. Inflammatory mediator-induced hypothalamic-

pituitary-adrenal activation is defective in streptococcal cell wall arthritis-susceptible Lewis rats. Proc Natl Acad Sci USA. 1989;86:2374–8.

27. McCall RD, Haskill JS, Sartor RB. Constitutive expression of TNFα and of an IL-8 like gene is associated with genetic susceptibility to chronic granulomatous enterocolitis in inbred rats. Gastroenterology. 1993;104:A740.

28. Sartor RB, Bender DE, Allen JB et al. Chronic experimental enterocolitis and extraintestinal inflammation are T lymphocyte dependent. Gastroenterology. 1993;104:775A.

29. Bristol LA, Durum SK, Eisenberg SP. Differential regulation of group A streptococcal peptidoglycan-polysaccharide (PG-APS)-stimulated macrophage production of IL-1 by rat strains susceptible and resistant to PG-APS-induced arthritis. Cell Immunol. 1993;149:130–43.

30. Isaacs KL, Sartor RB, Haskill JS. Cytokine mRNA profiles in inflammatory bowel disease mucosa detected by PCR amplification. Gastroenterology. 1992;103:1587–95.

31. Isaacs KL, Sartor RB, Haskill JS. Relative expression of IL-1 and IL-1 receptor antagonist in IBD. Gastroenterology. 1992;102:A729.

32. Beagley KW, Black DA, Elson CO. Strain differences in susceptibility to TNBS-induced colitis. Gastroenterology. 1991;100:A560.

33. Barthold SW, Osbaldiston GW, Jonas AM. Dietary, bacterial, and host genetic interactions in the pathogenesis of transmissible murine colonic hyperplasia. Lab Anim Sci. 1977;27:938–45.

34. Sartor RB. Role of the intestinal microflora in the pathogenesis and complications. In: Scholmerik J, Kruis W, Goebel H, Hohenberger W, Gross V, editors. Inflammatory bowel diseases: pathology as basis of treatment. Falk Symposium 67. Dordrecht: Kluwer; 1993:175–87.

3
Multifactorial control of autoimmune insulin-dependent diabetes in NOD mice: lessons for inflammatory bowel disease

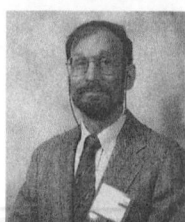

E. H. LEITER

INTRODUCTION

The mouse has been a favored organism for development of models of human genetic diseases. The mouse genome is over 85% homologous with the human genome. In contrast to the other nonhuman mammalian genomes, the mouse genome has been extensively characterized, and is readily amenable to manipulation by transgenic or gene targeting technologies. Inbred mice have been extensively employed to analyze the complex interplay between genes and environment in the development and control of immune responsiveness to antigens. A multiplicity of genes with known effects on immune responsiveness have been mapped. The use of gene targeting to elicit null mutations in specific interleukin genes (e.g. *Il2, Il4, Il10, Tgfb1*) or T cell receptor (TCR) genes render mice susceptible to intestinal inflammation. Indeed, in certain of these gene 'knockout' mice, mucosal inflammation is often the most profound lesion observed; perhaps because, unlike internal tissues, mucosal epithelium and attendant gut-associated lymphoreticular tissue (GALT) are under constant antigenic bombardment[1]. Cytokine imbalances elicited by targeting specific interleukin genes may lead to loss of T lymphocyte-mediated suppression of B lymphocyte responses to mucosal antigens[1]. Differential sensitivity of certain inbred strains to colonic inflammation induced by the macrophage-activating agent, dextran sulfate[2], affords a promising avenue for identifying major genes associated with acute inflammatory responsiveness leading to ulceration of the lower bowel. In addition, identification of a spontaneous, juvenile-onset colitis in C3H/HeJBir mice[3] affords yet another promising tool for dissecting the complex relationship between genes and environment that must underlie most instances of inflammatory bowel disease (IBD) in humans.

Genetic factors presumably comprise a major component of susceptibility to IBD in humans[4]. For example, first-degree relatives of Ashkenazi Jews are at higher risk for IBD development than are first-degree relatives of non-Jewish IBD patients in the same neighborhoods[5]. HLA-B27 is a human MHC class I allele associated with susceptibility to inflammation of joints, as well as the gastrointestinal and urogenital tracts. Lewis rats transgenically expressing both HLA-B27 and human β2-microglobulin (B2M) genes develop a variety of multi-organ inflammatory disorders, including IBD[6]. IBD is a genetically heterogeneous group of disorders, since susceptibility to ulcerative colitis (UC) and Crohn's disease (CD) are associated with different major histocompatibility complex (MHC) class II alleles (DR2 versus DR1/DQw5 respectively)[7]. Insulin-dependent diabetes mellitus (IDDM) is a prototypic example of another genetically heterogeneous, multifactorial disease that geneticists have been grappling with for many years. Until it was recognized that IDDM had an entirely different etiopathogenic basis than the more common forms of human diabetes, collectively referred to as non-insulin-dependent diabetes mellitus (NIDDM), little progress was made. Although advances in knowledge have made IDDM less of the 'geneticist's nightmare' that it formerly was, the polygenetic interactions underlying IDDM in humans are still only poorly understood. A common observation regarding IDDM inheritance in nonconsanguineous human pedigrees was that the disease did not appear in every generation. This underscores the multifactorial nature of this genetically complex disease. IDDM in affected probands likely reflects heterogeneous admixtures of polygenes reassorting throughout the pedigree. The penetrance of susceptibility genes within these changing polygenic combinations likely is responsive to different thresholds of intragenic as well as environmental influences. The importance of various MHC class II (HLA-DR and DQ) alleles as primary determinants of susceptibility in humans[8–10] is clearly established. What remains unclear is whether a finite set of non-MHC susceptibility genes are being segregated, or whether different combinations of polygenes can interact deleteriously with IDDM-predisposing HLA alleles in different environments.

Genetic analysis of IDDM susceptibility in NOD mice provides insight into this question. Currently the products of over 60 generations of brother × sister matings, NOD mice inherit the same gender-specific set of susceptibility genes through the germ line. The genetics and immunology of diabetes in NOD mice have been reviewed recently[11–14]. This chapter will attempt to distill some of the insights gained from genetic and immunologic analysis of NOD mice to project how mouse models of spontaneous IBD may compare to experimentally induced models. The complexity of the polygenetic control of IDDM in NOD mice will also be discussed in the context of the search for IBD susceptibility genes in humans.

MHC CONTROL OF DIABETOGENESIS IN NOD MICE

In mice, autoimmune diseases associated with a number of single gene mutations can be transferred into genetically normal mice following lethal irradiation and reconstitution with bone marrow from mutant mice[15]. In both the NOD mouse and the BB rat (another model of spontaneous IDDM), IDDM can also be transmitted via hematopoietic stem cells[13]. Two recent case reports indicate that IDDM etiopathogenesis in humans also originates as specific defects expressed at the level of bone marrow stem cells. In both case studies, autoimmune diabetes or its preclinical symptoms appear to have been inadvertently transferred by bone marrow transplantation from HLA-matched donors who themselves subsequently developed autoimmune IDDM[16,17]. Since marrow from the *HLA-B27/B2m* transgenic Lewis rat elicits IBD in irradiated hosts, this model clearly shares etiopathogenic features with autoimmune IDDM in NOD mice and BB rats. It was mentioned above that *HLA-DR* class II genes have been identified with risk for development of UC and CD, whereas *HLA-B27* is a class I gene. Presumably, a combination of genes including both MHC class I and class II alleles, and perhaps other intra-MHC loci, is necessary to confer high IBD risk. MHC control of diabetogenesis in the NOD mouse has provided insight into this issue.

The unique MHC haplotpe ($H2^{g7}$) of NOD mice represents the major component of IDDM susceptibility[18]. It should be noted that the uniqueness of this diabetogenic MHC distinguishes it from the relatively common MHC haplotype of IDDM-prone BB rats ($RT1^u$) and the relatively common HLA haplotypes associated with high IDDM risk in Caucasians. As reviewed in ref. 11, DNA sequence analysis shows that the NOD $A\beta$ gene (the homolog to human $DQ\beta$) has a 'diabetogenic' substitution of histidine and serine in place of proline and aspartic acid at residues 56–57[9]. This $A\beta^{g7}$ is quite rare in mice, and its diabetogenic potency has been verified by site-specific mutagenesis to restore either the proline or the aspartic acid codons. Transgenic insertion of either modified $A\beta$ construct into NOD zygotes prevented IDDM. As confirmed by transgenic insertion of a wild-type allele, another diabetogenic component of $H2^{g7}$ is a mutation in the $E\alpha$ gene (homolog to human $DR\alpha$) preventing expression of I-E molecules on the cell surface of antigen-presenting cells (APC). In addition to these two MHC class II alleles, diabetogenesis requires additional genes within the $H2^{g7}$. CTS is an NOD-related inbred strain sharing the same MHC class II and class III alleles as NOD, but differing at MHC class I loci. This MHC haplotype ($H2^{ct}$) is less diabetogenic than $H2^{g7}$ when transferred onto the NOD inbred strain background. Thus, while the MHC class I alleles expressed by the $H2^{g7}$ haplotype are not rare, they are diabetogenic when paired with the specific combination of MHC class II and class III alleles contained within the haplotype.

A locus encoding heat shock protein 70 (*Hsp70*) within the class III region, as well as a locus in the region between *H2K* and *Aβ* encoding a transporter associated with antigen processing (*Tap1*) are among the rare alleles associated with the $H2^{g7}$ haplotype. Although a null mutation preventing *Tap1* gene expression in NOD APC (leading to subsequent low levels of cell surface class I available to present (and tolerize) to self-antigens) has been proposed as the basis for $H2^{g7}$-induced susceptibility[19]; this proposition has not been supported[20-22]. Knockout of the mouse *Tap1* gene by homologous recombination produces mice lacking CD8$^+$ T cells[23]. Deficiency of CD8$^+$ T cells is not a phenotype descriptive of NOD mice. A strain-specific feature of NOD mice is T cell accumulation in the periphery, represented by increases in the percentages of both CD4$^+$ and CD8$^+$ T cells in lymphoid organs, with a coincident decrease in the percentage of B lymphocytes. Diabetogenesis in NOD mice is T cell-mediated. NOD/Lt mice homozygous for the severe combined immunodeficiency (*scid*) mutation cannot generate functional T or B lymphocytes. These mutant mice develop neither insulitis nor IDDM. Splenic T cells from wild-type NOD/Lt mice transfer insulitis and diabetes into unirradiated NOD-*scid/scid* recipients. Both MHC class II-restricted CD4$^+$ T cells and MHC class I restricted CD8$^+$ T cells are required to initiate β cell pathogenesis in this adoptive transfer model[24], NOD mice homozygous for a *B2m* gene inactivated by homologous recombination do not express MHC class I molecules on cell surfaces and, as expected, the thymus fails to positively select a peripheral CD8$^+$ T cell repertoire. Not surprisingly, these CD8$^+$ T cell-deficient mice are incapable of triggering the initial lesions required for development of destructive insulitis and IDDM development[25,26].

Transfer of the NOD$H2^{g7}$ haplotype onto the NON/Lt inbred strain background only rarely elicits IDDM, despite the fact that NON mice are closely related to NOD mice and are the product of selection for impaired glucose tolerance[11]. This clearly illustrates that the MHC component of diabetogenesis requires the presence of (and very likely interaction with) non-MHC susceptibility genes, referred to as *Idd* (insulin-dependent diabetes) loci. Non-MHC genes contribute to numerous defects in APC differentiation and function that reduce the stimulatory capacity of these cells[27]. Given the importance of normal APC function in development and maintenance of tolerance to autoantigens, the genetically controlled APC dysfunctions in NOD mice undoubtedly contribute to this strain's inability to prevent the generation and activation of autoreactive T cells. It has become clear that the NOD's immune system does not mount an isolated, organ-specific autoimmune attack only on the pancreatic β cells. Instead, a variety of tissues and organs are affected by immunoregulatory defects in NOD mice. Indeed, when IDDM is prevented in NOD mice by maintaining the mice on a semipurified diet instead of diabetogenic natural ingredient diets, a broad array of tissue infiltrates are observed. Affected organs and tissues include submandibular glands, thyroid, kidney, lacrimal and Harderian glands, central nervous system, and the large bowel.

The chromosomal locations of certain of the non-MHC *Idd* genes, and the influence of environment on the penetrance of these genes, has been reviewed recently[12]. An important insight gained from the genetic analysis of IDDM susceptibility in NOD mice is that the NOD genome contains but one subset of a much larger set of *potential Idd* genes predisposing to autoimmune disease. To illustrate, when NOD mice are outcrossed to inbred strains such as C57BL/6J (B6) or C57BL/10J (B10), F1 hybrids are uniformly IDDM-free. The conclusion is that the complex polygenic interactions between the specific set of NOD-derived MHC and non-MHC genes required for diabetogenesis have been disrupted. These F1 hybrids must be backcrossed to NOD mice to establish the minimum number of *Idd* genes required to mediate diabetogenesis and their chromosomal locations. When such a backcross is performed, and the genotypes of the diabetic probands determined, new diabetogenic combinations of polygenes distinct from the diabetogenic subset in the NOD genome are uncovered[28]. That is, the genome of the IDDM-resistant partner strain (B6 or B10) contains certain alleles that are even more diabetogenic than the NOD-derived alleles. Hypothetical examples of how susceptibility factors could derive from the 'resistant' strains are easy to provide. Natural killer (NK) activity is defective in NOD, but not in B6 or B10 mice. If more functional NK cells in an insulitic lesion could provide an additional cytopathic component, and if B6/B10 mice transmit an allele allowing normal NK function, then the resistant strain would be perceived as contributing to the penetrance of the diabetic phenotype in hybrid mice. Thus, the genome of the NOD mouse represents but one subset of a larger spectrum of potentially pathogenic gene combinations. When the NOD-specific diabetogenic interactions are disrupted by outcross, and then reassorted into diabetogenic combinations through intercross or backcross progeny, the same fixed set of IDDM susceptibility modifiers defining the NOD genome need not be fully reconstituted to elicit IDDM. In human terms this means that the genetic mechanisms underlying diabetogenesis in NOD mice might be applicable to IDDM in some human pedigrees, but not to others. Identification of the physical nature of the non-MHC *Idd* susceptibility genes in NOD mice will allow medical geneticists to search for the human homologs and assess their contribution to IDDM risk at both the population and family level. However, the evidence that IDDM is genetically heterogeneous in both mice and humans renders its unlikely that the same collection of *Idd* genes contributing to IDDM susceptibility in NOD mice would be faithfully mirrored in the randomly mating human population. This author would predict that a similar level of genetic heterogeneity will underlie susceptibility to IDB. Specifically, even if the genetic basis for UC or CD susceptibility were completely understood in a given animal model, the profile of the human homologs of these loci would fit only a subset of the individuals affected with the respective disease.

COMPARISON OF INDUCED VERSUS SPONTANEOUS MODELS OF IDDM

A number of models exist for experimentally inducing IBD in rodents by exposure to inflammatory or microbial agents. Since IDDM can be elicited in male mice by administration of multiple low doses of the fungal antibiotic stretozotocin (SZ), it is instructive to compare etiopathogenesis with the spontaneous IDDM developing in NOD mice. In males of certain inbred strains, IDDM induction by multi-dose SZ is associated with insulitis development. The issue has been whether or not the insulitis was a response to inflammation induced by the direct β cell cytotoxic effects of SZ, or whether it represented an autoimmune, T cell-mediated destruction as observed in NOD mice[29]. NOD-*scid* mice provide a useful means for testing the ability of leukocytes to adoptively transfer IDDM. Young NOD males treated with multi-dose SZ rapidly become hyperglycemic several months before the time spontaneous IDDM customarily develops. Yet splenic leukocytes from these SZ-diabetic males cannot adoptively transfer disease into NOD-*scid* mice. In contrast, splenic leukocytes from spontaneously diabetic NOD male donors rapidly transfer insulitis and diabetes into NOD-*scid* mice[30]. Thus, the immune system exerts a primary pathogenic role in the spontaneous model, but not in the chemically induced model. In IBD induced in mice by dextran sulfate feeding, leukocytic involvement also appears to be a secondary response to inflammatory damage rather than its cause, since the colonic lesions can also be elicited in *scid* mice (Dr Charles Elson, personal communication).

It is of further interest to compare the T cell-mediated diabetes developing in NOD mice to other induced inflammatory diseases, such as murine experimental allergic encephalomyelitis (EAE). Inbred strain sensitivity to EAE following injection of fragments of myelin basic protein in complete Freund's adjuvant (CFA) is MHC-dependent, and the T cell repertoire is oligoclonal[31]. In marked contrast, a diverse, polyclonal TCR Vβ gene usage by islet-infiltrating T cells has been demonstrated in the early stages of insulitis in NOD mice[32,33]. One other interesting distinction between the EAE model and spontaneous IDDM in mice is that whereas CFA is essential to prime T cells to the myelin basic protein fragments in the EAE model, administration of CFA to prediabetic NOD mice completely suppresses IDDM development[34]. Based upon differences in cytokine mRNA profiles of islet-infiltrating T cells in CFA-treated versus untreated NOD mice, it has been suggested that a predominance of T-helper 1 (Th1) subset of CD4$^+$ T cells expressing IL-2 and interferon-gamma (IFN-γ) are particularly diagnostic of a destructive T cell infiltration of pancreatic islets, whereas a shift in infiltrate composition to the Th2 phenotype (producing IL-4 and IL-10 mRNA) reflects a less pathogenic population[35]. However, recent studies in our laboratory, performed in association with Dr Ammon Peck and colleagues at the University of Florida, indicate that this view may be overly simplistic. We have analyzed by polymerase chain reaction the cytokine profiles in islet-infiltrating macrophages and T cells under conditions in which diabetogenesis was either retarded or accelerated. Reductions in macrophage and CD8-associated mRNA levels correlated with protective treatment (intrathymic islet cells presumably eliciting tolerance). Although both IL-2 and IFN-γ have been used to classify the Th1 phenotype, our data indicated protection was associated with up-regulated IL-2 while IFN-γ mRNA decreased. These results indicate that changes in the overall profiles of monokines and lymphokines can be used to describe the pathogenicity of inflammatory infiltrates.

In IBD, evidence from certain of the knockout mice suggests that cytokine imbalances lead to unregulated B lymphocyte production of cytopathic autoantibodies against mucosal antigens. In NOD mice, B lymphocytes and autoantibodies apparently play a secondary role in pathogenesis. As illustrated by the effect of CFA injection, immunostimulation, far from exacerbating the development of a destructive insulitic lesion, actually retards or prevents it (reviewed recently in ref. 14). One of the primary β cell autoantigens appears to be the enzyme glutamic acid decarboxylase (GAD). Tolerization of adolescent NOD mice with recombinant murine GAD by either intrathymic or i.v. injection prevents IDDM and reduces insulitis[36,37]; interestingly, 'split' tolerance is elicited in that humoral anti-GAD titers are increased in the protected mice.

DYSREGULATED CYTOKINE COMMUNICATION, CANDIDATE AUTOANTIGENS, AND THE ROLE OF THE ENVIRONMENT

The role of environmental factors remains a major unresolved question in the epidemiology of IDDM in humans. Compelling evidence that environmental factors are important modulators of genetic susceptibility to IDDM is provided by analysis of the NOD mouse model. Incidence of diabetes in NOD females is usually 80% or higher by 30 weeks of age, whereas male incidence is highly variable among colonies at different institutions. In one colony, male incidence is 100%, whereas it is as low as 0% in certain other colonies. The environment accounts for a major component of this variation[12]. Diabetes incidence in NOD males serves as a useful indicator of the presence of environmental factors affecting the penetrance of this strain's genetic susceptibility to IDDM. Transfer of NOD males from a conventional mouseroom in Japan into germ-free conditions raised the male diabetes incidence from 6% to 70%[38]. Exposure of NOD mice to variety of murine viruses (encephalomyocarditis virus, lymphocytic choriomeningitis virus, and murine hepatitis virus) prevents diabetes development[39–41]. These infectious agents apparently protect by providing general immunostimulation, since treatment of prediabetic NOD mice with various types of exogenous immunomodulators, including complete Freund's adjuvant[42], cytokines (IL-1, TNF-α, IL-2, IL-4), and poly I:C all circumvent diabetes development (reviewed in ref. 14). Diabetogenic catalysts are also present in natural ingredient diets which contain lipoidal moieties that are absent or present in low concentration in semipurified diets[43]. Thus, penetrance of the diabetic phenotype is strongly modified by the environment. Both mouse and rat models of IBD also appear to be strongly sensitive to environmental stimuli. The maintenance of HLA-B27/B2M rats, IL-2 knockout mice, and IL-10 knockout mice in a high specific-pathogen-free (SPF) state apparently suppresses IBD totally or, in the case of the IL-10 knockout, shifts the extent of the lesions from the small bowel and colon to the right colon only (Dr C. O. Elson, personal communication).

Certain peripheral immunoregulatory functions appear to be defective in NOD mice maintained in SPF environments as exemplified by defective T-suppressor cell functions measured *in vitro*, as well as in defects in the differentiation and maturation of APC developing from bone marrow progenitors (reviewed in ref. 18). Defects in the degree of cytokine-elicited differentiation of APC from bone marrow have been associated with inefficient presentation of 'self' antigens[27,44]. Inefficient presentation of self antigens by NOD APC may explain not only the defective tolerogenic functions of these cells, but also a number of the other dysregulated immune functions characteristic of NOD mice. These include the subnormal secretion of monokines by peripheral macrophages in response to lipopolysaccharide stimulation, the subnormal secretion of IL-2 and IL-4 by splenic and thymic T lymphocytes respectively, the depressed NK cell activity, the depressed thymocyte responses to mitogenic stimulation, and T lymphoaccumulation. Presumably, immunomodulatory effects mediated via environmental components serve to up-regulate certain of these defective APC functions, resulting either in more normal thymic elimination of autoreactive T lymphocytes, more potent activation of immunoregulatory T lymphocytes in the periphery, or both.

One might presume that the target antigens/autoantigens associated with IBD and IDDM would be quite distinct. If much of the inflammatory damage in IBD reflects the consequences of poorly regulated humoral respone to bacterial antigens, IBD would be seemingly distinguished from IDDM, where loss of tolerance to low-abundance β cell products, such as GAD, would be a key element in the pathogenetic process. Bacteria (*E. coli*) produce two GAD isoforms (52.6 kDa) immunologically cross-reactive with the two mouse isoforms (65 and 67 kDa). The recent demonstration[45] that bacterial (*E. coli*) GAD is recognized by GAD-reactive T cells from NOD mice raises the following question: do mice acquire tolerance to low-abundance β cell primary autoantigens such as GAD via exposure of the mucosal immune system to high levels of bacterial homologs or to other proteins introduced through the infant's diet? A small amount of homology has been found between a low-abundance β cell autoantigen (ICA69) and a putatively diabetogenic peptide in cow's milk comprising part of bovine serum albumin (the 'ABBOS' peptide)[46]. Potentially, tolerance to the β cell autoantigen is normally acquired by exposure to the 'molecular mimic' in milk. The observation that gnotobiotic (germ-free) environments increase the penetrance of diabetogenic genes in NOD mice clearly suggests that tolerance to a subset of β cell self antigens is acquired through GALT exposure to bacterially derived homologs or to food proteins processed through the digestive tract. Thus, although this chapter has illustrated as many differences as similarities between rodent models of IBD and IDDM, regulation of mucosal immunity will prove to be an important pathway of effecting therapy in both diseases.

Acknowledgements

The writing of this review was supported by NIH grants DK36175, DK27722, and grants from the Juvenile Diabetes Foundation, International. Dr John

Sundberg (the Jackson Laboratory) is thanked for providing information regarding large bowel histopathology, and Dr Charles Elson (University of Alabama, Birmingham) is thanked for helpful discussions.

References

1. Strober W, Ehrhadt R. Chronic intestinal inflammation: an unexpected outcome in cytokine or T cell receptor mutant mice. Cell. 1993;75:203–5.
2. Cooper H, Murthy S, Shah R, Sedergran D. Clinicopathologic study of dextran sulfate sodium experimental murine colitis. Lab Invest. 1993;69:238–49.
3. Sundberg J, Elson C, Bedigian H, Birkenmeier E. Spontaneous, heritable colitis in a new substrain of C3H/HeJ mice. Gastroenterology. 1994 (Submitted).
4. Yang H, Shohat T, Rotter J. The genetics of inflammatory bowel disease. In: MacDermott R, Stenson W, editors. Current topics in gastroenterology: inflammatory bowel disease. New York: Elsevier; 1992:17–51.
5. Yang H, McElree C, Roth M-P, Shanahan F, Targan S, Rotter J. Familial empirical risks for inflammatory bowel disease: differences between Jews and non-Jews. Gut. 1993;34:517–24.
6. Hammer R, Maika S, Richardson J, Tang J-P, Taurog J. Spontaneous inflammatory disease in transgenic rats expressing HLA-B27 and human β2-m: an animal model of HLA-B27-associated human disorders. Cell. 1990;63:1099–112.
7. Rotter J, Yang H. Resolving the genetics of IBD: the challenge for the 90's. Prog Inflamm Bowel Dis. 1993;14:1–7.
8. Sheehy MJ. HLA and insulin-dependent diabetes. Diabetes. 1992;41:123–9.
9. Todd JA, Acha-Orbea H, Bell JI et al. A molecular basis for MHC class II-associated autoimmunity. Science. 1988;240:1003–9.
10. Nepom GT. A unified hypothesis for the complex genetics of HLA associations with IDDM. Diabetes. 1990;39:1153–7.
11. Kikutani H, Makino S. The murine autoimmune diabetes model: NOD and related strains. In Dixon FJ, editor. Advances in immunology. New York: Academic Press; 1992:285–322.
12. Leiter E. The nonobese diabetic mouse: a model for analyzing the interplay between heredity and environment in development of autoimmune disease. ILAR News. 1993;35:4–14.
13. Serreze D, Leiter E. Insulin dependent diabetes mellitus (IDDM) in NOD mice and BB rats: origins in hematopoietic stem cell defects and implications for therapy. In: Shafrir E, editor. Lessons from animal diabetes. London: Smith-Gordon; 1994 (In press).
14. Bowman M, Leiter E, Atkinson M. Autoimmune diabetes in NOD mice: a genetic programme interruptible by environmental manipulation. Immunol Today. 1994:15:115–20.
15. Shultz LD, Sidman CL. Genetically determined murine models of immunodeficiency. Annu Rev Immunol. 1987;5:367–403.
16. Lampeter E, Homberg M, Quabeck K et al. Transfer of insulin dependent diabetes between HLA-identical siblings by bone marrow transplantation. Lancet. 1993;341:1243–4.
17. Vialettes B, Maraninchi D, San Marco MP et al. Autoimmune polyendocrine failure – type 1 (insulin-dependent) diabetes mellitus and hypothyroidism – after allogeneic bone marrow transplantation in a patient with lymphoblastic leukaemia. Diabetologia. 1993;36:541–6.
18. Leiter EH, Serreze DV. Antigen presenting cells and the immunogenetics of autoimmune diabetes in NOD mice. Reg Immunol. 1992;4:263–73.
19. Faustman D, Li X, Lin HY et al. Linkage of faulty major histocompatibility complex class I to autoimmune diabetes. Science. 1992;254:1756–61.
20. Gaskins HR, Monaco JJ, Leiter EH. Intra-MHC transporter (Ham) genes in diabetes susceptible NOD/Lt mice. Science. 1992;256:1826–8.
21. Wicker L, Podolin P, Fischer P, Sirotina A, Boltz R, Peterson L. Expression of intra-MHC transporter (Ham) genes and class I antigens in diabetes-susceptible NOD mice. Science. 1992;256:1828–30.
22. Pearce RB, Trigler L, Svaasand EK, Peterson CM. Polymorphism in the mouse Tap-1 gene.

J Immunol. 1993;15110:5338–47.

23. Van Kaer L, Ashton-Rickardt P, Ploegh J, Tonegawa S. TAP1 mutant mice are deficient in antigen presentation, surface class I molecules, and CD4$^-$8$^+$ T cells. Cell. 1993;71: 1205–14.

24. Christianson SW, Shultz LD, Leiter EH. Adoptive transfer of diabetes into immunodeficient NOD-scid/scid mice: relative contributions of CD4$^+$ and cD8$^+$ T lymphocytes from diabetic versus prediabetic NON.NON-Thy-1^a donors. Diabetes. 1993;42:44–55.

25. Wicker L, Leiter E, Todd J et al. β2 microglobulin-deficient NOD mice do not develop insulitis or diabetes. Diabetes. 1994;43:500–4.

26. Serreze DV, Leiter EH, Christianson GJ, Greiner D, Roopenian DC. MHC class I deficient NOD-$B2m^{null}$ mice are diabetes and insulitis resistant. Diabetes. 1994;43:505–9.

27. Serreze DV, Gaskins HR, Leiter EH. Defects in the differentiation and function of antigen presenting cells in NOD/Lt mice. J Immunol. 1993;150:2534–43.

28. Risch N, Ghosh S, Todd J. Statistical evaluation of multiple-locus linkage data in eperimental species and its relevance to human studies: application to nonobese diabetic (NOD) mouse and human insulin-dependent diabetes mellitus (IDDM). Am J Hum Genet. 1993;53: 702–14.

29. Wilson GL, Leiter EH. Streptozotocin interactions with pancreatic β cells and the induction of insulin dependent diabetes. In: Dyrberg T, editor. Current topics in microbiology and immunobiology. Berlin: Springer Verlag; 1990:27–54.

30. Gerling I, Freidman H, Greiner D, Shultz L, Leiter E. Multiple low dose streptozotocin-induced diabetes in NOD-scid/scid mice in the absence of functional lymphocytes. Diabetes. 1994;43:433–40.

31. Acha-Orbea H, Mitchell DJ, Timmerman L et al. Limited heterogeneity of T cell receptors from lymphocytes mediating autoimmune encephalomyelitis allows specific immune intervention. Cell. 1988;54:263–73.

32. Waters SH, O'Neill JJ, Melican DT, Appel MC. Multiple TCR Vβ usage by infiltrates of young NOD mouse islets of Langerhans: a polymerase chain reaction analysis. Diabetes. 1992;41:308–12.

33. Maeda T, Sumida T, Kurasawa K et al. T-lymphocyte-receptor repertoire of infiltrating T lymphocytes into NOD mouse pancreas. Diabetes. 1991;40:1580–5.

34. Singh B, Rabinovitch A. Influence of microbial agents on the development and prevention of autoimmune diabetes. Autoimmunity. 1993;15:209–13.

35. Shehadeh NN, LaRosa F, Lafferty KJ. Altered cytokine activity in adjuvant inhibition of autoimmune diabetes. J Autoimmun. 1993;6:291–300.

36. Kaufman D, Clare-Salzler M, Tlan J et al. Spontaneous loss of T-cell tolerance to glutamic acid decarboxylase in murine insulin-dependent diabetes. Nature. 1993;366:69–72.

37. Tisch R, Yang X-D, Singer S, Liblau R, Fugger L, McDevitt H. Immune response to glutamic acid decarboxylase correlates with insulitis in non-obese diabetic mice. Nature. 1993;366:72–5.

38. Suzuki T, Yamada T, Takao T et al. Diabetogenic effects of lymphocyte transfusion on the NOD or NOD nude mouse. In: Rygaard NBJ, Graem M, Sprang-Thomsen M, editors. Immune-deficient animals in biomedical research. Basel: Karger; 1987:112–16.

39. Oldstone MBA. Prevention of type 1 diabetes in nonobese diabetic mice by virus infection. Science. 1988;23:500–2.

40. Wilberz S, Partke HJ, Dagnaes-Hansen F, Herberg L. Persistent MHV (mouse hepatitis virus) infection reduces the incidence of diabetes mellitus in non-obese diabetic mice. Diabetologia. 1991;34:2–5.

41. Hermite L, Vialettes B, Naquet P, Atlan C, Payan M-J, Vague P. Paradoxical lessening of autoimmune processes in non-obese diabetic mice after injection with the diabetogenic variant of encephalomyocarditis virus. Eur J Immunol. 1990;20:1297–303.

42. Sadelain MWJ, Qin H-Y, Lauzon J, Singh B. Prevention of type 1 diabetes in NOD mice by adjuvant immunotherapy. Diabetes. 1990;39:583–9.

43. Coleman DL, Kuzava JE, Leiter EH. Effect of diet on the incidence of diabetes in non-obese diabetic (NOD) mice. Diabetes. 1990;39:432–6.

44. Serreze DV, Gaedeke JW, Leiter EH. Hematopoietic stem cell defects underlying abnormal macrophage development and maturation in NOD/Lt mice: defective regulation of cytokine receptors and protein kinase C. Proc Natl Acad Sci USA. 1993;90:9625–9.

45. Elliott J, Qin H-Y, Bhatti S *et al.* Immunological cross-reactivity between mouse and *E. coli* glutamic acid decarboxylase (GAD) in NOD mice: implications for induction and prevention of autoimmune diabetes. Diabetes. 1994 (In press).
46. Pietropaolo M, Castano L, Babu S *et al.* Molecular cloning, characterization, and chromosome localization of a novel type 1 diabetes-related neuroendocrine autoantigen. J Clin Invest. 1993;92:359–71.

4
Genetics of complex diseases: from mouse to man and back

C. H. WARDEN, J. I. ROTTER and A. J. LUSIS

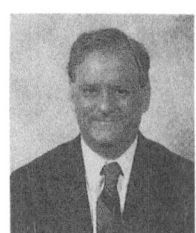

C. H. WARDEN

INTRODUCTION

Identification of genes underlying complex (non-Mendelian) traits, which include diseases such as IBD, has been an important and difficult problem in genetics. However, new tools and methods have brought on a new era in the genetic analysis of complex traits. While identification of the genes underlying common diseases will never be easy, we believe that general approaches to analysis of common diseases are practical now. An outline of the approaches to analysis of complex diseases is given in Fig. 1. The numbers shown for each step correspond to the six sections of this chapter:

1. The role of rare monogenic syndromes in the analysis of complex diseases.
2. Candidate gene and biochemical approaches to complex diseases.
3. Complete linkage maps in humans and animal models.
4. Positional cloning of genes underlying complex diseases in animal models.
5. Testing hypotheses by genetic modifications in animals.
6. Testing whether genes identified in animal models also cause human complex disease.

We plan to illustrate theories and methods recently developed to detect novel genes underlying complex traits using our own studies of the genes underlying atherosclerosis[1-3]. The primary general conclusion of these studies is that

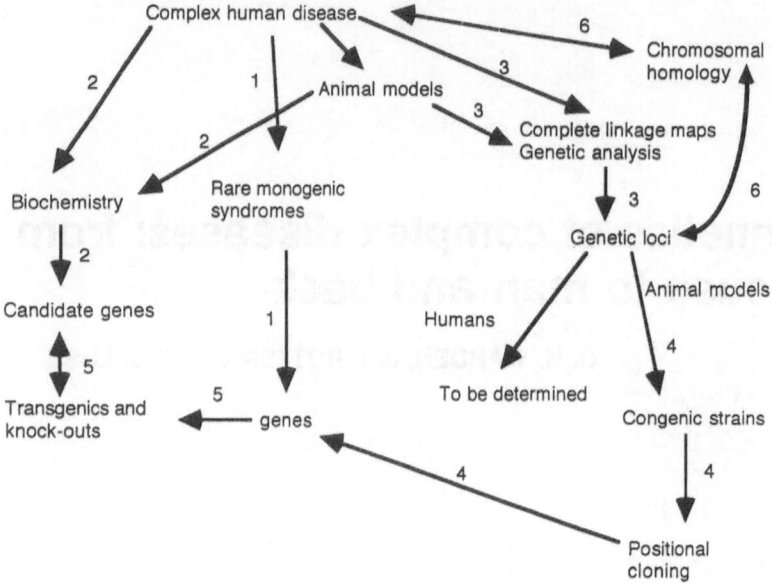

Fig. 1 Outline of the steps involved in the analysis of complex diseases. Numbers in the figure correspond to the numbers of each step in the outline

systematic linkage maps are a particularly powerful approach to the study of complex diseases.

RARE MONOGENIC SYNDROMES

Rare genetic syndromes can provide biochemical and genetic information that leads to the identification of genes underlying complex human diseases. As one example, severe hypercholesterolemia found in familial hypercholesterolemia led to the identification of the role of the low-density lipoprotein receptor (LDLR) in atherosclerosis and facilitated the cloning of the LDLR gene[4,5]. Several recent papers have reported the use of rare genetic syndromes to clone genes involved in colon cancer.

Several rare genetic syndromes are associated with IBD. These syndromes include Hermansky-Pudlak, albinism and glycogen storage disease type Ib[6]. Families exhibiting these diseases provide an opportunity to clone genes involved in IBD. One concern is that these genes may underlie only a very small percentage of the total cases of IBD, as is the case for the LDLR gene and atherosclerosis.

CANDIDATE GENE AND BIOCHEMICAL APPROACHES

We will illustrate the role of biochemical and candidate gene approaches to a complex disease with studies from atherosclerosis[7]. The identification of genes underlying susceptibility to atherosclerosis and its risk factors has thus far involved two direct approaches. The first is a biochemical approach, involving the direct isolation and characterization of products of the responsible gene. In the area of atherosclerosis, an outstanding example is the identification of the LDLR defects in familial hypercholesterolemia[4,8]. Success with a biochemical approach generally requires that the effects of the genetic alteration are substantial rather than subtle, that tissues or cells expressing the altered gene product are accessible, and that some clues about the nature of the alteration can be deduced.

A second direct approach has been termed the 'candidate gene' approach. It involves testing whether polymorphisms of genes that mechanistically may be responsible for disorders (therefore the term 'candidate') correlate in population or family studies with susceptibility to the disorder[9]. Polymorphisms of DNA, such as restriction fragment length polymorphisms (RFLP), or microsatellite polymorphisms, are used to type the individuals involved in the population or family study. The first striking example of the utility of the candidate gene approach was the demonstration that structural polymorphisms of apolipoprotein E (apoE) affect cholesterol levels and are associated with type III hyperlipidemia. Subsequent work revealed the biochemical basis of the polymorphisms: altered binding of apoE containing lipoproteins to LDLR[10].

It has recently been estimated that 35 of the 41 genes underlying diseases in mice, that have been identified at a molecular level, were identified by a candidate gene approach[11]. The candidate gene approach can also be applied to complex traits. Studies of the non-obese diabetic (NOD) mouse have used comprehensive linkage maps constructed in genetic crosses to demonstrate that there is linkage of a defective Fc receptor for IgG to autoimmune diabetes in NOD mice[12].

There are a large number of candidate genes for IBD. They include genes coding for the HLA complex, complement proteins, immunoglobulins, cytokines and additional molecules. These candidate genes could be tested for their association and linkage to IBD by using specific assays in human families and in association studies. The role of each of these many candidate genes in IBD could be tested more quickly by using complete linkage maps in family studies.

COMPLETE LINKAGE MAPS

Animal models

A method has recently been developed for mapping of quantitative trait loci in animal models (QTL)[13,14]. QTL mapping is a general method that does not require any previous knowledge regarding the underlying physiology of the disease being studied.

QTL mapping involves four steps: (a) two different inbred strains are crossed to produce F2 or backcross progeny; (b) the progeny are individually genotyped for markers which span the genome at 10–20 centiMorgan (cM) intervals (a centiMorgan is a measure of genetic linkage distance, indicating frequency of recombination between the genetic loci of 1%); (c) each of the progeny is phenotyped for the traits of interest; and (d) QTLs are located by a statistical approach, such as that provided by Mapmaker/QTL[14].

Mice have many advantages for studies of the genetics of complex traits that have made them a useful resource [7]; (a) many diverse inbred strains are available; (b) mice can be used for hypothesis testing by construction of transgenics and knockout mice; (c) the genetic map of the mouse is second only to that of humans; (d) finally, many powerful genetic resources are available, such as congenics and recombinant inbred strains.

Example of mapping complex traits in a mouse model: apoA-II

The principles of QTL mapping can be illustrated with a mouse backcross that has been analyzed for genes underlying obesity and atherosclerosis. A backcross was performed by crossing F1 females, resulting from the cross of female C57BL/6J with male *M. spretus* mice, with male C57BL/6J mice. We have designated these backcross progeny as BSB mice[15]. Linkage of these genes with the quantitative traits has been determined by analysis of variance (ANOVA) and by LOD score analysis with the Mapmaker/QTL program[2].

We have measured plasma apolipoprotein A-II (apoA-II) levels in the BSB mice. A peak LOD score of 4.0 was revealed on mouse chromosome 1 centered around the Apoa2 gene locus. This QTL includes approximately 10 cM in the 90% confidence interval and thus includes many diverse genes. However, the coincidence of the QTL for plasma apoA-II levels and the Apoa2 gene, suggests that the Apoa2 gene directly controls plasma apoA-II levels. This hypothesis was subsequently tested successfully in transgenic mice and in humans (see below).

Animal models for IBD

There are several animal models that might be used for studies of IBD. For instance, peptidoglycan-polysaccharide injection of Lewis rats leads to granulomatous hepatitis and anemia. However, Buffalo and F344 rats are genetically resistant to this injection. Thus, crosses of Lewis rats with Buffalo or F344 rats could be used to identify genes involved in this response.

Complete linkage maps in humans

Theories and methods to detect novel genes underlying complex traits with systematic linkage maps in humans have been developed[13,16]. The major requirement of these methods is the generation of systematic linkage maps. Systematic linkage maps will require that hundreds of markers be typed in each member of families with IBD. The simple sequence repeat PCR markers are ideal for this purpose. There are currently more than 2000 simple sequence repeat PCR markers available for human linkage mapping[17,18]. These markers can be typed rapidly, at low cost, are highly polymorphic, and are spaced at an average of 1.5 cM (since there are 3000 cM in the human genome).

Studies with the Apoa2 locus, to be discussed below, suggest that random genetic markers may exhibit significant linkage to quantitative traits at 5–20 cM distances from the genes underlying quantitative traits. For instance, we have found that D1S74, 5.7 cM from the apolipoprotein A-II structural locus, can detect a highly significant linkage ($p < 0.045$) to serum levels of free fatty acids (FFA), in multiplex coronary artery disease families[1]. A complete linkage map capable of detecting novel genes underlying quantitative traits could then be constructed by genotyping just 150 markers. The actual number of markers needed will depend on the complexity of the disease, the heterozygosity of the markers, the number of families, and the number of affected in each family[16].

Positional cloning

Positional cloning (also known as reverse genetics) is a powerful approach for identification and characterization of genes for monogenic disorders in which no biochemical or candidate gene can be identified. Positional cloning involves: first, the identification of genetic markers linked to a disease gene by testing for cosegregation of the disease phenotype with genetic markers spanning various parts of the genome; second, physically cloning regions of the genome surrounding the genetic markers; and third, testing whether genes present in the cloned regions have properties consistent with the disease gene, such as lack of recombination with the disease gene or alterations in expression in affected individuals. Thus, a reverse genetics approach is not dependent upon an understanding of the molecular mechanisms contributing to the disease. Recent years have witnessed the cloning of several genes causing human disease by a 'positional genetics' approach, including those for familial adenomatous polyposis[19,20] and colon cancer.

Unfortunately, reverse genetic approaches are difficult to use in human studies of multifactorial disorders such as atherosclerosis and IBD. First, it is difficult to identify the responsible genetic loci, since multiple independently segregating loci contribute to the disorders. This problem is exacerbated by the problem of genetic heterogeneity (in which a similar disorder is caused in different individuals by different genetic defects). Other problems with human genetic studies include: incomplete penetrance, and gene interactions (synthetic traits).

Use of congenics to facilitate positional cloning

Identification of QTLs is just the first step in the study of genes underlying atherosclerosis in mice. Biochemical and physiological studies will require that identification of the specific genes underlying complex traits. One method to identify the specific gene underlying a QTL is to use, or to produce, congenic mouse strains. A congenic mouse strain is genetically identical to a background strain, except for a small chromosomal region derived from a donor strain. Thus, one can study the effects of a single donor gene on the background of a second strain, isolated from the effects of other donor strain

Mouse chromosome 7

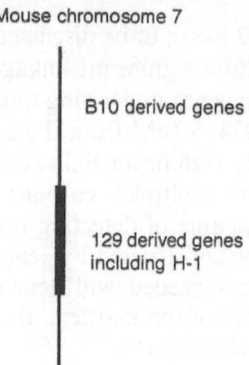

B10 derived genes

129 derived genes
including H-1

Fig. 2 Approximate appearance of the B10.129 (H-1) congenic mouse strain. All other chromosomes in this congenic strain would be derived from the C57BL/10SnJ background strain

genes[21]. For example, a congenic with C57BL10/J as the background strain and strain 129 as the donor strain for the mouse chromosome 7 H-1 locus would then have this very approximate appearance (Fig. 2).

Congenic strains can be bred to their background strain and the resulting F2 progeny used to isolate the underlying genes. For instance, positional cloning of atherosclerosis genes could be guided by progeny of a cross between a congenic strain containing a single atherosclerosis susceptibility gene with the background strain. This can work because a single gene would now be responsible for genetic variation in the trait. Several methods are also available that specifically identify restriction fragment length variants (RFLVs) for the donor strain of a congenic[22]. These RFLVs could aid in the positional cloning of the underlying genes.

Testing hypotheses by genetic modification in animals

As shown above, we have demonstrated a QTL for serum apoA-II levels at the locus surrounding the mouse Apoa2 gene. We next used transgenic mice to test the hypothesis that the Apoa2 gene controls plasma apoA-II levels. We have generated mice that are transgenic for the mouse Apoa2 gene[23]. Transgenic mice were constructed using a genomic clone of the mouse Apoa2 gene containing several kb of 5' flanking and 3' flanking DNA. Southern blot analysis revealed that approximately 10 copies of the Apoa2 gene were integrated into the genome in this line.

The studies revealed that transgenic mice that overexpress mouse apoA-II had elevated HDL-cholesterol concentrations but, nevertheless, exhibited increased atherosclerotic lesion development as compared to normal mice[3]. Laboratory strains of mice do not develop significant aortic fatty streak lesions when maintained on chow diets. ApoA-II transgenic mice developed aortic lesions on a chow diet despite the fact that they had high concentrations of HDL and low concentrations of LDL and VLDL. Lesion development was observed in transgenic mice of both sexes. The HDL in the transgenic mice was larger and had an increased ratio of apoA-II to apoA-I. Thus, both the composition and amount of HDL appear to be important determinants of atherosclerosis. These results clearly suggest that the Apoa2 gene underlies the QTL observed in the BSB cross.

Testing whether genes contribute to human disease

Extension of mouse mapping results to humans is possible because comparative gene mapping has demonstrated that linked homologous genes are found in 101 conserved autosomal segments[11]. To test whether variations of the Apoa2 gene influence plasma lipid metabolism in humans, we studied 306 individuals in 25 families enriched for coronary artery disease. The segregation of the Apoa2 gene was followed using an informative simple sequence repeat in the second intron of the gene[24] as well as two nearby genetic markers. Robust sib-pair linkage analysis was performed on members of these families using the SAGE linkage programs[25].

The results demonstrated linkage between the human Apoa2 gene and a gene controlling plasma apoA-II levels. Plasma apoA-II levels were also significantly correlated with plasma free fatty acid levels. Moreover, the Apoa2 gene exhibited significant linkage with a gene controlling free fatty acid levels. Evidence for nonrandom segregation was seen with markers as far as 6–12 cM from the Apoa2 structural locus[1].

SUMMARY

Animal models are useful to identify genes underlying complex diseases and for testing hypotheses and studying functions of proteins involved in complex traits (Fig. 1). Thus, transgenic models have been recently used to examine questions relating to atherosclerosis. Targeted disruption of genes in mice are potentially very informative. Similarly, several novel models of IBD have been identified by targeted mutagenesis in mice. Many studies have suggested that IBD patients have hyperresponsiveness to normal gut constituents; however, they have failed to define the reasons at cellular or molecular levels[26]. Thus, the discovery of ulcerative colitis-like disease in mice with a disrupted interleukin-2 gene suggested a primary role for the immune system in the etiology of ulcerative colitis[27]. Spontaneous development of IBD has also been reported in mice with mutations in the T cell receptor (TCR) a mutant, TCR β mutant, or class II major histocompatibility mutant mice[28]. These results suggested that dysfunction of the immune system may underlie pathogenesis of IBD. Finally, it has also been reported that interleukin-10-deficient mice suffer from chronic enterocolitis[29]. The results suggest that bowel inflammation results from uncontrolled immune responses and that interleukin-10 is an essential regulator[29]. All totaled, these gene targeted mice represent novel models of IBD. The presumed final common pathway is a disorder in the normal control mechanisms that normally down-regulate responses to mucosal antigens. Finally, it seems possible that these models can be used to develop therapeutic strategies for IBD, even though the pathogenesis of the mouse and human diseases are not identical[26].

CONCLUSIONS

Our work with mice strongly suggests that complete linkage maps are very likely to identify genes underlying complex traits, such as IBD. One of the biggest advantages of the systematic linkage approach is that one can narrow the list of candidate genes for a disease to those that are present in the loci underlying complex traits. Furthermore, systematic linkage maps may also identify novel genes or loci that are important in the etiology of the disease.

Acknowledgements

This work was supported in part by grants from the Crohn's and Colitis Foundation of America, NIH Program project grant DK46763, the Stuart foundation, and the Cedars-Sinai Board of Governors' Chair in Medical Genetics (JIR).

References

1. Warden CH, Daluiski A, Bu X *et al*. Evidence for linkage of the apolipoprotein A-II locus to plasma apolipoprotein A-II and free fatty acid levels in mice and humans. Proc Natl Acad Sci USA. 1993;90:10886–90.
2. Warden CH, Fisler JS, Pace MJ, Svenson KL, Lusis AJ. Coincidence of genetic loci for plasma cholesterol levels and obesity in a multifactorial mouse model. J Clin Invest. 1993;92:773–9.
3. Warden CH, Hedrick CC, Qiao JH, Castellani LW, Lusis AJ. Atherosclerosis in transgenic mice overexpressing apolipoprotein A-II. Science. 1993;261:469–72.
4. Goldstein JL, Brown MS. Familial hypercholesterolemia. In: Stanbury JB, Wyngaarden JB, Frederickson DS, Goldstein JL, Brown MS, editors. The metabolic basis of inherited disease. New York: McGraw-Hill; 1983;672–712.
5. Hobbs HH, Russell DW, Brown MS, Goldstein JL. The LDL receptor locus in familial hypercholesterolemia: mutational analysis of a membrane protein. Annu Rev Genet. 1990;24:133–70.
6. Yang H, Rotter JI. The genetics of inflammatory bowel disease: genetic predispositions, disease markers, and genetic heterogeneity. In: Targan SR, Shanahan F, editors. Inflammatory bowel disease: from bench to bedside. Baltimore: Williams & Wilkins; 1994:32–64.
7. Warden CH, Daluiski A, Lusis AJ. Identification of new genes contributing to atherosclerosis: the mapping of genes contributing to complex disorders in animal models. In: Lusis AJ, Rotter JI, Sparkes RS, editors. Monographs in human genetics: molecular genetics of coronary artery disease. Basel: Karger; 1992:419–41.
8. Brown MS, Goldstein JL. A receptor-mediated pathway for cholesterol homeostasis. Science. 1986;232:34–47.
9. Mehrabian M, Lusis AJ. Genetic markers for studies of atherosclerosis and related risk factors. In: Lusis AJ, Rotter JI, Sparkes RS, editors. Monographs in human genetics: molecular genetics of coronary artery disease. Basel: Karger; 1992:363–418.
10. Rall SC Jr, Mahley RW. The role of apolipoprotein E genetic variants in lipoprotein disorders. J Intern Med. 1992;231:653–9.
11. Copeland NG, Jenkins NA, Gilbert DJ *et al*. A genetic linkage map of the mouse: current

applications and future prospects. Science. 1993;262:57–66.

12. Prins J-B, Todd JA, Rodrigues NR *et al*. Linkage on chromosone 3 of autoimmune diabetes and defective Fc receptor for IgG in NOD mice. Science. 1993;260:695–8.

13. Lander ES, Botstein D. Mapping Mendelian factors underlying quantitative traits using RFLP linkage maps. Genetics. 1989;121:185–99.

14. Paterson AH, Damon S, Hewitt JD *et al*. Mendelian factors underlying quantitative traits in tomato: Comparison across species, generations, and environments. Genetics. 1991;127:181–97.

15. Warden CH, Mehrabian M, He K *et al*. Linkage mapping of 40 randomly isolated liver cDNA clones in the mouse. Genomics. 1993;18:295–307.

16. Lander ES, Botstein D. Mapping complex genetic traits in humans: new methods using a complete RFLP linkage map. Cold Spring Harb Symp Quant Biol. 1986;LI:49–62.

17. Weissenbach J, Gyapay G, Dib C *et al*. A second-generation linkage map of the human genome. Nature. 1992;359:794–801.

18. Hudson TJ, Engelstein M, Lee MK *et al*. Isolation and chromosomal assignment of 100 highly informative human simple sequence repeat polymorphisms. Genomics. 1992;13:622–9.

19. Groden J, Thilveris A, Samowitz W *et al*. Identification and characterization of the familial adenomatous polyposis coli gene. Cell. 1991;66:589–600.

20. Kinzler KW, Nilbert MC, Su L-K *et al*. Identification of FAP locus genes from chromosome 5q21. Science. 1991;253:661–5.

21. Mehrabian M, Quiao J-H, Human R, Ruddle D, Laughton C, Lusis AJ. Influence of the ApoA-II gene locus on HDL levels and fatty streak development in mice. Arterioscler Thromb. 1993;13:1–10.

22. Lisitsyn NA, Segre JA, Kusumi K *et al*. Direct isolation of polymorphic markers linked to a trait by genetically directed representational difference analysis. Nature Genet. 1994;6:57–63.

23. Hedrick CC, Castellani LW, Warden CH, Puppione DL, Lusis AJ. Influence of mouse apolipoprotein A-II on plasma lipoproteins in transgenic mice. J Biol Chem. 1993;268:20676–82.

24. Weber JL, May PE. Abundant class of human DNA polymorphisms which can be typed using the polymerase chain reaction. Am J Hum Genet. 1989;44:388–96.

25. Wilson AF, Elston RC, Tran LD, Siervogel RM. Use of the robust sib-pair method to screen for single-locus, multiple-locus, and pleiotropic effects: application to traits related to hypertension. Am J Hum Genet. 1991;48:862–72.

26. Strober W, Ehrhardt RO. Chronic intestinal inflammation: an unexpected outcome in cytokine or T cell receptor mutant mice. Cell. 1993;75:203–5.

27. Sadlack B, Merz H, Schorle H, Schimpl A, Feller AC, Horak I. Ulcerative colitis-like disease in mice with a disrupted interleukin-2 gene. Cell. 1993;75:253–61.

28. Mombaerts P, Mizoguchi E, Grosby MJ, Glimcher LH, Bhan AK, Tonegawa S. Spontaneous development of inflammatory bowel disease in T cell receptor mutant mice. Cell. 1993;75:275–82.

29. Kühn R, Löhler J, Rennick D, Rajewsky K, Müller W. Interleukin-10-deficient mice develop spontaneous chronic enterocolitis. Cell. 1993;75:263–74.

Section II
Predisposing factors in the etiology of IBD: bugs, drugs and leaks

5
Crohn's disease: the pathogenesis of a granulomatous vasculitis: a hypothesis

A. J. WAKEFIELD

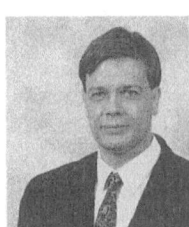

INTRODUCTION

Crohn's disease, considered by many authorities to be a disease primarily of the intestinal mucosa[1,2], is characterized both histologically and immunologically by a cell-mediated immune response to an as yet unidentified antigen(s)[3].

In 1987, based upon macroscopic similarities between rejecting experimental intestinal allografts and Crohn's disease, the hypothesis was formulated that common pathogenetic factors may be operating in these two otherwise distinct disease entities. In allograft rejection, microvascular activation and injury are early events, initiated by host immune recognition of alloantigen on graft vascular endothelium[4]. In Crohn's disease there were clues to suggest that microvascular injury might be involved in the pathogenesis of intestinal inflammation: in biopsies of patients with inflammatory bowel disease, mucosal capillary thrombi can be seen[5] and vasculitis, including granulomatous vasculitis, is a recognized feature of Crohn's disease[6,7]. Regarded previously as a secondary phenomenon, however, vasculitis was seen only occasionally in routinely processed histological sections, and was considered to be of little pathological significance[6,7]. In parallel with this apparent dismissal of the potential significance of granulomatous vasculitis in Crohn's disease was a disregard, with notable exceptions[8,9], for the tissue origins of the granuloma, an early and hallmark lesion of this condition. The granuloma represents a localizing reaction to persistent and potentially causative antigen:

47

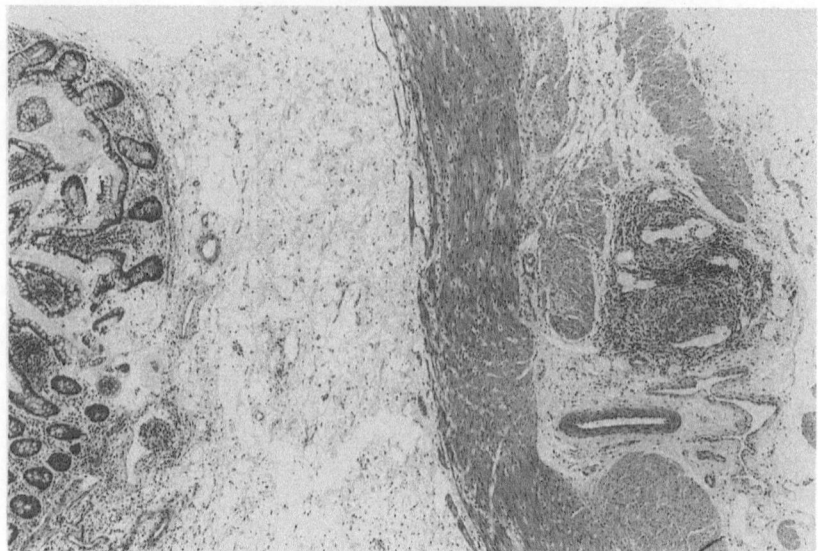

Fig. 1   Focus of serosal granulomatous vasculitis in Crohn's disease. (Magnification × 250)

therefore, the tissue relationships of this lesion assumed great importance in progressing our own understanding of Crohn's disease.

GRANULOMATOUS VASCULITIS IN CROHN'S DISEASE

Based upon the hypothesis that foci of both granulomatous and lymphocytic vasculitis in Crohn's disease may have evolved from blood vessels that contain foreign antigen, clarifying the interrelationship of these two tissue elements was a priority. This was aided by overcoming vascular artefacts produced by routine immersion–fixation of tissues, and immunostaining for specific vascular and granulomatous elements in tissue sections[10,11].

Perfusion–fixation at mean arterial pressure not only produced excellent tissue preservation, but also prevented vascular collapse and blood clot obscuring the relationship of blood vessels to foci of inflammation. Immunostaining for vascular elements and macrophages on serial sections facilitated the recognition that the great majority of granulomas in Crohn's disease arise from blood vessels – predominantly thin-walled veins. This process is associated with thrombosis, vascular occlusion and likely ischemia of the dependent tissues (Fig. 1). We have since shown that vasculitis and a chronic ischemic injury of the intestine may help to explain many of the idiosyncrasies of this condition, including 'skip' lesions and transmural inflammation[12,13], aphthoid ulceration[14], anastomotic recurrence[15] and thrombogenesis[16–19].

Of greater importance, perhaps, was the observation that many granulomas were associated intimately with pathologically altered endothelium. In view of the capacity of activated endothelium to present antigen in association

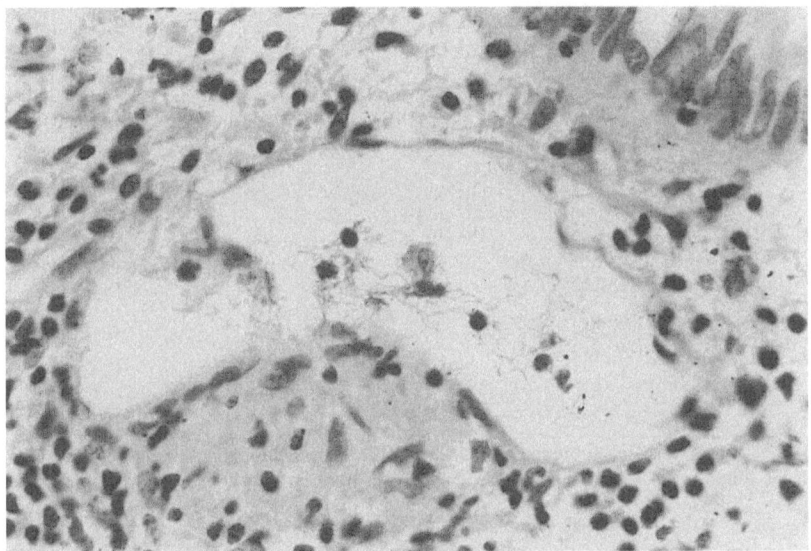

Fig. 2 Crohn's disease: intravascular mucosal granuloma surrounded by fibrin thrombus immunostained for fibrinogen (arrowed) (Dako). (Magnification × 300)

with class II determinants[20], the hypothesis that the mesenteric microvascular endothelium is a reservoir for the persistent antigen that induces Crohn's disease, seemed increasingly attractive. The hypothesis did not maintain that the vasculature, or indeed the endothelium, was the only site of primary antigen presentation. These elements did, however, provide a target for further detailed studies.

MEASLES VIRUS AND MICROVASCULAR ENDOTHELIUM

The hypothesis proposed that persistent viral infection of the mesenteric endothelium is necessary for the development of Crohn's disease. Certain criteria were considered when selecting candidate viruses for further study: enterotropism during the primary infection, the capacity to infect and persist within microvascular endothelium, and the capacity to induce a profound cellular immune response that is associated with giant cell formation.

Measles virus – a common, highly infectious agent recognized for its capacity to persist within, and induce chronic inflammation of, cerebral tissues – appeared to fulfill these criteria[21]. A number of other viruses were studied in detail, but were not found to be implicated[22].

Subsequent detailed examination of 24 cases of Crohn's disease and 22 inflammatory and non-inflammatory intestinal controls identified measles virus in the endothelium, lymphocytes and macrophages of inflammatory foci in Crohn's disease, but this was not seen in controls[23]. Transmission electron microscopy identified paramyxovirus-like nucleocapsids within

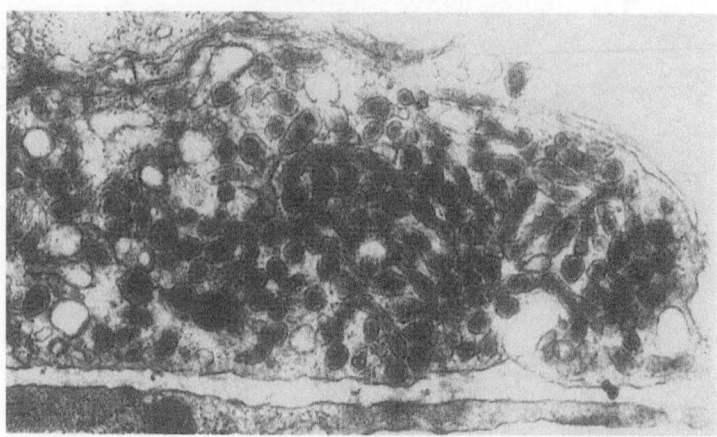

Fig. 3 Crohn's disease: submucosal microvascular endothelium containing discrete pleomorphic tubular and vesicular virus particles 70–100 nm diameter consistent with paramyxoviridae

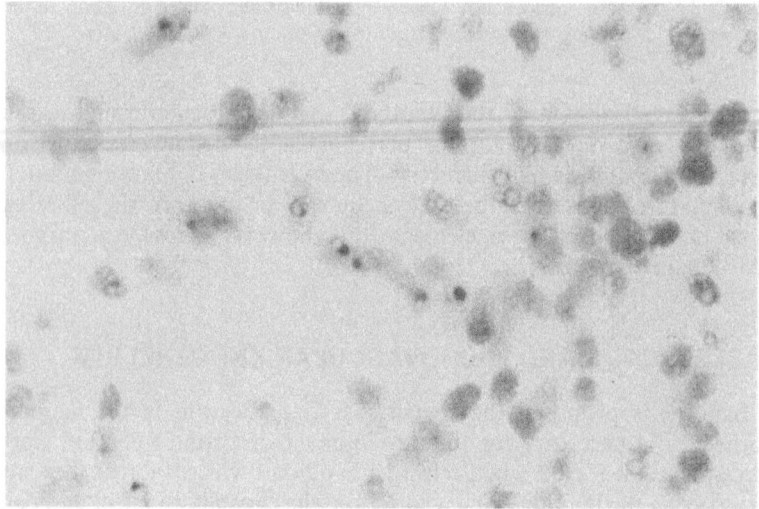

Fig. 4 Crohn's disease: *in-situ* hybridization for measles virus N-gene (arrowed) in the centre of a granuloma. (Magnification × 320)

endothelial cells in areas of granulomatous vasculitis: endothelial cells, apparently infected with virus, were participating actively in the inflammatory process (Fig. 3). *In-situ* hybridization for measles virus genomic RNA gave positive signals in the same cellular location (Fig. 4). Hybridization signals were also strongly positive in the centers of secondary lymphoid follicles in a pattern identical to that described previously in the appendix, in association with persistent measles virus infection[24]. Immunocytochemistry using both

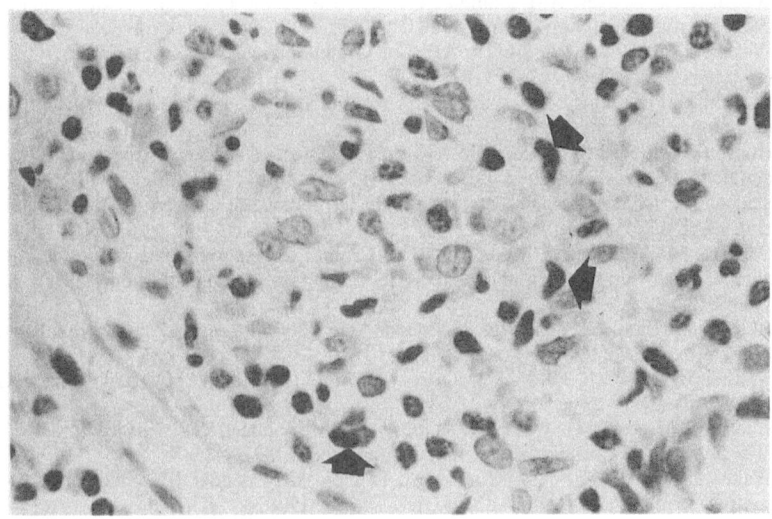

Fig. 5 Crohn's disease: immunohistochemistry for measles virus N-protein (arrowed) in a small submucosal granuloma. (Magnification × 320)

measles virus-specific monoclonal and polyclonal antibodies was positive in these lesions in 13 of 15 cases (Fig. 5) and was not seen in intestinal tuberculosis, studied as a granulomatous control.

Other groups have now obtained independent evidence, from both basic science and epidemiological studies, of a role for persistent measles virus infection in the etiology of Crohn's disease[25,26]. Although much work remains to be done these data are interesting and merit further study.

References

1. Price A, Talbot IC, Thompson H, Williams GT. Pathogenesis of Crohn's disease. Lancet. 1990;1:804.
2. Morson BC. The earliest histological lesion of Crohn's disease. Proc R Soc Med. 1972;65: 71–2.
3. Jewell DP, Snook JA. Immunology of ulcerative colitis and Crohn's disease. In: Allan RN, Keighley MRB, Alexander-Williams J, Hawkins C, editors. Inflammatory bowel diseases. 2nd edn. Edinburgh: Churchill-Livingstone; 1990;12:127–46.
4. Bishop GA, Waugh GA, Landers DV, Krensky AM, Hall BM. Microvascular destruction in renal transplant rejection. Transplantation. 1989;48:408–14.
5. Dhillon AP, Anthony A, Sim R *et al*. Mucosal capillary thrombi in rectal biopsies. Histopathology. 1992;21:127–33.
6. Knutson H, Lunderquist A. Vascular changes in Crohn's disease. Am J Roentgenol. 1968;103:380–5.
7. Geller SA, Cohen A. Arterial inflammatory infiltration in Crohn's disease. Arch Pathol Lab Med. 1983;107:473–7.
8. Lockhart-Mummery HE, Morson BC. Crohn's disease of the large intestine. Gut. 1964;5: 493–509.
9. Morson BC. Pathology of Crohn's disease. In: Brooke BB, editor. Clinics in gastroenterology, 1(2); Crohn's disease. London: WB Saunders; 1972:265–77.

10. Wakefield AJ, Sawyerr AM, Dhillon AP et al. Pathogenesis of Crohn's disease: multifocal gastrointestinal infarction. Lancet. 1989;1:1057–62.
11. Wakefield AJ, Sankey EA, Dhillon AP et al. Granulomatous vasculitis in Crohn's disease. Gastroenterology. 1990;100:1279–87.
12. Hudson M, Piasecki C, Sankey EA et al. A ferret model of acute multifocal gastrointestinal infarction. Gastroenterology. 1992;102:1591–6.
13. Hudson M, Piasecki C, Wakefield AJ et al. A vascular hypersensitivity model of acute multifocal intestinal infarction. Dig Dis Sci. 1994 (In press).
14. Sankey EA, Dhillon AP, Wakefield AJ et al. Early mucosal changes in Crohn's disease. Gut. 1993;34:375–81.
15. Osborne MJ, Hudson M, Piasecki C et al. Crohn's disease and anastomotic recurrence: microvascular ischaemia and anastomotic healing in an animal model. Br J Surg. 1993;80:226–9.
16. Hudson M, Chitole A, Wakefield AJ, Pounder RE. Thrombogenic risk factors in inflammatory bowel disease. 1994 (Submitted).
17. Hudson M, Wakefield AJ, Hutton RA et al. Factor XIIIA subunit in Crohn's disease. Gut. 1993;34:75–9.
18. Hudson M, Hutton RA, Wakefield AJ, Sawyerr AM, Pounder RE. Evidence for activation of coagulation in Crohn's disease. Blood Coag Fibrin. 1992;3:773–8.
19. Wakefield AJ, Sawyerr AM, Hudson M, Dhillon AP, Pounder RE. Smoking, the oral contraceptive pill and Crohn's disease. Dig Dis Sci. 1991;36:1147–50.
20. Petty RG, Pearson JD. Endothelium – the axis of vascular health and disease. J Roy Coll Phys. 1989;23:92–102.
21. Norby E, Oxman MN. Measles virus. In: Fields BN, editor. Virology. New York: Raven Press; 1990;37:1013–44.
22. Wakefield AJ, Fox JD, Sawyerr AM et al. Detection of herpesvirus DNA in the large intestine of patients with ulcerative colitis and Crohn's disease using the nested polymerase chain reaction. J Med Virol. 1992;38:183–90.
23. Wakefield AJ, Pittilo RM, Sim R et al. Evidence of persistent measles virus infection in Crohn's disease. J Med Virol. 1993;39:345–53.
24. Fournier JG, Lebon P, Bouteille M, Goutiers F, Rozenblatt S. Subacute sclerosing panencephalitis: detection of measles virus RNA in appendix lymphoid tissue before clinical signs. Br Med J. 1986;293:523–4.
25. Knibbs DR, Van Kruiningen HJ, Colombel JF, Cotort A. Ultrastructural evidence of paramyxovirus in two French families with Crohn's disease. Gastroenterology. 1993;104:A726.
26. Ekbom A, Wakefield AJ, Zack M, Adami HO. The role of perinatal measles infection in the aetiology of Crohn's disease: a population based epidemiological study. 1994 (Submitted).

6
Intestinal permeability: the basics

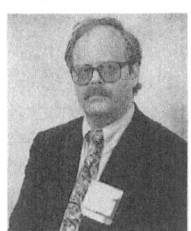

I. BJARNASON, A. MACPHERSON and
I. S. MENZIES

I. BJARNASON

INTRODUCTION

Twenty years ago it became possible, with the introduction of nonmetabolized sugars as test substances, to assess intestinal permeability reliably and non-invasively in humans[1]. Acceptance of the technique was initially slow, mainly because of the confusion that the use of polyethylene glycol (PEG 400) brought with it[2,3], but in the past few years there has been a proliferation of published studies, from a wide range of research workers, using these tests to assess various aspects of gastrointestinal diseases. Tests of intestinal permeability may relate to at least five purposes; these are:

1. Diagnostic screening for intestinal disease.
2. Confirming diagnosis; indication of therapeutic response and prognosis.
3. Evaluation of drug-related, dietary and environmental factors upon the intestine.
4. The effect of various physiological factors on intestinal barrier function; for instance, related to diet (e.g. level of food intake and osmolar content), level of nutrition and state of blood flow.
5. To assess the importance of the intestinal barrier function in the etiology, pathophysiology and pathogenesis of intestinal and systemic disease.

A detailed discussion of all of the above is beyond the scope of this chapter. However, a noticeable feature of many publications involving tests of intestinal permeability is a frequent failure to realize the importance of factors relating to the preparation of test solutions and conduct of test procedures. Furthermore, many practical problems encountered when setting up the necessary clinical and laboratory procedures require attention to special details. It is important to discuss these issues to ensure that such non-invasive test procedures might be successfully exploited to assess intestinal permeability and related aspects of intestinal function.

CHOICE OF MARKER: PRINCIPLE OF THE URINARY EXCRETION OF ORALLY ADMINISTERED TEST SUBSTANCES

Testing intestinal permeability sounds simple! The subject fasts overnight, drinks a solution containing test substances the following morning and the subsequent timed recovery of test substances in the urine indicates intestinal permeation of the administered probes.

The choice of probe employed for assessing intestinal permeability has changed somewhat through the years. Initially a single probe such as lactulose or other non-metabolized disaccharide (melibiose), trisaccharide (raffinose) or polysaccharide (dextrans), was used by itself[1,4-6]. Properties with respect to molecular size, water/lipid solubility, susceptibility to metabolic degradation, affinity for transport systems and toxicity are important, and require careful definition to ensure that renal excretion of the probe was determined mainly by the state of intestinal permeability[7-12]. However, even when recovery in urine following intravenous administration was complete – indicating minimal systemic loss – recovery of the probe following ingestion (usually expressed as a percentage of the dose) was, as indicated in Table 1, influenced by a number of factors in addition to intestinal permeability.

To increase specificity the principle of 'differential urinary excretion' of several simultaneously ingested test substances was then formulated. Table 1 details the basis of this principle, which proposes that two test substances, for instance a monosaccharide (L-rhamnose) and a disaccharide (lactulose), the behavior of which differ only in respect to the pathway of permeation across the intestinal mucosa, should be used together. In these circumstances the differential urinary excretion of disaccharide/monosaccharide after simultaneous ingestion provides a much more specific indication of the state of mucosal permeability, in this instance specifically large/small pore incidence[13], than would be indicated by the urinary recovery of either probe by itself. Usually either lactulose, melibiose or raffinose have been employed in combination with either L-rhamnose or mannitol. Cellobiose has also been proposed, but the suitability of this probe has been questioned because of the presence of some intestinal cellobiase activity[14]. [51Cr]EDTA which, apart from resistance to bacterial degradation, has almost identical properties to that of lactulose, can be substituted for lactulose, but this is not ideal as small intestinal bacterial overgrowth (causing degradation of L-rhamnose and mannitol) or a particularly rapid intestinal transit (reducing the effective mucosal contact time of L-rhamnose) may give rise to an increased [51Cr]EDTA/monosaccharide urinary excretion ratio in the absence of a genuine alteration of permeability.

The place of PEG 400 in testing for intestinal permeability is clear in our minds. It should be avoided – and for a number of reasons!

1. The PEG 400 polymers, despite physicochemical similarities with respect

Table 1 Factors affecting the urinary excretion of orally administered test substances. The principle of the differential urinary excretion of ingested test substances

Factors affecting the urinary excretion of orally administered test substances		Monosaccharide	Non-hydrolysed disaccharide	Hydrolysed disaccharide
Premucosal	Completeness of ingestion	=	=	=
	Gastric dilution	=	=	=
	Gastric emptying	=	=	=
	Intestinal dilution	=	=	=
	Intestinal transit	=	=	=
	Bacterial degradation	=	=	=
	Unstirred water layer	=	=	=
	Digestion-hydrolysis	0	0	+
Mucosal	Route of permeation	A	B	B
	Intestinal blood flow	=	=	=
Postmucosal	Metabolism	0	0	0
	Endogenous production[a]	0	0	0
	Tissue distribution	C	D	D
	Renal function	=	=	=
	Timing and completeness of urinary collection[b]	=	=	=
	Bacterial degradation	=	=	=
	Analytical performance[c]	=	=	=

=: Identical or affects all test substances equally.

0: Does not take place.

+: Determined mainly by intestinal disaccharidase activities.

A, B: Indicate different routes of permeation; C, D: mono- and disaccharides have a different volume of distribution following intravenous administration and hence there is a slight difference in the speed and completeness of their urinary excretions. This is for practical purposes not of major importance.

[a]There may be some but minimal endogenous production of mannitol.

[b]Roughly equal for the mono- and disaccharides, but see C and D above.

[c]Equal if thin-layer chromatography is used.

When a non-hydrolyzed disaccharide (i.e. lactulose) and a monosaccharide (L-rhamnose or mannitol) are ingested together all the above factors will contribute to their (percentage of oral dose) excretion in urine. However, as all the pre- and postmucosal determinants of their excretion affect the two test substances equally, the urinary excretion ratio (lactulose/L-rhamnose) will only be minimally or not at all affected by these variables. The two probes differ significantly only in their routes of permeation across the intestine. The permeation pathways are affected to a different extent in small intestinal disease and are subject to specific modification to physiological stress (hyperosmolarity), damage by drugs (i.e. nonsteroidal anti-inflammatory drugs) and inflammation. The urinary excretion ratio of lactulose/L-rhamnose thereby becomes a specific index of intestinal permeability which is not affected to an appreciable extent by nonmucosal factors. The simultaneous administration of a nonhydrolyzed (lactulose) and a hydrolyzed disaccharide (lactose, sucrose or palatinose), with subsequent analysis in urine, to assess the efficacy of intestinal disaccharidase activities (lactase, sucrase and isomaltase, respectively) is an extension of the above principle. The disaccharides differ only in respect of their rate of hydrolyses in the intestine, which in turn governs the amount of intact disaccharide available for transport across the mucosa. In normal subjects the urinary excretion (percentage of dose) ratios of hydrolyzable to non-hydrolyzable disaccharides is < 0.3, but with increasing severity of disaccharide deficiency (primary or secondary) this ratio approaches 1.0, at which time there are no disaccharide hydrolyses to size and solubility to non-metabolized di- and monosaccharides, permeate the small intestine 10/50 times more readily than saccharides of similar mass. The precise reason for such atypical permeation is uncertain, but discussion has centered on the question of molecular shape or lipid solubility[10,15-19]. In any case a readily permeating test substance is inappropriate for assessing a barrier function.

2. Recovery of PEG 400 in human urine following intravenous administration is incomplete, and varies between 26% and 72% of the administered dose excreted within $5\,h$[13]. As PEG 400 is not known to be metabolized it is surprising that recovery in the urine is so low, and ceases within 10 h of intravenous administration. Such a brief and incomplete recovery suggests that these polymers must be retained in the tissues.

3. PEG 400 is not appropriate for assessing the profile of intestinal permeability as this range of polymers all appear to use the same diffusion pathway. Diagnostically meaningful alterations in permeation ratio have not yet been described.

4. Altered permeation of PEG 400 recorded in various diseases does not correlate in a logical fashion with any aspect of intestinal physiology or pathology.

5. The PEG 400 test lacks sensitivity, and only a marginal improvement is achieved by mathematical manipulation (filter function or N1/2)[20-23].

TEST DOSE COMPOSITION

The purpose of the investigation determines test dose composition. It is informative to review the main developments of test dose composition in a historical context: first, with respect to the use of 'osmotic fillers' the effects of which have been responsible for considerable confusion, and then test marker composition.

Effects of poorly absorbed solute on intestinal absorption

Inclusion of slowly absorbed solutes such as lactulose, mannitol and L-rhamnose in the preparation of test solutions, inducing retention of fluid within the intestinal lumen and stimulating peristaltic activity, will, by reducing concentration gradients and duration of contact with the absorptive surfaces, reduce absorptive uptake (otherwise permeation) of all test substances present[24]. In the presence of small intestinal malabsorption it should be remembered that solutes normally well absorbed often become poorly absorbed and behave in a similar way.

Effects of hyperosmolar solutions: 'hyperosmolar stress'

Early investigators indicated the importance of controlling the osmolarity of ingested test solutions in relation to urinary excretion of lactulose and other oligosaccharides[1]. 'Hyperosmolar stress', represented by ingestion of a solution of 100 ml volume above 1500 mOsm/l, was found to increase intestinal permeation of disaccharide but not monosaccharide in healthy human subjects[1,4-6,25]. The observation that 'hyperosmolar stress' at the 1500 mOsm/l threshold produced no significant effect upon the normal intestine, whereas patients with villous atrophy demonstrated a significant rise in permeability, led to the use of hyperosmotic test solutions in the belief that this would increase diagnostic discrimination. Several osmotic fillers were used: a mixture of sucrose and lactose, glycerol, glucose, etc. Unfortunately osmotic fillers tend to differ in their behavior in the intestine, and hence vary in their osmotic effect. Furthermore, the osmolarity of test solutions employed by different workers varied widely[26-34] and, as a consequence, results obtained failed to correspond. This problem is well illustrated in Table 2.

The choice of osmotic filler needs very careful attention if additional unwanted variables are to be avoided. Variations in hydrolysis of lactose and sucrose are particularly liable to complicate the action of these sugars, which are best avoided as osmotic fillers. The absorption of D-glucose, which is sodium coupled, may also represent a variable which is best avoided. Though the effect of osmotic fillers, so far as they might be poorly absorbed would not alter disaccharide/monosaccharide permeation ratios, the percentage of monosaccharide recovery in urine, which provides a valuable assessment of absorptive capacity, is certainly reduced. Probes in use for the latter purpose (3-O-methyl-D-glucose, D-xylose and L-rhamnose), are critically dependent on test dose composition as well as the completeness and accurate timing of urine collections. Perhaps the best current advice would be to avoid osmotic fillers as their use has not in general achieved a better diagnostic discrimination.

Test markers

[51Cr]EDTA can be used by itself, but the 24-h urinary excretion includes a substantial amount of the probe passing across the colon, as well as the small intestine, and its use by itself does not allow the specific assessment of intestinal permeability. Nevertheless increased urinary excretion of this marker in diseases has almost invariably been shown to be associated with increased disaccharide/monosaccharide urinary excretion ratios[29,35-41]. Lactulose is the most widely used disaccharide in tests of intestinal permeability. It resists action of small intestinal disaccharidases and is not widely distributed in foods, although commonly used as a laxative and in the treatment of hepatic encephalopathy. Prohibitively expensive when purchased as powder, it is available as a reasonably priced syrup. The additional osmolarity of the syrup should be noted when preparing test solutions. Melibiose also resists intestinal disaccharidase and has been successfully employed as an alternative to lactulose, particularly in liver failure patients, many of whom take lactulose. Raffinose, a trisaccharide, can equally be used. There is little to choose between the two monosaccharides L-rhamnose or mannitol. The latter has theoretical advantages, as urinary

Table 2 Content of lactulose/mannitol test solutions employed by various authors. Comparison of urine lactulose, mannitol and lactulose/mannitol with test solution osmolarity and poorly absorbed solute (PAS) content of test solution

	Ukabam et al.	Murphy et al.	Andre et al.	Wyatt et al.	Elia et al.	Kabembwa et al.	van der Hulst et al.	Juby et al.	Blomquist et al.
Content of test solution									
Lactulose	10.0g	5.0g	5.0g	10g	10g	10g	10g	5.0g	5.0g
Other solutes	nil	nil	nil	glucose 22 g	lactose 1.5 g	nil	xylose 5.0 g	glucose 22.3 g	glycerol 2.0 g
Volume (ml)	100	65	65	150	50	50	65	100	50
Duration of urine save	6 h	5 h	5 h	5 h	6 h	6 h	6 h	5 h	6 h
Number of subjects	33	42	100	30	35	19	12	12	28
Osmolarity of test solution (mOsm/l)	320	580	658	1300	1300	1350	1474	1500	1700
Urinary excretion									
Lactulose (percentage of dose)	0.16	0.26	0.30	0.22	0.26	0.28	0.4	0.44	0.60
Mannitol (percentage of dose)	15.6	13.2	14.3	12.7	13.3	11.4	17.6	28.5	15.7
PAS content (mOsm) per test dose	32	42	42	57	57	57	32	26	35
Lactulose/mannitol	0.16	0.26	0.30	0.22	0.26	0.28	0.40	0.44	0.60

excretion following intravenous administration simulates that of [⁵¹Cr]EDTA and lactulose more closely than L-rhamnose[13,42–45], but mannitol is present in certain foodstuffs and cannot be quantitatively estimated by thin-layer chromatography as the color reaction lacks sufficient sensitivity.

Lactulose and monosaccharide probes should be administered in low dosage, as these substances have limited intestinal permeation and therefore cause osmotic fluid retention within the bowel, as already described[24].

For routine assessment of small intestinal permeability in man a 100 ml test solution should include: lactulose (or equivalent non-hydrolyzable oligosaccharide): not more than 5 g, L-rhamnose (1.0 g) or mannitol (not more than 2 g). A 5-h urine collection should be made into a container with sufficient preservative (e.g. merthiolate 100 mg) to prevent bacterial degradation of sugars. For the combined assessment of intestinal permeability and absorptive capacity the following should be added to the above test solution: (a) 3-O-methyl-D-glucose (0.2 g), which assesses an active carrier-mediated process in the enterocytes; (b) D-xylose (0.5 g), which assesses a passive carrier-mediated transport system.

A complete and accurate urine recovery is essential as an incomplete collection will give an erroneous underestimate of absorptive capacity. The adequacy of both renal function and urine collection can be confirmed by estimating serum and urine creatinine concentrations and calculating a creatinine clearance index.

ANALYSES OF TEST MARKERS

Reliable analysis of these sugar markers in urine requires great care and experience. Column chromatography (GLC and HPLC) have both proven to be difficult techniques to control, but quantitative thin-layer chromatography has proved a reliable method, enabling samples to be 'batched', although requiring adequate experience and manual skill. Introduction of a technique of 'multiple application' enables precise analysis of the very low urine disaccharide concentrations obtained with these tests[46,47]. Enzyme analyses for lactulose have had some proponents. Stability and specificity of the enzyme preparation is important, and a 'control' analysis to make due allowances for pre-existing monosaccharides present in urine is essential. For estimation of lactulose it should be remembered that it is necessary to estimate fructose rather than the galactose generated by incubation with β-galactosidase, otherwise any lactose present will be mistakenly included!

Radiolabeling the probes is yet another possibility. However, as these sugars are inert the radiolabel needs to be incorporated into its basic structure. ¹⁴C-labeled L-rhamnose and mannitol are available. There is a substantial problem if [⁵¹Cr]EDTA is used concomitantly with ¹⁴C, because both isotopes have a similar β-radiation spectrum which is difficult to separate. Whatever technique is used the analytical performance (accuracy and sensitivity) should be clearly stated.

EXPANDING THE PRINCIPLE OF URINARY EXCRETION OF ORALLY ADMINISTERED TEST PROBES

Assessment of colonic permeability

By attention to details of the principle of the urinary excretion of orally administered test probes it is possible to combine the use of the commonly used markers of intestinal permeability with specially selected ones, which allows various other intestinal functions to be assessed noninvasively. One such modification is to administer [^{51}Cr]EDTA with lactulose and L-rhamnose followed by a 5 and 24 h urine collection for marker analyses[48,49]. The principle is that lactulose and L-rhamnose are both rapidly degraded by colonic bacteria whilst [^{51}Cr]EDTA is not. Additionally in most aspects [^{51}Cr]EDTA has identical physicochemical properties to that of lactulose, apart from the bacterial degradability of the latter. Certainly in ileostomy patients equal amounts appear in urine following their simultaneous oral administration. However when [^{51}Cr]EDTA, lactulose and L-rhamnose are ingested together and urine collected for the first 5 h period there is always a bit more of [^{51}Cr]EDTA than lactulose[13]. This is almost certainly due to presence and availability of [^{51}Cr]EDTA to permeate across part of the intestine where the concentration of lactulose has been eliminated by bacterial degradation, namely the colon. When the total 24-h urinary excretion of lactulose is subtracted from that of [^{51}Cr]EDTA the difference represents what has permeated through the colon (or more precisely that part of the intestine containing an active bacterial flora, which may also include the lower ileum). The technique has only been used in a limited number of diseases, but its simplicity suggests that it may have a much wider application.

Localizing intestinal permeability changes

The above technique allows the simultaneous assessment of small and large bowel permeability. A more labor-intensive and accurate technique has been used which may be useful for assessing the precise intestinal location of various absorptive processes (such as iron and calcium absorption) and perhaps to assess the efficacy of drug delivery systems.

The principle of the technique is that a range of test substances, whose absorptive site is well defined to a particular region of the intestine, are given orally, with subsequent serum analyses[50]. The absorptive profile of the test substance, in this case [^{51}Cr]EDTA, is then compared with that of the other markers, which allows the site of increased intestinal permeability to be assessed. The test substances are:

1. 3-O-methyl-D-glucose, absorbed predominantly from the jejunum.
2. [^{51}Co]Vitamin B_{12}, absorbed from the terminal ileum.
3. Sulphasalazine, which passes unchanged into the cecum where it is cleaved into 5-aminosalicylic acid and sulphapyridine by azoreductase-containing bacteria. Sulphapyridine is rapidly absorbed and its appearance in serum indicates when the test solution enters the cecum.

The absorption profile from patients with untreated celiac disease shows in increased serum levels of $[^{51}Cr]$EDTA corresponding to the 3-O-methyl-D-glucose absorption curve. Similarly the peak serum levels of $[^{51}Cr]$EDTA in patients with ileal Crohn's disease correspond to the appearance of the ileal and colonic marker, while patients with severe total colitis have peak levels following the appearance of these markers. This is in keeping with the idea that the main site of increased intestinal permeability in patients with celiac and inflammatory bowel disease is indeed the diseased intestinal mucosa itself.

Assessment of intestinal disaccharidase activities

By careful attention to the details of the principle of the differential urinary excretion of orally administered test substances it is possible to design noninvasive tests which specifically quantify intestinal disaccharidase activities[51-53]. Table 1 shows the variables that determine the amount of intact disaccharide excreted in urine following oral administration.

Simultaneous ingestion of lactulose and melibiose, which both resist mucosal hydrolysis, gives a urine excretion (percentage of dose) ratio of melibiose/lactulose of 1.0, as these oligosaccharides do not differ in their properties and permeation pathways. However if a hydrolyzable disaccharide is substituted for melibiose all the variables in Table 1 will affect the two test substances equally, except for the enzymatic degradation of the hydrolyzable disaccharide. The amount available for permeation in this case is determined by the rate of intestinal hydrolysis (disaccharidase activities) relevant for that sugar. Based on the above, sucrose, lactose and palatinose can (being substrates for sucrase, lactase and iso-maltase) be given with lactulose. Normal urinary excretion ratios of sucrose, lactose, and palatinose to that of lactulose in 5 or 10 h urines following their oral administration are 0.3 or below in subjects with active intestinal disaccharidase hydrolysis. Ratios of 0.3–1.0 indicate increasing impairment of intestinal hydrolysis. Clinically relevant impairment of lactase activity is usually associated with lactose/lactulose urinary excretion ratios of 0.45 or greater in 10 h urine. The technique has been used to demonstrate transient lactase deficiency following Rotavirus enteritis in children[54], combined sucrase and palatinase deficiency in asucrasia[51,52,54], effectiveness of α-glucosidase inhibitors on sucrose hydrolysis and to quantitate total small intestinal hydrolytic activity in patients with celiac disease[53]. The technique would seem to have potential as a routine noninvasive screening test for intestinal disaccharidase deficiency, and may discriminate between isolated, usually genetically determined disaccharidase deficiency and acquired pan-disaccharidase deficiency associated with smal intestinal disease. A point of great importance is that, since excretion of dietary lactose and sucrose is a natural phenomenon in normal subjects, it is necessary to exclude all dietary sources of lactose and sucrose for at least 18 h before and during the whole period of urine collection.

INTESTINAL PERMEABILITY IN CROHN'S DISEASE

The intriguing question is whether altered intestinal permeability plays an etiologic or pathogenic role in Crohn's disease[55-57]. The problem here is familiar to clinical investigators interested in inflammatory bowel disease: deciding whether the abnormalities are the cause or result of pathology[40]. In this case the problem is not so much to do with the interpretation of data as the importance of looking at the problem from a different perspective and in context of results obtained in other diseases – a feature sadly lacking from much recent, uncritical and high profile work.

Pathogenic importance of increased intestinal permeability

Tests of intestinal permeability were specifically designed to assess the intestinal barrier function, and it is the integrity of this barrier which is thought to be important for limiting macromolecular permeation. Increased macromolecular permeation, it is suggested, may play a role in systemic disease as well as local[58,59]. In the latter situation it is important to assess and integrate all available data to assess whether a story is emerging.

Essentially it is suggested that increased intestinal permeability allows mucosal exposure of luminal aggressive factors, and an inflammatory reaction consequentially sets in because of the generation of, or exposure to, neutrophil chemotactic factors[60-62]. We have suggested that this is a central pathophysiological mechanism in a number of small intestinal diseases. Indeed there may be three ways of initiating intestinal damage, all of which lead to increased intestinal permeability – the prerequisite for an intestinal inflammatory reaction. The three mechanisms are broadly classified as primary permeability breakers, factors or disease associated with enhanced luminal aggressiveness, or diminished mucosal defense. It is of interest to compare the changes in intestinal permeability and quantitate intestinal inflammation in these diseases.

Intestinal permeability breakers

NSAID-induced small intestinal damage.   Following ingestion of NSAIDs there is a uniform and consistent increase in intestinal permeability. This occurs within 12 h of ingestion of the drugs and occurs predominantly during drug absorption when the enterocytes are exposed to the highest concentration of the drugs[40,63-67].

Quantitatively the increased intestinal permeability in response to NSAID ingestion does not differ from that seen in other small intestinal disorders such as Crohn's or celiac disease. Moreover there is no significant difference in the permeability changes following short- or long-term ingestion of NSAIDs.

Three lines of evidence show that NSAIDs cause small intestinal inflammation: namely; indium-111-labeled leukocytes, enteroscopy and post-mortem studies[62,68-71]. Collectively the data show that 65% of patients on long-term NSAIDs develop small intestinal inflammation. The fecal excretion of indium-111 shows that most patients have a low-grade enteropathy with a fecal excretion of 1–6% (normal < 1%). Once the inflammation is present patients bleed from the inflammatory site and lose protein, both of which are clinically relevant in patients with arthritis as they are prone to iron deficiency and hypoalbuminemia.

In short, NSAIDs have a specific detrimental biochemical action on enterocytes which is not evident to the same extent in other tissue because of lower drug concentrations. The ultrastructural–biochemical alterations lead to increased intestinal permeability, resulting in a low-grade enteropathy or substantial inflammation when normal intestinal defense mechanisms are intact or disrupted, respectively.

Alcohol-induced intestinal damage. Only a few studies have assessed intestinal permeability in alcoholic patients. The permeability changes were comparable with that found in Crohn's and celiac disease[38]. Increased intestinal permeability, unlike that observed with NSAIDs, is not seen following single doses of alcohol[1,72].

Very few data are available on possible intestinal inflammation in these patients. In a group of eight heavy drinkers we found (unpublished) a low-grade enteropathy in five with fecal excretions ranging from 1.2% to 4.3%.

Enteropathy of chronic renal failure. There are formidable difficulties associated with the noninvasive measurement of intestinal permeability in patients with chronic renal failure. We have found (unpublished) increased intestinal permeability (lactulose/L-rhamnose) in a small group of patients. The same patients had an enteropathy with a fecal excretion of indium-111 ranging from 2% to 9%. It is suggested that the uremia or other circulating toxins somehow interfere directly with enterocyte function or alter mucosal defense processes (specific or nonspecific) resulting in increased intestinal permeability with its consequences.

Miscellaneous. Antineoplastic agents increase intestinal permeability[73–76] and increased intestinal permeability is also evident in diabetes mellitus[77], patients undergoing major surgery or experiencing intestinal ischemia[78–80], following major burns or abdominal radiation[81–83]. Apart from abdominal radiation, where there is evidence of an inflammatory reaction (Qvist, personal communication) of comparable severity to that of NSAID enteropathy, it remains to a large extent to be explored whether the increased intestinal permeability in these situations leads to an inflammatory response.

Luminal aggressive factors

Various exogenous microbial infections increase intestinal permeability to a similar extent to that seen with the permeability breakers and in Crohn's and celiac disease[54]. The increased intestinal permeability may be an essential component in the pathogenesis of the intestinal infection, allowing mucosal exposure of the microbe, or it could be the consequence of neutrophil-induced tissue damage as detailed above, or due to cytokine release. Whatever the mechanism there is a moderately severe inflammatory response evident in these patients with indium-111 leukocyte excretion levels between 1% and 9%[84].

Patients with cystic fibrosis have striking increases in intestinal permeability[85-88]. The possible reason for this is that the viscous mucus provides a nidus for small intestinal microbial proliferation. Again the possibility that these patients develop an enteropathy remains to be examined.

Altered mucosal defense

Patients with hypogammaglobulinemia have been studied in some detail. Increased intestinal permeability is a universal feature and the fecal excretion of indium-111 leukocytes in these patients is in the range of 1.1–14.5% with a mean of 6.9%[89].

Patients with the acquired immunodeficiency syndrome (AIDS) have increased intestinal permeability regardless of subgrouping[90,91]. When studied with indium-111 leukocytes all those with increased intestinal permeability had a low-grade enteropathy, similar in severity to that found in NSAID enteropathy (unpublished).

The above data conform to a central importance to intestinal barrier function. They show that, by whatever means one disrupts the integrity of this barrier, there is a uniform inflammatory response, presumably and predominantly to luminal factors. It is now appropriate to re-examine the situation in Crohn's disease.

INTESTINAL PERMEABILITY AND INFLAMMATION IN CROHN'S DISEASE

Tests of intestinal permeability provide noninvasive functional assessment of the small intestine in patients with Crohn's disease[36,92] and ulcerative colitis. Most patients with small intestinal involvement of Crohn's disease, who have not undergone intestinal resection, have increased intestinal permeability, as assessed by the differential urine excretion of disaccharides/monosaccharides and [^{51}Cr]EDTA, and 50% of patients with colonic Crohn's disease are abnormal[28,31,36,92-106]. The permeability changes relate to extent of disease as well as activity. Of particular importance is the fact that the permeability changes are of equal magnitude to that of the above-mentioned diseases.

Similar studies with indium-111 leukocytes show all patients with active Crohn's disease to have increased fecal excretion of neutrophils. However, unlike that seen in NSAID-induced enteropathy and other diseases, the fecal excretion of labeled neutrophils is almost an order of magnitude higher, averaging 18% with a range between 10% and 60%, all depending on disease activity. It is the intensity of the neutrophil response which needs explanation.

Most feel confident that preliminary reports of increased intestinal permeation of PEG 400 in first-degree relatives of patients with Crohn's disease are incorrect[107-109]. Intestinal permeability is normal in relatives when tested with the differential urinary excretion of sugars or [^{51}Cr]EDTA[107,110] with the occasional subject[12,107,110-112] being abnormal, presumably because of alcohol, NSAIDs, etc.

Recent evidence shows that normal intestinal permeability in patients with Crohn's disease predicts well-being[34,100,103] and as permeability improves following treatment[99,100] it has been suggested that the main importance of increased intestinal permeability in patients with inflammatory bowel disease is that it is the central mechanism of relapse of the disease. This would then expose them to the same luminal aggressive factors as in the other enteropathies, but the severity of the neutrophil response, which may relate to the underlying immune derangement of the disease itself, is what distinguishes Crohn's disease clinically and pathophysiologically from the otherwise low-grade enteropathies. The relapse of Crohn's disease is then not an activation of the disease process itself, but a nonspecific unchecked acute inflammatory response to normal intestinal flora, caused by a breach in intestinal permeability and amplified by the disease itself. It certainly provides for a comprehensive, logical and testable framework for further investigations.

CONCLUSIONS

Tests of intestinal permeability have come a long way in the 20 years since they were introduced. Their use is simple, they are accurate and sensitive and provide information which is not obtainable noninvasively by the use of single markers. There are nevertheless many practical aspects of their use that need special attention, lest unpublishable data are obtained and time is wasted. We have outlined many of the common pitfalls involved when deciding on test dose composition and the method of urinary analyses of the markers. Most importantly prospective workers would be well advised to confer with established workers before embarking on their projects.

By exploiting the details of the underlying principles of the differential urinary excretion of orally administered test markers new tests have been introduced which allow the specific assessment of regional permeability changes and the noninvasive assessment of disaccharidase activities of the whole of the small intestine. It seems clear that further development of other noninvasive techniques for assessing other intestinal functions is limited only by the ingenuity of the investigator. An integrated approach to the study of intestinal permeability and inflammation in various diseases, and in classic inflammatory bowel disease, is providing insight into the basic mechanisms of a common final pathway for an intestinal inflammatory response.

References

1. Menzies IS. Absorption of intact oligosaccharide in health and disease. Biochem Soc Trans. 1974;2:1040–46.
2. Chadwick VS, Phillips SF, Hofman AF. Measurements of intestinal permeability using low molecular weight polyethylene glycols (PEG 400). I. Chemical analysis and biological properties of PEG 400. Gastroenterology. 1977;73:241–6.

3. Chadwick VS, Phillips SF, Hofman AF. Measurements of intestinal permeability using low molecular weight polyethylene glycols (PEG 400). II. Application to study of normal and abnormal permeability states in man and animals. Gastroenterology. 1977;73:247–51.

4. Laker MF, Menzies IS. Increase in human intestinal permeability following ingestion of hypertonic solutions. J Physiol (Lond.). 1977;273:881–94.

5. Laker MF. The effect of hypertonic solutions on intestinal permeability. MD thesis, University of London, 1978.

6. Wheeler PG, Menzies IS, Creamer B. Effect of hyperosmolar stimuli and coeliac disease on the permeability of the human gastrointestinal tract. Clin Sci Mol Med. 1978;54: 495–501.

7. Bjarnason I, Peters TJ, Levi AJ. Intestinal permeability: clinical correlates. Dig Dis. 1986;4:83–92.

8. Hamilton I. Small intestinal permeability. In: Pounder RE, editor. Recent advances in gastroenterology, 6. Edinburgh: Churchill Livingstone; 1986:73–91.

9. Cooper BT. The small intestinal permeability barrier. In: Losowski MH, Heatley RV, editors. Gut defences in clinical practice. Edinburgh: Churchill Livingstone; 1986:117–32.

10. Menzies IS. Transmucosal passage of inert molecules in health and disease. In: Skadhauge E, Heintze K, editors. Intestinal absorption and secretion. Falk Symposium 36. Lancaster: MTP Press; 1984:527–43.

11. Hollander D. The intestinal permeability barrier. A hypothesis as to its regulation and involvement in Crohn's disease. Scand J Gastroenterol. 1992;27:721–6.

12. Hollander D. Permeability in Crohn's disease – altered barrier function in healthy relatives? Gastroenterology. 1993;104:1848–51.

13. Maxton DG, Bjarnason I, Reynolds AP, Catt SD, Peters TJ, Menzies IS. Lactulose, ^{51}CrEDTA, L-rhamnose and polyethylene glycol 400 as probe markers for 'in vivo' assessment of human intestinal permeability. Clin Sci. 1986;71:71–80.

14. Dahlqvist A. Specificity of human intestinal disaccharidases and implications for hereditary disaccharide intolerance. J Clin Invest. 1962;41:463–70.

15. Hollander D, Rickets D, Boyd CAR. Importance of 'probe' molecular geometry in determining intestinal permeability. Can J Gastroenterol. 1988;2(Suppl. A):35–8A.

16. Ma TY, Hollander D, Krugliak P, Katz K. PEG 400, a hydrophillic molecular probe for measuring intestinal permeability. Gastroenterology. 1990;98:39–46.

17. Krugilak P, Hollander D, Ma TY et al. Mechanism of polyethylene glycol 400 permeability of perfused rat intestine. Gastroenterology. 1989;97:1164–70.

18. Krugliak P, Hollander D, Le K, Ma T, Dadufalza VD, Katz KD. Regulation of polyethylene glycol 400 intestinal permeability by endogenous and exogenous prostanoids. Influence of non-steroidal anti-inflammatory drugs. Gut. 1990;31:417–21.

19. Iqbal TH, Lewis KO, Cooper BT. Diffusion of polyethylene glycol-400 across lipid barriers in vitro. Clin Sci. 1993;85:111–15.

20. Magnusson KE, Sundqvist T. Mathematical modelling for determining intestinal permeability using polyethylene glycol. Gut. 1983;25:428–9.

21. Magnusson KE, Sundqvist T. Modelling of intestinal permeability in man to polyethylene glycols (PEG 400 and PEG 1000). Acta Physiol Scand. 1985;125:289–96.

22. Sundqvist T, Tageson C, Magnusson KE. Simulation of a multicompartment model for the intestinal permeability to low-molecular-weight probes (polyethylene glycol 400). Math Biosci. 1981;56:287–309.

23. Irving CS, Lifschitz CH, Marks LM, Nichols BC, Klein PD. Polyethylene glycol polymers of low molecular weight as probes of intestinal permeability. I. Innovations in analyses and quantitation. J Lab Clin Med. 1986;107:290–8.

24. Menzies IS, Jenkins AP, Heduan E, Catt SD, Segal MB, Creamer B. The effect of poorly absorbed solute on intestinal absorption. Scand J Gastroenterol. 1990;25:1257–64.

25. Menzies IS, Pounder R, Heyer S et al. Abnormal intestinal permeability to sugars in villus atrophy. Lancet. 1979;2:1107–09.

26. Blomquist L, Bark T, Hedenborg G, Svenberg T, Norman A. A comparison between the lactulose/mannitol and ^{51}CrEDTA/14C-mannitol methods for intestinal permeability. Scand J Gastroenterol. 1993;28:274–80.

27. Elia M, Beherens R, Northrop C, Wraight P, Neale G. Evaluation of mannitol, lactulose and 51Cr labelled ethylenediaminetetraacetate as markers of intestinal permeability in

man. Clin Sci. 1987;73:197–204.

28. Andre F, Andre C, Emery Y. Assessment of the lactulose–mannitol test in Crohn's disease. Gut. 1988;29:511–15.

29. Judby LD, Rothwell J, Axon ATR. Lactulose/mannitol test. An ideal screening test for coeliac disease. Gastroenterology. 1989;96:79–85.

30. Kapembwa MS, Fleming SC, Sewankambo N et al. Altered small-intestinal permeability associated with diarrhoea in human-immunodeficiency-virus-infected Caucasian and African subjects. Clin Sci. 1991;81:327–34.

31. Murphy MS, Eastham EJ, Nelson R, Pearson ADJ, Laker MF. Intestinal permeability in Crohn's disease. Arch Dis Child. 1989;64:321–5.

32. Ukabam SO, Homeda MA, Cooper BJ. Small intestinal permeability in Sudanese subjects: evidence of tropical enteropathy. Trans R Soc Trop Med Hyg. 1986;40:204–7.

33. van der Hulst PRWJ, Kreel BK, Meyenfelt MF et al. Glutamine and the preservation of gut integrity. Lancet. 1993;341:1363–5.

34. Wyatt J, Vogelsang H, Hubl W, Waldhoer T, Lochs H. Intestinal permeability and the predictor of relapse in Crohn's disease. Lancet. 1993;341:1437–9.

35. Bjarnason I, Peters TJ, Veall N. A persistent defect of intestinal permeability in coeliac disease as demonstrated by a ^{51}Cr-labelled EDTA absorption test. Lancet. 1983;1:323–5.

36. Bjarnason I, O'Morain C, Levi AJ, Peters TJ. The absorption of ^{51}Cr EDTA in inflammatory bowel disease. Gastroenterology. 1983;85:318–22.

37. Bjarnason I, Williams P, So A et al. Intestinal permeability and inflammation in rheumatoid arthritis; effects of non-steroidal anti-inflammatory drugs. Lancet. 1984;2:1171–4.

38. Bjarnason I, Ward K, Peters TJ. The leaky gut of alcoholism: possible route of entry for toxic compounds. Lancet. 1984;1:179–82.

39. Bjarnason I, Goolamali SK, Levi AJ, Peters TJ. Intestinal permeability in patients with atopic eczema. Br J Dermatol. 1985;112:291–7.

40. Bjarnason I, Peters TJ. Helping the mucosa make sense of macromolecules. Gut. 1987;28:1057–61.

41. Hamilton I, Fairris GM, Rotherwell J, Cunliffe WJ, Dixon MF, Axon ATR. Small intestinal permeability in dermatological disease. Q J Med. 1985;56:559–67.

42. Laker MF, Bull HJ, Menzies IS. Evaluation of mannitol for use as a probe marker of gastrointestinal permeability in man. Eur J Clin Invest. 1982;12:485–91.

43. Cobden I, Hamilton I, Rothwell J, Axon ATR. Cellobiose/mannitol test: Physiological properties of probe molecules and influence of extraneous factors. Clin Chim Acta. 1985;148:53–62.

44. Dominguez R, Corcoran AC, Page IH. Mannitol: kinetics of distribution, excretion and utilization in human beings. J Lab Clin Med. 1947;32:192–202.

45. Newman EV, Bordlay J, Winternitz J. The interrelationship of glomerular filtration rate (mannitol clearance), extracellular fluid volume, surface area of the body, and plasma concentration of mannitol. Bull Johns Hopkins Hosp. 1944;75:253–68.

46. Menzies IS. Quantitative estimation of sugars in blood and urine by paper chromatography using direct densitometry. J Chromatogr. 1983;81:109–27.

47. Menzies IS, Mount JN, Wheeler MJ. Quantitative estimation of clinically important monosaccharides in plasma by rapid thin layer chromatography. Ann Clin Biochem. 1978;15:65–76.

48. Jenkins AP, Nukajam WS, Menzies IS, Creamer B. Simultaneous administration of lactulose and 51Cr-ethylenediaminetetraacetic acid. A test to distinguish colonic from small-intestinal permeability change. Scand J Gastroenterol. 1992;27:769–73.

49. Jenkins AP, Trew DR, Crump BJ, Menzies IS, Creamer B. Do nonsteroidal anti-inflammatory drugs increase colonic permeability? Gut. 1991;32:66–9.

50. Teahon K, Smith T, Smethurst P, Bjarnason I. A technique for localizing alterations of intestinal permeability in man. Gastroenterology. 1991;100:A251.

51. Maxton DG, Catt SD, Menzies IS. Intestinal disaccharidases assessed in congenital asucrasia by differential urinary disaccharide excretion. Dig Dis Sci. 1989;34:129–31.

52. Maxton DG, Catt SD, Menzies IS. Combined assessment of intestinal disaccharidases in congenital asucrasia by differential urinary disaccharide excretion. J Clin Pathol. 1990;43:406–9.

53. Bjarnason I, Smethurst P, Batt R, Catt S, Maxton D, Menzies IS. Differential urine

excretion of disaccharides for the non-invasive assessment of intestinal disaccharidase activities: effects of α-glucosidase inhibitors and primary hypolactasia, and the correlation between in vivo and in vitro measurements of sucrase, lactase and isomaltase activity in patients with coeliac disease. 1994 (Submitted).

54. Ford RPK, Menzies IS, Phillips AD, Walker-Smith JA, Turner MW. Intestinal sugar permeability: Relationship to diarrhoeal disease and small bowel morphology. J Pediatr Gastroenterol Nutr. 1985;4:568–74.

55. Hollander D. Crohn's disease – a permeability disorder of the tight junctions? Gut. 1988;26:1621–4.

56. Hollander D, Vadheim C, Brettholz E, Pattersen GM, Delahunty T, Rotter JI. Increased intestinal permeability in patients with Crohn's disease and their relatives. Ann Intern Med. 1986;105:883–5.

57. Shorter RG, Huizenga GA, Spencer RJ. A working hypothesis for the etiology and pathogenesis of nonspecific inflammatory bowel disease. Dig Dis Sci. 1972;17:1024–31.

58. Walker AW, Isselbacher KJ. Uptake and transport of macromolecules by the intestine. Possible role in clinical disorders. Gastroenterology. 1974;67:531–50.

59. Walker WA. Mechanisms of antigen handling by the gut. Clin Immunol Allergy. 1982;2: 15–34.

60. Bjarnason I, Macpherson A, Somasundaram S, Teahon K. Nonsteroidal anti-inflammatory drugs and inflammatory bowel disease. Can J Gastroenterol. 1993;7:160–9.

61. Bjarnason I, Macpherson AS, Somasundaram S, Teahon K. Non-steroidal anti-inflammatory drugs and Crohn's disease. In: Scholmeric J, Kruis W, Goebbell H, Hohenberger W, Gross V, editors. Inflammatory bowel diseases: pathophysiology as basis of treatment. Falk Symposium No. 67. Lancaster: Kluwer; 1993:208–22.

62. Bjarnason I, Hayllar J, Macpherson AJ, Russell AS. Side effects of nonsteroidal anti-inflammatory drugs on the small and large intestine. Gastroenterology. 1993;104: 1832–47.

63. Auer IO, Habscheid W, Hiller S, Gerhards W, Eilles C. Nicht-steroidale antiphlogistika erhohen die darmpermeabilitat. D Med Wochenschr. 1987;112:1032–7.

64. Bjarnason I, Williams P, Smethurst P, Peters TJ, Levi AJ. The effect of NSAIDs and prostaglandins on the permeability of the human small intestine. Gut. 1986;27:1292–7.

65. Bjarnason I, Smethurst P, Clarke P, Menzies IS, Levi AJ, Peters TJ. Effect of prostaglandins on indomethacin induced increased intestinal permeability in man. Scand J Gastroenterol. 1989;29(Suppl.164):97–103.

66. Bjarnason I, Fehilly B, Smethurst P, Menzies IS, Levi AJ. The importance of local versus sytemic effects of non-steroidal anti-inflammatory drugs to increase intestinal permeability in man. Gut. 1991;32:275–7.

67. Bjarnason I, Smethurst P, Macpherson A et al. Glucose and citrate reduce the permeability changes caused by indomethacin in humans. Gastroenterology. 1992;102:1546–50.

68. Bjarnason I, Zanelli G, Smith T et al. Nonsteroidal antiinflammatory drug induced intestinal inflammation in humans. Gastroenterology. 1987;93:480–9.

69. Morris AJ, Wasson LA, Mackenzie JF. Small bowel enteroscopy in undiagnosed gastrointestinal blood loss. Gut. 1992;33:887–9.

70. Rooney PJ, Jenkins RT, Smith KM, Coates G. 111-Indium-labelled polymorphonuclear scans in rheumatoid arthritis – an important clinical cause of positive results. Br J Rheumatol. 1986;15:167–70.

71. Allison MC, Howatson AG, Torrance CJ, Lee FD, Russell RI. Gastrointestinal damage associated with the use of nonsteroidal anti-inflammatory drugs. N Engl J Med. 1992;327:749–54.

72. Smethurst P, Menzies IS, Levi AJ, Bjarnason I. Is alcohol directly toxic to the small bowel mucosa? Clin Sci. 1988;75:50–1P.

73. Parrilli G, Iaffaioli RV, Matorano M et al. Effects of anthracycline therapy on intestinal absorption in patients with advanced breast cancer. Cancer Res. 1989;49:3689–91.

74. Pledger JV, Pearson ADJ, Craft AW, Laker MF, Eastham EJ. Intestinal permeability during chemotherapy for childhood tumors. Eur J Pediatr. 1988;147:123–7.

75. Pearson ADJ, Craft AW, Pledger JV, Eastham EJ, Laker MF, Pearson CS. Small bowel function in acute lymphoblastic leukemia. Arch Dis Child. 1984;59:460–5.

76. Selby PJ, Lopes N, Mundy J, Crofts M, Millar JL, McElwain TJ. Cyclophosphomide

priming reduces intestinal damage in man following high dose melphalan chemotherapy. Br J Cancer. 1987;55:531-3.

77. Cooper BT, Ukabam SO, O'Brien IAD, Hara JPO, Corrall RJM. Intestinal permeability in diabetic diarrhoea. Diabet Med. 1987;4:49-52.

78. Ohri SK, Somasundaram S, Koak Y et al. The effect of intestinal hypoperfusion during cardiopulmonary bypass surgery on saccharide permeation and intestinal permeability in man. Gastroenterology. 1994;106:318-23.

79. Otamiri T, Sjodahl R, Tagesson C. An experimental model for studying reversible intestinal ischemia. Acta Chir Scand. 1987;153:51-6.

80. Roumen RM, van der Vliet JA, Wevers RA, Goris RJ. Intestinal permeability is increased after major vascular surgery. J Vasc Surg. 1993;17:734-7.

81. Coltart RS, Howard GC, Wraight EP, Bleehen NM. The effect of hyperthermia and radiation on small bowel permeability using ^{51}Cr EDTA and ^{14}C mannitol in man. Int J Hyperthermia. 1988;4:467-77.

82. Ruppin H, Hotze A, During A et al. Reversible funktionsstorungen des intestinaltraktes durch abdominelle strahlentherapy. Z Gastroenterol. 1987;25:261-9.

83. Yeoh EK, Horowitz M, Russo A, Muecke T, Robb T, Chatterton BE. Gastrointestinal function in chronic radiation enteritis-effects of loperamide-N-oxide. Gut. 1993;34:476-82.

84. Kardossis T, Joseph AEA, Gane JN, Bridges CE, Griffin GE. Fecal leucocytosis. Indium-111-labelled autologous polymorphonuclear leucocyte abdominal scanning, and quantitative fecal indium-111 excretion in acute gastroenteritis and enteropathogen carriage. Dig Dis Sci. 1988;33:1383-90.

85. Leclerc-Foucart J, Forget P Sodoyez-Gouffaux F, Zappitelli A. Intestinal permeability to ^{51}CrEDTA in children with cystic fibrosis. J Pediatr Gastroenterol Nutr. 1986;5:384-7.

86. Leclercq-Foucart J, Forget P, Van Cutsem JL. Lactulose-rhamnose intestinal permeability in children with cystic fibrosis. J Pediatr Gastroenterol Nutr. 1987;6:66-70.

87. Dalzell AM, Freestone NS, Billington D, Heaf PH. Small intestinal permeability and orocaecal transit time in cystic fibrosis. Arch Dis Child. 1990;65:585-8.

88. Escobar H, Perdomo M, Vasconez F, Camarero C, del Olmo MT, Suarez L. Intestinal permeability to ^{51}Cr-EDTA and orocecal transit time in cystic fibrosis. J Pediatr Gastroenterol Nutr. 1992;14:204-7.

89. Teahon K, Webster AD, Price AB, Bjarnason I. Studies of gastrointestinal structure and function in patients with primary hypogammaglobulinaemia. Gut. 1994 (In press).

90. Keating J, Bjarnason I, Somasundaram S et al. Intestinal absorptive capacity, intestinal permeability and jejunal histology in HIV infected patients and their relation to diarrhoea. Gastroenterology. 1994 (In press).

91. Lim SG, Menzies IS, Lee CA, Johnson MA, Pounder RE. Intestinal permeability and function in patients infected with human immunodeficiency virus. Scand J Gastroenterol. 1993;28:573-80.

92. Ukabam SO, Clamp JR, Cooper BT. Abnormal intestinal permeability to sugars in patients with Crohn's disease of the terminal ileum and colon. Digestion. 1982;27:70-4.

93. Casellas F, Aguade S, Soriano B, Accarino A, Molero J, Guarner L. Intestinal permeability to 99mTc diethylene-tetraaminopentaacetic acid in inflammatory bowel disease. Am J Gastroenterol. 1986;81:767-70.

94. Resnick RH, Royal H, Marshall W, Barron R, Werth T. Intestinal permeability in gastrointestinal disorders. Dig Dis Sci. 1990;35:205-11.

95. O'Morain C, Abelon AC, Chervli LR, Fleischner GM, Das KM. ^{51}CrEDTA a useful test in the assessment of inflammatory bowel disease. J Lab Clin Med. 1986;108:430-5.

96. Jenkins RT, Jones DB, Goodacre RL et al. Reversibility of increased intestinal permeability to ^{51}CrEDTA in patients with gastrointestinal inflammatory bowel disease. J Rheumatol. 1987;82:1159-64.

97. Turck D, Ythier H, Maquet E et al. Increased intestinal permeability to ^{51}CrEDTA in children with Crohn's disease and coeliac disease. J Pediatr Gastroenterol Nutr. 1987;6:535-7.

98. Pironi L, Miglioli M, Ruggeri E et al. Relationship between intestinal permeability to (51Cr)EDTA and inflammatory activity in asymptomatic patients with Crohn's disease. Dig Dis Sci. 1990;35:582-8.

99. Sanderson IR, Boulton P, Menzies IS, Walker-Smith JA. Improvement of abnormal

lactulose/rhamnose permeability in active Crohn's disease of the small bowel by an elemental diet. Gut. 1987;28:1073–6.

100. Teahon K, Smethurst P, Levi AJ, Bjarnason I. The effect of elemental diet on intestinal permeability and inflammation in Crohn's disease. Gastroenterology. 1991;101:84–9.

101. Jenkins RT, Ramage JK, Jones DB, Collins SM, Goodacre RL, Hunt RH. Small bowel and colonic permeability to ^{51}CrEDTA in patients with active inflammatory bowel disease. Clin Invest Med. 1988;11:151–5.

102. Pearson AD, Eastham EJ, Laker ME, Craft AW, Nelson R. Intestinal permeability in children with Crohn's disease and coeliac disease. Br Med J. 1982;285:20–1.

103. Teahon K, Smethurst P, Macpherson AJ, Levi AJ, Menzies IS, Bjarnason I. Intestinal permeability in Crohn's disease and its relation to disease activity and relapse following treatment with elemental diet. Eur J Gastroenterol Hepatol. 1993;5:79–84.

104. Adenis A, Colombel JF, Lecouffe P et al. Increased pulmonary and intestinal permeability in Crohn's disease. Gut. 1992;33:678–82.

105. Howden CW, Robertson C, Duncan A, Morris AJ, Russel RI. Comparison of different measurements of intestinal permeability in inflammatory bowel disease. Am J Gastroenterol. 1991;86:1445–9.

106. Wallaert B, Colombel JF, Adenis A et al. Increased intestinal permeability in active pulmonary sarcoidosis. Am Rev Respir Dis. 1992;145:1440–5.

107. Teahon K, Smethurst P, Levi AJ, Menzies IS, Bjarnason I. Intestinal permeability in patients with Crohn's disease and their first degree relatives. Gut. 1992;33:320–3.

108. Ruttenberg D, Young GO, Wright JP, Isaacs S. PEG 400 excretion in patients with Crohn's disease, their first degree relatives, and healthy volunteers. Dig Dis Sci. 1992;37:705–8.

109. Munkholm P, Langholz E, Hollander D et al. Intestinal permeability in patients with Crohn's disease and ulcerative colitis and their first degree relatives. Gut. 1994;35:68–72.

110. Ainsworth M, Eriksen J, Rasmussen JW, Schaffalitzkydemuckadel OB. Intestinal permeability of ^{51}Cr-labelled ethylenediaminetetraacetic acid in patients with Crohn's disease and their first degree relatives. Scand J Gastroenterology. 1989;24:993–8.

111. Katz KD, Hollander D, Vadheim CM et al. Intestinal permeability in patients with Crohn's disease and their healthy relatives. Gastroenterology. 1989;97:927–31.

112. May GR, Sutherland LR, Meddings JB. Is small intestinal permeability really increased in relatives of patients with Crohn's disease? Gastroenterology. 1993;104:1627–32.

Section III
Predisposing factors in the etiology of IBD: is there a primary immune defect?

7
Etiology of organ-specific autoimmunity

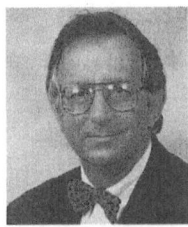

G. S. EISENBARTH

Fundamental questions concerning autoimmune disorders include:

1. What genetic elements determine disease susceptibility?
2. What activates/suppresses autoimmunity in genetically susceptible individuals?
3. What are the target autoantigens (initiating, perpetuating, secondary)?
4. What are the effector mechanisms?
5. What are the clinical sequelae of answers to the above questions in terms of disease prevention with, in particular, antigen-specific therapies?

Answers to the above questions are now available in humans and spontaneous autoimmune animal models for a subset of the above questions in a subset of autoimmune disorders. For no disease are answers to all questions available. Nevertheless, the clear answers which are selectively available for a few disorders will almost certainly be relevant to many autoimmune diseases. The linking of autoimmune disorders into characteristic disease syndromes affecting many target tissues provides evidence for the interrelatedness of disease pathogenesis. In particular, the polyendocrine autoimmune syndromes[1-3] indicate that disease susceptibility can lead over time to multiple organ-specific autoimmune diseases (Table 1). This chapter will review selected organ-specific autoimmune diseases and syndromes where specific answers to the above questions are available with an emphasis on type I diabetes.

Table 1 Autoimmune polyendocrine syndromes

Type I syndrome	Type II syndrome
Mucocutaneous candidiasis	
Hypoparathyroidism	
Addison's disease	Addison's disease
Type I diabetes (5%)	Type I diabetes (50%)
Chronic active hepatitis	
Graves' disease/thyroiditis	Graves' disease/thyroiditis
Vitiligo	Vitiligo
Asplenism	
	Celiac disease
	Serositis
Pernicious anemia	Pernicious anemia
	Stiff man syndrome/Parkinson's disease
	Myasthenia gravis
IgA deficiency[5]	IgA deficiency[6]

GENETIC ELEMENTS

For most (but not all) organ-specific autoimmune syndromes, genes within the major histocompatibility complex (MHC) contribute to susceptibility[4]. An interesting exception is the polyendocrine autoimmune syndrome type I, with its mucocutaneous candidiasis, Addison's disease and hypoparathyroidism. This syndrome is inherited in an autosomal recessive manner. In contrast to Addison's disease of the type II autoimmune polyendocrine autoimmune syndrome, which is strongly associated with DR3 and DR4 haplotypes, the type I syndrome with Addison's disease has no class II HLA association[7]. In addition, approximately 5% of individuals with this syndrome develop type I diabetes. The DQ molecule DQA1*0102,DQB1*0602 is usually dramatically protective for type I diabetes[8,9]. This molecule occurs in approximately 20% of Caucasians, but among approximately 250 patients with type I diabetes we have observed only one individual with this allele, and that individual has the autoimmune polyendocrine syndrome (APS) type I. DQA1*0102,DQB1*0602 is associated with protection from type I diabetes even in the presence of cytoplasmic islet cell autoantibodies. Approximately 12% of ICA-positive first-degree relatives of patients with type I diabetes express this allele, but we have yet to observe one such relative progress to diabetes. One hypothesis is that protection by this class II allele requires an active immune response, and this response cannot be generated in the presence of the immunodeficiency associated with APS type I. The molecule DQA1*0102,DQB1*0602 does not protect from all autoimmunity as, for example, this molecule is associated with multiple sclerosis. Protection from diabetes by class II alleles is most dramatically demonstrated by transgenic NOD mice, in which replacement of the missing functional DRalpha allele (I-E alpha of mouse) protects from diabetes. To date the mechanism underlying this protection is unknown.

The insulin autoimmune syndrome is characterized by high levels of insulin autoantibodies and is almost always associated with methimazole therapy for Graves' disease. Essentially 100% of individuals with this syndrome are

DR4-positive with the specific DRB1*0406 allele[10]. In patients developing type I diabetes, lower levels of anti-insulin autoantibodies are usually present, and in this case the autoantibodies are associated with lineage 1 DQalpha alleles (01* to 04*)[11]. In particular, DR3 homozygous prediabetic and islet cell autoantibody-positive individuals homozygous for DQA*0501 rarely express anti-insulin autoantibodies.

Celiac disease is of particular interest in that the disorder appears to be associated with a specific DQalpha and DQbeta heterodimer (DQA1*-0501,DQB1*0201), produced either in *trans* with DR5 (DQA1*0501, DQB1*0301) and DR7 (DQA1*0201,DQB1*0201)) or *cis* with DR3 (DQA1*-0501,DQB1*0201) containing haplotypes[4].

Finally, myasthenia gravis is associated with different HLA haplotypes, depending upon disease-initiating factors. Idiopathic myasthenia gravis is associated with DR3, while myasthenia gravis developing after ingestion of penicillamine is associated with DR7[12].

The class II alleles within the major histocompatibility complex have received the most attention relative to disease pathogenesis. As these molecules are essential for antigen presentation, this emphasis is likely to be appropriate. Nevertheless, with more than 100 genes within this region, and extensive linkage disequilibrium between alleles, other genes important for immunologic function may contribute to disease susceptibility[13–15].

In addition to genes within the major histocompatibility complex, intense efforts are under way to identify other loci contributing to disease suscepti-bility. To date most of these efforts have not been successful, or not confirmed, including intense study of T cell receptor genes. For type I diabetes, polymorphisms of the insulin gene are clearly associated with risk for type I diabetes[16,17]. In addition several repositories are now available with DNA and EBV lines available from hundreds of families with type I diabetes. With the availability of appropriate family resources and polymorphic microsatellite markers spanning the human genome, it is very likely that additional important loci will be identified. We hypothesize that such loci, similar to mutations of the Fas (apoptosis) gene in Ipr mice[18], will globally influence ability to maintain tolerance and prevent autoimmunity. In associ-ation with such 'global' autoimmune genes, it is likely that alleles within the major histocompatibility complex contribute to targeting specific organs.

DISEASE ACTIVATION

Factors which trigger autoimmunity have been elegantly defined for a small number of autoimmune disorders such that an etiologic classification of autoimmunity can be proposed (Table 2). It is noteworthy that, for several forms of oncogenic autoimmunity, specific molecules are expressed only by the tumors associated with the remote autoimmunity[19–23]. Several of these triggering molecules have been identified and sequenced[24]. The existence of oncogenic autoimmunity suggests that presentation of self antigens within inflammatory lesions can abrogate self-tolerance. It is clear from experimen-tally induced autoimmune disorders that immunization with self antigens[25–27]

Table 2 Etiologic classification of autoimmunity

Etiology	Example
Oncogenic	Cerebellar degeneration – ovarian cancer
Drug-induced	Myasthenia gravis – penicillamine
Diet-induced	Celiac disease – gluten
Infectious	Streptotocci – rheumatic fever
Idiopathic	Type I diabetes – unknown

and self peptides can lead to autoimmunity and tissue destruction. Thus, lymphocytes reacting with self are present in normal animals.

The ability to 'break tolerance' to a series of molecules within inflammatory lesions may also contribute to the existence of linked autoimmune disorders such as Graves' thyroid disease associated with Graves' ophthalmopathy, and ovarian autoimmunity associated with myasthenia gravis. A recent report demonstrates that T cells recognize relatively few amino acids within peptides[27]. Thus, T cell lines can react with peptides of both the acetylcholine receptor and ZP3, the ovarian sperm receptor sharing less than five of nine amino acids. Thus immunization with the appropriate peptide of the acetylcholine receptor can induce ovarian destruction[27].

Studies of type I diabetes have to date failed to identify a crucial environmental factor triggering type I diabetes. To date the three factors receiving the majority of study include congenital rubella infection[28], Coxsackie viral infection[29], and ingestion of milk within the first 3 months of life[30].

Congenital rubella infection is associated with a marked increase in diabetes risk. One hypothesis relates a 52 kDa islet protein recognized by diabetic sera (with homology to heat-shock protein 60) to a specific rubella capsid protein[31]. The rubella and islet protein are both recognized by an anti-rubella monoclonal antibody. Rubella infection increases the risk of diabetes only with fetal infection. Thus an alternative hypothesis is that rubella infection increases the risk of diabetes secondary to lifelong T cell abnormalities[32]. These T cell abnormalities may also contribute to the frequent occurrence of thyroiditis in such patients.

Coxsackie viral infections were originally associated with type I diabetes when it was assumed that the disorder was of acute onset. With accumulating data that type I diabetes develops slowly in the great majority of individuals it is likely that acute infections at the time of disease onset are not of direct pathogenic significance. Recently one of the most studied autoantigens associated with type I diabetes, namely glutamic acid decarboxylase (GD)[33-36], was found to have homology with a peptide sequence of a Coxsackie protein. This region of homology is being studied for relevance to disease induction.

A large number of epidemiologic studies suggest that either decreased breast feeding or early introduction of cow's milk products increase diabetes risk[37-40]. These epidemiologic data are surprisingly consistent, given the less than two-fold increased risk. The risk ascribed to cow's milk ingestion may be higher in individuals with genetic susceptibility for type I diabetes. Trials to test the elimination of cow's milk from diets of infants are being designed.

One hypothesis relating cow's milk to type I diabetes is that bovine albumin shares several small regions of homology with an islet molecule termed ICA69 or p69. Pietropaolo and co-workers recently cloned, sequenced and expressed ICA69. Though there is considerable controversy as to whether antibodies to albumin are associated with type I diabetes, several laboratories have now demonstrated that ICA69 autoantibodies are present in more than 50% of individuals developing type I diabetes[41,42], and less than 5% of normal controls[43]. A number of studies are now addressing T cell responses to albumin and ICA69.

AUTOANTIGENS

During the past 3 years investigators have characterized a large series of islet autoantigens. Similar to other organ-specific autoimmune disorders[44], islet enzymes are prominent islet autoantigens. Autoantigens include glutamic acid decarboxylase[45], carboxypeptidase H[46], and a novel tyrosine phosphatase termed ICA512. In addition, the hormone insulin[47-51] and ICA69[52] (unknown function) is recognized by autoantibodies and T cells. Gangliosides, and in particular a GM2-1 islet ganglioside[53], are also recognized by anti-islet autoantibodies.

With an increasing number of islet autoantigens, the question as to whether any given autoantigen is primary to the disease process, and the related question as to whether any given autoantigen is primary for any individual developing type I diabetes, is not answered. I favor the hypothesis that if there is a primary autoantigen it will be insulin. To date insulin is the only beta cell-specific target molecule. All other characterized autoantigens are expressed in non-islet cells (particularly neuroendocrine cells) or within the alpha and delta cells of islets which are not destroyed in patients with type I diabetes. For example, GAD in the rat is beta cell-specific, but in humans it is expressed by non-beta cells[36].

Criteria to distinguish primary from 'secondary' autoantigens are just being developed. The most important evidence that insulin plays an important role in the pathogenesis of type I diabetes comes from studies of insulin-reactive T cell clones and therapy of NOD mice and humans with insulin. Wegmann and co-workers have recently isolated from NOD islets, T cell clones which react with an insulin peptide (Wegmann and co-workers, unpublished observations). T cells reacting with a peptide of the B chain of insulin are a major component of intra-islet T cells, and most importantly such T cells are capable of transferring diabetes to NOD SCID mice. NOD SCID mice are unable to generate B and T lymphocytes; Wegmann's studies indicate that insulin-reactive T cells are both present in the islet lesion of NOD mice and capable of producing beta cell destruction and type I diabetes. In our studies, and those of Ziegler and co-workers[50] of the chronology of autoimmunity in humans, insulin autoantibodies frequently precede autoantibodies to other autoantigens, including GAD. Oral ingestion of insulin can delay or prevent diabetes in NOD mice[54], and pilot studies suggest that parenteral insulin administration may prevent type I diabetes in a subset of islet cell autoantibody-positive first-degree relatives of patients with type I diabetes[55]. This pilot trial has been followed by a large multicenter NIH trial for the prevention of type I diabetes with parenteral insulin therapy.

With a series of characterized autoantigens, identification of susceptibility, alleles, and two spontaneous animal models, studies concerning the pathogenesis of type I diabetes are accelerating. It is hoped that, with increased knowledge, type I diabetes mellitus will be preventable and the lessons learned for this illness will positively impact studies of other autoimmune disorders.

Acknowledgements

This work was supported by grants from the National Institutes of Health (DK32083, DK43279), the Juvenile Diabetes Foundation, the American Diabetes Association, the Blum-Kovler Foundation and the Children's Diabetes Foundation. The Children's Hospital CRC was essential for the clinical studies described.

References

1. Muir A, Maclaren NK. Autoimmune diseases of the adrenal glands, parathyroid glands, gonads, and hypothalamic-pituitary axis. Endocrinol Metab Clin N Am. 1991;20:619–44.
2. Riley WJ. Autoimmune polyglandular syndromes. Horm Res. 1992;38(Suppl.2):9–15.
3. Eisenbarth GS, Jackson RA. The immunoendocrinopathy syndromes. In: Wilson JD, Foster DW, editors. Williams textbook of endocrinology, 8th edn. Philadelphia: W.B. Saunders; 1992:1555–66.
4. Nepom GT, Erlich H. MHC class-II molecules and autoimmunity. Annu Rev Immunol. 1991;9:493–525.
5. Garty BZ, Kauli R. Alopecia universalis in autoimmune polyglandular syndrome type I [letter, comment]. West J Med. 1990;152:76–7.
6. Torrelo A, Espana A, Balsa J, Ledo A. Vitiligo and polyglandular autoimmune syndrome with selective IgA deficiency. Int J Dermatol. 1992;31:343–4.
7. Maclaren NK, Riley WJ. Inherited susceptibility to autoimmune Addison's disease is linked to human leukocyte antigens DR3 and/or DR4, except when associated with type 1 autoimmune polyglandular syndrome. J Clin Endocrinol Metab. 1986;62:455–9.
8. Baisch JM, Weeks T, Giles R, Hoover M, Stastny P, Capra JD. Analysis of HLA-DQ genotypes and susceptibility in insulin-dependent diabetes mellitus. N Engl J Med. 1990;322:1836–41.
9. Erlich HA, Griffith RL, Bugawan TL, Ziegler R, Alper C, Eisenbarth GS. Implication of specific DQB1 alleles in genetic susceptibility and resistance by identification of IDDM siblings with novel HLA-DQB1 allele and unusual DR2 and DR1 haplotypes. Diabetes. 1991;40:478–81.
10. Uchigata Y, Kuwata S, Tsushima T et al. Patients with Graves' disease who developed insulin autoimmune syndrome (hirata disease) possess HLA-Bw62/Cw4/DR4 carrying DRB1*0406. J Clin Endocrinol Metab. 1993;77;249–54.
11. Pugliese A, Bugawan T, Moromisato R et al. Two subsets of HLA-DQA1 alleles mark phenotypic variation in levels of insulin autoantibodies in first degree relatives at risk for insulin-dependent diabetes. J Clin Invest. 1994 (In press).
12. Garlepp MJ, Dawkins RL, Christiansen FT. HLA antigens and acetylcholine receptor antibodies in penicillamine induced myasthenia gravis. Br Med J. 1983;286:338–40.
13. Awdeh ZL, Raum D, Yunis EJ, Alper CA. Extended HLA/complement allele haplotypes:

evidence for T/t like complex in man. Proc Natl Acad Sci USA. 1983;80:259–63.

14. French MAH, Dawkins RL. Central MHC genes, IgA deficiency and autoimmune disease. Immunol Today. 1990;11:271–4.

15. Li X, Golden J, Faustman DL. Faulty major histocompatibility complex class II I-E expression is associated with autoimmunity in diverse strains of mice. Diabetes. 1993;42:1166–72.

16. Julier C, Hyer RN, Davis J et al. Insulin-IGF2 region encodes a gene implicated in HLA-DR4-dependent diabetes susceptibility. Nature. 1991;354:155–9.

17. Lucassen A, Julier C, Beressi J-P et al. Susceptibility to insulin dependent diabetes mellitus maps to a 4.1 kb segment of DNA spanning the insulin gene and associated VNTR. Nature Genet. 1993;4:305–10.

18. Watanabe-Fukunaga R, Brannan CI, Copeland NG, Jenkins NA, Nagata S. Lymphoproliferation disorder in mice explained by defects in Fas antigen that mediate apoptosis. Nature. 1992;356:314–17.

19. Anhalt GJ, Kim S-C, Stanley JR et al. Paraneoplastic pemphigus. An autoimmune mucocutaneous disease associated with neoplasia. N Engl J Med. 1990;323:1729–35.

20. Hetzel DJ, Stanhope R, O'Neill BP, Lennon VA. Gynecologic cancer in patients with subacute cerebellar degeneration predicted by anti-Purkinje cell antibodies and limited in metastatic volume. Mayo Clin Proc. 1990;65:1558–63.

21. Kornguth SE. Neuronal proteins and paraneoplastic syndromes. N Engl J Med. 1989; 321:1607–8.

22. Grunwald GB, Simmonds MA, Klein R, Kornguth SE. Autoimmune basis for visual paraneoplastic syndrome in patients with small-cell lung carcinoma. Lancet. 1985;1658–61.

23. Anhalt GJ, SooChan K, Stanley JR et al. Paraneoplastic pemphigus: an autoimmune mucocutaneous disease associated with neoplasia. N Engl J Med. 1990;323:1729–35.

24. Dropcho EJ, Chen Y-T, Posner JB, Old LJ. Cloning of a brain protein identified by autoantibodies from a patient with paraneoplastic cerebellar degeneration. Proc Natl Acad Sci USA. 1987;84:4552–6.

25. Massacesi L, Joshi N, Le-Parritz D, Rombos A, Letvin NL, Hauser SL. Experimental allergic encephalomyelitis in cynomolgus monkeys: Quantitation of T cell responses in peripheral blood. J Clin Invest. 1992;90:399–404.

26. Rhim SH, Millar SE, Robey F et al. Autoimmune disease of the ovary induced by a ZP3 peptide from the mouse zona pellucida. J Clin Invest. 1992;89:28–35.

27. Luo A-M, Garza KM, Hunt D, Tung KSK. Antigen mimicry in autoimmune disease sharing of amino acid residues critical for pathogenic T cell activation. J Clin Invest. 1993;92:2117–23.

28. Ginsberg-Fellner F, Witt ME, Yagihashi S et al. Congenital rubella syndrome as a model for type I (insulin-dependent) diabetes mellitus: increased prevalence of islet cell surface antibodies. Diabetologia. 1984;27:87–9.

29. Frisk G, Friman G, Tuvemo T, Fohlman J, Diderholm H, Coxsackie B virus IgM in children at onset of Type I (insulin-dependent) diabetes mellitus: evidence for IgM induction by a recent or current infection. Diabetologia. 1992;35:249–53.

30. Kostraba JN, Cruickshanks KJ, Lawler-Heavner J et al. Early exposure to cow's milk and solid foods in infancy, genetic predisposition and risk of IDDM. Diabetes. 1993;42:288–95.

31. Karounos DG, Wolinsky JS, Thomas JW. Monoclonal antibody to rubella virus capsid protein recognizes a B-cell antigen. J Immunol. 1993;150:3080–5.

32. Rabinowe SL, George KL, Laughlin R, Soeldner JS, Eisenbarth GS. Congenital rubella: monoclonal antibody defined T cell abnormalities in young children. Am J Med. 1986;81: 779–82.

33. Atkinson A, Kaufman DL, Campbell L et al. Response of peripheral-blood mononuclear cells to glutamate decarboxylase in insulin-dependent diabetes. Lancet. 1992;339:458–9.

34. Kaufman DL, Erlander MG, Clare-Salzler M, Atkinson MA, Maclaren NK, Tobin AJ. Autoimmunity to two forms of glutamate decarboxylase in insulin dependent diabetes mellitus. J Clin Invest. 1992;89:283–92.

35. Rowley MJ, Mackay IR, Chen Q, Knowles WJ, Zimmet PZ. Antibodies to glutamic acid decarboxylase discriminate major types of diabetes mellitus. Diabetes. 1992;41:548–51.

36. Petersen JS, Russel S, Marshall MO et al. Differential expression of glutamic acid decarboxylase in rat and human islets. Diabetes. 1993;42:484–95.

37. Martin JM, Trink B, Daneman D, Dosch H, Robinson B. Milk proteins in the etiology of insulin-dependent diabetes mellitus (IDDM). Ann Med. 1991;23:447–52.
38. Borch-Johnson K, Joner G, Mandrup-Poulsen T et al. Relation between breast-feeding and incidence rates of insulin-dependent diabetes mellitus. Lancet. 1984;2:1083–6.
39. Vialettes B, Zevaco-Mattel C, Thirion X et al. Acute insulin response to glucose and glucagon in subjects at risk of developing type I diabetes. Diabetes Care. 1993;16:973–7.
40. Gerstein HC. Cow's milk exposure and type I diabetes mellitus. Diabetes Care. 1994;17:13–19.
41. Karjalainen J, Martin JM, Knip M et al. A bovine albumin peptide as a possible trigger of insulin-dependent diabetes mellitus. N Engl J Med. 1992;327:302–7.
42. Handwerger S, Capel WD. Differences in the cell surface antigens of prolactin-producing cells of human decidual and pituitary tissues. J Clin Endocrinol Metab. 1985;61:830–3.
43. Pietropaolo M, Castano L, Babu S, Powers A, Eisenbarth GS. Molecular cloning and characterization of a novel neuroendocrine autoantigen (PM-1) related to type I diabetes. Diabetes. 1992;41(Suppl. 1):98A(abstr.).
44. Winqvist O, Gustafsson J, Rorsman F, Karlsson FA, Kampe O. Two different cytochrome P450 enzymes are the adrenal antigens in autoimmune polyendocrine syndrome type I and Addison's disease. J Clin Invest. 1993;92:2377–85.
45. Baekkeskov S, Aanstoot H, Christgau S et al. Identification of the 64K autoantigen in insulin dependent diabetes as the GABA-synthesizing enzyme glutamic acid decarboxylase. Nature. 1990;347:151–6.
46. Castano L, Russo E, Zhou L, Lipes MA, Eisenbarth GS. Identification and cloning of a granule autoantigen (carboxypeptidase H) associated with type I diabetes. J Clin Endocrinol Metab. 1991;73:1197–201.
47. Palmer JP, Asplin CM, Clemons P et al. Insulin antibodies in insulin-dependent diabetics before insulin treatment. Science. 1983;222:1337–9.
48. Vardi P, Ziegler AG, Matthews JH et al. Concentration of insulin autoantibodies at onset of Type I diabetes: inverse log-linear correlation with age. Diabetes Care. 1988;11:736–9.
49. Ziegler AG, Ziegler R, Vardi P, Jackson RA, Soeldner JS, Eisenbarth GS. Life table analysis of progression to diabetes of anti-insulin autoantibody-positive relatives of individuals with Type I diabetes. Diabetes. 1989;38:1320–5.
50. Ziegler AG, Hillebrand B, Rabl W et al. On the appearance of islet associated autoimmunity in offspring of diabetic mothers: a prospective study from birth. Diabetologia. 1993;36:402–8.
51. Castano L, Ziegler A, Ziegler R, Shoelson S, Eisenbarth GS. Characterization of insulin autoantibodies in relatives of patients with insulin-dependent diabetes mellitus. Diabetes. 1993;42:1202–9.
52. Zielasek J, Jackson RA, Eisenbarth GS. The potentially simple mathematics of Type I diabetes. Clin Immunol Immunopathol. 1989;52:347–65.
53. Dotta F, Previti M, Tiberti C, Lenti L, Pugliese G, DiMario U. Identification of the GM2-1 islet ganglioside: similarities with a major neuronal autoantigen. Diabetes. 1992;41:365A.
54. Zhang JZ, Davidson L, Eisenbarth GS, Weiner HL. Suppression of diabetes in nonobese diabetic mice by oral administration of porcine insulin. Proc Natl Acad Sci USA. 1991;88:10252–6.
55. Keller RJ, Eisenbarth GS, Jackson RA. Insulin prophylaxis in individuals at high risk of type I diabetes. Lancet. 1993;341:927–8.

8
Regulation of mucosal immune responses – the missing link in IBD?

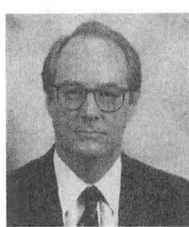

C. O. ELSON, R. P. McCABE, Jr, K. W. BEAGLEY,
A. SHARMANOV, S. L. BRANDWEIN,
B. U. RIDWAN, C. WEAVER, R. P. BUCY,
J. R. McGHEE, J. SUNDBERG and
E. BIRKENMEIER

C. O. ELSON

The intestine is quite distinct from other organs which are involved in chronic inflammatory/autoimmune diseases. Mucosal surfaces, in particular the intestinal mucosa, represent the major interface between the immune system and the antigens and microbes of the external environment. In order to deal with this challenge a specialized mucosal immune system has evolved, which is marked by certain features distinct to this system[1]. The massive antigenic challenge and the specialized features of the mucosal immune system add further complexity to our potential understanding of the mechanisms of inflammatory bowel disease (IBD) compared to diseases such as autoimmune diabetes or multiple sclerosis, which affect organs that are largely sequestered from antigenic challenge.

An understanding of the mucosal immune system and how it is regulated is thus very important to our eventual understanding of IBD. There are a number of important aspects or concepts of mucosal immune regulation that provide a context or framework for the understanding of IBD (Table 1). The first of these is the enormous and continuous IgA response in the mucosa. Some 60% of all the immunoglobulin made daily is IgA; quantitatively this

Table 1 Concepts of mucosal immune regulation

Enormous S-IgA response
Th1 vs Th2: gut mucosa a preferential Th2 site
Environment differs at various mucosal sites
Mucosal tolerance prevents response to many antigens
Potent regulatory mechanisms restore homeostasis after injury

represents some 3000–4000 mg per day of IgA, produced predominantly in the gut[2]. The number of gut lymphoid cells producing IgA has been estimated at 10^{10}/meter of small intestine in humans[3]. Secondly, and consistent with this strong humoral response in the mucosa, the intestinal mucosa appears to be a preferential site for Th2-type T cell responses. Thus, an antigen encounter in the gut mucosa tends to generate predominantly a Th2 response, whereas that same antigen given systemically tends to elicit a predominantly Th1 response[4]. The Th1 and Th2 pathways of T cell responses are important in the outcome of the host response to various microbial pathogens, and disturbance of the balance between these pathways might well result in chronic inflammatory disease[5,6]. Third, the environmental exposure of different regions of the mucosa varies tremendously. For example, the antigenic environment in the small bowel is quite different from that in the colon. Perhaps related to this, cells comprising the mucosal immune system in the mouse colon are quite distinct from those of the small bowel[7]. These differences may relate to a need to respond to a different assortment of food and microbial antigens at these different sites. Whether similar differences exist in humans is unknown. Fourth, the mucosal immune system does not respond to every antigen which transits the bowel: many antigens elicit tolerance rather than immunity. This is demonstrated readily by feeding an antigen prior to systemically immunizing with the same antigen. Animals fed the antigen prior to immunization have a markedly reduced response. Mechanisms underlying such 'oral tolerance' remain unclear, but clonal anergy and $CD8^+$ T cells secreting the inhibitory cytokine TGF-β have both been reported[8]. Lastly, there are potent mechanisms in place that rapidly restore homeostasis following injury to the bowel[9]. For example, after enemas of irritant chemicals these mechanisms rapidly restore the epithelial barrier, repair the tissue matrix, and down-regulate the potentially deleterious immune cell populations. Each of these various aspects of mucosal immune regulation is germane to, and important in the understanding of, potential abnormalities occurring during IBD.

Although the pathogenesis of IBD remains obscure, these clearly are complex disorders with immune, genetic, and environmental components. It has been difficult to study the early events and interactions among these components leading to chronic intestinal inflammation; however, there have been a number of recent developments which now make such studies possible. A number of new mouse models of chronic colitis have recently become available, several due to advances in genetic technology that allows targeted gene inactivation in mice. As shown in Table 2, deletions of certain genes of the immune system has resulted in mice which spontaneously develop chronic intestinal inflammation. Interestingly, certain of these genes encode cytokines that are involved in maintaining the Th1/Th2 balance[5]. Although deletion of certain of these genes such as IL-2[10] and IL-10[11] has resulted in mice that develop colitis, deletions of others such as IL-4 and IFN-γ that are also involved in maintaining the Th1/Th2 balance, have not. Likewise, mice rendered deficient in TCR-$\alpha\beta$-bearing T cells by deletion of the T cell receptor α chain has resulted in colitis[12], but colitis has not been reported to occur in nude mice which also lack T cells. Although a unifying theory has been

Table 2 Mouse genetic mutants relevant to IBD

Mice that get IBD
C3H/HeJBir
IL-2 knockout
IL-10 knockout
TCR-α knockout
Mice that do not get IBD
SCID mice
RAG knockout
IL-4 knockout
IFN-γ knockout

advanced to explain the pathogenesis of colitis in these knockout mice, it seems more likely that there are multiple different pathways that can result in chronic intestinal inflammation. Whether these immune gene deletions are causing disease by disrupting the normal regulation of mucosal immune responses is an attractive hypothesis which will require further experimental study.

Some insights into the importance of immune regulation relative to chronic intestinal inflammation has come from the adaptation of the TNBS/ethanol model to mice. This model originated in Canada and was applied initially to studies in rats[13]. Trinitrobenzenesulfonic acid (TNBS) is one of a group of contact-sensitizing allergens which have been used for years to study the mechanisms of delayed hypersensitivity. These compounds are covalently reactive chemicals which attach to tissue proteins and induce a CD4$^+$ T cell reaction to the resulting hapten-modified self antigens[14]. One advantage of this system is that the antigen or agent is known and well defined; thus both the specific and non-specific response to it can be measured and their regulation studied. We have recently adapted this system to the mouse. One of the interesting observations made in adapting this system to mice is that there are major differences in susceptibility among inbred strains. For example, C3H/HeJ and BALB/C strains are quite susceptible, whereas C57Bl/6 and DBA/2 are very resistant. Mice of the resistant strains develop skin test reactivity to the allergen but rapidly down-regulate the inflammation in the colon, such that within days of the challenge enema the mucosa looks quite normal. Moreover, spontaneous production of cytokines by lymph node cells draining the distal colon is found in susceptible mice, but not at all in mice of the resistant strains. Despite this being a lesion mediated by CD4$^+$ T cells, there are dramatic changes in the B cell compartment during TNBS-induced colitis. This B cell response includes a prominent shift of B cells from spleen and Peyer's patch into the lesions, the draining lymph node, and the mesenteric lymph node. Only about half of this B cell response can be attributed to the anti-TNP response, indicating that there is a large concomitant polyclonal response[15]. The antibody response to the hapten is mainly of the IgG2a subclass, which would be consistent with a predominant Th1 T cell immune reaction[16].

It has been known for some time that the feeding of contact allergens to mice results in a state of oral tolerance[17]. We recently completed a series of

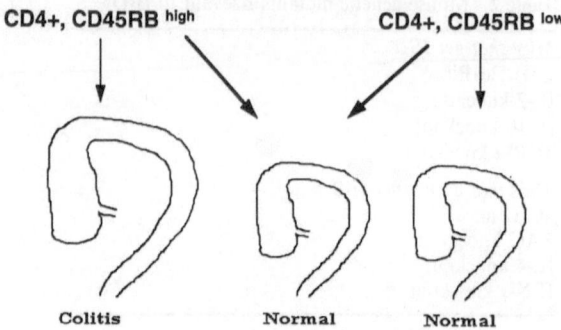

Fig. 1 Outcome of autologous CD4$^+$, CD45RB cell transfers to SCID recipients. Adoptive transfer of CD4$^+$, CD45RB^{high} T cells results in a striking colitis after 5–10 weeks. Transfer of CD4$^+$ CD45RB^{low} T cells does not cause disease. Co-transfer of both subsets abrogates the disease seen after transfer of only the CD4$^+$ CD45RB^{high} subset

experiments addressing whether the induction of oral tolerance with TNBS would affect the anti-TNP immune response or the severity of TNBS-induced colitis. Mice were fed 10 mg of soluble TNBS on two occasions prior to the sensitizing and challenge enema with TNBS and ethanol. The anti-TNP response in various tissues was analyzed in tolerized mice vs. control mice using the ELISPOT technique. The prior feeding of TNBS abrogated the IgG anti-TNP response, although the local mucosal IgA anti-TNP response was maintained. More interestingly, the induction of oral tolerance to TNBS significantly ameliorated the severity of the inflammation in subsequent TNBS-induced colitis[16]. These results indicate that it may be possible to exploit the intrinsic regulatory mechanisms of the mucosal immune system in the treatment of chronic intestinal inflammation.

A second mouse model has recently been described that is highly relevant to the present discussion. In this model, a subset of CD4$^+$ T cells which express a high level of the CD45RB surface antigen are transferred into syngeneic SCID recipients[18,19]. Mice with the SCID mutation lack B cells or T cells but have intact innate immunity consisting of macrophages, neutrophils and NK cells. After a lag phase of some weeks the recipients begin to lose weight due to the development of a prominent colitis. In the colon of such mice there is infiltration of CD4$^+$ T cells and macrophages, crypt hyperplasia, mucin depletion, and scattered crypt abscesses. The clinical course of these animals is that of progressive weight loss, inanition and death. This pathology is very similar to that which was seen in a cyclosporin A-induced colitis that was previously reported[20]. If the reciprocal CD4$^+$ subset, which expresses low levels of the CD45RB surface marker, is transferred to SCID mice, or if whole CD4$^+$ T cells are given, no colitis ensues, although the animals become populated with these T cells. If both CD4$^+$ T cell subsets are given together (CD45RB^{high} plus CD45RB^{low}), no colitis occurs (Fig. 1). There are two major lessons from these experiments. First, T cells are present in normal mice that are capable of causing chronic colitis. One can detect the presence of these cells only in an environment lacking immune regulatory mechanisms. The second lesson is that regulatory

T cells are present also in normal mice that prevent the induction of colitis by the former effector T cells.

A question that immediately jumps to mind is 'What is the antigen driving chronic colitis in this model?' The same question could be asked in human IBD. The antigens have yet to be identified in the CD45RB transfer model; however, there is information from some of the other genetic models. The IL-2 knockout mouse does not develop colitis when rendered germ-free[10], implicating the normal enteric bacterial flora in this disease. Interestingly, the bowel lesions in the IL-2 knockout mouse are limited to the colon and do not affect the small bowel. This indicates that the localization of the enteric flora mainly in the colon is what limits the disease to this segment of the intestine. The IL-10 knockout mouse has a greatly reduced pathology when rendered specific pathogen-free[11]. The HLAB27/β2-microglobulin transgenic rat does not develop enteritis or arthritis when made germ-free[21]. Lastly, spontaneous colitis in C3H/HeJBir mice is associated with a strong response to antigens of the normal enteric flora[22,23]. A reasonable unifying hypothesis that would fit all of these observations is that chronic colitis is the result of a dysregulated mucosal immune response to enteric bacterial antigens normally present in the colon. This hypothesis has been advanced for a number of years, but until recently there has been a relative dearth of experimental models in which to test it. These newer models of colitis should allow a definitive answer to it, as well as allowing the definition of the cellular and molecular mechanisms involved.

Irun Cohen has advanced a novel hypothesis which he has termed the 'cognitive paradigm', in which preformed internal images of external antigens guide and restrict the process of clonal activation[24]. Thus, the immune system is seen as representing an 'immunological homunculus', i.e. the immune system exists to protect us against microbes, and the receptors of the immune system in essence are the mirror-image of the microbial antigen universe. Under this paradigm, autoimmunity is seen as the price that humans pay for effective protection against microbes, e.g. via microbe–autoantigen crossreactivity. When one considers that the major interface between microbial antigens and the immune system resides in the intestine, this paradigm has interesting implications for our understanding of chronic intestinal inflammation, e.g. is IBD the price that humans pay for effective mucosal immunity against microbes?

In summary, an understanding of mucosal immune regulation is crucial to understanding IBD. T cells can mediate chronic colitis in at least two mouse models, and will likely be found to do so in others. Genetic susceptibility plays a major role in disease expression in such models, and probably in humans. The possibility of mapping genetic loci responsible for such susceptibility in mice is an exciting prospect due to the strong homology between mouse and human genomes. These newer mouse models provide a good deal of support for the hypothesis that a dysregulation of the mucosal immune response to common enteric bacterial antigens may be the fundamental underlying defect in the pathogenesis of chronic intestinal IBD.

References

1. MacDermott RP, Elson CO, editors. Mucosal Immunology, vol. 1. Philadelphia: W.B. Saunders; 1991.
2. Mestecky J, McGhee JR, Elson CO. Intestinal IgA system. Immunol Allergy Clin N Am. 1988;8:349–68.
3. Brandtzaeg P. Overview of the mucosal immune system. In: Mestecky J, McGhee JR, editors. New strategies for oral immunization. New York: Springer-Verlag; 1989:13–25.
4. Xu-Amano J, Jackson RJ, Staats HF et al. Helper T cell subsets for IgA responses. Oral immunization with tetanus toxoid and cholera toxin as adjuvant selectively induces Th2 cells in mucosa-associated tissues. J Exp Med. 1993;178:1309–20.
5. Mosmann TR, Coffman RL. TH1 and TH2 cells: different patterns of lymphokine secretion lead to different functional properties. Annu Rev Immunol. 1989;7:145–73.
6. Heinzel FP, Sadick MD, Holoday BJ, Coffman RL, Locksley RM. Reciprocal expression of interferon gamma or interleukin 4 during the resolution or progression of murine leischmaniasis. Evidence for expansion of distinct helper T cell subsets. J Exp Med. 1989;169:59–72.
7. Beagley KW, Fujihashi K, Lagoo AS, Elson CO. Regional differences in mucosal lymphoid cells of murine small vs. large bowel. Gastroenterology. 1992;102:A593.
8. Miller A, Lider O, Roberts AB, Sporn MB, Weiner HL. Suppressor T cells generated by oral tolerization to myelin basic protein suppress both in vitro and in vivo immune responses by the release of transforming growth factor beta after antigen-specific triggering. Proc Natl Acad Sci USA. 1992;89:421–5.
9. Dielemann LA, Elson CO, Tennyson GS, Beagley KW. Cytokine expression during acute colonic injury in mice. Gastroenterology. 1992;102:A616.
10. Sadlack B, Merz H, Schorle H, Schimpl A, Feller AC, Horak I. Ulcerative colitis-like disease in mice with a disrupted interleukin-2 gene. Cell. 1993;75:253–61.
11. Kuhn R, Lohler J, Rennick D, Rajewsky K, Muller W. Interleukin-10-deficient mice develop chronic enterocolitis. Cell. 1993;75:263–74.
12. Mombaerts P, Mizoguchi E, Grusby MJ, Glimcher LH, Bhan AK, Tonegawa S. Spontaneous development of inflammatory bowel disease in T cell receptor mutant mice. Cell. 1993;75: 1–20.
13. Morris GP, Beck PL, Herridge MS, Depew WT, Szewczuk MR, Wallace JL. Hapten-induced model of chronic inflammation and ulceration in the rat colon. Gastroenterology. 1989;96:795–803.
14. Miller SD, Butler LD, Cleveland RP, Moorhead JW, Claman HN, Chiller JC. T-cell responses induced by the parenteral injection of antigen-modified syngeneic cells. II. Mechanisms, specificity, and cellular analysis of 2,4,6-trinitrophenol (TNP)-specific cytolytic response priming by intravenous versus subcutaneous injection with TNP-modified syngeneic cells. Cell Immunol. 1983;82:378–93.
15. Beagley KW, Tennyson GS, Black CA, Sharmanov A, Cummings OW, Elson CO. Hapten-induced colitis in mice. Differences in susceptibility among mouse strains. 1994 (Submitted).
16. Sharmanov AT, Elson CO, Kiyono H et al. Murine hapten-induced colitis: antibody response analysis and protection after oral tolerance induction. 1994 (Submitted).
17. Asherson GL, Zembala M, Perera MACC, Mayhew B, Thomas WR. Production of immunity and unresponsiveness in the mouse by feeding contact sensitizing agents and the role of suppressor cells in the Peyer's patches, mesenteric lymph nodes and other lymphoid tissues. Cell Immunol. 1977;33:145–55.
18. Powrie F, Leach MW, Mauze S, Caddle LB, Coffman RL. Phenotypically distinct subsets of CD4+ T cells induce or protect from chronic intestinal inflammation in C.B-17 scid mice. Eur J Immunol. 1993;5:1461–71.
19. Morrissey PJ, Charrier K, Braddy S, Liggitt D, Watson JD. CD4+ T cells that express high levels of CD45RB induce wasting disease when transferred into congenic severe combined immunodeficient mice. Disease development is prevented by cotransfer of purified CD4+ T cells. J Exp Med. 1993;178:237–44.
20. Bucy RP, Xu XY, Li J, Huang GQ. Cyclosporin A-induced autoimmune disease in mice. J Immunol. 1993;151:1039–50.
21. Taurog JD, Richardson JA, Hadavand R et al. The germfree state protects HLA-B27

transgenic rats from gut and joint inflammation. FASEB J. 1994;8 (In press).
22. Sundberg JP, Elson CO, Bedigian H, Birkenmeier EH. Spontaneous, heritable colitis in a new substrain of C3H/HeJ mice. Gastroenterology. 1994 (in press).
23. Brandwein SL, McCabe RP, Dadrat A et al. Immunologic reactivity of colitic C3H/BejBir mice to enteric bacteria. Gastroenterology. 1994;106:A656.
24. Cohen IR. The cognitive paradigm and the immunological homunculus. Immunol Today. 1992;13:490–4.

9
T cell repertoire and IBD

K. CROITORU, D. K. H. WONG and
M. E. BACA-ESTRADA

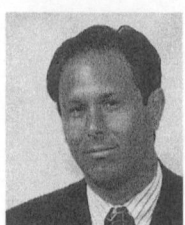

K. CROITORU

INTRODUCTION

Crohn's disease and ulcerative colitis are characterized by chronic intestinal inflammation of unknown etiology. It has been proposed that, in an individual with the appropriate genetic background, exposure to environmental agents or organisms leads to activation of intestinal immune cells and chronic inflammation. Whether or not this results in autoreactivity, it is proposed that the activation of intestinal T cells is critical to the initiation and perpetuation of IBD.

T cells recognize antigen via the surface T cell receptor (TCR). Signals initiated through the TCR lead to a functional response that may be characterized by proliferation, cytotoxicity or cytokine production. Under certain conditions there is a lack of response (anergy) or activation of programmed cell death (apoptosis). A number of cellular processes and molecular signals serve to influence the outcome of TCR-mediated T cell activation[1]. These processes can serve to turn off a T cell response, i.e. induce anergy. The mechanisms of anergy induction are related to inappropriate signals or lack of accessory signals.

T lymphocyte responses are also controlled by selection processes that shape the TCR repertoire, so that reactivity to foreign antigens is permitted and reactivity to self-antigens prevented, i.e. distinguishing self from non-self. Although selection occurs predominantly in the thymus a significant element of extrathymic T cell development has been shown to occur in mice[2]. In the intestine these may serve to limit reactivity to self-antigens and possibly dampen responses to dietary and bacterial antigens presented to the gut. Therefore, the study of the TCR repertoire provides the context in which to consider the role of T cell activation in IBD. If IBD is an autoimmune disease it is possible that the control of T cell responses to foreign and self-antigens may be dysfunctional. Therefore, in the context of IBD, it is possible that the environment in which antigen is encountered, i.e. the intestine, can have an important influence on the T cell repertoire and the nature of T cell responses. Identifying the changes in such control mechanisms will help clarify the role of T cells in IBD, and may provide clues regarding the nature of disease-specific antigen.

To explore the mechanisms that control the induction of T cell tolerance in the intestine we have studied the function of mucosal T cells in mice. In addition, we have examined the cytotoxic function of T cell subsets in patients with Crohn's disease to determine if TCR-restricted changes in function may reflect exposure to superantigens.

MUCOSAL T CELL DIFFERENTIATION

Significant differences exist between the mucosal and systemic immune system[3]. The mucosal immune system is compartmentalized into distinct anatomic regions. Lymphocytes from mesenteric lymph nodes (MLN), Peyer's patches (PP), lamina propria (LPL) and the epithelium each differ in morphology, phenotype and function. Collectively these sites are referred to as the gut-associated lymphoid tissue or GALT. Antigens and bacterial products within the intestinal lumen all serve to activate mucosal T lymphocytes, as reflected by the unique phenotypes[4]. For example, in humans a majority of mucosal lymphocytes express surface markers associated with 'memory' or activated T cells, e.g. CD45RA-low, CD45RO-high[5]. In addition to the 'activated' state of mucosal lymphocytes there is evidence that mucosal T cells in the mouse can develop extrathymically. The positive and negative selection of the TCR repertoire of thymic-independent intestinal intraepithelial lymphocytes (IEL) is thought to occur, to some degree, within the intestine itself[6-8]. It is therefore possible that the local TCR repertoire is shaped to accommodate local antigen exposure.

These issues have been studied best in the IEL, which make up 10–15% of the cells in the epithelium[9]. Most of these cells express the T cell marker CD8 and either the α/β or γ/δ TCR[10,11]. T cells in IEL are unusual in that half lack pan-T cell markers such as Thy1 and CD5[11,12] and CD8 is expressed as an α/α homodimer rather than the usual α/β heterodimer[11]. It has been suggested that these unusual phenotypes identify the extrathymic lineage of T cells[6,7] that can express the γ/δ TCR or 'autospecific' α/β TCR. In mice, autoreactive T cells of either the α/β and γ/δ TCR subsets somehow escape thymic deletion. We have shown that IEL expressing the autoreactive Vβ6 TCR in MIs-1^a mice fail to proliferate or secrete interleukin-2 (IL-2) in response to TCR stimulation. Importantly, this anergic response can be reversed by the addition of exogenous IL-2, suggesting a mechanism by which tolerance in autoreactive mucosal T cells can be overcome. If such a mechanism serves to control the response of autoreactive T cells *in vivo* then loss of such control could lead to intestinal damage and inflammation.

IEL in humans are similar to those found in mice in that they have cytoplasmic granules, and can express the CD5⁻CD8⁺ phenotype[13,14]. Although some express the γ/δ TCR, the majority of human IEL express α/β TCR[15]. It is not known if human IEL contain 'autospecific' TCR or if they can develop extrathymically.

T CELL RECEPTOR-TRIGGERED ACTIVATION

The TCR molecules are composed of variable (V), diversity (D), joining (J) and constant (C) elements, analogous to the immunoglobulin molecule. During T cell differentiation noncontiguous gene segments undergo somatic rearrangement, randomly generating the diversity necessary to deal with the infinite number of foreign Ag[16,17]. The self-reactive T cell clones that could emerge during such a random process are eliminated by deletion or functional inactivation. The T cell receptor, which is a disulfide-linked heterodimer, associated with monomorphic CD3 molecules, is responsible for the recognition of antigen[18].

Antigen or anti-CD3 activation of the TCR/CD3 complex leads to T cell proliferation and cytokine production. Since it is difficult in humans to study antigen-specific cytotoxic T cells (CTL), anti-CD3 stimulation allows one to bypass the need for antigen or MHC-restriction to study T cell reactivity. Cytotoxicity generated through anti-CD3 stimulation has been used to demonstrate that mucosal T cells have CTL activity[19]. The target or physiological role of such cytotoxic cells is unknown[20]; however, the ability to study the nature of these T cells can provide new information about T cell function in IBD.

T cell function and response to TCR-mediated activation in the mucosa differs from that seen in PBL. In an infectious model of intestinal inflammation, James *et al.* showed that lymphocytes isolated from non-human primates infected with *Chlamydia trachomatis* did not proliferate in response to Ag, but rather showed an increase in cytokine production[21]. In a second study, anti-CD3 stimulation failed to induce proliferation of LPL or PBL cultured with mucosal tissue supernatants, suggesting that intestinal factors serve to dampen this response[22,23], possibly explaining the low proliferative reseponse of IEL[24]. Alternate pathways of mucosal T cell signalling such as anti-CD2 stimulation exist for both IEL and LPL[24,25]. Therefore, T cell proliferation alone may not adequately reflect mucosal T cell responses. In addition T cell responses require appropriate accessory signals such as co-stimulation of CD28[26].

Furthermore, under appropriate conditions, TCR activation of immature T cells leads to apoptosis or programmed cell death; a part of the negative selection process in the thymus[27,28]. Mature peripheral T cells can also be activated to undergo apoptosis[29,30]; for example, antigen stimulation of T cells preactivated with IL-2 can lead to programmed cell death[30]. Intestinal γ/δ and α/β TCR IEL can undergo apoptosis after TCR stimulation[31] and, under certain conditions, anti-CD2 stimulation of activated peripheral T cells can lead to apoptosis[32]. Therefore, the outcome of T cell activation by the TCR is dependent on the circumstances surrounding the stimulating event, and there are a number of factors that can influence T cell reactivity.

ALTERATIONS OF MUCOSAL T LYMPHOCYTES IN IBD

Although a number of alterations of the humoral and cellular immune responses have been described in IBD[33,34] it is not clear which is directly related to the pathogenesis or etiology of the disease. Nonetheless, immune activation is a necessary part of the disease. What is known about changes in human T cells in IBD is for the most part nonspecific. Increases in IEL numbers have only rarely been described[35]. IEL and LPL phenotypes are not overly altered and although total lamina propria T cells are increased, the CD4:CD8 ratio is unchanged[33]. Data on LPL function are contradictory, in that some studies have shown that IL-2 production is decreased[36] and others increased[37]. No disease-specific cytotoxic function has been identified[4,33,34]. As discussed, antigen-specific T cell responses in IBD are difficult to study. In PBL of IBD patients there is an increase in anti-CD3-induced cytotoxicity[38]; however, in LPL there have been conflicting data regarding changes of this activity in IBD[19,39].

With the availability of molecular probes and monoclonal antibodies (MAb) to the TCR, changes in TCR expression have been examined as a means of trying to identify a specific antigenic stimulus. This includes the use of MAb to TCR variable-gene products and the use of reverse transcriptase–polymerase chain reaction (PCR) analysis for V-gene mRNA in chronic inflammatory and autoimmune diseases[40–42]. Early studies in IBD failed to show clonal rearrangements at either the α/β or γ TCR loci in LPL[43]. More recent work indicates that normal human IEL undergo oligoclonal expansion based on TCR V-region gene expression[44], but there are few data regarding IBD-specific changes in mucosal lymphocytes[45]. Increases in the proportion of T cells expressing TCR Vβ-gene product in different chronic inflammatory diseases suggest that superantigens may be involved in the pathogenesis of some of these diseases[40,46].

Superantigens activate T cell subsets through binding to a particular V-region gene product, usually on the β-chain of the TCR[47–49]. In mice, in-vivo stimulation with the superantigen, staphylococcal enterotoxin, causes proliferation and alterations in function in V gene-restricted T cell subsets[50]. In Crohn's disease a subgroup of patients have an increased number of TCR Vβ8 PBL, raising the possibility that superantigens may be involved in activating T cells in IBD[51].

Since the initiation of CD disease may be far removed in time from when most patients are diagnosed, it is possible that remnants of the initiating event may be found in changes in the expression of the TCR repertoire. It is also possible that changes may be detectable in the function of T cell subsets with or without changes in TCR V-gene expression. Studies of the effect of superantigens on T cells in mice indicate that after initial proliferation of a restricted T cell subset there is loss of function and subsequent elimination through clonal deletion and apoptosis[50,52,53]. Furthermore, in the initial stages of disease, patients with Kawasaki's disease show a short-lived expansion of Vβ2 and Vβ8 TCR that, with time, is followed by the deletion of these T cell subsets[54]. Therefore, measuring alterations in the proportion of T cells expressing different TCR V-gene products may fail to detect significant changes relevant to the pathogenesis of Crohn's disease. Further insight into the possibility that a superantigen may be involved in these disorders would be discernible through examining changes in the function of the different T cell subsets as well as changes in TCR expression.

We have examined the cytotoxic activity of T cells bearing specific TCR V-gene products using MAb specific for individual TCR variable gene products. This redirected cytotoxicity assay reflects the cytotoxic potential of the T cell subset identified by the MAb used to crosslink the TCR and induce activation[55,56]. Our findings indicate that little difference could be detected in the cytotoxic function between normal and Crohn's disease patients using MAb that recognize five different T cell subsets. On the other hand the cytotoxic activity of Vβ8 T cells in PBL was significantly decreased in patients with Crohn's disease. This was not due to changes in the total cytotoxic activity measured with anti-CD3 or to a decrease in the proportion of the CD8$^+$ T cells expressing the Vβ8 TCR. Therefore, whatever the factor(s) involved in this change, it seems to selectively affect a common TCR V-gene expression. This suggests these patients may have been exposed to a stimulus that behaves like a superantigen. To explore this possibility we examined the effect of staphylococcal enterotoxins B (SEB) and E (SEE) on the cytotoxic activity of Vβ8 T cells. The Vβ8 selective, SEE, failed to increase the cytotoxicity of Vβ8 T cells in Crohn's patients in spite of an appropriate proliferative response. Recently, intestinal epithelial cells have been shown to present superantigens to mucosal T cells[57], although the degree to which this was V-region selective was not indicated. Staphylococcal enterotoxins have been shown to affect human T cell function[48,58,59], and can induce anergy, without interfering in the cytotoxic function of T cell lines[60,61]. Therefore, TCR activation can influence these effector functions independently of one another. The mechanism by which alterations in cytotoxic function of Vβ8$^+$ T cells might contribute to the pathogenesis of Crohn's disease is unclear. The 'superantigen' responsible for such changes in CD is not necessarily of bacterial origin, although it is tempting to suggest that the increased intestinal permeability associated with chronic inflammation allows for exposure to bacterial products. Alternatively, in autoimmune disease, T cells have been shown to be resistant to tolerance induction[62]. It is possible that the presence of Vβ8 T cells with altered cytotoxic function may represent a clone of T cells that have escaped tolerance induction, leaving only these functional changes as a marker of this abrogated attempt at tolerance[62].

CONCLUSION

The causes of inflammatory bowel diseases, Crohn's disease and ulcerative colitis, are unknown. It is likely that the intestinal immune system plays an important role in the pathogenesis and possibly the etiology of IBD. T lymphocytes, which are an intrinsic part of the immune response, would therefore be a critical component of the chronic inflammation of IBD. The intestinal lymphocytes, in particular, may hold the clues that will explain the cause of these diseases. Knowing where to search for these clues in the study of T cells still remains a challenge.

Advances in the cellular and molecular biology of T cells continue to open new avenues for the investigation of the role of T cells in the pathogenesis of autoimmune diseases. In particular, the identification and isolation of the T cell receptor molecules and their genes, and the specific MAb that allow us to detect these products, provide new tools that can be used in dissecting T-cell specificity in diseases of unknown etiology. As new advances are being made in our understanding of mucosal T cell function and differentiation in animal models, opportunities to explore new avenues in human mucosal T cells will emerge.

Acknowledgements

The author acknowledges the efforts of Paula Deschamps and Darlene Steele-Norwood in these studies. This work has been supported by the Medical Research Council of Canada and the Crohn's and Colitis Foundation of Canada. Dr Croitoru is a recipient of an Ontario Ministry of Health Career Scientist Award.

References

1. Schwartz RH. A cell culture model for T lymphocyte clonal anergy. Science. 1990;248: 1349–55.
2. Rocha B, von Boehmer H. Peripheral selection of the T cell repertoire. Nature. 1991;251:1225–8.
3. Croitoru K, Bienenstock J. Characteristics and functions of mucosa-associated lymphoid tissue. In: Ogra PL, Strober W, Mestecky J, McGhee JR, Lamm ME, Bienenstock J, editors. Handbook of mucosal immunology. San Diego: Academic Press; 1994:141–9.
4. James SP, Zeitz M. Human gastrointestinal mucosal T cells. In: Ogra PL, Strober W, Mestecky J, McGhee JR, Lamm ME, Bienenstock J, editors. Handbook of mucosal immunology. San Diego: Academic Press; 1994:275–85.
5. Schieferdecker HL, Ullrich R, Weiss-Breckwoldt AN et al. The HML-1 antigen of intestinal lymphocytes is an activation antigen. J Immunol. 1990;144:2541–9.
6. Rocha B, Vassalli P, Guy-Grand D. The $V\beta$ repertoire of mouse gut homodimeric α CD8$^+$ intraepithelial T cell receptor α/β^+ lymphocytes reveals a major extrathymic pathway of T cell differentiation. J Exp Med. 1991;173:483–6.
7. Poussier P, Edouard P, Lee C, Binnie M, Julius M. Thymus-independent development and negative selection of T cells expressing T cell receptor α/β in the intestinal epithelium: evidence for distinct circulation patterns of gut- and thymus-derived T lymphocytes. J Exp Med. 1992;176:187–99.
8. Mosley RL, Klein JR. Peripheral engraftment of fetal intestine into athymic mice sponsors T cell development: direct evidence for thymopoietic function of murine small intestine. J Exp Med. 1992;176:1365–73.
9. Ferguson A. Intraepithelial lymphocytes of the small intestine. Gut. 1977;18:921–37.
10. Goodman T, Lefrancois L. Expression of the gamma-delta T-cell receptor on intestinal CD8+ intraepithelial lymphocytes. Nature. 1988;333:855–8.
11. Croitoru K, Ernst PB. Leukocytes in the intestinal epithelium: An unusual immunological compartment revisited. Reg Immunol. 1992;4:63–9.

12. Ernst PB, Befus AD, Bienenstock J. Leukocytes in the intestinal epithelium. An unusual immunological compartment. Immunol Today. 1985;6:50–5.
13. Selby WS, Janossy G, Goldstein G. T lymphocytes subsets in human intestinal mucosa. The distribution and relationship to MHC-derived antigens. Clin Exp Immunol. 1981;44:453–8.
14. Cerf-Bensussan N, Griscelli C. Intraepithelial lymphocytes of human gut. Isolation, characterization and study of natural killer activity. Gut. 1985;26:81–8.
15. Spencer J, Choy MY, MacDonald TT. T cell receptor Vβ expression by mucosal T cells. J Clin Pathol. 1991;44:915–18.
16. Jorgensen JL, Reay PA, Ehrich EW, Davis MM. Molecular components of T-cell recognition. Annu Rev Immunol. 1992;10:835–73.
17. Haas W, Pereira P, Tonegawa S. Gamma/delta cells. Annu Rev Immunol. 1993;11:637–85.
18. Weiss A, Imboden J, Hardy K, Manger B, Terhorst C, Stobo J. The role of the T3/antigen receptor complex in T-cell activation. Annu Rev Immunol. 1986;4:593–619.
19. Shanahan F, Deem R, Nayersina R, Leman S, Targan S. Human mucosal T-cell cytotoxicity. Gastroenterology. 1988;94:960–7.
20. Croitoru K, Ernst PB. Intraepithelial lymphocyte lineage and function: the interactions between the intestinal epithelium and the IEL. In: Kiyono H, McGhee JR, editors. Mucosal immunology: intraepithelial lymphocytes (IELs). New York: Raven Press; 1993 (In press).
21. Zeitz M, Quinn TC, Graeff AS, James SP. Mucosal T cells provide helper function but do not proliferate when stimulated by specific antigen in Lymphogranuloma venerium proctitis in non-human primates. Gastroenterology. 1988;94:353–66.
22. Qiao L, Schürmann G, Betzler M, Meuer SC. Down-regulation of protein kinase C activation in human lamina propria T lymphocytes: influence of intestinal mucosa on T cell reactivity. Eur J Immunol. 1991;21:2385–9.
23. Qiao L, Schürmann G, Autschbach F, Wallich R, Meuer SC. Human intestinal mucosa alters T-cell reactivities. Gastroenterology. 1993;105:814–19.
24. Ebert EC. Proliferative responses of human intraepithelial lymphocytes to various T-cell stimuli. Gastroenterology. 1989;97:1372–81.
25. Qiao L, Schürmann G, Betzler M, Meuer SC. Functional properties of human lamina propria T lymphocytes assessed with mitogenic monoclonal antibodies. Immunol Res. 1991;10:218–25.
26. June CH, Ledbetter JA, Linsley PS, Thompson CB. Role of the CD28 receptor in T-cell activation. Immunol Today. 1990;11:211–16.
27. Zacharchuk CM, Mercep M, Ashwell JD. Thymocyte activation and death: a mechanism for molding the T cell repertoire. Ann NY Acad Sci. 1991;636:52–70.
28. Cohen JJ. Apoptosis. Immunol Today. 1993;14:126–30.
29. Groux H, Monte D, Plouvier B, Capron A, Ameisen J-C. CD3-mediated apoptosis of human medullary thymocytes and activated peripheral T cells: respective roles of interleukin-1, interleukin-2, interferon-gamma and accessory cells. Eur J Immunol. 1993;23:1623–9.
30. Lenardo MJ. Interleukin-2 programs mouse αβ T lymphocytes for apoptosis. Nature. 1991;353:858–61.
31. Viney JL, MacDonald TT. Selective death of T cell receptor gamma/delta + intraepithelial lymphocytes by apoptosis. Eur J Immunol. 1990;20:2809.
32. Wesselborg S, Prüfer U, Wild M, Schraven B, Meuer SC, Kabelitz D. Triggering via the alternative CD2 pathway induces apoptosis in activated human T lymphocytes. Eur J Immunol. 1993;23:2707–10.
33. Croitoru K, Bienenstock J, Ernst PB. Immunological alterations associated with inflammatory bowel disease. In: Freeman HJ, editor. Inflammatory bowel disease. Boca Raton: CRC Press; 1989:40–58.
34. Elson CO. The immunology of inflammatory bowel disease. In: Kirnser JB, Shorter RG, editors. Inflammatory bowel disease. Philadelphia: Lea & febiger; 1988:97–164.
35. Hirata I, Berrebi G, Austin LL. Immunohistochemical characterization of intraepithelial and lamina propria lymphocytes in control ileum and colon and in inflammatory bowel disease. Dig Dis Sci. 1986;31:593–603.
36. Kusugami K, Matsuura T, West GA, Youngman KR, Rachmilewitz D, Fiocchi C. Loss of interleukin-2-producing intestinal CD4 + T cells in inflammatory bowel disease. Gastroenterology. 1991;101:1594–605.
37. Brynskov J, Tvede N, Andersen CB, Vilien M. Increased concentrations of interleukin 1β,

interleukin-2, and soluble interleukin-2 receptors in endoscopical mucosal biopsy specimens with active inflammatory bowel disease. Gut. 1992;33:55–8.

38. Shanahan F, Leman B, Deem R, Niederlehner A, Brogan M, Targan S. Enhanced peripheral blood T-cell cytotoxicity in inflammatory bowel disease. J Clin Immunol. 1989;9:55–64.

39. Rüthlein J, Heinze G, Auer IO. Anti-CD2 and anti-CD3 induced T cell cytotoxicity of human intraepithelial and lamina propria lymphocytes. Gut. 1992;33:1626–32.

40. Drake CG, Kotzin BL. Superantigens: biology, immunology, and potential role in disease. J Clin Immunol. 1992;12:149–62.

41. Moss PAH, Rosenberg WMC, Bell JI. The human T cell receptor in health and disease. Annu Rev Immunol. 1992;10:71–96.

42. Wigzell H, Grunewald J, Tehrani M et al. T cell V-gene usage in man in some normal and abnormal situations. Ann NY Acad Sci. 1991;636:9–19.

43. Kaulfersch W, Fiocchi C, Waldmann TA. Polyclonal nature of the intestinal mucosal lymphocyte populations in inflammatory bowel disease. A molecular genetic evaluation of the immunoglobulin and T-cell antigen receptors. Gastroenterology. 1988;95:364–70.

44. Blumberg RS, Yockey CE, Gross GG, Ebert EC, Balk SP. Human intestinal intraepithelial lymphocytes are derived from a limited number of T cell clones that utilize multiple Vβ T cell receptor genes. J Immunol. 1993;150:5144–53.

45. Duchmann R, Strober W, Fiocchi C, James SP. TCR Vβ gene expression is selective in control but not in IBD lamina propria lymphocytes. Gastroenterology. 1992;102:A617.

46. Posnett DN. Do superantigens play a role in autoimmunity? Sem Immunol. 1993;5:65–72.

47. White J, Herman A, Pullen AM, Kubo R, Kappler JW, Marrack P. The Vb-specific superantigen staphylococcal enterotoxin B: stimulation of mature T cells and clonal deletion in neonatal mice. Cell. 1989;56:27–35.

48. Kappler J, Kotzin B, Herron L et al. Vβ-specific stimulation of human T cells by staphylococcal toxins. Science. 1989;244:811–13.

49. Choi Y, Kotzin B, Herron L, Callahan J, Marrack P, Kappler J. Interaction of *Staphylococcus aureus* toxin 'superantigens' with human T cells. Proc Natl Acad Sci USA. 1993;86:8941–5.

50. Rellahan BL, Jones LA, Kruisbeek AM, Fry AM, Matis LA. *In vivo* induction of anergy in peripheral Vβ8+ T cells by staphylococcal enterotoxin B. J Exp Med. 1990;172:1091–100.

51. Posnett DN, Schmelkin I, Burton DA, August A, McGrath H, Mayer LF. T cell antigen receptor V gene usage. Increases in Vβ8 + T cells in Crohn's disease. J Clin Invest. 1990;85:1770–6.

52. Kawabe Y, Ochi A. Programmed cell death and extrathymic reduction of Vβ8+ CD4+ T cells in mice tolerant to *Staphylococcus aureus* enterotoxin B. Nature. 1991;349:245–8.

53. Macdonald HR, Baschieri S, Lees RK. Clonal expansion precedes anergy and death of Vb8+ peripheral T cells responding to staphylococcal enterotoxin B *in vivo*. Eur J Immunol. 1991;21:1963–6.

54. Abe J, Kotzin BL, Jujo K et al. Selective expansion of T cells expressing T-cell receptor variable regions Vβ2 and Vβ8 in Kawasaki disease. Proc Natl Acad Sci USA. 1992;89:4066–70.

55. Phillips JH, Lanier LL. Lectin-dependent and anti-CD3 induced cytotoxicity are preferentially mediated by peripheral blood cytotoxic T lymphocytes expressing Leu-7 antigen. J Immunol. 1986;136:1579–85.

56. Grant MD, Smaill FM, Laurie K, Rosenthal KL. Changes in the cytotoxic T-cell repertoire of HIV-1 infected individuals: Relationships to disease progression. Viral Immunol. 1993;6:85–95.

57. Aisenberg J, Ebert EC, Mayer L. T-cell activation in human intestinal mucosa: the role of superantigens. Gastroenterology. 1993;105:1421–30.

58. Irwin MJ, Gascoigne NRJ. Interplay between superantigens and the immune system. J Leukocyte Biol. 1993;54:495–503.

59. O'Hehir RE, Lamb JR. Induction of specific clonal anergy in human T lymphocytes by *Staphylococcus aureus* enterotoxins. Proc Natl Acad Sci USA. 1990;87:8884–8.

60. Otten GR, Germain RN. Split anergy in a CD8+ T cell: receptor-dependent cytolysis in the absence of interleukin-2 production. Science. 1991;251:1228–31.

61. Go C, Lancki DW, Fitch FW, Miller J. Anergized T cell clones retain their cytolytic ability. J Immunol. 1993;150:367–76.

62. Dayan CM, Chu NR, Londei M, Rapoport B, Feldman M. T cells involved in human autoimmune disease are resistant to tolerance induction. J Immunol. 1993;151:1606–13.

10
On the pathogenesis trail: what marker B cell clones tell us about IBD

J. BRAUN, Y. VALLES-AYOUB, L. BERBERIAN, M. EGGENA, L. K. GORDON and S. TARGAN

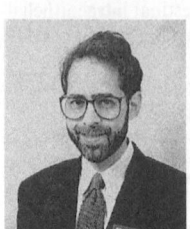

J. BRAUN

INTRODUCTION

The pathogenesis of Crohn's disease (CD) and ulcerative colitis (UC) is incompletely understood, but ultimately involves immune-mediated tissue damage. These diseases are associated with various immunologic abnormalities, many of which are probably secondary to inflammation[1-5]. CD4 T cells are widely believed to serve as key regulatory cells in tissue-destructive immune responses. In the case of inflammatory bowel disease (IBD), the response occurs in a mucosal site interfacing with the intestinal lumen. Consequently, an obvious source of target antigens are microbial products, although the identification of their role, or that of other lumenal or intrinsic mucosal cellular antigens, has yet to be established. A key step in the resolution of IBD pathogenesis and eventual treatment is the resolution of the target antigens initiating the disease. The cells which would most directly reveal the identity of these antigens are T cells. However, the low avidity of the T cell antigen receptor, and the complicated peptide/MHC II structure of its natural ligand, render these cells unsuitable for analytic studies of this important issue.

DETECTING IMMUNE RESPONSE TARGET ANTIGENS WITH THE B LYMPHOCYTE

In contrast, immunoglobulin, both in its membrane form as the B cell antigen receptor and as soluble antibody, is a high-avidity receptor ideally suited for

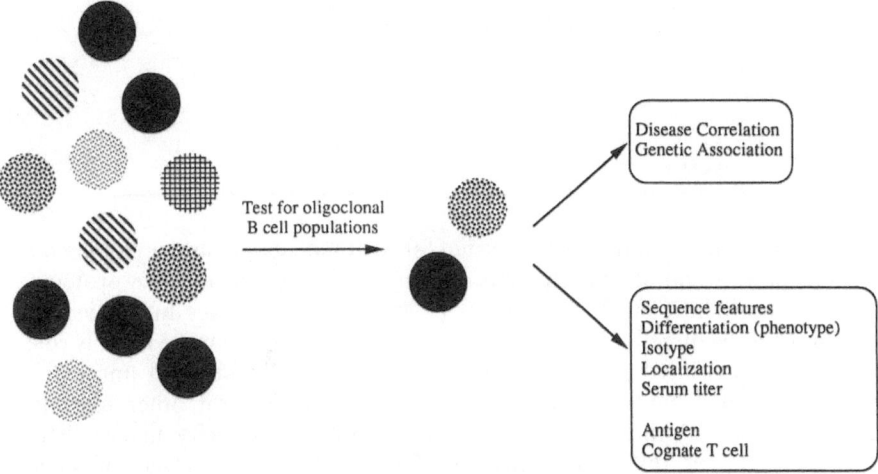

Fig. 1 Proposed genesis of B cells expressing disease markers. In mucosal sites of an IBD lesion, immunologic activity is regulated by 'autoreactive' T cells specific for local target antigens (which may include food, microbial or intrinsic mucosal peptides). B cells expressing antibodies which share this specificity efficiently capture and present these antigens, resulting in their preferential activation by IBD T cells. Antibody secretion by these activated B cells is detected in serum using adventitious crossreactive antigens (ANCA and AEA)

use in isolation and characterization of antigens. *In vivo*, B cells have the predominant role of capturing antigens, and creating the peptide/MHC II ligand ('antigen presentation') for the T cell antigen receptor[6]. Moreover, in this role B cells may serve a pivotal immunologic role in the abridgement of tolerance to self-antigens and in the activation of pathogenic T cells (as suggested for the NOD murine model of type 1 diabetes mellitus[7]).

Conversely, B cell activation and clonal expansion is dependent on interaction with T cells through antigen presentation. Thus, in sites of an immune response, B and T cells sharing the same antigenic specificity activate and expand in parallel. Consequently, if one can identify such selected B cells, their antibodies offer a tool to characterize the target antigen driving the immune response. Since preferential antigen presentation by B cells reflects the exceptional avidity of membrane Ig for specific antigen, this suggests that the antibodies produced by at least a subgroup of B cells in autoimmune lesions may actually identify the target antigen of the pathogenic T cell (Fig. 1).

ANTIBODIES AS DISEASE MARKERS, AND THE pANCA PARADIGM

Certain immune-mediated disorders, such as systemic lupus erythematosus, primary biliary cirrhosis and chronic active hepatitis, are closely associated with distinctive patterns of autoantibodies. In the case of IBD, various autoantibodies and antimicrobial agents have been reported: lymphocyto-

Table 1 Marker antibodies in IBD

Marker	UC	CD	Disease activity	References
pANCA	+ + +	±	−	16–18
AEA-15	+	+ + +	−	
Anti-HSP70	+	+ +	+	13–15
AECA	+ +	+	+	12
Anti-42 kDa	+ + +	−	+	11

toxic antibodies; antibodies specific for colonic epithelium, cytoplasmic neutrophil or endothelial antigens, certain erythrocyte membrane proteins, and bacterial heat shock proteins[8–19] (Table 1). These marker antibodies are unlikely to be directly pathogenic, although interesting evidence for this role has been presented in the case of a 42 kDa colonic epithelial antigen[11]. However, they have demonstrated importance for several other reasons. First, from the practical standpoint, their disease specificity makes them useful tools for diagnostic purposes. Second, the serum levels of some antibodies correlate with disease activity, and thus may be useful in titrating or modifying treatment regimens. Finally, from the conceptual standpoint, these markers may represent the antibodies produced by activated B cells in sites of the disease-specific immune response. If so, their avidity for 'laboratory' antigens (e.g. cytoplasmic neutrophil or endothelial components) is likely to reflect a serendipitous but idiosyncratic crossreactivity.

One marker antibody, pANCA, provides a revealing example relating the marker B cell clone to the immunobiology of the underlying disease. Elevated serum levels of pANCA are a sensitive marker for individuals with UC. The marker is specific for this disease process, since it is not observed in individuals with a variety of other acute and chronic colitides. Serum titers of ANCA are elevated regardless of clinical status, and are thus not useful to monitor disease activity. However, while individuals with elevated pANCA are rare among healthy children and adults, an elevated frequency is observed among healthy relatives of UC patients, and in the related syndrome of sclerosing cholangitis. In view of such observations, pANCA is hypothesized to reflect an immunogenetic susceptibility trait for UC. This idea is supported by the unique HLA-D alleles associated with pANCA-positive individuals with UC (and the uncommon, pANCA-positive CD subset)[18]. It thus appears that secretory B cells expressing pANCA may be closely associated with the genetic predisposition and primary immunopathophysiology of UC.

DISTINCTIVE CLONAL B CELL POPULATIONS IN NORMAL AND UC LAMINA PROPRIA

The most logical place to find such marker B cells is in the mucosal lesions, which in both CD and UC are associated with abundant B cells (many at the plasma cell stage). Intralesional B cells are notable for high frequency of IgG expression, and skewed towards IgG2 and IgG1 subclasses in CD and UC, respectively[4]. These IgG subclass patterns may largely reflect, at least in part, the immunoregulatory action of a distinct pattern of local lymphokine

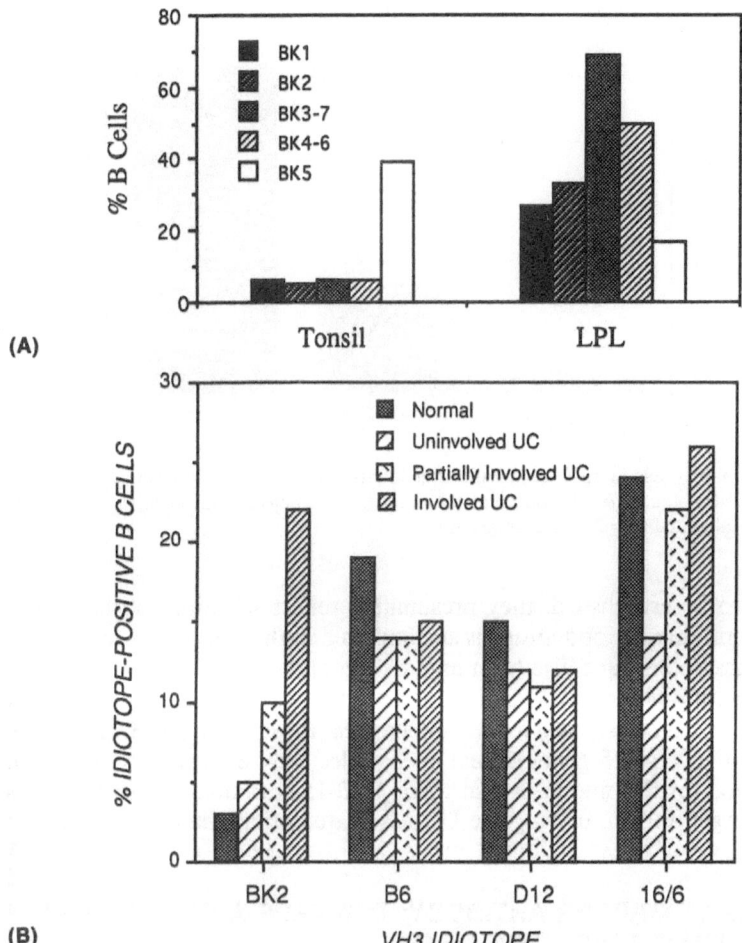

Fig. 2 Abundance of VH3 idiotope positive LPL B cells in normal and UC. Lamina propria mononuclear cells were isolated from endoscopic colonic biopsies, and stained with fluorescent antibodies for CD19 (a pan-B cell marker), and anti-idiotype reagents specific for various VH genes. A: Frequency of B cells expressing various BK anti-idiotopes (specific for various VH3 family epitopes) in tonsil and colonic lamina propria. B: Frequency of B cells expressing VH3 family idiotopes: B6 and D12 (anti-VH3-30); 16/6 (anti-VH3-23); BK2 (anti-VH3-15)

production and activity of the corresponding T cell subpopulations. Clonal characterization of these intralesional B cells has been previously limited to Southern analysis, which has shown that these subpopulations are not monoclonal or oligoclonal[19].

Using a set of reagents (anti-idiotopes) which detect specific antibody VH genes, we have had the opportunity to readdress the frequency of B cell clonal subsets in blood and colonic lamina propria B cells (Fig. 2A). Compared to the blood B cell population, cells in the mucosa are distinguished by their profile of VH gene idiotopes. While the basis of these differences

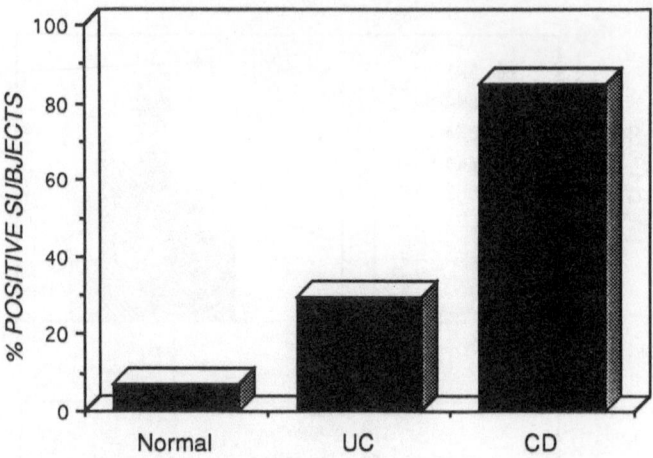

Fig. 3 AEA-15 levels in IBD. Sera from individuals with UC, CD, or healthy adults were tested by ELISA for AEA-15 levels, and the frequency of subjects with positive sera in each group was tabulated ($n = 27$ for each group)

remains to be established, they presumably reflect selection by the unique set of microbial and food antigens accumulated in the colonic mucosa. These clonal parameters have also been used to compare mucosal B cells from UC patients with different levels of disease activity (Fig. 2B). Interestingly, while several clonal B cell subsets remain unchanged, those using the BK2 idiotope (defining the VH3-15 gene) appear to be selectively expanded. One simple explanation for this finding is that these VH3-15 antibodies share specificity for the target antigen driving the UC-associated inflammatory response.

THE AEA-15 MARKER ANTIBODY: TOWARDS A LABORATORY DIFFERENTIAL DIAGNOSIS OF IBD

Since VH3-15 antibodies appear to be informative for UC-related inflammation, we have recently searched for corresponding crossreactive autoantibodies which could serve as serum disease-specific markers[20]. Individuals with UC were found to commonly express an anti-erythrocyte VH3-15 antibody, designated AEA-15, reactive with a novel erythrocyte membrane protein. Like pANCA, the presence of the antibody was not related to disease activity, and was detectable even in postcolectomy UC patients. Further investigation revealed an even higher frequency and titer of this antibody in individuals with Crohn's disease (Fig. 3). This marker antibody was selective for IBD, since it was rarely observed in healthy individuals, or those with other forms of inflammatory or infectious colitis. An unexpected and interesting exception was *Campylobacter jejuni* enterocolitis, in which the marker antibody was also prevalent[20].

There are two implications of this finding. First, AEA-15 represents a new serum marker for a novel subset of inflammatory colitides, notably CD.

Table 2 A candidate diagnostic panel for UC and CD. AEA-15 and pANCA levels in patient sera are tested by a standard microtiter plate enzyme-linked immunoassay

pANCA	AEA-15	Diagnosis
Neg	Neg	Non-IBD
Pos	Neg	Ulcerative colitis
Neg	Pos	Crohn's disease
Pos	Pos	Mixed IBD

Moreover, initial studies comparing AEA-15 and pANCA reveal that they are independent parameters. As a combined set of markers they may thus allow a tool for provisional laboratory diagnosis of UC versus CD (Table 2). Second, the association of *C. jejuni* with IBD is provocative from the standpoint of IBD pathogenesis. Work during the past few years has advanced the concept of microbial pathogens as initiating agents in chronic mucosal inflammation (notably *Helicobacter pylori* in peptic ulcer disease[21]). This paradigm prompts the hypothesis that *C. jejuni* has a similar pathogenic role in IBD. In this line of thinking, individuals with UC and CD are distinguished from normals by immunogenetic traits which cause inefficient resolution of this bacterial infection, and inflammatory responses to it which are necrotizing and granulomatous, respectively. While the presence of conventional active *C. jejuni* infection has been refuted by a careful study by Blaser and colleagues[22], the role of this pathogen deserves re-evaluation in this new context of pathogenesis.

STRATEGIES ON THE HORIZON

The preceding examples reflect some of the opportunities presented by the systematic analysis of clonal B cell activity in IBD. Thus far, such clonal B cell analysis is restricted to direct studies of antibody V gene usage at the nucleic acid level, or by detection with the relatively small number of anti-V gene reagents. Conceptually, a much more ideal approach would be to comprehensively evaluate lesional B cells for those reactive with disease-specific target antigens. Recently, the technology for such investigation has appeared in the form of phage display antibody libraries[23]. Using small amounts of RNA (obtainable even from endoscopic biopsy specimens), recombinant methods allow the creation of libraries of cloned antibody genes, in which each antibody gene is not only carried by the phage vector, but also expressed as part of its coat protein. The power of this system is that complete libraries of antibodies representative of a B cell population can be readily created, and rapidly selected by direct binding to mucosal antigens (Fig. 4). Using this technology it is for the first time feasible to comprehensively select and characterize the antibody repertoire of lesional B cells. There is much activity in the autoimmunity field to identify representative lesional antibodies, and to use them in searching for the pathogenic antigenic targets of the disease-specific immune response. The

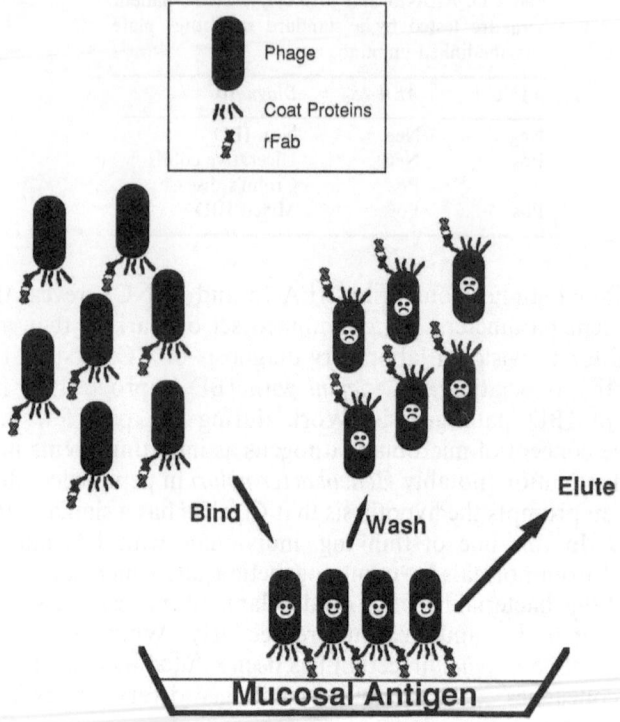

Fig. 4 Strategy for selection of phage expressing recombinant antibodies (rFab) on microwells coated with mucosal antigen

outcome of such research will be an important test of this concept of autoimmune pathogenesis and, if successful, a source of candidate antigens for disease-specific immune therapies.

References

1. Tan EM. Interactions between autoimmunity and molecular and cell biology. Bridges between clinical and basic sciences. J Clin Invest. 1989;84:1–6.
2. Strober W, James SP. The immunologic basis of inflammatory bowel disease. J Clin Immunol. 1986;6:414–32.
3. Targan SR, Kagnoff MF, Brogan MD, Shanahan F. Immunologic mechanisms in intestinal diseases. Ann Intern Med. 1987;106:853–70.
4. MacDermott RP, Stenson WF. Alterations of the immune system in ulcerative colitis and Crohn's disease. Adv Immunol. 1988;42:285–328.
5. Elson CO. The immunology of inflammatory bowel disease. In: Kirsner JB, Sorter R, editors. Inflammatory bowel disease, 3rd edn. Philadelphia: Lea & Febiger; 1988:97–164.
6. Lin R-W, Mamula MJ, Hardin JA, Janeway CA. Induction of autoreactive B cells allows priming of autoreactive T cells. J Exp Med. 1991;173:1433–9.
7. McInerney MF, Rath S, Janeway CA. Exclusive expression of MHC class II proteins on CD45+ cells in pancreatic islets of NOD mice. Diabetes. 1991;40:648–51.
8. Korsmeyer SJ, Williams Jr, RC, Wilson AO, Strickland RG. Lymphocytotoxic antibody in

inflammatory bowel disease. A family study. N Engl J Med. 1975;293:1117–20.

9. Lagercrantz R, Perlman P, Hammersstrom S. Immunological studies in ulcerative colitis. Gastroenterology. 1971;60:381–9.

10. Fiocchi C, Roche JK, Michener WM. High prevalence of antibodies to intestinal epithelial antigens in patients with inflammatory bowel disease and their relatives. Ann Intern Med. 1989;110:786–94.

11. Das KM, Vecchi M, Sakamaki S. A shared and unique epitope(s) on human colon, skin, and biliary epithelium detected by a monoclonal antibody. Gastroenterology. 1990;98:464.

12. Stevens TR, Harley SL, Groom JS et al. Anti-endothelial cell antibodies in inflammatory bowel disease. Dig Dis Sci. 1993;38:426.

13. Lindberg E, Magnusson KE, Tysk C, Jarnerot G. Antibody (IgG, IgA, and IgM) to baker's yeast (Saccharomyces cerevisiae), yeast mannan, gliadin, ovalbumin, and betalactoglobulin in monozygotic twins with inflammatory bowel disease. Gut. 1992;33:909.

14. O'Mahony S, Anderson N, Nuki G, Ferguson A. Systemic and mucosal antibodies to Klebsiella in patients with ankylosing spondylitis and Crohn's disease. Ann Rheum Dis. 1992;51:1296.

15. Elsaghier A, Prantera C, Moreno C, Ivanyi J. Antibodies to Mycobacterium paratuberculosis-specific protein antigens in Crohn's disease. Clin Exp Immunol. 1992;90:503.

16. Saxon A, Shanahan F, Landers C, Ganz T, Targan S. A distinct subset of antineutrophil cytoplasmic antibodies is associated with inflammatory bowel disease. J Allergy Clin Immunol. 1990;86:202.

17. Duerr RH, Targan SR, Landers CJ, Sutherland LR, Shanahan F. Anti-neutrophil cytoplasmic antibodies in ulcerative colitis. Comparison with other colitides/diarrheal illnesses. Gastroenterology. 1991;100:1590.

18. Yang H, Rotter JI, Toyoda H et al. Ulcerative colitis: a genetically heterogeneous disorder defined by genetic (HLA class II) and subclinical (antineutrophil cytoplasmic antibodies) markers. J Clin Invest. 1993;92:1080.

19. Kaulfersch W, Fiocchi C, Waldman TA. Gastroenterology. 1988;95:364–70.

20. Berberian LS, Valles-Ayoub Y, Gordon LK, Targan SR, Braun J. Expression of a novel autoantibody defined by the VH3-15 gene in inflammatory bowel disease and Campylobacter jejuni enterocolitis. J Immunol. 1994;153:(in press).

21. Graham DY. Campylobacter pylori and peptic ulcer disease. Gastroenterology. 1989;96:615.

22. Blaser MJ, Hoverson D, Ely IG, Juncan DJ, Wang WL, Brown WR. Studies of Campylobacter jejuni in patients with inflammatory bowel disease. Gastroenterology. 1984;86:33.

23. Persson MA, Caothien RH, Burton DR. Generation of diverse high-affinity human monoclonal antibodies by repertoire cloning. Proc Natl Acad Sci USA. 1991;88:2432–6.

Section IV
Pathophysiology of intestinal inflammation: intracellular and intercellular signalling

11
Growth factors in IBD

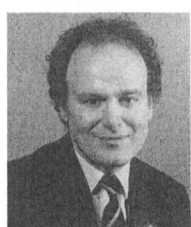

N. A. WRIGHT

INTRODUCTION

There are several morphological changes which can be discerned in the spectrum of inflammatory bowel disease (IBD), encompassed by the general processes of cell proliferation and differentiation. Examples which spring immediately to mind are the mucosal hyperplasia which accompanies ulcerative colitis, where colonic crypts lengthen and undergo increased crypt fission, the mucin cell depletion also found in ulcerative colitis, and the several metaplasias, such as pyloric metaplasia in Crohn's disease, and Paneth cell metaplasia, commonest in ulcerative colitis. It is therefore relatively easy to manufacture a slot for the study of growth control in understanding the pathogenesis of IBD.

Knowledge of the regulation of growth in the intestine is at an interesting stage: we have come a long way in our understanding of how the intestinal renewal system is organized. However, the molecular processes which control this integrated proliferative system have only now begun to be identified, and while we are able to write a list of molecules which we believe are involved in growth control, we are not able to appreciate how these molecules interplay to produce an organized and responsive proliferative system.

The organization of crypt systems in the gut is relatively well known[1] (Fig. 1). Each small intestinal or colonic crypt is a clonal population derived, ultimately at least, from a single stem cell. The 'unitarian hypothesis' of intestinal cytogenesis, which states that all cell lineages emanate from a single stem cell, was conceived long ago by Cheng and Leblond[2] for the small bowel and by Chang and Leblond[3] for the colon, but definitive proof was lacking until the advent of tetraparental allophenic chimeric mice[4] and

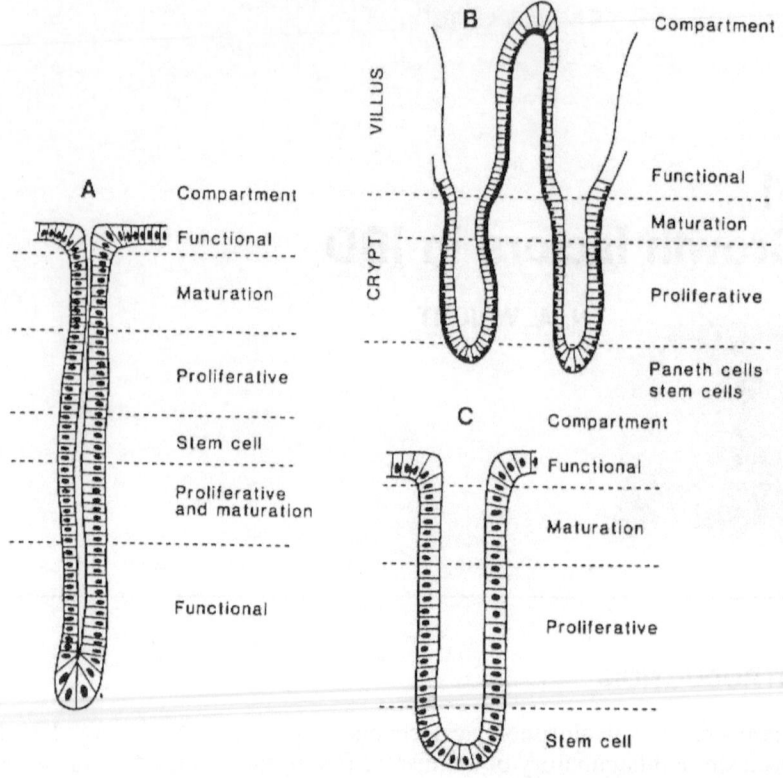

Fig. 1 Classical concept of the organization of cell proliferation in the crypt systems of the gut

associated crypt-restricted lectin binding, and of mice heterozygous for an X-chromosome-linked enzyme defect (glucose-6-phosphate dehydrogenase)[5]. Such crypt-restricted markers in these models show that Paneth, columnar and goblet cell lineages were clonal, but the clonality of gut endocrine cells was shown only by using male:female allophenic chimeric mice[6], in effect the final nail in the neural crest component of the all-encompassing APUD cell hypothesis[7].

The crypt stem cell feeds the proliferative compartment of the crypt, where the stem cell efflux is amplified, and subsequently cells cease division and migrate onto the surface – to clothe the villi in the small intestine and the surface of the colon, as functional enterocytes and colonocytes.

Intestinal cells are well known for their rapid rate of proliferation, one of the highest in the human body. Nevertheless, the system remains adaptive, undergoing circadian variation (see ref. 1 for review) and responding to different physiological and, of course, pathological conditions. Intestinal adaptation has perhaps been best studied by partial resection, after which the remnant undergoes considerable hyperplasia (see ref. 1 for review). As well as hyperplastic phenomena the intestine also adapts to decreased workload during starvation or total parenteral nutrition, by reducing its rate of cell production.

GROWTH PHENOMENA IN IBD

In ulcerative colitis there is an increase in the rate of crypt cell proliferation, not only in the mucosa surrounding the ulcers, but also in the mucosa between the ulcers[8]. This results in lengthening of the colonic crypts. There is also an increase in the rate of crypt fission which, in ulcerative colitis, can result in as many as 30% of crypts dividing. There are also changes in the cytology of the crypts themselves, with a reduction in the numbers of mucin-secreting goblet cells; while in experimental colitis with goblet cell depletion there is an increased rate of production of goblet cells; there is also an increased rate of mucin discharge so that goblet cells cannot be recognized in tissue sections[8]. Later in the condition, of course, there is also an increased risk of dysplasia and of carcinoma, both in ulcerative colitis and Crohn's disease[9].

Other changes in crypt cytology include the Paneth cell 'metaplasia' which is found in the colon, especially in ulcerative colitis. Also in ulcerative colitis, but especially in Crohn's disease and particularly in the small bowel, cells resembling pyloric cells appear in the mucosa, earning these cells the appellation 'pyloric' or 'pseudopyloric' metaplasia. The life history and function of these cells has recently been traced, and they are a source of several modulating peptides which have considerable trophic effects in the regenerating mucosa[10] (see below).

In IBD there is also a considerable infiltrate of both mononuclear and polymorphonuclear cells in the lamina propria, and associated hyperplasia of mucosal lymphoid tissue.

SOURCES OF GROWTH FACTORS

Circulating hormones

There is little doubt that circulating hormones can modulate growth responses in the gut. The older literature documents effects of 'classical' hormones such as corticosteroids, thyroxine, growth hormone and insulin on cell proliferation in the intestine; however, how important these are in the pathogenesis of IBD is difficult to say, apart from the obvious statement that the reduction in proliferative rate induced by corticosteroids may be important therapeutically[11]. However, there is a considerable body of evidence which supports the hypothesis that circulating hormones, probably of intestinal origin, are important in inducing adaptive responses in the gut. The minutiae of this complex field are summarized by Williamson[12,13], but the critical experiments are probably:

1. Partial intestinal resection of one animal in a pair of rats joined in cross-circulation (not parabiosis) results in induced cell proliferation in the intestine of the unoperated partner[14].
2. Thiry-Vella loops, isolated from the normal fecal stream, show proliferative responses: (a) when the animals are fed orally but not when fed by total parenteral nutrition[15], and (b) after resection of the intestine in continuity[16].

3. Infusion of hypertonic glucose into the rectum of rats leads to the induction of cell proliferation in the small intestine[17].

The identity of the circulating hormone, and its source, is not yet clear. However, suspicion has fallen on enteroglucagon as the candidate hormone[18]. Definitive proof of this is, however, lacking.

Luminal factors

There is no doubt that, in some way, food in the lumen of the gut is a potent stimulus to cell proliferation. The exact nature of this so-called 'luminal nutrition' has defied explanation for some considerable time: whether the epithelial cells need a constant supply of absorbed nutrients for sustained proliferation[19], whether some nutrients, for example polyamines, glutamine and short-chain fatty acids (SCFA, the fermentation products of soluble fibre, themselves influence growth, see below), or whether the induction of a 'functional demand' in the form of increased mucosal workload by absorption/secretion[19] is operative, or indeed whether luminal contents themselves evoke trophic gut hormone or growth factor release, is as yet unclear.

Certainly, absence of food in the lumen leads to prominent mucosal atrophy; that this is not due to overall calorie malnutrition can be shown by the observation that such atrophy still occurs when animals are fed intravenously[20]. There is also evidence that individual nutrients, when infused into isolated loops or Thiry-Vella fistulae, induce local cell proliferation, viz. elemental diets, glucose, disaccharides and amino acids. Such induction may be independent of substrate, and thus transport alone may be the inducer of cell proliferation[19].

Specific luminal molecules may act as growth factors for the epithelium. Polyamines have a potent effect on the growth of the intestinal mucosa[21,22]. The production of polyamines is rate-limited by the enzyme ornithine decarboxylase (ODC), and inhibition of ODC leads to abrogation of EGF-induced cell proliferation in the small intestine[23], and also leads to hypoplasia, as well as reducing the proliferative response to other hyperplastic stimuli[23,24]. Polyamines in the lumen may increase expression of ODC, increasing the production of spermine and spermidine, which stimulate cell proliferation[24]. Epithelial cells in the small intestine can utilize polyamines[25], and infusions of putrescine, a further polyamine, also increase mucosal growth rate[26]. Other molecules which have designated trophic actions include SCFA and glutamine. The well-known stimulation of cell proliferation in the rat colon caused by dietary fibre has been shown to be due to its fermentation, producing SCFAs[27], and direct luminal infusions of SCFA also increase cell proliferation in the rat colon[27].

Hormones/growth factors induced by luminal contents

There remains the possibility that the presence of food in the lumen induces secretion of gut hormones and/or growth factors, which stimulate growth

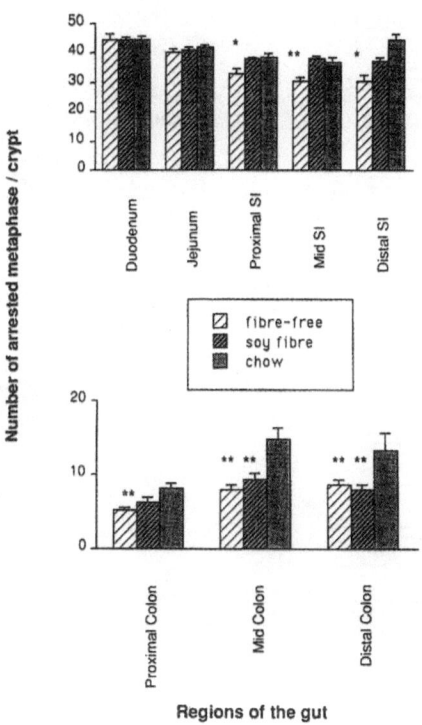

Fig. 2 Relationship between rate of crypt cell production in the rat colon, here represented by the crypt cell production rate, and ingestion of different types of dietary fiber

and hence maintain mucosal mass. There is no doubt, for example, that feeding induces secretion of enteroglucagon, the candidate enterotrophin, in both animals and humans[28], as well as other candidate hormones. The direct trophic action of these hormones is yet to be determined, however.

Perhaps more reliable is the report that luminal contents can induce the expression of genes which encode for growth factors known to stimulate cell proliferation in the gut[29]. Dietary fiber has been shown to stimulate rat colonic cell proliferation[27]; Fig. 2 shows the relationship between dietary fiber type and cell proliferation in the rat colon, and Fig. 3 shows that this induction of cell proliferation is associated with increased TGF-α gene expression. It is thus clear that luminally-directed growth responses in the gut are associated with growth factor gene expression.

This naturally leads us to a consideration of these growth factors in gut growth responses.

EGF/TGF-α

These growth factors are members of a growing group of molecules which include EGF, TGF-α, amphiregulin and heparin-binding EGF; there are

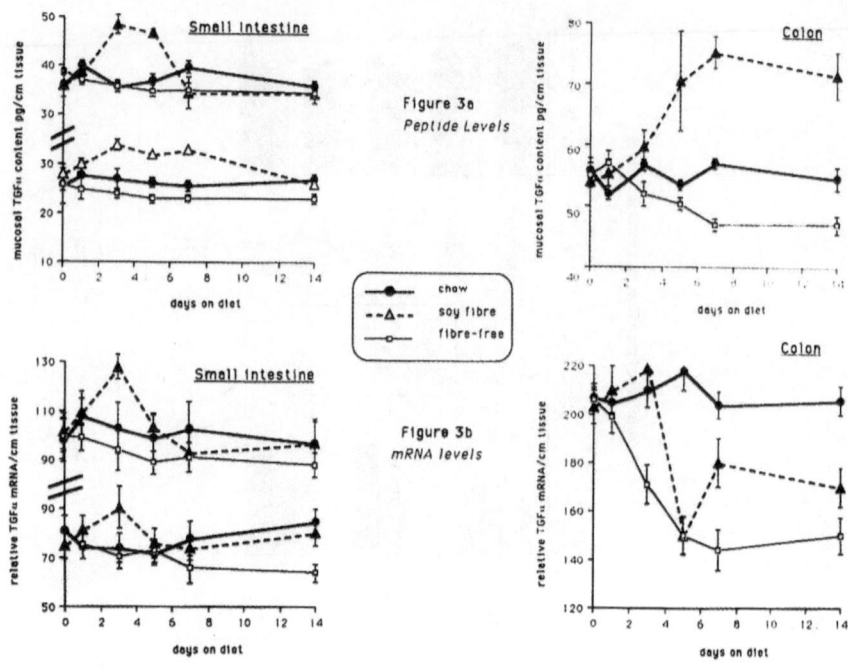

Fig. 3 Effects of different types of fiber on TGF-α mRNA and peptide levels in the small intestine and colon of the rat

other homologs such as cripto. Their commonality lies in the possession of six cysteine residues which form three disulfide bonds, resulting in highly stable molecules. Both EGF and TGF-α are initially elaborated as membrane-bound molecules; pre-proEGF has a 24-amino acid signal peptide on its amino terminal, and a 25-residue hydrophobic domain on the C-terminal end which is membrane-bound. TGF-α also has this membrane-spanning domain, and it is clear that both EGF and TGF-α have to be enzymically released from the membrane-bound state to be secreted. However, TGF-α can certainly act in a juxtacrine manner when still attached to the membrane, although the evidence for EGF acting in this manner is scant. There is little known about the regulation of EGF gene expression, but the upstream elements of the TGF-α gene show SP1 and AF2 binding sites.

Both EGF and TGF-α bind the EGF receptor (EGFR), a 150 000 kDa membrane-spanning molecule, with a ligand-binding extracellular domain, a hydrophobic transmembrane domain and an intracellular domain with tyrosine kinase activity. Ligand–receptor binding results in autophosphorylation and possible nuclear translocation. While there are some differences between EGF and TGF-α in their affinities for the EGFR, their functional effects are remarkably similar.

EGF is a secreted molecule in the gastrointestinal tract, being found in upper gastrointestinal secretions, and can be localized to the salivary glands, the mucous neck cells of the gastric mucosa, and the mucus-secreting acini of Brunner's glands; there is little evidence for EGF secretion elsewhere in the gut. EGF is also present in maternal milk[30]. It is therefore important to ask whether EGF acts luminally. EGF receptors are found both on the apical enterocyte surface and on the basolateral surface. In the neonate there are certainly EGF-modulated effects evoked by luminally administered EGF[31]. While in the calf there is evidence that apical EGFR are not phosphorylated by EGF ligand–receptor binding, although the basolateral receptors are, Thompson[31] has recently shown that luminal EGF binds EGFR and *neu* on the apical surface in neonatal rat intestine, resulting in phosphorylation of both these receptors. Nevertheless, certainly in the adult animal[32], and possibly in the neonate[40], EGFR are concentrated on the basolateral surface. This distribution implies that EGF would have to be transported intact across the mucosa to have an effect. While there is limited evidence for intact EGF being taken up by the neonatal rat ileum[33], in these studies most is degraded. It has also been anticipated that EGF would be degraded in the mature intestine[34], but it has been suggested that pancreatic secretory trypsin inhibitor, secreted not only by the pancreas but also by the mucous neck cell lineage in the stomach, and evoked by luminal contents, protects EGF in the intestinal lumen.

However, the evidence for luminal activity of EGF in mature animals is mixed: certainly infusion into defunctionalized colonic segments also stimulated cell proliferation[35]. Goodlad and colleagues failed to show any action of luminal EGF in animals maintained on total parenteral nutrition, even in high dosage, whereas lower doses given intravenously were able to replicate levels of cell proliferation seen in intact, fed control animals[36]. Moreover, the acid-inhibitory action of EGF, while seen after intravenous infusion, is not evoked by intragastric or intrajejunal infusion[37].

These studies evoke the view that EGF may need mucosal damage to bind its receptor; certainly orally administered iodinated EGF does not bind to intact rat gastrointestinal mucosa, but does bind locally around areas of mucosal damage. In IBD, especially Crohn's disease, EGF can be produced by a cell lineage, the so-called 'ulcer-associated cell lineage' (UACL), which grows adjacent to the chronic ulcers[10].

TGF-α on the other hand, is found throughout the gastrointestinal mucosa[38], although occupying the differentiated cell compartment – in the small intestine, the villus epithelium. Nevertheless, there is evidence that TGF-α does stimulate gut epithelial cell proliferation. There is little information on how TGF-α localizes to and binds the EGFR.

While the growth-promoting properties of EGF/TGF-α are concentrated upon by investigators, non-cell cycle-related genes are also regulated. For example EGF stimulates electrolyte and nutrient transport in the gut[39], up-regulating brush-border enzyme activity[40], and EGF also enhances pS2 (a trefoil peptide, see below), gene expression[41].

TGF-β

First described as a 'transforming activity' that induced anchorage-independent growth in a non-neoplastic cell line[42,43], there are now a series of related molecules, the TGFβ molecules, TGF-β1–5. In mammals the main TGF-β are TGF-β1–3. These are again synthesized as large precursor molecules, and processed to yield 12.5 kDa mature monomers. However, the sequence of events which leads to the secretion of the homodimeric peptide has not yet been fully discovered. There are at least three classes of TGF-β receptor.

TGF-β has several functions which make it potentially a very important molecule in IBD; it inhibits epithelial cell proliferation[44], has effects on the differentiation of colorectal carcinoma cells[45,46], and has important actions on the synthesis of extracellular matrix proteins, increasing synthesis of the collagens, fibronectin, tenascin and elastin, decreasing synthesis of collagenases, stromelysin, and plasminogen activators, and increasing synthesis of protease inhibitors such as TIMP and plasminogen activator inhibitor (see ref. 47 for review). Thus, in a very complex manner, TGF-β induces formation of extracellular matrix and affects its composition. Moreover, TGF-β can act as an 'indirect mitogen' for mesenchymal cells, possibly upregulating PDGF expression[48].

TGF-β also acts on immune function, inhibiting both T and B cell growth, reducing immunoglobulin production, natural killer cell activity, and also modulates cytokine production, reducing the synthesis of interleukin 1, 2 and 3 (see ref. 47 for review). TGF-β is also a powerful attractant for monocytes, fibroblasts and neutrophils[47], in femtomolar concentrations. In this respect TGF-β also stimulates cell migration in IEC-6 cells, an intestinal cell line, after 'wounding' a monolayer of these cells *in vitro*, while cell proliferation was inhibited[49]; this was inhibited by anti-TGF-β antiserum. This suggests a role for TGF-β in promoting epithelial restitution after mucosal damage.

TGF-β1–3 are found in the intestine, both in crypt epithelial cells and in the lamina proprial cell populations. Thus these molecules have a potentially important role to play in IBD.

TREFOIL PEPTIDES

These are a series of related molecules which are characteristically secreted by mucus-secreting cells. Their common characteristic is the possession of a three-looped structure strongly held by disulphide bonds based on six intramolecular cysteine residues. The three-dimensional structure of these molecules has recently been calculated using a combination of X-ray crystallographic and NMR methods[50,51]. Trefoil peptides exist in mammalian tissues as single trefoil domain peptides, such as pS2, which is found in the gastric epithelium, and ITF (intestinal trefoil factor) which is usually localized to the intestinal goblet cells, and also as two-domain molecules, such as SP (spasmolytic polypeptide), first described by Thim *et al.*[52] in pig pancreas, but in humans localized in mucous neck and foveolar cells of the gastric mucosa, antral mucus-secreting glands, and also Brunner's gland acini and ducts.

The functions of these peptides are not yet clear; pSP has been reported to inhibit gastric acid secretion and also intestinal muscular activity (see ref. 53 for review); however, recent results have not confirmed this latter action (M. Parsons, unpublished). There have been reports that pSP stimulates the growth of colorectal carcinoma cells *in vitro*, but in this action it is singular in being glutathione-dependent (W. Otto, unpublished), and there does not appear to be any effect when infused into rats maintained on total parenteral nutrition (R. Goodlad, unpublished). However, ITF does appear to have an action on electrogenic chloride transport in the rat small intestine, and also to be a powerful stimulant of cell migration in epithelial monolayers 'wounded' *in vitro* (H. Cox and R. Chinery, unpublished). Moreover, hSP has been shown to stimulate epithelial restitution after indomethacin-induced damage in the rat stomach (R. Playford, unpublished). The possibility also exists that these molecules are involved in the organization of the viscoelastic mucus layer. These molecules are abundant and very resistant to degradation, and their function in the gut is therefore important to resolve.

OTHER GROWTH FACTORS

There are several other growth factor families which are indeed produced in the gut, whose role in the control of homeostasis is less well known. Thus the insulin-like growth factors (IGF) do have a minor proliferative effect on the intestine, and the fibroblast growth factor family has major effects on angiogenesis, actions which may be very important in the healing of ulcers.

THE ROLE OF GROWTH FACTORS IN IBD

While it must be very tempting to speculate, it is not yet possible to say which growth factors are responsible for the several growth phenomena noted in IBD and listed above. Certainly the EGF/TGF-α molecules are very likely to be involved in the mucosal hyperplasia which accompanies ulcerative colitis. However, direct evidence of this is lacking. On the other hand, IGF-1 expression is up-regulated in fibroblast-like cells of granulation tissue in an animal model of enterocolitis, pointing to a potential role for IGF-1 in the fibrogenic complications associated with IBD[54]. A preliminary report describing TGF-β mRNA levels in patients with varying levels of IBD activity did not find statistically significant differences[55].

However, one phenomenon which does give some insight into the potential role of growth factors in the repair of ulcerative intestinal disease is the formation of the ulcer-associated cell lineage (UACL)[10]. In the crypts surrounding chronic ulcers in the gastrointestinal tract, small buds of cells appear with a distinctive phenotype, mucus-secreting cells which elaborate D/PAS-positive neutral mucin rather than the alcianophilic acid mucin usually found in indigenous goblet cells. These buds grow into tubules, which ramify in the lamina propria and form new glandular complexes. A duct then grows upwards through the lamina propria to make contact with the

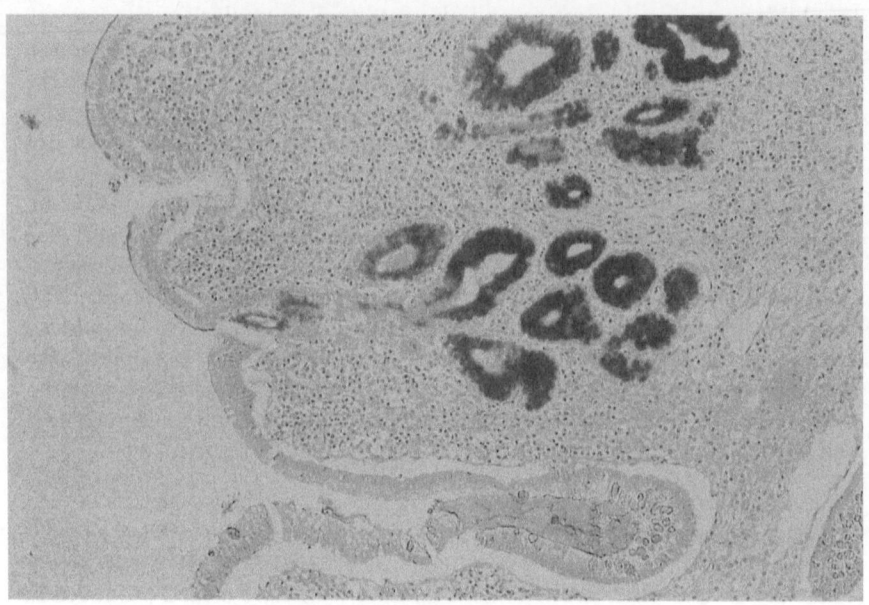

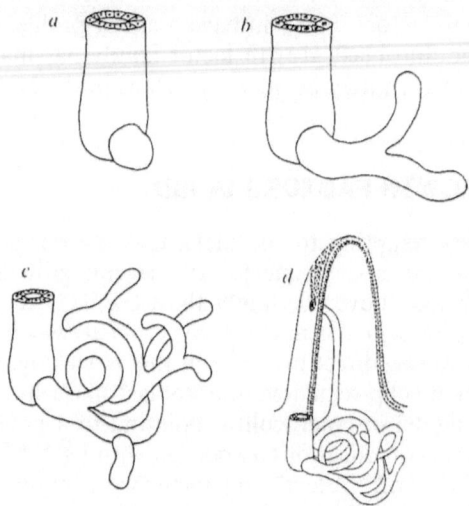

Fig. 4 (a) A mature UACL system. The condition is Crohn's disease. Note the acini, the duct, and the cells emerging onto the villus surface replacing the indigenous cell lineages. (b) A diagrammatic representation of the histogenesis of the UACL

surface via a pore. Figure 4 shows a photomicrograph of the mature UACL, together with a diagram of the proposed histogenesis. The system is presumably fed by cells from the parent crypt(s) but, in the mature UACL a proliferative zone develops in the duct, which probably feeds cells upwards towards the surface, and also downwards into the acinar area[56].

The range of regulatory peptides elaborated by the UACL is really quite

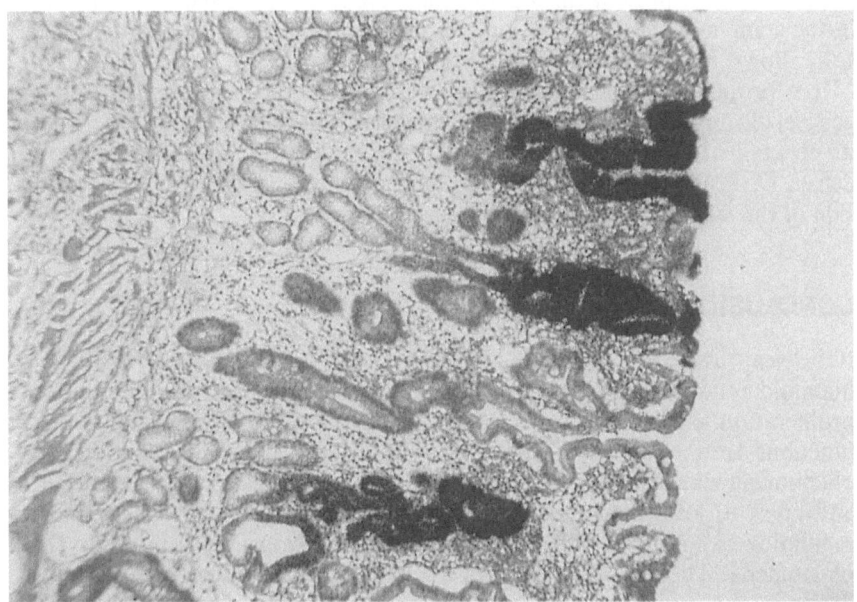

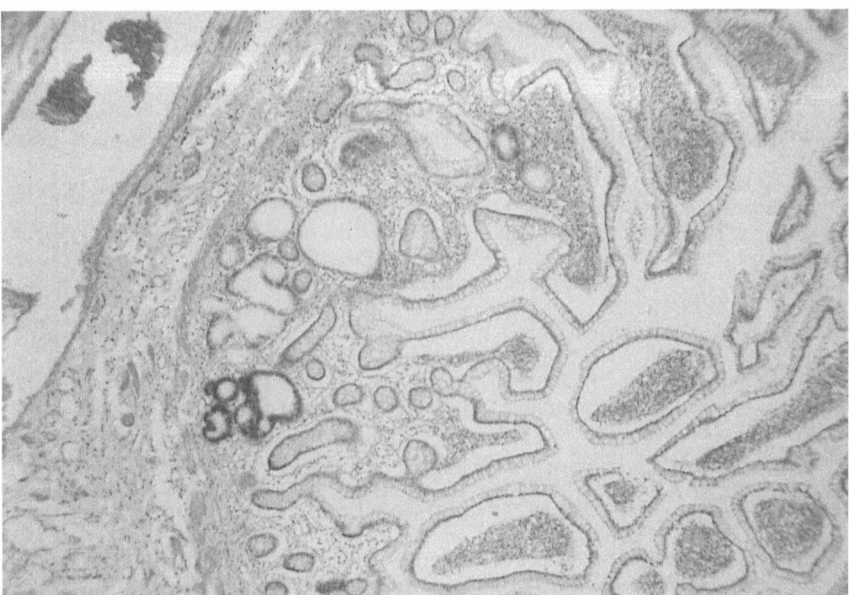

Fig. 5 Distribution of (**a**) pS2 mRNA and (**b**) hSP mRNA in the UACL, as demonstrated by *in situ* hybridization using ^{35}S riboprobes

extensive. The basal acini contain quantities of immunoreactive EGF, while the whole lineage contains immunoreactive TGF-α. The acini and the lower duct contain hSP protein and mRNA (Fig. 5), while pS2 mRNA and peptide are concentrated in considerable amounts in the upper duct and surface cells

(Fig. 5); hITF is present throughout the UACL[53]. Lysozyme is also present in the acini, and the UACL is singular in the intestine for expressing MUC 1, as shown by HMFG1 and HMFG2 staining[10].

It is proposed that this lineage grows adjacent to intestinal (and indeed gastric) ulcers and, once access to the mucosal surface has been gained, pours its cocktail of growth factors into the local milieu; because of the mucosal defect, EGF and TGF-α at least can bind their receptors on the basolateral side of the surrounding enterocytes or colonocytes.

CONCLUSION

It is clear from this short chapter that growth factors have many and manifold influences on the gastrointestinal tract; not just modulating cell proliferation, but also acting on other aspects of physiology. Several of these functions are incriminated, by implication, in the pathogenetic and healing phenomena which accompany IBD. Now that we can recognize the molecules and know at least their potential functions, it is time to study their genetic regulation, and how their expression and functions contribute to IBD phenomena. Thereby, perhaps, lies the avenue to future therapeutic intervention.

References

1. Wright NA, Alison MR. The biology of epithelial populations. Oxford: Clarendon Press; 1984.
2. Cheng H, Leblond CP. Origin, differentiation and renewal of the four main cell types in the mouse small intestine. V. The unitarian hypothesis. Am J Anat. 1974;141:537–62.
3. Chang WWL, Leblond CP. A unitarian theory of the origin of the three main types of epithelial cells in the mouse small intestine. Anat Rec. 1971;269:293.
4. Winton DJ, Ponder BA. Stem cell organisation in the mouse small intestine. Proc R Soc Lond B. 1990;241:13–18.
5. Griffiths DR, Davies SJ, Williams D, Williams GT, Williams ED. Demonstration of somatic mutation and crypt clonality by X-linked histochemistry. Nature (Lond.). 1988;333:461.
6. Thompson M, Fleming K, Evans D, Wright NA. Clonal origin of gut endocrine cells in male:female chimaeras demonstrated by combined in situ hybridisation and immunocytochemistry. Development. 1990;110:477–81.
7. Pearse AGE, Tabor Tabor T. Neuroendocrine embryology and the APUD cell concept. Clin Endocrinol Suppl. 1976;5:299–344.
8. Kaftan, Wright NA. Studies on the mechanism of goblet cell depletion in experimental colitis. J Pathol. 1989;159:75–85.
9. Riddell R. The precancerous phase of ulcerative colitis. In: Morson B, editor. Topics in pathology. Berlin: Springer; 1978:179–219.
10. Wright NA, Pike C, Elias G. Ulceration induces a novel epidermal growth factor-secreting cell lineage in human gastrointestinal stem cells. Nature. 1990;343:82–5.
11. Wright NA, Al-Dewachi HF, Watson AJ, Appleton DR. The effect of single and multiple injections of prednisolone on cell population kinetics in the small bowel of the rat. Virch Arch Cell B. 1978;28:1339–50.
12. Williamson R. Intestinal adaptation. 1. Structural, functional and cytokinetic aspects. N Engl J Med. 1978;298:1398–402.
13. Williamson R. Intestinal adaptation. 2. Mechanisms of control. N Engl J Med. 1978;298:1444–50.

14. Williamson R, Bucholtz TN, Malt RA. Humoral stimulation in small bowel after transection and resection. Gastroenterology. 1978;75:249–54.

15. Feldman EJ, Dowling RH, McNaughton J, Peters TJ. Effect of oral versus intravenous nutrition on intestinal adaptation after small bowel resection in the dog. Gastroenterology. 1976;70:712.

16. Hanson WR, Rijke RPC, Plaiier HM et al. The effect of intestinal resection on Thiry-Vella fistula of jejunal and ileal origin in the rat; evidence for a systemic control mechanism of cell renewal. Cell Tissue Kinet. 1975;8:135.

17. Miazza et al. The effects of intrarectal installation of hypertonic glucose on cell proliferation in the small intestine. Gut. 1985;26:518–24.

18. Al-Mukhtar MYT, Sagor G, Ghatei M et al. The relationship between endogenous gastrointestinal hormones and cell proliferation in models of intestinal adaptation. In: Robinson J, Dowling RH, Ricken EO, editors. Mechanism of intestinal adaptation. Lancaster: MTP Press; 1989:243–53.

19. Clarke RM. 'Luminal nutrition' versus 'functional workload' as controllers of mucosal morphology and epithelial cell replacement in the rat small intestine. Digestion. 1977;68: 83–93.

20. Jacobs LR, Taylor BR, Dowling R. Effect of luminal nutrition on the intestinal adaptation following Thiry-Vella fistula in the dog. Clin Sci Mol Med. 1975;49:26.

21. Hosomi M, Stace ME, Larussi F, Smith SM, Murphy GM, Dowling RH. Role of polyamines in intestinal adaptation in the rat. Eur J Clin Invest. 1987;375:375–85.

22. Goodlad RA, Gregory H, Wright NA. Is polyamine synthesis in the proliferative response of the intestinal epithelium to urogastrone-epidermal growth factor. Clin Sci Mol Med. 1989;64:595–8.

23. Yarrington JT, Sprinkle DJ, Loude DE, Diekema KA, MaCann PP, Gibson JP. Intestinal changes caused by DL-α-difluomethylornithine (DFMO), an inhibitor of ornithine decarboxylase. Exp Mol Pathol. 1983;39:300–16.

24. Yang P, Baylin SB, Luk GD. Polyamines and intestinal growth: absolute requirement for ODC activity in adaptation during lactation. Am J Physiol. 1984;247:G553–7.

25. McCormack SA, Johnson LR. Role of polyamines in gastrointestinal growth. Am J Physiol. 1991;260:G695–806.

26. Seidel ER, Haddox MK, Johnson LR. Ileal mucosal growth during intraluminal infusion of ethylamine or putrescine. Am J Physiol. 1985;249:G434–8.

27. Ratcliffe B, Lee CY, Wright NA, Goodlad RA. Dietary fibre and the gastrointestinal epithelium; differential response in the stomach small intestine and colon of conventional and germ-free rats. In: Waldron KW, editors. Food and cancer prevention. Royal Society of Chemistry; 1991:364–8.

28. Bloom S, Polak J. Hormonal pattern of intestinal adaptation. In: Polak J, Bloom SR, Daly M, Wright NA, editors. Structure of the gut. London: Glaxo; 1984:409–19.

29. Chinery R, Goodlad RA, Wright NA. The effects of fibre on the expression of growth factors in the colon. J Nutr. 1991;

30. Schaudies P, Grines J, Wray HL, Koldovsky O. Identification and partial characterisation of multiple forms of biologically active EGF in rat milk. Am J Physiol. 1990;Suppl.69: G1056–61.

31. Thompson JF. Specific receptors for epidermal growth factor in rat intestinal microvillus membranes. Am J Physiol. 1988;254:G429–35.

32. Scheving LA, Shiurba RA, Nyguyen TD, Gray GM. Epidermal growth factor receptor of the intestinal enterocyte. Localization to laterobasal but not brush border membrane. J Biol Chem. 1989;264:1735–41.

33. Weaver LT, Gonnella PA, Israel EJ, Walker WA. Uptake of epidermal growth factor by the small intestinal epithelium of the fetal rat. Endocrinology. 1990;98:828–37.

34. Rao RK, Thornburg W, Korc M, Matrisian SM, Magun BE, Koldovsky O. Processing of epidermal growth factor by suckling and adult rat intestinal cells. Am J Physiol. 1986;250:G850–5.

35. Reeve JR, Richards RC, Cooke T. The effects of intracolonic EGF on mucosal growth and experimental carcinogenesis. Br J Cancer. 1991;63:223–6.

36. Goodlad RA, Wilson TJ, Lenton W, Gregory H, Wright NA. Intravenous but not intragastric urogastrone-EGF is trophic to the intestine of parenterally-fed rats. Gut. 1987;28:573–82.

37. Konturek SJ, Ciezkowski M, Jaworek J. Effects of epidermal growth factor on gastroduo-denal secretions. Am J Physiol. 1984;246:G580–6.
38. Koyama D, Podolsky DK. Differential expression of transforming growth factors α and β in rat intestinal cells. J Clin Invest. 1989;83:1768–73.
39. Opleta-Madsen K, Hardin J, Gall DG. Epidermal growth factor upregulates intestinal electrolyte transport. Am J Physiol. 1991;260:G807–14.
40. Goodlad RA, Raja KB, Peters TJ, Wright NA. Effects of urogastrone-epidermal growth factor on intestinal brush border enzymes and mitotic activity. Gut. 1991;32:994–8.
41. Tomasetto C, Rio M-C, Gautier C, Wolf C, Hareuvenu M, Chambon P, Lathe R. hSP, the domain-duplicated homologue of pS2 protein, is expressed with pS2 in the stomach but not in the breast. EMBO J. 1990;92:407–14.
42. Delarco JE, Todaro GJ. Growth factors from murine sarcoma virus-induced cells. Proc Natl Acad Sci USA. 1978;75:4001–5.
43. Moses HL, Branum EB, Proper JA, Robinson RA. Transforming growth factor production by chemically-transformed cells. Cancer Res. 1981;41:2842–8.
44. Coffey RJ, Snipes NH, Bascom CC et al. Growth modulation of mouse keratinocytes by transforming growth factors. Cancer Res. 1988;48:1596–602.
45. Hoosein NM, Brattain DE, MacKight MK, Levine AE, Brattain MG. Characterisation of the inhibitory effects of transforming growth factor-β on a human colon carcinoma cell line. Cancer Res. 1987;47:2950–4.
46. Chakrabarty S, Fan D, Varani G. Modulation of differentiation and proliferation in human carcinoma cells by transforming growth factor β1 and β2. Int J Cancer. 1990;46:493–9.
47. Barnard JA, Coffey RJ. Transforming growth factor β. In: Walsh JH, Dockray GJ, editors. Gut peptides; biochemistry and physiology. New York: Raven Press; 1993;615–31.
48. Leof EB, Proper JA, Goustin AS, Shipley GD, DiCorleto PE, Moses HL. Induction of c-sis mRNA and activity similar to platelet derived growth factor by transforming growth factor-b; a proposed model for indirect mitogenesis involving autocrine activity. Proc Natl Acad Sci USA. 1986;83:2453–7.
49. Suemori S, Ciacci C, Podolsky DK. Regulation of transforming growth factor expression in rat intestinal epithelial cell lines. J Clin Invest. 1991;67:2216–21.
50. Freemont P et al. The three-dimensional structure of PSP as shown by X-ray crystallography. Proc Natl Acad Sci USA. 1994 (In press).
51. Carr M, Lane A et al. The solution structure of PSP demonstrated by 2D NMR. Proc Natl Acad Sci USA. 1994 (In press).
52. Thim L, Thomsen J, Christensen M, Jorgensen KH. The amino acid sequence of pancreatic spasmolytic polypeptide. Biochim Biophys Acta. 1985;285:410–18.
53. Poulsom R, Wright NA. The trefoil peptide family. Am J Physiol. 1993;
54. Zimmerman EM, Sartor RB, McCall RD, Pardo M, Spencer EM, Lund PK. Insulin-like growth factor 1 and interleukin 1b mRNA in a rat model of granulomatous enterocolitis and hepatitis. Gastroenterology. 1993;105:399–409.
55. Rossiter G, Podolsky DK. Expression of transforming growth factor α and β in colonic mucosa in ulcerative colitis. Gastroenterology. 1990;98:A471.
56. Ahnen D et al. The ulcer-associated cell lineage shows the histogenetic programme of Brunners glands but evolves the proliferative organisation of the gastric gland. J Pathol. 1994 (In press).

12
Nitric oxide and chronic colitis

M. B. GRISHAM, S. AIKO and T. E. ZIMMERMAN

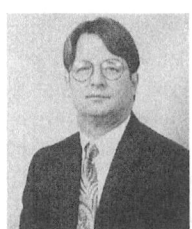

M. B. GRISHAM

INTRODUCTION

There is a growing body of both experimental and clinical data to suggest that chronic inflammation of the colon is associated with enhanced production of nitric oxide (NO)[1-3]. NO is thought to play an important role in modulating the inflammatory response by virtue of its ability to affect blood flow and leukocyte function[4]. Furthermore, this reactive nitrogen intermediate will rapidly and spontaneously interact with molecular oxygen or superoxide to yield potentially injurious oxidizing and nitrosating agents. Although the sources of this enhanced NO production *in vivo* have not been definitively identified, it is very probable that the phagocytic leukocytes (neutrophils, monocytes, macrophages), known to accumulate within the colonic interstitium are primary candidates[5]. We have demonstrated that extravasated, but not circulating, neutrophils produce much larger amounts of NO via the up-regulation of both mRNA and inducible No synthase (iNOS) enzymatic activity[6]. Intestinal inflammation induced in experimental animals or in human IBD is associated with increases in one or more tissue-derived cytokines such as tumor necrosis factor (TNF), interferon-γ (IFN-γ) and interleukin-1β (IL-1)[7]. Some of these cytokines are potent inducers of NO synthase in macrophages, neutrophils and endothelial cells[4]. In addition we, as well as others, have found that incubation of IL-1, TNF and/or IFN-γ with cultured rat intestinal epithelial cells[8,9] for 24 h promotes the release of large quantities of NO_2^- and NO_3^-. Several groups of investigators have demonstrated that NO produced from activated macrophages is capable of injuring microorganisms, tumor cells and some normal cells such as hepatocytes, pancreatic islet cells and lymphocytes[10-14]. In view of the potential injurious and proinflammatory properties of NO produced by iNOS, we wished to assess whether NO plays a role in mediating the mucosal injury and inflammation in a model of immunologically induced chronic granulomatous colitis. The objective of this study was to assess the role of NO or NO-derived metabolites as mediators of the mucosal injury and inflammation observed in a model of chronic granulomatous colitis in rats[2].

METHODS

Induction of colitis

Female specific pathogen-free Lewis rats (150–175 g) were housed in wire-mesh bottomed cages and given free access to water and standard laboratory rat chow. A total of 44 rats were randomized into four major groups consisting of a control group ($n = 7$), a peptidoglycan/polysaccharide (PG/PS) treated group ($n = 15$), a PG/PS + L-NAME (N^G-nitro-L-arginine methyl ester) group ($n = 15$) and a PG/PS + aminoguanidine (AG) group ($n = 7$). The animals were anesthetized via inhalation of isofluorane and their descending colons were exposed by laparotomy using aseptic technique. Colitis was induced via nine or 10 intramural (subserosal) injections (50–60 μl/injection) of PG/PS (12.5 μg rhamnose/g body weight) into the distal colon (4 cm) using a 30G needle[2]. Control animals were treated identically using nine or 10 injections (50–60 μl/injection) of a sterile saline solution. The NO synthase (NOS) inhibitors (L-NAME; 15 μmol/kg per day and AG; 15 μmol/kg per day) were administered to the colitic animals in their drinking water beginning 3 days prior to the induction of colitis and continuing for the entire 3-week period. Assuming that each drug freely equilibrates with the entire extracellular volume (30% of body weight), steady-state concentrations of L-NAME and AG would approximate 50 μmol/l, respectively. This concentration of L-NAME would produce near-maximal inhibition of constitutive NO synthase (cNOS) as measured by its ability to increase mean arterial pressure (MAP) but would have little or no effect on phagocytic leukocyte (PMNs, macrophage)-associated iNOS[15,16]. Fifty micromolar AG, on the other hand, has been demonstrated to inhibit phagocyte iNOS completely, but to have little or no effect on cNOS as judged by its lack of effect on MAP *in vivo*[17].

Quantitative indices of colonic injury and inflammation

Macroscopically visible injury and inflammation, colonic myeloperoxidase (MPO) activity and colon dry weight were quantified and used as indices of colonic inflammation, granulocyte infiltration and interstitial fibrosis, respectively[2]. Plasma nitrate and nitrite levels were used as indirect indices of NO metabolism *in vivo* and quantified by converting nitrate to nitrite using *E. coli* nitrate reductase and then measuring total nitrite using the Griess reagent[10].

RESULTS

Subserosal (intramural) injection of PG/PS into the distal colon results in an acute and spontaneously reactivating chronic colitis characterized by leukocyte infiltration, colonic granulomas, adhesions and bowel wall thickening at 3 weeks post PG/PS injection[2]. We found that chronic NOS inhibition by L-NAME or AG attenuated the PG/PS-induced increases in macroscopic colonic inflammation scores (2.5 ± 0.2 and 3.0 ± 0.4 vs 4.4 ± 0.4, respectively; $p < 0.05$) and colonic MPO activity (1.7 ± 0.2 and 1.6 ± 0.1 vs 6.1 ± 0.8 units/cm, respectively; $p < 0.01$). Only AG and not L-NAME attenuated the PG/PS-induced increases in colon dry weight (0.0135 ± 0.002 vs 0.022 ± 0.002 g dry weight/cm; $p < 0.05$). Both L-NAME and AG significantly attenuated the PG/PS-induced increases in spleen weight (3.8 ± 0.7 and 2.8 ± 0.2 vs 6.6 ± 2 mg/g body weight, respectively, $p < 0.05$), whereas neither drug was effective at significantly attenuating the PG/PS-induced increases in liver weight. Although both L-NAME and AG inhibited NO production *in vivo*, as measured by decreases in plasma nitrite and nitrate levels, only AG was found to produce significantly lower values (38 ± 3 vs 83 ± 8 μmol/l, respectively; $p < 0.05$). Finally, L-NAME but not AG administration significantly increased mean arterial pressure (MAP) from 83 mmHg in colitic animals to 105 mmHg in the PG/PS + L-NAME-treated animals ($p < 0.05$).

DISCUSSION

We have found that the intramural injection of PG/PS induces an acute and chronic granulomatous inflammation of the distal colon[2]. In contrast to other models of colitis induced by the intrarectal administration of noxious organic acids and/or solvents, this model produces a chronic colonic inflammation via one injection of a nontoxic biopolymer. Although injections of the bacterial cell wall polymer were made into the distal colon, the animals developed systemic inflammation, including arthritis, hepatic and splenic granulomas. It is known that certain inflammatory mediators, cytokines and bacterial products such as LPS and PG/PS activate monocytes, macrophages and neutrophils[4]. This activation may be expressed in a variety of different ways including synthesis and release of certain cytokines, proinflammatory mediators (e.g. PAF, LTB4), protease secretion, and the release of reactive oxygen metabolites (e.g. superoxide, hydrogen peroxide)[4]. The L-arginine-dependent production of NO has been shown to be induced in phagocytic leukocytes by these mediators[4]. Macrophages and neutrophils contain a Ca-independent NO synthase that is transcriptionally activated by LPS and IFN-γ[4]. Since histological inspection of colonic and hepatic tissue revealed the presence of acute and chronic inflammatory cells such as neutrophils, macrophages and monocytes in inflamed intestine and liver 3–4 weeks after PG/PS injection, we quantified the plasma levels of nitrite and nitrate as an index of regulation of NO synthase *in vivo*[2]. We found that the intramural administration of PG/PS enhanced plasma levels of these nitrogen oxides by 4-fold at 3 weeks, suggesting that this bacterial polymer may induce NO synthase in one or more populations of cells *in vivo*. These data suggest that hepatic and colonic macrophages and neutrophils may be major sources of these nitrogen oxides in the chronically inflamed animal. This suggestion is supported by our observations that elicited rat peritoneal macrophages and neutrophils produce relatively large amounts of nitrite in an L-arginine-dependent manner when cultured with PG/PS at concentrations calculated to be achieved *in vivo*[2]. It should be emphasized that although the major source of nitrite and nitrate *in vivo* in response to inflammatory mediators is assumed to be macrophages (and possibly neutrophils) it is possible that other cells such as endothelial cells, smooth muscle cells, fibroblasts, hepatocytes and/or mast cells may contribute to the overall production of nitrogen oxides *in vivo*[4].

Several recent studies have reported that L-NAME is a much more selective inhibitor for cNOS whereas AG is much more selective for iNOS[15-17]. A dose of 15 μmol/kg per day of either L-NAME or AG would produce steady-state concentrations of 50 μmol/l each, assuming that each drug freely equilibrates with the entire extracellular volume (30% of body weight). This concentration of L-NAME would produce near-maximal inhibition of cNOS as measured by its ability to cause substantial increases in mean arterial pressure (MAP), but would have little or no effect on phagocytic leukocyte (PMNs, macrophage)-associated iNOS[15,16]. A steady-state concentration of 50 μmol/l AG, on the other hand, has been demonstrated to completely inhibit phagocyte iNOS but have little or no effect on cNOS as judged by its lack of effect on MAP *in vivo*[17]. We have found in the present study that chronic NOS inhibition using 15 μmol/kg per day of either L-NAME or AG attenuated colonic injury and inflammation as judged by similar reductions in macroscopically visible lesions and colonic MPO activity. Histologic inspection of the colons revealed similar anti-inflammatory activities of L-NAME and AG as judged by the lack of leukocyte infiltration and maintenance of epithelial and crypt integrity.

Interestingly, only AG and not L-NAME significantly attenuated the PG/PS-induced increases in the dry weight of the colon and plasma levels of nitrate and nitrite, suggesting differences in the ability of L-NAME and AG to inhibit protein (collagen) deposition in the inflamed colon and NOS inhibition *in vivo*. The precise mechanisms for these differences are not known; however, it has been demonstrated that L-NAME, at the concentration calculated to be present *in vivo* in our model of colitis, would be much more effective at inhibiting cNOS than would be AG. Indeed, L-NAME but not AG was found to significantly increase MAP by 30 mmHg. These data are consistent with the idea that the enhanced levels of nitrate and nitrite observed during chronic gut, liver and spleen inflammation are a result of the up-regulation of iNOS. Because cNOS is regulated by the small and transient increases in intracellular Ca^{2+}, this isoenzyme produces only small amounts of NO for short periods of time, whereas iNOS produces much larger amounts during times of chronic inflammation. Thus, the overall contribution of systemic NO made by cNOS would be expected to be minimal. One would predict that selective inhibition of cNOS by L-NAME would be expected to increase MAP but have little effect on circulating levels of nitrate and nitrite. Indeed, this is exactly what we find. Selective inhibition of iNOS by AG, on the other hand, would be expected to produce no effect on blood pressure but to substantially inhibit systemic nitrate and nitrite levels. Again, this is observed. The mechanisms responsible for L-NAME or AG-dependent inhibition of leukocyte accumulation in the PG/PS-treated colons is not clear. As in other models of inflammation-induced vascular injury, it could be argued that inhibition of cNOS by L-NAME would reduce blood flow to the colon, thereby delivering circulating leukocytes to the tissue[18]. This explanation is unlikely in our model, since AG appears not to alter cNOS, but it does inhibit leukocyte accumulation.

Enhanced and sustained production of NO may alter the normal physiology of the colon and possibly other tissues such as the liver and spleen. NO, known as endothelial-derived relaxing factor, is a potent vasodilator that will increase tissue blood flow quite dramatically[4]. Clinical and experimental studies demonstrate that the blood flow of the inflamed colon increases quite dramatically during active episodes of gut inflammation. Furthermore, NO is known to reversibly and/or irreversibly injure parenchymal and leukocytic cells such as hepatocytes, pancreatic islet cells and lymphocytes[12-14]. This may be an important mechanism by which PG/PS mediates injury and fibrosis to the gut, liver and spleen in our model. More recent data suggest that enhanced production of NO has the potential to induce mutagenic and possibly carcinogenic alterations in the gut epithelium via the formation of potent N-nitrosating agents derived from the spontaneous decomposition of NO in oxygenated solutions[19].

Acknowledgements

Some of the work reported in this chapter was supported by grants from the National Institutes of Health (DK47663 and DK47385; Project 6).

References

1. Roediger WEW, Lawson MJ, Radcliffe BC. Nitrite from inflammatory cells – a cancer risk factor in ulcerative colitis? Dis Colon Rectum. 1990;33:1034–6.
2. Yamada T, Sartor RB, Marshall S, Specian RD, Grisham MB. Mucosal injury and inflammation in a model of granulomatous colitis in rats. Gastroenterology. 1993;104: 759–77.
3. Boughton-Smith NK, Evans SM, Hawkey CJ et al. Nitric oxide synthase activity in ulcerative colitis and Crohn's disease. Lancet. 1993;342:338–40.
4. Moncada S, Higgs A. The L-arginine–nitric oxide pathway. N Engl J Med. 1993;329: 2002–12.
5. Grisham MB, Ware K, Yamada T. Neutrophil-mediated nitrosamine formation: role of nitric oxide in rats. Gastroenterology. 1992;103:1260–6.
6. Grisham MB, Miles AM, Owens M, Johnson GG. Molecular, biochemical and cellular characterization of the inducible nitric oxide synthase in circulating vs. extravasated polymorphonuclear leukocytes (PMNs). FASEB J. 1994;9:A682.
7. Sartor RB. Pathogenic and clinical relevance of cytokines in inflammatory bowel disease. Immunol Res. 1991;10:465–71.

8. Grisham MB. Nitric oxide production by intestinal epithelial cells. Gastroenterology. 1993;104:A710.

9. Tepperman BL, Brown JF, Whittle BJR. Nitric oxide synthase induction and intestinal epithelial cell viability in rats. Am J Physiol. 1993;265:G214–18.

10. Granger DL, Hibbs JB, Perfect JR, Durack DT. Metabolic fate of L-arginine in relation to microbiostatic capability of murine macrophages. J Clin Invest. 1990;85:264–73.

11. Stuehr DJ, Nathan CF. Nitric oxide: a macrophage product responsible for cytostasis and respiratory inhibition in tumor target cells. J Exp Med. 1989;169:1543–55.

12. Stadler J, Billiar TR, Curran RD, Stuehr DJ, Ochoa JB, Simmons RL. Effect of exogenous and endogenous nitric oxide on mitochondrial respiration of rat hepatocytes. Am J Physiol. 1991;260:C910–16.

13. Kroncke KD, Rodriguez ML, Kolb H, Kolb-Bachofen V. Cytotoxicity of activated rat macrophages against syngeneic islet cells is arginine-dependent, correlates with citrulline and nitrite concentrations and is identical to lysis by the nitric oxide donor nitroprusside. Diabetologia. 1993;36:17–24.

14. Kroncke KD, Brenner HH, Rodriguez ML et al. Pancreatic islet cells are highly susceptible towards the cytotoxic effects of chemically generated nitric oxide. Biochim Biophys Acta. 1993;1182:221–9.

15. McCall TB, Feelisch M, Palmer RMJ, Moncada S. Identification of N-iminoethyl-L-ornithine as an irreversible inhibitor of nitric oxide synthase in phagocytic cells. Br J Pharmacol. 1991;102:234–8.

16. Rees DD, Palmer RMJ, Schulz R, Hodson HF, Moncada S. Characterization of three inhibitors of endothelial nitric oxide synthase in vitro and in vivo. Br J Pharmacol. 1990;101:746–52.

17. Corbett JA, Tilton RG, Chang K et al. Aminoguanidine, a novel inhibitor of nitric oxide formation, prevents diabetic vascular dysfunction. Diabetes. 1992;41:552–6.

18. Antunes E, Mariano M, Cirino G, Levi S, De Nucci G. Pharmacological characterization of polycation-induced rat hind-paw oedema. Br J Pharmacol. 1990;101:986–90.

19. Wink DA, Darbyshire JF, Nims RW, Saavedra JE, Ford PC. Reactions of the bioregulatory agent nitric oxide in oxygenated aqueous media: determination of the kinetics for oxidation and nitrosation by intermediates generated in the NO/O_2 reaction. Chem Res Toxicol. 1993;6:23–7.

Section V
Pathophysiology of intestinal inflammation: symptom generation in IBD

13
Cytokine interactions with epithelium

K. E. BARRETT

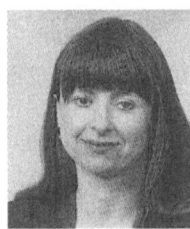

INTRODUCTION

Cytokines are a family of proteins that serve as intracellular messengers within the immune system, and as growth factors for several cell types. Recent studies indicate that intestinal inflammation is accompanied by increases in a wide variety of such cytokines and growth factors (reviewed in ref. 1). Since the intestinal epithelium is a frequent target of the inflammatory process in diseases such as Crohn's disease and ulcerative colitis, it has been logical to examine whether epithelial functions are modulated by cytokines. Indeed, many cytokines and growth factors have been shown to alter a spectrum of epithelial functions (Table 1). Another area of research receiving considerable attention of late is the possibility that the epithelium acts not only as a target of intestinal inflammation, but also as an active participant in the overall inflammatory response. In part this participation may result from the ability of epithelial cells to express adhesion and accessory molecules, and to synthesize inflammatory mediators such as eicosanoids. Both of these

Table 1 Epithelial functions subject to regulation by cytokines and growth factors

Function	Implicated cytokines
Ion transport	IL-1, IL-3, TGF-β, EGF
Paracellular permeability	IFN-γ, IGF-1
Restitution and proliferation	IL-1, EGF, TGF-α, TGF-β
Viability	TNF-α, IFN-γ
Expression of adhesion and accessory molecules	IL-1, IL-6, TNF-α, IFN-γ
Production of cytokines and other inflammatory mediators	IL-1, IL-6, TGF-β, TNF-α, IFN-γ

properties may be subject to cytokine regulation. Other recent data suggest that the epithelium itself can act as a source of some cytokines. The ability of the epithelium to produce both eicosanoids and proinflammatory cytokines may represent one segment of an autocrine loop whereby inflammatory dysfunction of the epithelium is amplified. This chapter will review recent progress in the area of cytokine–epithelial interactions, with particular reference to the involvement of such interactions in intestinal inflammation. I will draw on the findings of a number of laboratories, as well as our own, to provide an integrated overview of the epithelial functions that may be subject to regulation by cytokines and growth factors.

EPITHELIAL FUNCTIONS SUBJECT TO MODULATION BY CYTOKINES

Effects of cytokines on epithelial transport properties

A primary function of the intestinal epithelium is to control the movement of electrolytes and other solutes[2]. This function, which is responsible for the control of luminal water content, is achieved via the regulation of two main pathways: transcellular transport, whereby electrolytes and nutrients are actively transported across cells, and the paracellular pathway, controlled by intercellular tight junctions. A classical view of the regulation of active ion transport across the intestinal epithelium recognized three main regulatory systems: paracrine regulation by adjacent endocrine cells located within the epithelium itself; endocrine regulation involving blood-borne hormones from distant sites; and neurocrine regulation, via the release of stimulatory and inhibitory neurotransmitters by nerves within the enteric nervous system. However, over the past 10 years it has become apparent that a fourth regulatory system should be added to this list, that of the intestinal immune system[3]. Studies both *in vivo* and *in vitro*, and in humans and experimental animals, have revealed that the release of inflammatory and immune mediators can be a prominent stimulus leading to transepithelial chloride secretion in the mammalian gastrointestinal tract. Since active secretion of chloride is the primary driving force for secretory diarrhea, the hypothesis has arisen that the ability of various immune and inflammatory mediators to evoke chloride secretion, perhaps in concert with agonists from other regulatory systems (such as the enteric nervous system[3]), is the primary pathophysiological mechanism underlying diarrhea associated with intestinal inflammation. In this context a number of investigators have examined the ability of various cytokines to modify chloride secretory responses of the epithelium.

There is evidence that chloride transport may be stimulated by various cytokines. However, in contrast to the secretory effects of various other inflammatory mediators (including histamine, adenosine, prostaglandins and certain reactive oxygen species), the stimulatory effects of cytokines on chloride secretion appear to be primarily indirect, and to require the participation of secondary mediators released from nonepithelial cell types.

This conclusion is based on the fact that cytokines examined to date do not appear to evoke chloride secretion directly when added acutely to intestinal epithelial cell lines. Secretory effects have been noted, however, when certain cytokines are added to intact intestinal preparations. Addition of interleukin-1 (IL-1) or interleukin-3 (IL-3) to segments of chicken intestine mounted in Ussing chambers led to a rapid increase in chloride secretion[4]. This effect, however, was blocked by a cyclooxygenase inhibitor, suggesting that it involved the secondary generation of prostaglandins, which then acted as the final stimulus for chloride secretion acting at the level of the secretory epithelial cells. Similarly, the stimulatory effects of cytokines on chloride secretion may not be acute, but rather may involve delayed up-regulation of responsiveness to other neurohormonal stimuli. This was found to be the case for a stimulatory effect of transforming growth factor-β (TGF-β) on chloride secretion by the T_{84} intestinal epithelial cell line, where the effect of the cytokine was to potentiate responses to vasoactive intestinal polypeptide (VIP) after a 24-h preincubation[5]. Further, as discussed in more detail in Chapter 14, IL-1 can chronically up-regulate the ability of fibroblasts to deliver a paracrine signal for the stimulation of chloride secretion by the epithelium[6].

Cytokines and growth factors may also have negative effects on chloride secretion and/or positive effects on absorptive mechanisms. In the case of TGF-β, an inhibitory effect of chronic exposure on responses to the cAMP-dependent agonist VIP, or direct elevation of intracellular cAMP levels with a cell-permeant cAMP analogue, was noted in some T_{84} cell monolayers; this contrasts with the stimulatory effect of this cytokine described above[5]. Whether a stimulatory or an inhibitory effect was observed appeared to depend, at least to some extent, on the overall level of responsiveness of the monolayers. Thus, when cells displayed an inhibition of chloride secretion after TGF-β treatment, other monolayers examined in parallel were more likely to have a higher level of responsiveness to VIP under control conditions. These findings indicate that factors intrinsic to the epithelium may quantitatively or even qualitatively define the response of the epithelium to a given cytokine. Another cytokine capable of acting as an anti-secretagogue is epidermal growth factor (EGF). This factor has been shown to enhance nutrient absorptive mechanisms in the small intestine[7], apparently by rapidly increasing the surface area of absorptive cells via an effect directed to the microvilli[8]. EGF also specifically down-regulates calcium-dependent chloride secretion, an action that may be related to the prolonged generation of a putative second messenger for this process, inositol-(3,4,5,6)-tetrakisphosphate[9]. Overall, these antisecretory effects of TGF-β and EGF may represent an adaptive response of the epithelium. Conversely, diarrhea might result if a normal inhibitory tone, provided by the influence of agonists such as EGF, is lost in the setting of disease.

In addition to the regulation of active transport mechanisms in the intestinal epithelium, intestinal fluid and electrolyte balance is also modulated by the dynamic regulation of paracellular permeability pathways, via the regulation of intercellular tight junctions. Cytokines may also regulate these paracellular transport pathways. Interferon-γ (IFN-γ), insulin, and insulin-like growth factors significantly reduce transepithelial resistance and thus enhance permeability to small solutes[10-14]. The effect of these substances on epithelial resistance is slow in onset, and appears to require the synthesis of new proteins within the epithelial cell. In general, the effects of these agents appear to be limited to increasing epithelial permeability to small solutes and electrolytes. No evidence has been presented to date to suggest that cytokines such as IFN-γ provide the mechanism whereby epithelial macromolecular permeability is up-regulated in intestinal inflammation[15].

Effects of cytokines on epithelial damage, restitution and proliferation

Intestinal inflammation is frequently characterized by frank damage to the epithelium. This effect itself could partially result from the actions of cytokines. Supernatants from activated mucosal T lymphocytes were shown to be cytotoxic for HT29 intestinal epithelial cells grown in culture[16]. This effect has been ascribed to the synergistic action of the cytokines tumor necrosis factor-α (TNF-α) and interferon-γ (IFN-γ). While almost all of the cytotoxicity of supernatants appeared due to the presence of TNF-α, when the effects of recombinant TNF-α on cell viability were assessed the cytokine was capable of causing significant cell death only when given simultaneously with IFN-γ. Overall, these results point to the potential for cytokine release from activated lymphocytes, and other inflammatory cells in the lamina propria, to contribute to the epithelial damage seen in inflammatory bowel disease.

The epithelium can respond to inflammatory damage in two ways. The first of these is a rapid repair mechanism, and involves a process referred to as restitution. In this process, epithelial cells adjacent to damaged areas flatten and migrate to seal epithelial discontinuities. There is evidence that cytokines and growth factors may be regulators of this process. For example, IL-1 has been shown to induce ornithine decarboxylase (ODC) activity in intestinal epithelial cells[17]. ODC is a key initial enzyme involved in both restitution and epithelial proliferation[18]. Likewise, both EGF and TGF-β stimulate migration of epithelial cells over extracellular matrix components[19,20]. The effect of EGF appears attributable, in part, to the up-regulation of epithelial integrins[19].

The second means by which the epithelium can respond to damage is by increasing its rate of proliferation. Ultimately, this may lead to the crypt hyperplasia which is a common feature of inflammatory bowel disease, since it is reasonable to propose that the rate at which enterocytes differentiate might not be able to keep pace with a larger increase in epithelial proliferative capacity. It is beyond the scope of this chapter to review in detail the complex networks thought to be responsible for the control of epithelial dynamics in both the normal and diseased intestine (the reader is referred to an excellent recent review of this area[21]). However, it is pertinent to make a few remarks concerning the peptide growth factors that are thought to be primarily responsible for control of this process. The overall rate of proliferation of the intestinal epithelium appears to reflect a balance between the growth-stimulatory factor TGF-α, and the growth-inhibitory TGF-β[21]. EGF may also play a stimulatory role in the control of epithelial proliferation, though the importance of this growth factor relative to the transforming growth factor is not yet clearly defined. This is because the majority of EGF is secreted into the intestinal lumen where it is subject to significant proteolytic cleavage; moreover, EGF receptors on intestinal epithelial cells appear to be confined to the basolateral membrane domain[22].

Effects of cytokines on the ability of the epithelium to express immune accessory and adhesion molecules

The intestinal epithelium is becoming increasingly recognized as a constituent of the mucosal immune system[23]. Intestinal epithelial cells have the capability to present antigen to helper lymphocytes, a property that appears to be specifically up-regulated during inflammation[24]. Conversely, epithelial cells from inflamed tissues fail to effectively present antigen to antigen nonspecific suppressor T cells[24]. Stimulated intestinal lymphocytes release a cytokine, identified as IFN-γ, that can induce major histocompatibility class II molecule (HLA-DR) expression on HT29 cultured intestinal epithelial cells[25]. Similarly, recombinant IFN-γ induces HLA-DR on the surface of the T_{84} epithelial cell line[26]. These findings may relate to the changes in antigen presentation seen in inflammatory bowel disease, since it was shown that lamina propria lymphocytes from patients with either Crohn's disease or ulcerative colitis displayed significantly higher rates of IFN-γ secretion upon stimulation[27].

Cytokines may also be responsible for the regulation of adhesion molecule expression on intestinal epithelial cells. For example, intercellular adhesion molecule-1 (ICAM-1) expression can be induced on cultured epithelial cells by IFN-γ, IL-1, TNF-α and IL-6[28,29]. This may again have implications for the ability of epithelial cells to orchestrate mucosal immune responses, in that increased ICAM-1 expression promotes the adhesion of activated T cells via the LFA-1 ligand for this molecule[30]. The expression of adhesion molecules on the epithelial surface may also be important for their interaction with other inflammatory cell types. Neutrophils have been shown to adhere to and migrate through T_{84} epithelial cell monolayers when driven by a chemotactic gradient[31]. Neutrophil migration across epithelial monolayers is subject to modulation by IFN-γ, although the effects seen are qualitatively different depending on the direction of cell migration examined. Thus IFN-γ pretreatment markedly up-regulated transmigration of neutrophils in the apical to basolateral direction[32]. However, in the physiologically more relevant basolateral to apical direction for migration, IFN-γ actually reduced transmigration[32]. Rather, the cytokine appeared to up-regulate an adhesive interaction between the neutrophils and the basolateral surface of the epithelial cells that enhanced the retention of the inflammatory cell type in the subepithelial space. The authors speculated that this may result in the

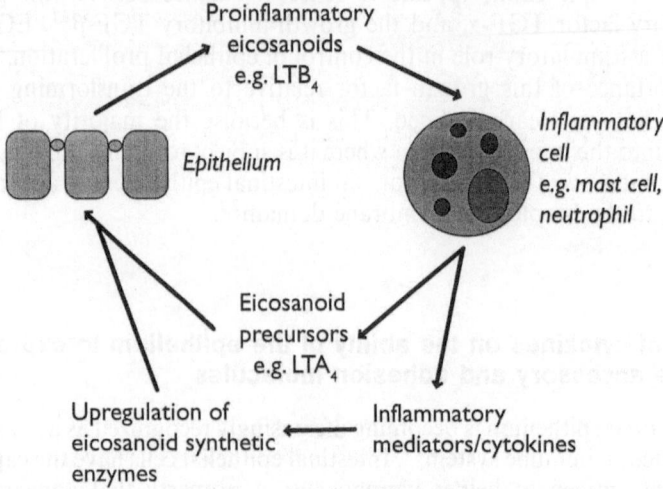

Fig. 1 Example of a potential eicosanoid synthetic pathway, involving transcellular cooperation between the epithelium and inflammatory cell types, that might be subject to up-regulation by cytokines. Inflammatory cells can supply LTA_4 to the epithelium for conversion to the chemotactic lipid, LTB_4, which would then stimulate further inflammatory cell migration and activation. Inflammatory cells could also supply cytokines capable of specifically upregulating enzyme (e.g. LTA_4 hydrolase) expression, thereby amplifying the loop and providing for a vicious cycle of inflammation

accumulation of neutrophils in a location where they would be poised to participate in host defense responses[32].

Effect of cytokines on the production of inflammatory mediators by the epithelium

Finally, the ability of the epithelium to itself synthesize proinflammatory mediators and, indeed, cytokines, has recently been recognized, and is the subject of much active research. These abilities themselves may also be subject to regulation by the cytokine milieu. The epithelium has, for example, been recognized as a potential supplier of proinflammatory eicosanoids. In some cases synthesis may involve a transcellular metabolic route, where infiltrating inflammatory cells supply the intermediate substrate, leukotriene A_4, for conversion to the proinflammatory LTB_4 by the intestinal epithelial LTA_4 hydrolase (Barrett and Bigby, unpublished observations). This ability of the epithelium could contribute to a vicious cycle of inflammation, contributing to tissue damage by amplifying inflammatory cell migration (Fig. 1). In other cases the complete enzymatic machinery for the generation of an eicosanoid product may be present within the epithelial cell. It has been shown that the enzyme 12-lipoxygenase is specifically induced in the epithelium of tissue specimens from patients suffering from inflammatory bowel disease[33]. Similarly, epithelial cells express phospholipase A_2 enzymes responsible for the initial release of arachidonic acid from membrane phospholipids, which then supplies downstream eicosanoid synthetic pathways[34]. Arachidonic acid metabolites have also been implicated as second messengers for chloride secretion[35], and an increase in their synthesis might thus contribute to inflammatory diarrhea. By analogy with other epithelial and nonepithelial systems, it seems reasonable to predict that these various eicosanoid metabolic enzymes may be subject to regulation by cytokines and growth factors. However, with the exception of the observation that TNF-α appears to up-regulate phospholipase A_2 activity in the cultured human intestinal cell line INT 407[34], the precise cytokine signals responsible for modulating arachidonic acid metabolism in the epithelium, *in vivo* or *in vitro*, remain to be established.

The intestinal epithelium may also serve as a local source of complement components. *In vitro* analyses of Caco-2 cells showed that these cells were capable of synthesizing biologically active C3, C4 and factor B under control conditions[36]. Moreover, the synthesis of each of these molecules was selectively up-regulated by cytokines. C3 production was enhanced by IL-1 and TNF-α, C4 by IL-6 and IFN-γ, and factor B by IL-1, IL-6 and, to a small extent, by IFN-β[36]. Given the numerical significance of epithelial cells in the intestine, the findings suggest that the epithelium might act as the primary source for complement components involved in mucosal host defense and/or local inflammation.

Epithelial cells have also been shown, at least in *in-vitro* models, themselves to act as a source of proinflammatory and chemotactic cytokines, such as IL-1, IL-6 and IL-8. IL-8 secretion may represent a primitive immune response to a cellular insult, such as that provided by bacterial colonization with invasive bacteria such as *Salmonella*[37]. Similarly, mucosal cytokines derived from lamina propria mononuclear cells may also signal the epithelium to produce additional cytokines. In the rat intestinal epithelial cell line IEC-6, TGF-β and IL-1 have been shown to synergistically promote the secretion of IL-6[38,39]. Likewise, in four human intestinal epithelial cell lines, TNF-α, IL-1 and bacterial lipopolysaccharide all serve to up-regulate the synthesis of IL-8[40]. In sum, the ability of the epithelium to secrete chemokines and other proinflammatory cytokines may provide a mechanism whereby phagocytes are recruited to a specific mucosal location (Fig. 2). This may be a highly appropriate response if evoked in response to bacterial invasion. However, inappropriate triggering of cytokine secretion might lead to an uncontrolled inflammatory response, perhaps also involving some of the other cytokine regulatory loops described above.

SUMMARY AND CONCLUSIONS

In summary, the intestinal epithelium appears to act as both a target for, and a supplier of, cytokines – properties that may be of particular relevance in the setting of inflammation. In some cases the precise response displayed by the epithelium to a given cytokine may depend on the intrinsic functional properties of the epithelial cell. Thus, significant information remains to be elucidated regarding the exact details of the highly integrated and redundant

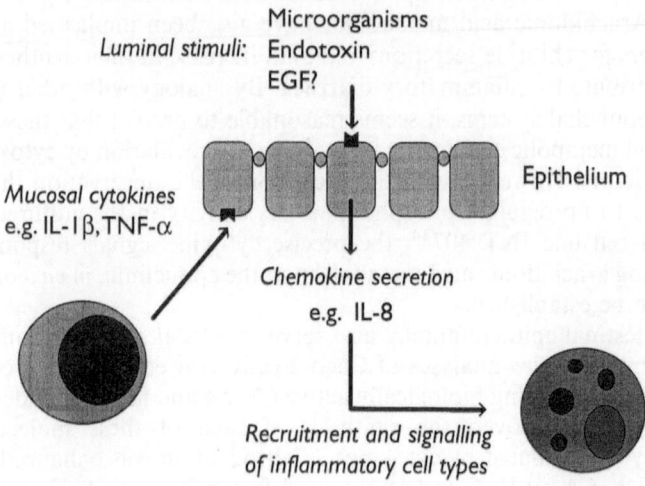

Fig. 2 The epithelium acts as a source of cytokines. In response to luminal stimuli, such as invasive microorganisms or endotoxin (or possibly EGF), or in response to mucosal cytokines, intestinal epithelial cells can synthesize the chemotactic cytokine IL-8. This likely results in the recruitment of inflammatory cell types to the site of initial injury or insult, and their subsequent activation

network of cytokine–epithelial interactions. Similarly, despite considerable progress in identifying the cytokines that are elevated in the inflamed tissue of inflammatory bowel disease patients[1], details of the precise cytokine milieu (both qualitatively and quantitatively) at different stages of the disease process, or in patients who are being treated with various therapeutic modalities, remain to be determined. Nevertheless, information obtained to date regarding the interaction of cytokines with epithelial cells suggests that increased knowledge in these areas may have clinical implications for the management of inflammatory bowel disease. Elucidation of the precise regulatory loops involved may aid our ability to modulate processes such as secretory diarrhea, epithelial restitution and mucosal immunity.

Acknowledgements

I thank Julie Lessem for help with manuscript preparation. I am also grateful to the following former and present colleagues and collaborators for their contributions to the studies from my laboratory that are outlined in this chapter, and for helpful discussions: Timothy Bigby, MD, Cornelia Gelbmann, MD, Alexis Traynor-Kaplan, PhD, Jorge Uribe, MS, and Mana Vajanaphanich, MD. Studies from the author's laboratory have been supported by grants from the National Institutes of Health (AI 24992 and DK 28305).

References

1. Sartor RB. Cytokines in intestinal inflammation: pathophysiological and clinical considerations. Gastroenterology. 1994;106:533–9.
2. Barrett KE, Dharmsathaphorn K. Secretion and absorption: small intestine and colon. In: Yamada T, editor. Textbook of gastroenterology. Philadelphia: Lippincott; 1991:265–94.
3. Stead RH, Perdue MH, Cooke H, Powell DW, Barrett KE (editors). Neuro-immuno-physiology of the gastrointestinal mucosa: implications for inflammatory diseases. New York: New York Academy of Sciences; 1992.
4. Chang EB, Musch MW, Mayer L. Interleukins 1 and 3 stimulate anion secretion in chicken intestine. Gastroenterology. 1990;98:1518–24.
5. Gelbmann C, Eckmann L, Vajanaphanich M, Kagnoff MF, Barrett KE. Dual effects of TGF-β_1 on epithelial chloride secretion. Gastroenterology. 1992;102:A211.
6. Hinterleitner TA, Berschneider HM, Powell DW. Fibroblast-mediated Cl$^-$ secretion by T_{84} cells is amplified by interleukin-1β. Gastroenterology. 1991;100:A690.
7. Opleta-Madsen K, Hardin J, Gall DG. Epidermal growth factor upregulates intestinal electrolyte and nutrient transport. Am J Physiol. 1991;260:G807–14.
8. Hardin JA, Buret A, Meddings JB, Gall DG. Effect of epidermal growth factor on enterocyte brush-border surface area. Am J Physiol. 1993;264:G312–18.
9. Uribe JM, Gelbmann CM, Traynor-Kaplan AE, Barrett KE. Epidermal growth factor inhibits Ca^{++} dependent Cl$^-$ secretion in T_{84} cells. Gastroenterology. 1994;106:A1053.
10. Hiribarren A, Heyman M, 'Helgouac'h AL, Desjeux JF. Effect of cytokines on the epithelial function of the human colon carcinoma cell line HT29 cl 19A. Gut. 1993;34:616–20.
11. Adams RB, Palnchon SM, Roche JK. IFN-γ modulation of epithelial barrier function. Time course, reversibility, and site of cytokine binding. J Immunol. 1993;150:2356–63.
12. McRoberts JA, Riley NE. Regulation of T_{84} cell monolayer permeability by insulin-like growth factors. Am J Physiol. 1992;262:C207–13.
13. Madara JL, Stafford J. Interferon-γ directly affects barrier function of cultured intestinal epithelial monolayers. J Clin Invest. 1989;83:724–7.
14. McRoberts JA, Aranda R, Riley N, Kang H. Insulin regulates the paracellular permeability of cultured intestinal epithelial cell monolayers. J Clin Invest. 1990;85:1127–34.
15. May GR, Sutherland LR, Meddings JB. Is small intestinal permeability really increased in relatives of patients with Crohn's disease? Gastroenterology. 1993;104:1627–32.
16. Deem RL, Shanahan F, Targan SR. Triggered human mucosal T cells release tumour necrosis factor-α and interferon-α which kill human colonic epithelial cells. Clin Exp Immunol. 1991;83:79–84.
17. Chung DH, Evers BM, Townsend CM et al. Cytokine regulation of gut ornithine decarboxylase gene expression and enzyme activity. Surgery. 1992;112:364–9.
18. McCormack SA, Viar MJ, Johnson LR. Polyamines are necessary for cell migration by a small intestinal crypt cell line. Am J Physiol. 1993;264:G367–74.
19. Basson MD, Modlin IM, Madri JA. Human enterocyte (Caco-2) migration is modulated in vitro by extracellular matrix composition and epidermal growth factor. J Clin Invest. 1992;90:15–23.
20. Ciacci C, Lind SE, Podolsky DK. Transforming growth factor β regulation of migration in wounded rat intestinal epithelial monolayers. Gastroenterology. 1993;105:93–101.
21. Podolsky DK. Regulation of intestinal epithelial proliferation: a few answers, many questions. Am J Physiol. 1993;264:G179–86.
22. Scheving LA, Shiurba RA, Nguyen TD, Gray GM. Epidermal growth factor receptor of the intestinal enterocyte. Localization to laterobasal but not brush border membrane. J Biol Chem. 1989;264:1735–41.
23. Mayer L, Shlien R. Evidence for function of Ia molecules on gut epithelial cells in man. J Exp Med. 1987;166:1471–83.
24. Mayer L, Eisenhardt D. Lack of induction of suppressor T cells by intestinal epithelial cells from patients with inflammatory bowel disease. J Clin Invest. 1990;86:1255–60.
25. Lowes JR, Radwan P, Priddle JD, Jewell DP. Characterisation and quantification of mucosal cytokine that induces epithelial histocompatibility locus antigen-Dr expression in inflammatory bowel disease. Gut. 1992;33:315–19.
26. Mayer L, Eisenhardt D, Salomon P, Bauer W, Plous R, Piccinini L. Expression of class II

molecules on intestinal epithelial cells in humans. Gastroenterology. 1991;100:3–12.

27. Salomon P, Pizzimenti A, Panja A, Reisman A, Mayer L. The expression and regulation of class II antigens in normal and inflammatory bowel disease peripheral blood monocytes and intestinal epithelium. Autoimmunity. 1991;9:141–9.
28. Kvale D, Krajci P, Brandtzaeg P. Expression and regulation of adhesion molecules ICAM-1 (CD54) and LFA-3 (CD58) in human intestinal epithelial cell lines. Scand J Immunol. 1992;35:669–76.
29. Kaiserlian D, Rigal D, Abello J, Revillard J-P. Expression, function and regulation of the intercellular adhesion molecule-1 (ICAM-1) on human intestinal epithelial cell lines. Eur J Immunol. 1991;21:2415–21.
30. Springer TA. Adhesion receptors of the immune system. Nature. 1990;346:425–34.
31. Nash S, Stafford J, Madara JL. Effects of polymorphonuclear leukocyte transmigration on the barrier function of cultured intestinal epithelial monolayers. J Clin Invest. 1987;80:1104–13.
32. Colgan SP, Parkos CA, Delp C, Arnaout MA, Madara JL. Neutrophil migration across cultured intestinal epithelial monolayers is modulated by epithelial exposure to IFN-γ in a highly polarized fashion. J Cell Biol. 1993;120:785–98.
33. Shannon VR, Stenson WF, Holtzman MJ. Induction of epithelial arachidonate 12-lipoxygenase at active sites of inflammatory bowel disease. Am J Physiol. 1993;264:G104–11.
34. Gustafson-Svard C, Tagesson C, Boll R-M, Kald B. Tumor necrosis factor-α potentiates phospholipase A_2-stimulated release and metabolism of arachidonic acid in cultured intestinal epithelial cells (INT 407). Scand J Gastroenterol. 1993;28:323–30.
35. Barrett KE, Bigby TD. Involvement of arachidonic acid in the chloride secretory response of intestinal epithelial cells. Am J Physiol. 1993;264:C446–52.
36. Andoh A, Fujiyama Y, Bamba T, Hosoda S. Differential cytokine regulation of complement C3, C4, and factor B synthesis in human intestinal epithelial cell line, Caco-2. J Immunol. 1993;151:4239–47.
37. Eckmann L, Kagnoff MF, Fierer J. Epithelial cells secrete the chemokine interleukin-8 in response to bacterial entry. Infect Immun. 1993;61:4569–74.
38. McGee DW, Beagley KW, Aicher WK, McGhee JR. Transforming growth factor-β and IL-1β act in synergy to enhance IL-6 secretion by the intestinal epithelial cell line, IEC-6. J Immunol. 1993;151:970–8.
39. McGee DW, Beagley KW, Aicher WK, McGhee JR. Transforming growth factor-β enhances interleukin-6 secretion by intestinal epithelial cells. Immunology. 1992;77:7–12.
40. Eckmann L, Jung HC, Schurer-Maly C, Panja A, Morzycka-Wroblewska E, Kagnoff MF. Differential cytokine expression by human intestinal epithelial cell lines: regulated expression of interleukin 8. Gastroenterology. 1993;105:1689–97.

14
Immunomodulation of epithelium

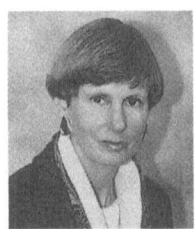

M. H. PERDUE

INTRODUCTION

Over recent years many studies have provided evidence that the immune system is a key regulatory system of intestinal function. Immunophysiology has been coined as a term to describe the control of physiology by immune cells and their chemical mediators. The interaction of immune cells with the gut epithelium plays an important role in host defense, acting to eliminate pathogens, antigens and other noxious material from the lumen of the gastrointestinal tract.

In the intestine the epithelium is a layer of single cells extending over the mucosal surface and down into the crypts. The main cells in the epithelium are the transporting enterocytes that are joined together at their apical surfaces by tight junctions and supported beneath the basal lamina by a fibroblast sheath. The lamina propria contains nerves and a large variety of immune cells including T and B lymphocytes, plasma cells, macrophages, mast cells, eosinophils and neutrophils. These cells can react to an antigenic stimulus either specifically via self-generated receptors, or by virtue of their ability to bind antibodies, or non-specifically to bacterial products such as endotoxin or other activators. Antigenic stimulation results in expansion of resident immune cell populations. Therefore, during inflammatory conditions of the gut, the mucosa becomes packed with immune cells in close proximity to the enterocytes. Mediators released from these cells have profound effects on epithelial functions.

The two main functions of the intestinal epithelium are: (a) a transport function for nutrients, ions and water and (b) a barrier function to prevent unimpeded uptake of antigenic material and microbes from the lumen. Our work indicates that both these functions are altered by immune reactions in response to various stimuli. We have used several experimental systems to demonstrate these effects, including *in-vivo* studies in rodent models of intestinal hypersensitivity or inflammation, isolated segments of intact intestine studied in Ussing chambers and *in-vitro* co-culture systems of immune cells with epithelial cell monolayers. Although our studies have examined the role of mast cells and T cells as effector cells, it is obvious from the studies of others that activation of immune cells such as neutrophils, macrophages and eosinophils also results in abnormalities of epithelial physiology.

MAST CELLS AND EPITHELIAL FUNCTION

Our early studies examined the effect of immune stimulation on intestinal transport. Rats sensitized to ovalbumin (with adjuvants that stimulate IgE production such as pertussis vaccine and/or alum) studied 14 days later demonstrated reduced net absorption of Na^+, K^+, Cl^- and water beginning within minutes of addition of antigen to the buffer perfusing the small intestine[1]. These transport changes were associated with histamine release and were inhibited by mast cell stabilization[2].

Subsequent experiments examined the mechanisms of the response using isolated segments of intestine studied in Ussing chambers where an increase in the short-circuit current (I_{sc}) indicates anion secretion (mainly Cl^-). Specific immune stimulation with ovalbumin antigen initiated a rapid (beginning within $\sim 2\,min$) secretory response that involved an increased short-circuit current, increased net Cl^- secretion and decreased net absorption[3] of Na^+ and Cl^-. Mast cell mediators were implicated resulting in enhanced production of cAMP in enterocytes immediately preceding the rise in intestinal I_{sc}. These findings resulted in the schema shown in Fig. 1A to explain the pathophysiology.

More direct evidence that specific immune stimulation of mast cells alters ion secretion came from studies of genetic mutant W/W^v mice. Mutations of the *ckit* locus result in an abnormal tyrosine kinase receptor for stem cell growth factor, necessary for the differentiation of functional mast cells from their precursors[4]. These mice have $< 0.3\%$ of the normal number of mast cells in skin and none at all in the gut[5]. W/W^v mice and $+/+$ congenic controls were sensitized in a similar manner to that described for rats. Studies of antigen-induced ion secretion in sensitized W/W^v mice demonstrated a small I_{sc} response to secondary antigen compared with the large response observed in intestine from congenic $+/+$ controls. However, mast cell reconstitution after adoptive transfer of congenic bone marrow cells restored the normal secretory response[6], demonstrating the important role of mast cells as effectors. In support of this hypothesis, antagonists of the mast cell mediators histamine and serotonin produced inhibition in $+/+$ mice but none in W/W^v.

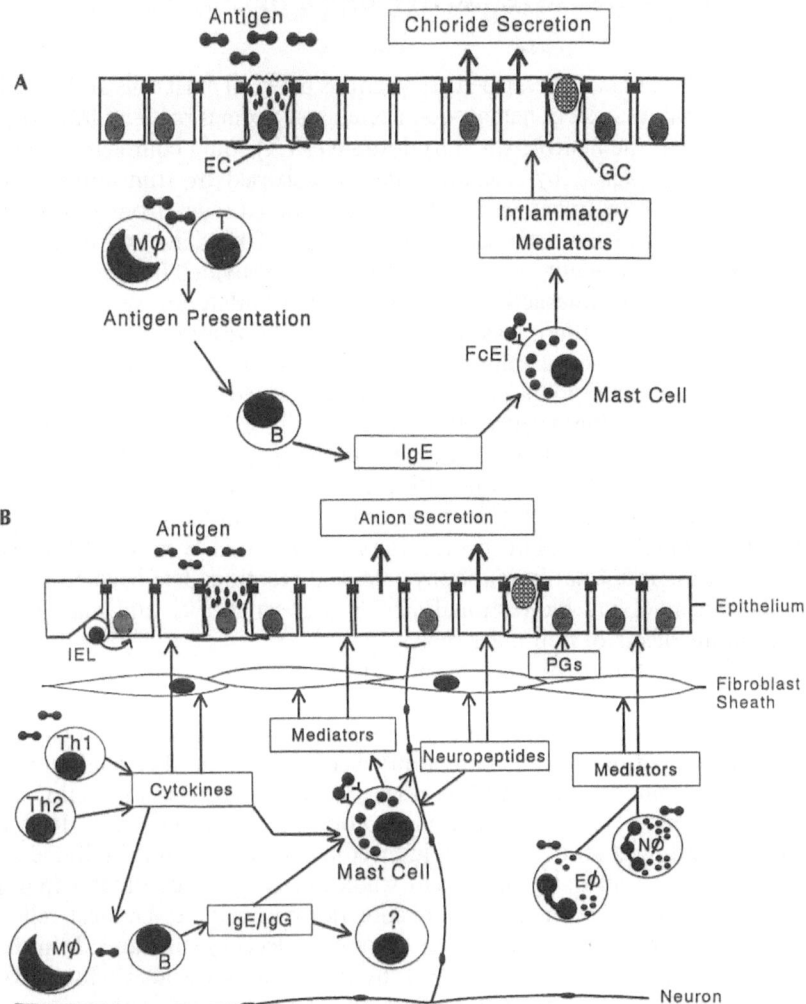

Fig. 1 **A**: Traditional schema for intestinal hypersensitivity reactions. Primary exposure to antigen results in the formation of IgE antibodies by β cells. Secondary exposure to antigen results in crosslinking of IgE bound to the mast cell surface and subsequent release of mediators that act on epithelial cells to stimulate secretion of chloride ions. **B**: Revised schema for intestinal hypersensitivity reactions. Primary exposure to antigen results in T cell activation, clonal expansion and cytokine release leading to β cell stimulation of antibody production, specifically IgE and subclasses of IgG. These antibodies bind to mast cells and other effector cells. Secondary exposure to antigen causes release of mediators and cytokines that attract other inflammatory cells to the site and stimulate nerves. Anion secretion from epithelial cells is the final outcome of the direct and indirect (via prostaglandin production from fibroblasts) effects of various cytokines, neuropeptides and mediators

MAST CELL–NERVE INTERACTIVE UNITS REGULATE PHYSIOLOGY

Anatomical studies have described associations between mast cells and nerves in the intestinal mucosa of nematode-infected and normal rats and humans[7]. We showed that the neurotoxin, tetrodotoxin (TTX) could completely block increases in I_{sc} caused by neurotransmitters released by transmural field stimulation[8]. Pretreatment with TTX of intestinal tissues from sensitized $+/+$ mice reduced the response to antigen by $> 50\%$. The fact that such inhibition was not evident in sensitized W/W^v mice provided further evidence that mast cells were interacting with nerves to stimulate ion secretion[6]. In the presence of TTX there was no difference in the response to antigen in mast cell-deficient vs mast cell-containing intestine. Therefore, the effects of mast cells to stimulate ion secretion appear to be mediated through nerves. However, some residual effects were still evident in mast cell-deficient mice, suggesting the participation of another effector cell or cells. In addition, stimulating nerves with field stimulation caused an increase in I_{sc}, and that response was significantly less in mast cell-deficient mice. Therefore, some of the effects of release of neurotransmitters are mediated by mast cells. Thus, the schema for intestinal immunophysiological reactions has become more complicated involving bidirectional signals between nerves and mast cells and separate effects of non-mast cells.

More direct studies of nerves and neural activity have demonstrated specific effects of inflammatory mediators on nerves. Histamine depolarizes neurons in the submucosal plexus and causes recurrent cyclical Cl^- secretion for prolonged periods via H_2 receptors[9]. Serotonin is another mediator of mast cells in some species, and has been shown to induce ion secretion by acting both on 5-HT$_2$ and 5-HT$_3$ receptors on enteric nerves[10]. It is a significant finding that the secretion induced by cholera toxin is inhibited by blocking these receptors[11], and recent studies in W/W^v mice suggest that a major source of serotonin released by cholera toxin may be the mast cell[12]. In addition, there is evidence that the secretory effects of substance P in the intestine are mediated, at least in part, by mast cell activation[13]. Intestinal responses to toxin A (from *Clostridium difficile*) associated with mast cell activation have been shown to be inhibited by substance P antagonists[14]. We also reported that the I_{sc} response to luminal antigen was reduced by $\sim 50\%$ by treating rats with capsaicin (depletes substance P and other neuropeptides from afferents)[15]. These latter studies provide support for mast cells interacting with substance P containing nerves in an axon reflex.

Prostaglandins and leukotrienes are released from mast cells and other immunocytes and may also affect neurons[16-18]. Sensitization itself alters the regulation of epithelial ion transport, particularly by LTB$_4$ interacting with enteric nerves[19]. Other studies have demonstrated that epithelial permeability to macromolecular antigens and inert probe molecules is influenced by neural factors in that antigen uptake both *in vivo* and *in vitro* is inhibited by tetrodotoxin[20,21].

Table 1 Mast cell mediators

Stored	
Amines	Histamine, serotonin
Cytokines	TNF-α
Enzymes	Tryptase; chymotryptase; RMCP-I, RMCP-II; carboxypeptidase
Proteoglycans	Heparin; chondroitin-di-β sulphate
Rapidly formed	
Lipid	Prostaglandins; leukotrienes; platelet-activating factor
Reactive species	Nitric oxide; oxygen radicals
Slowly formed	
Cytokines	IL-1, IL-3, IL-5, IL-6, IL-10; TNF-α; GM–CSF

ADDITIONAL CONSIDERATIONS RELATED TO MAST CELL ACTIVATION

Mast cells release biologically active products in addition to the well-known mediators of hypersensitivity such as histamine, serotonin, proteases and leukotrienes. Among these are a vast array of multifunctional cytokines, and other active compounds such as platelet-activating factor (PAF) and nitric oxide[22,23] (Table 1). Many of these compounds can stimulate ion secretion from intestinal preparations or epithelial monolayers (reviewed in ref. 24).

One mast cell cytokine that has been demonstrated to have significant biological effects is TNF-α, since it is stored and released from mast cells with prolonged kinetics following activation[25]. Recruitment of neutrophils following cutaneous anaphylaxis was significantly impaired in W/W^v mice and in congenic controls by treatment with an anti-TNF-α antibody[26]. TNF-α, like IFN-γ (see Chapter 13), may be responsible for epithelial pathophysiology[27]. Mast cells are also one source of TGF-β that is important in repair of epithelial injury[28]. Therefore, it is likely that mast cell activation contributes to a phenotypic change in epithelial cells during inflammation that may affect its transport function. These findings are relevant in a clinical setting, as mast cells have been implicated in the pathophysiology of diseases such as inflammatory bowel disease (IBD), celiac disease and food allergy, where debilitating diarrhea is a common symptom (reviewed in ref. 29).

NEUTROPHILS, EOSINOPHILS AND MACROPHAGES

Neutrophils, eosinophils and macrophages have all been implicated either directly or indirectly in affecting epithelial function. These phagocytes have some common properties in that when they are activated (by bacterial products or phagocytosis) they release potent chemicals such as reactive oxidant species (nitric oxide, hydrogen peroxide, N-chloramines), proteases and arachidonic acid metabolites[27]. These cells also synthesize and react to various cytokines. The release of inflammatory mediators has beneficial effects in removing particulate antigens and infected or transformed cells; however, epithelial injury and/or dysfunction can occur as a result. Ongoing activation of these cells in chronic diseases may account for significant intestinal pathophysiology. There is some evidence that monocytes in Crohn's disease are primed by bacterial endotoxin (lipopolysaccharide, LPS) for accentuated release of toxic oxygen metabolites[30].

LPS is a general activator of phagocytes, and has provided a significant amount of information regarding the potential contribution of these cells in inflammatory reactions. LPS injection into animals leads to nitric oxide production by phagocytic leukocytes that is required for the tumoricidal, tumoristatic and antimicrobial activity of macrophages[31].

Direct experimental studies have provided evidence for the effects of neutrophils on epithelial functions. Neutrophils stimulated to cross monolayers of the T84 human colonic cell line in response to gradients of chemotactic bacterial peptides such as f-met-leu-phe (fMLP)[32], cause a dramatic fall in transepithelial resistance and increased fluxes of inert probes as well as protein antigens. The translocation is facilitated by the expression of the $\beta2$ integrin (CD11b/CD18) on the surface of the neutrophil, binding with the appropriate ligand on the enterocytes[33]. Madara and colleagues report that treatment with IFN-γ elicits enhanced neutrophil transepithelial migration[34]. Activated neutrophils in the intestinal lumen (as in the case of crypt abscesses) can evoke Cl^- secretion from the epithelium by the release of a molecule originally termed neutrophil-derived cAMP[34].

Eosinophils isolated from human blood evoke Cl^- scretion from T84 monolayers by the release of cAMP[35]. The effects of other eosinophil products such as major basic protein and eosinophil-derived neurotoxin have not been tested in the gut, but they have deleterious effects on the epithelial lining of the airways. In addition, release of eosinophil cationic protein has been demonstrated in response to allergen in food-allergic individuals[36] and in response to gliadin in patients with celiac disease[37]. Eosinophils have been shown to contribute to the inflammatory response in other systems[38] and demonstrate an altered appearance in inflamed intestine in Crohn's disease[39].

T CELLS

The gastrointestinal tract is the largest immune organ in the body, and represents a major T cell compartment where the cells are located in the lamina propria or epithelium (intraepithelial lymphocytes, IEL). T cells are further classified by the presence of surface markers into helper or suppressor/cytotoxic cells, T_h or $T_{s/c}$. Studies in the early 1970s implicated T cells in causing villus atrophy/crypt hyperplasia. Subsequent studies examining transfer of T cells from normal donors to irradiated or immuno-compromised recipients helped consolidate the fact that T cells influence intestinal morphology by affecting epithelial proliferation (reviewed in ref. 40). Using human fetal intestinal explants it was shown that in-situ specific T cell stimulation led to a crypt cell hyperplasia that preceded villus atrophy[41]. We confirmed that this sequence of events also occurred when T cells were stimulated during intestinal inflammatory reactions by nematode parasitic infection[42,43]. It is clear that T cell activation can result in increased epithelial proliferation rates in the crypt mediated by the release of cytokines from T_h cells.

The impact of T cells on the two main roles of the intestinal epithelium has not been extensively studied. To address this question we have established an *in-vitro* co-culture model of inflammation consisting of confluent T84 epithelial cell monolayers and peripheral blood mononuclear cells (PBM) from human volunteers, in which the T cell component is stimulated via the T cell receptor. We have presented preliminary findings showing that such activation in mixed lymphocyte/monocyte populations can alter epithelial physiology[44]. Monolayers that are exposed to activated T cells demonstrate a reduced ion secretory capacity to several known secretagogues and increased permeability. Transepithelial resistance is also decreased across monolayers exposed to non-activated PBM, as well as to PBM in which T cells are activated. In support of these findings, co-culture of T84 monolayers with lamina propria lymphocytes isolated from intestine surgically removed from ulcerative colitis patients increased epithelial permeability[45]. These *in-vitro* approaches provide the opportunity to accumulate data on the mechanism whereby immunocytes affect various aspects of epithelial function.

PROSTAGLANDINS AND IMMUNE CELL ACTIVATION

Other findings that have been of great importance in developing our understanding of immunophysiology are those that described the role of prostaglandins in mediating the effects of inflammatory mediators[46]. Since epithelial cells generate small amounts of prostaglandins relative to cells of the lamina propria, and since activation of isolated immune/inflammatory cells initiates the metabolism of arachidonic acid, the participation of accessory cells has been suggested. Elegant co-culture studies of T84 epithelial monolayers with fibroblasts demonstrated that prostaglandin production by fibroblasts is responsible for a large component of the secretory response to inflammatory mediators originating from immune cells[47]. These studies demonstrated that fibroblasts generate PGE_2 and prostacyclin that act directly or indirectly via enteric nerves to cause secretion in rat colon[48].

SUMMARY AND CONCLUSIONS

As a result of our studies, and those of others, there is no longer a controversy regarding immune regulation of epithelial functions. In addition, in many cases the effects of immune activation are amplified by nerves. Thus, it would appear that an effective system has evolved to detect and react to antigenic challenge of the gut via neural reflex mechanisms. The information accumulated over the recent past has resulted in a modification of our original schema of hypersensitivity reactions (Fig. 1B). The benefit of this system to the organism in acute situations must be weighed against its deleterious effects when continuous activation results in ongoing release of mediators leading to chronic inflammatory diseases. Our knowledge is now probing the mechanisms that turn off such responses. However, it is clear that the concepts of immunophysiology are essential for deciphering the pathophysiology of IBD and identifying targets for therapeutic agents.

References

1. Perdue MH, Chung M, Gall DG. The effect of intestinal anaphylaxis on gut function in the rat. Gastroenterology. 1984;86:391–7.
2. Perdue MH, Gall DG. Transport abnormalities during intestinal anaphylaxis in the rat. Effect of anti-allergic agents. J Allergy Clin Immunol. 1985;76:498–503.
3. Perdue MH, Gall DG. Intestinal anaphylaxis in the rat: jejunal response to in vitro antigen exposure. Am J Physiol. 1986;250:G427–31.
4. Galli SJ, Kitamura Y. Genetically mast cell-deficient W/W^v and SI/SI^d mice. Their value for the analysis of the roles of mast cells in biologic responses in vivo. Am J Pathol. 1987;127:191–8.
5. Wershil BK, Galli SJ. Gastrointestinal mast cells. New approaches for analyzing their function in vivo. Gastroenterol Clin N Am. 1991;20:613–27.
6. Perdue MH, Masson S, Wershil BK, Galli SJ. Role of mast cells in ion transport abnormalities associated with intestinal anaphylaxis. Correction of the diminished secretory response in genetically mast cell-deficient W/Wv mice by bone marrow transplantation. J Clin Invest. 1991;87:687–93.
7. Stead RH, Perdue MH, Blennerhassett G, Kakuta Y, Sestini P, Bienenstock J. The innervation of mast cells. In: Freir S, editor. Neuroendocrine-immune network. Boca Raton: CRC Press; 1990:19–37.
8. Perdue MH, Davison JS. Response of jejunal mucosa to electrical transmural stimulation and two neurotoxins. Am J Physiol. 1986;251:G642–8.
9. Cooke HJ, Wang Y, Rogers R. Coordination of CL⁻ secretion and concentration by a histamine H2-receptor agonist in guinea pig distal colon. Am J Physiol. 1993;265:G973–8.
10. Frieling T, Cooke HJ, Wood JD. Serotonin receptors on submucous neurons in guinea pig colon. Am J Physiol. 1991;261:G1017–23.
11. Sjöqvist A, Cassuto J, Jodal M, Lundgren O. Actions of serotonin antagonists on cholera-toxin-induced intestinal fluid secretion. Acta Physiol Scand. 1992;145:229–37.
12. Wang L, Savedia S, Benjamin M, Perdue MH. The role of mast cells in intestinal immunophysiology. In: Mestecky J, editor. Advances in experimental medicine and biology. New York: Plenum Press, 1994 (In press).
13. Wang L, Stanis AM, Perdue MH. Activation of mast cells by substance P in the regulation of ion secretion in the mouse intestine. Gastroenterology. 1994 (In press) (Abstr.).
14. Pothoulakis C, Castagliuolo I, LaMont JT et al. CP 96,345, a substance P antagonist, inhibits rat intestinal responses to Clostridium difficile toxin A but not cholera toxin. Proc Natl Acad Sci. 1994 (In press).
15. Crowe SE, Sestini P, Perdue MH. Allergic reactions of rat jejunal mucosa. Ion transport responses to luminal antigen and inflammatory mediators. Gastroenterology. 1990;99:74–82.
16. Levine JD, Lam D, Taiwo YO, Donatoni P, Goetzl EJ. Hyperalgesic properties of 15-lipoxygenase products of arachidonic acid. Proc Natl Acad Sci. 1986;83:5331–4.
17. Diener M, Bridges RJ, Knoblock SF, Rummel W. Neuronally mediated and direct effects of prostaglandins on ion transport in rat colon descendens. Naunyn-Schmiedeberg's Arch Pharmacol. 1989;337:74–8.
18. Hammerbeck DM, Brown DR. Neurally mediated actions of leukotrienes on ion transport in guinea pig distal colon. J Pharmacol Exp Ther. 1993;264:384–90.
19. Javed NH, Barrett KE, Wang YZ, Bidinger J, Cooke HJ. Enhanced tissue responsiveness in colonic ion transport of cow's milk-sensitized guinea pigs. Agents Actions. 1994 (In press).
20. Crowe SE, Soda K, Stanisz AM, Perdue MH. Intestinal permeability in allergic rats: nerve involvement in antigen-induced changes. Am J Physiol. 1993;264:G617–23.
21. Kimm MH, Curtis GH, Hardin JA, Gall DG. Transport of bovine serum albumin across rat jejunum: The role of the enteric nervous system. Am J Physiol. 1994;266:G186–93.

22. Galli SJ, Gordon JR, Wershill BK. Cytokine production by mast cells and basophils. Curr Opin Immunol. 1991;3:865–73.
23. Serafin WE, Austen KF. Mediators of immediate hypersensitivity reactions. N Engl J Med. 1987;317:30–4.
24. Powell DW. Epithelial secretory responses to inflammation. Platelet activating factor and reactive oxygen metabolites. Ann NY Acad Sci. 1992;664:232–47.
25. Payan DG. Neuropeptides and inflammation: the role of substance P. Annu Rev Med. 1989;40:341–52.
26. Wershil BK, Wang Z-K, Gordon JR, Galli SJ. Recruitment of neutrophils during IgE-dependent cutaneous late phase responses in the mouse is mast cell dependent: partial inhibition of the reaction with antiserum against tumor necrosis factor-α. J Clin Invest. 1991;87:446–53.
27. McKay DM, Perdue H. Intestinal epithelial function: the case for immunophysiological regulation. Cells and mediators. (Part 1 of 2). Dig Dis Sci. 1993;38:1377–87.
28. Ciacci C, Lind SE, Podolsky DK. Transforming growth factor-beta regulation of migration in wounded rat intestinal epithelial monolayers. Gastroenterology. 1993;105:93–101.
29. Crowe SE, Perdue MH. Gastrointestinal food hypersensitivity: basic mechanisms of pathophysiology. Gastroenterology. 1992;103:1075–95.
30. Baldassano RN, Schreiber S, Johnston RB, Fu RDJ, Muraki T, MacDermott RP. Crohn's disease monocytes are primed for accentuated release of toxic oxygen metabolites. Gastroenterology. 1993;105:60–6.
31. Grisham MB, Yamada T. Neutrophils, nitrogen oxides, and inflammatory bowel disease. Ann NY Acad Sci. 1992;664:103–15.
32. Nash S, Parkos C, Nusrat A, Delp C, Madara JL. In vitro model of intestinal crypt abscess. J Clin Invest. 1991;87:1474–7.
33. Parkos CA, Delp C, Arnaout MA, Madara JL. Neutrophil migration across a cultured intestinal epithelium. J Clin Invest. 1991;88:1605–12.
34. Colgan SP, Parkos CA, Delp C, Arnaout MA, Madara JL. Neutrophil migration cross cultured intestinal epithelial monolayers is modulated by epithelial exposure to IFN-gamma in a highly polarized fashion. J Cell Biol. 1993;120:785–98.
35. Resnick MB, Colgan SP, Patapoff TW et al. Activated eosinophils evoke chloride secretion in model intestinal epithelia primarily via regulated release of 5'-AMP. J Immunol. 1993;151:5716–23.
36. Knutson TW, Bengtsson U, Dannaeus A et al. Intestinal reactivity in allergic and nonallergic patients: an approach to determine the complexity of the mucosal reaction. J Allergy Clin Immunol. 1993;91:553–9.
37. Lavö B, Knutson L, Lööf L, Odlind B, Venge P, Hällgren R. Challenge with gliadin induces eosinophil and mast cell activation in the jejunum of patients with celiac disease. Am J Med. 1989;87:655–60.
38. Denburg JA, Otsuka H, Ohnisi M, Ruhno J, Bienenstock J, Dolovich J. Contribution of basophil/mast cell and eosinophil growth and differentiation to the allergic tissue inflammatory response. Int Arch Allergy Appl Immunol. 1987;82:321–6.
39. Dvorak AM, Monahan RA, Osage JE, Dickersin GR. Crohn's disease: transmission electron microscopic studies. II. Immunologic inflammatory response. Alterations of mast cells, basophils, eosinophils, and the microvasculature. Hum Pathol. 1980;11:606–19.
40. MacDonald TT, Spencer J. Cell-mediated immune injury in the intestine. Gastroenterol Clin N Am. 1992;21:367–86.
41. MacDonald TT, Spencer J. Evidence that activated mucosal T cells play a role in the pathogenesis of enteropathy in human small intestine. J Exp Med. 1988;167:1341–9.
42. Perdue MH, Ramage JK, Burget D, Marshall JS, Masson S. Intestinal mucosal injury is associated with mast cell activation and leukotriene generation during Nippostrongylus-induced inflammation in the rat. Dig Dis Sci. 1989;34:724–31.
43. D'Inca R, Ernst P, Hunt RH, Perdue MH. Role of T lymphocytes in intestinal mucosal injury. Inflammatory changes in athymic nude rats. Dig Dis Sci. 1992;37:33–9.
44. McKay DM, Croitoru K, Perdue MH. Activation of T lymphocytes causes increased permeability of T84 epithelial monolayers and reduces responses to secretagogues. Gastroenterology. 1993;104:A741 (abstr.).
45. Roche JK, Planchon S, Lai J, Fiocchi C. Effect of ulcerative colitis immune mucosal cells

upon epithelial barrier function. Gastroenterology. 1993;104:A771 (abstr.).

46. Powell DW. Immunophysiology of intestinal electrolyte transport. In: Schultz SG, editor. Handbook of physiology: the gastrointestinal system. IV. Rockville, MD: American Physiologic Society; 1991:591–641.

47. Berschneider HM, Powell DW. Fibroblasts modulate intestinal secretory response to inflammatory mediators. J Clin Invest. 1992;89:484–9.

48. Bern MJ, Sturbaum CW, Karaylcin SS, Berschneider HM, Wachsman JT, Powell DW. Immune system control of rat and rabbit colonic electrolyte transport. Role of prostaglandins and enteric nervous system. J Clin Invest. 1989;83:1810–20.

15
The enteric nervous system in intestinal inflammation

K. A. SHARKEY and E. J. PARR

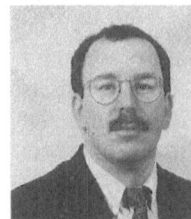

K. A. SHARKEY

INTRODUCTION

For about 40 years, nerves in the wall of the intestine have been postulated to play a role in the pathogenesis of inflammatory bowel disease (IBD). Storsteen and colleagues[1] were the first to demonstrate that enteric neurons were involved in this process, by providing histological evidence for an increased number of myenteric ganglion cells in chronic ulcerative colitis. Similar observations were also made in Crohn's disease[2]. Extrinsic nerves innervating the bowel have also been implicated in these diseases, based not only on the common observation of abdominal pain in IBD but also on clinical observations that vagotomy and pelvic nerve lesions could modify, and in some cases 'improve', the outcome of IBD[3-5]. Additionally, autonomic neuropathy has been described in IBD and might contribute to the symptoms of these diseases[6,7]. Though surgical denervation is no longer used for the therapeutic management of IBD, the role of nerves in this multifactorial disease has become established. This review will focus on human and animal studies on the role of nerves in intestinal inflammation. Consideration will be given to two possible ways that nerves are involved in IBD. First, through the local release of transmitters nerves may play a role in the development or maintenance of inflammation. Second, once initiated (by whatever means), the processes of inflammation could cause disruption of the normal pattern of innervation and the interactions of nerves and their target tissues. Finally, acknowledgement of the role of the central nervous system in modulation of immune function must be made, but it is outside the scope of this review to consider this aspect of the nervous regulation of inflammation.

INNERVATION OF THE GASTROINTESTINAL TRACT

The GI tract is innervated by extrinsic sympathetic and parasympathetic autonomic nerves, primary afferent fibers that follow the course of the autonomic nerves and by enteric nerves[8]. Though thought of as largely efferent, it is clear that the majority of extrinsic nerves innervating the bowel are afferents[9]. These nerves respond to noxious mechanical and chemical stimulation and are mostly sensitive to the selective sensory neurotoxin capsaicin[9-11]. They contain a number of biologically active peptides, in particular substance P and calcitonin gene-related peptide (CGRP)[12]. The local release of these peptides from the peripheral terminals of primary afferents gives rise to *neurogenic inflammation*[13]. This is manifested as local vasodilatation, the extravasation of plasma proteins and mast cell degranulation, among other effects. The contribution that primary afferents make to inflammatory processes in the GI tract is not clear, in part due to the complexity of intestinal innervation and the fact that many transmitters found in primary afferents are also present in enteric nerves.

The enteric nervous system (ENS) consists of two interconnected ganglionated plexuses and an extensive fiber and terminal network that innervates all components of the bowel wall[8]. The ganglionated plexuses lie between the longitudinal and circular muscle layers (myenteric plexus) and in the submucosa (submucous plexus). One feature that has come to light in recent years is the observation that a single enteric neuron may contain more than one transmitter or neuron-specific marker. This has led to the concept of chemical coding of enteric neurons[14]. Indeed, so successful has this been in the guinea-pig ileum that the groups of Furness and Costa have apparently accounted for 100% of neurons in both plexuses[14-16]. However, it should be noted that this detailed coding has not been fully explored in many other regions or in other species, so its true value or applicability is currently limited. Chemical coding has recently been extended further by combining studies based on the projections of identified neurons and coupling this with their electrophysiological classification[15-17]. Taken together, a structural and functional mapping of the guinea-pig ileum has been achieved. Thus, by visualizing identified cell types, inferences can be made about their function and changes in the number or proportion of given cells might then be indicative of altered function.

Neurons in the ENS are in a unique environment: they are regularly distorted by peristaltic contractions, the wall of the gut contains a resident population of inflammatory cells which contribute to a physiological state of basal (low-level) inflammation and there is a constant remodeling of the mucosa, due to epithelial sloughing, which includes remodeling of the neural connections. This environment leads to a cell phenotype that differs substantially from other autonomic neurons. For example, work from my laboratory has recently shown that enteric neurons constitutively express high levels of the protein B-50[18] and certain proto-oncogene products such as Fos and Myc[19,20].

ENTERIC INNERVATION IN INFLAMMATION – ANIMAL STUDIES

Peptides

In animal models of GI inflammation much of the work to date has focused on substance P, because of its role as a mediator of neurogenic inflammation[21]. Using a hapten-induced model of ileitis (intraluminal injection of trinitrobenzene sulfonic acid [TNBS]) it is clear that the pattern of substance P immunoreactivity in the submucosa of the guinea pig ileum is modified[22]. Substance P in the ileum is in primary afferent and enteric nerves, and the former (detected on the basis of their location around blood vessels) appeared particularly affected. There is an initial reduction in substance P (by 24 h, Fig. 1) consistent with a sustained release, followed by a gradual increase in the intensity and density of immunoreactive nerves and an increased quantity of substance P, first in enteric and later in primary afferent nerves, until by 21–30 days the pattern of innervation has returned to normal. When substance P and CGRP were measured in rabbit colitis or ferret jejunitis/ileitis models, they were found to be reduced up to 48 h after induction of the inflammation[23,24]. In the rabbit it was also found that the density and intensity of immunoreactivity were reduced, though the overall pattern of nerves was similar in inflamed and control animals[24].

In jejunitis due to *Trichinella spiralis* infection, Collins' group showed substance P levels were increased in the myenteric plexus up to 6 days postinfection[25]. This increase was abolished in capsaicin-treated rats, indicating a primary afferent origin of the substance P. It was also abolished in congenitally athymic rats, suggesting that T lymphocytes play some role in the increase, probably through release of cytokines. Together, we have followed up that observation and demonstrated that interleukin-1β is involved in the increase in substance P which was found to be exclusively neuronal[26]. The cellular mechanisms and inflammatory cell types underlying this neuroimmune interaction in the myenteric plexus have yet to be elucidated, and whether similar mechanisms apply to the submucous plexus is also unknown. In contrast to substance P, we have preliminary evidence that the number of vasoactive intestinal polypeptide (VIP)-immunoreactive neurons in the submucous plexus of the guinea pig were not affected in TNBS-induced ileitis, but VIP-containing neurons in the myenteric plexus were actually increased[27]. Similarly, Kishimoto *et al.* observed an increased VIP immunoreactivity in neurons and fibers in both plexuses of the colon, and an elevated content of VIP in dextran sulfate-induced colitis in rats[28]. Interestingly, these increases are consistent with preliminary reports of increased VIP mRNA in IBD in humans[29].

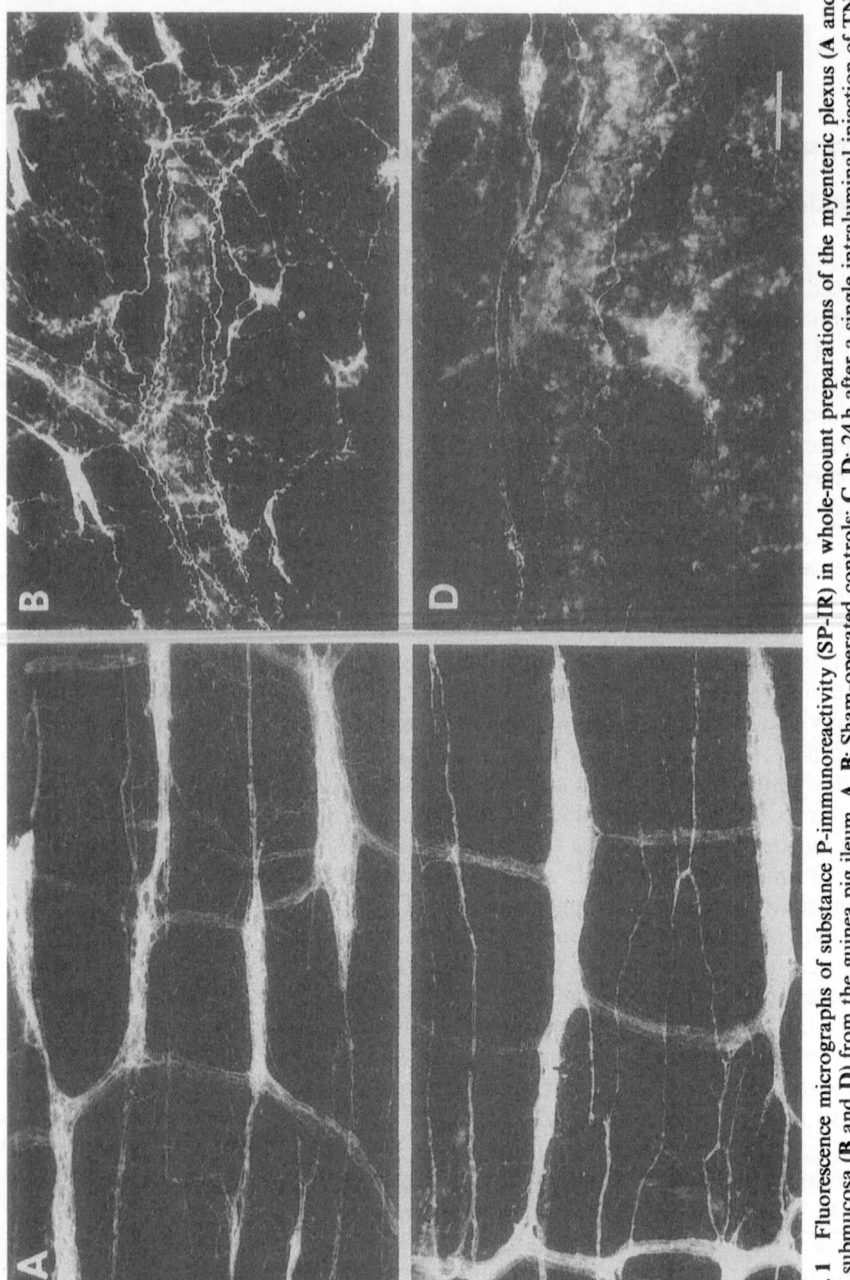

Fig. 1 Fluorescence micrographs of substance P-immunoreactivity (SP-IR) in whole-mount preparations of the myenteric plexus (**A** and **C**) and submucosa (**B** and **D**) from the guinea pig ileum. **A**, **B**: Sham-operated controls; **C**, **D**: 24 h after a single intraluminal injection of TNBS. Note that 24 h after the induction of inflammation there was a substantial reduction in SP-IR in the submucosa, particularly that associated with blood vessels. No reduction, and possibly a slight increase, in SP-IR was observed in the myenteric plexus. Full details can be found in ref. 22, from which the figure is taken (with permission) (Scale bar: 100 μm)

Capsaicin-sensitive nerves

In intestinal inflammation only a few studies have examined the role of capsaicin-sensitive nerves[12]. In rats with colitis induced with TNBS, acetic acid or dextran sulfate sodium, neonatal capsaicin treatment augments damage at various times after induction of inflammation[30-33]. This suggests that primary afferent nerves are involved in aspects of the restoration of mucosal integrity in 'chronic' inflammation; however, further confirmation and extension of these data are required.

In rats sensitized to egg albumin, neonatal capsaicin treatment reduced the short-circuit current responses (an indicator of active chloride secretion) to antigen challenge by about 50%[34]. This implies a role for these nerves in the regulation of secretory events in inflammation. Since a mast cell stabilizer also blocked secretion induced by antigen challenge, it is conceivable that some of the effects of nerves are mediated through a nerve–mast cell interaction[34]. Secretion is an important physiological defense mechanism to luminal irritants (or inflammatory agents). Because of this we have examined some aspects of the neural control of secretory events. We have recently shown that mast cells are essential for nerve-mediated chloride secretion in the rat ileum in uninflamed tissues[35]. Another important secretory product is mucin, which acts as a physical defense mechanism, and whose release is enhanced in inflammation[36]. It has now been demonstrated, by us and others, that capsaicin-sensitive nerves are involved in the neural regulation of mucin secretion[37,38].

Transmitters and receptors

An area that has lacked attention until recently has been neurotransmitter receptors in inflammation. A recent study has corrected this by examining the regulation of adrenergic receptors on smooth muscle/myenteric plexus preparations of guinea-pig jejunum[39]. In this report, α_1- and α_2-adrenergic receptors were up-regulated 10 days after induction of jejunitis with TNBS, whereas β-adrenergic receptors were down-regulated. The authors suggested that motility disturbances seen in small bowel inflammation might be related to this inverse receptor regulation.

Finally, a few studies have investigated transmitter release from the ENS or its electrophysiological consequences. Both acetylcholine and noradrenaline release are depressed in *Trichinella*-infected rats[40,41]. The depression observed in infected animals was mimicked in both cases by preincubation of tissues with interleukin-1β, suggesting that it may be the inflammatory mediator of this effect[42]. This is further supported by studies in which an interleukin-1 receptor antagonist was given to infected rats. In this case noradrenaline release was enhanced compared to infected controls[42]. In contrast to the depressed release of acetylcholine seen in rats, neurons in the myenteric plexus of *Trichinella*-infected guinea pigs were found to have an enhanced sensitivity to applied acetylcholine – potentially compensating for the reduced release[43]. Although it appears that this is not due to marked changes in electrical properties of the neurons, there was a trend towards enhanced excitability of neuronal membranes. In addition, neurons from infected animals also showed a marked increase in responsiveness to histamine[43]. This has led Wood and his colleagues to suggest that histamine, released from mast cells, is responsible for many of the observed pathophysiological effects of inflammation through actions at the level of the enteric plexuses[44,45].

ENTERIC INNERVATION IN INFLAMMATION – HUMAN STUDIES

The original observation of increased ganglion cells in the ENS in IBD not only established a neural involvement in these diseases but also initiated a controversy: how can there be more enteric neurons if they are postmitotic? This has not been resolved to date, but evidence suggests that adult enteric neurons (at least in animals) have a remarkable plasticity of form, and the capacity for growth and active DNA synthesis[46,47]. Though cell division in adult neurons seems unlikely, it cannot be completely excluded as a possibility since, in a study in humans, the number of centrioles in neurons of the submucous plexus was reported to be increased in Crohn's disease[48], which is potentially indicative of mitosis. Another possible explanation for the observed enteric neuronal hyperplasia is that this disorder is established early in development, but does not become clinically apparent until much later in life. This would imply that IBD is directly related to a developmental defect that results in abnormal proliferation and/or survival of enteric neuronal precursors. A third possible explanation is that there are precursor cells in enteric ganglia capable of proliferation into neurons. Whether or not this is likely is not known, but it should be considered as a possibility in the light of observations of the presence of stem cells in the adult CNS[49].

In addition to neuronal hyperplasia, ganglion cell and axonal degeneration and necrosis have also been observed in IBD[50-52]. The pathological abnormalities of IBD appear to be dependent on the disease (Crohn's vs ulcerative colitis), the region of the intestinal wall (mucosa vs muscle) and whether or not the tissue was from a site of active disease[50-52]. The damage observed might be immunologically mediated, since it has been shown that neurons (and glia) in tissues from Crohn's disease display the major histocompatibility class II antigen on their surface[53]. Since this is important for antigen presentation to T lymphocytes it seems likely that it is in some way linked to the response of nerves to these inflammatory cells; however, its significance is at present not clear. Also at the cellular level in Crohn's disease, it appears that there is an up-regulation of nerve growth factor in coarse nerve fibers in actively inflamed regions of bowel[54]. This may reflect remodeling or regrowth of nerves, or their response to inflammatory stimuli, but at present this also is not known.

There have been a number of studies that have examined neuropeptides in the bowel in IBD, and these have found both quantitative and qualitative changes in the innervation. The best-studied peptides have been VIP and substance P. In the earliest reports VIP-immunoreactive fibers were found to be coarser, thicker and more intensely stained in Crohn's disease compared to tissues from ulcerative colitis or controls[55,56]. Associated with this was an increase in VIP content in full-wall thickness and biopsy specimens from Crohn's disease. Later studies have not been able to confirm these findings. In one study VIP-immunoreactive nerves were found to be coarser in Crohn's disease compared to controls, but the levels of VIP were not found to be elevated in the ileum and were significantly reduced in the colon[57]. In other studies VIP-immunoreactive nerves were reduced in the colon in Crohn's disease[58-60] and ulcerative colitis[60], as was the content of VIP measured by radioimmunoassay (RIA)[61]. Why such differences have been found between studies is not completely clear, but regional variation, disease state and sampling may all contribute. However, real differences may exist, because in some of these studies substance P was also assessed and far fewer discrepancies were noted. In support of the studies that show a reduction in VIP, one report has measured plasma levels of VIP and shown a significant positive correlation between VIP levels and disease activity[62]. In active disease VIP levels nearly doubled. This may indicate a massive and sustained release of VIP in active disease which is consistent with reduced levels detected in tissues, though it should be noted that other explanations are possible.

In the case of substance P, it appears to be increased in the mucosa in ulcerative colitis as determined by RIA[61,63,64] and by immunohistochemistry[58]. In one study this was shown to correlate with the extent of inflammation, indicating a potential role of this peptide in contributing to the pathogenesis of this state[64]. On the other hand, substance P appears to be relatively unaffected in Crohn's disease[57,61]. However, it has been demonstrated that receptors for substance P were up-regulated on blood vessels and lymphoid follicles in Crohn's disease and ulcerative colitis[65].

A few studies have also examined other peptidergic neuronal systems. Enkephalin and bombesin appear to be reduced in Crohn's disease but increased in ulcerative colitis[61]. Calcitonin gene-related peptide was reported to be reduced in the muscle layers of resected specimens in Crohn's disease[30]. Somatostatin-containing neurons in the submucous plexus were found to be reduced in Crohn's disease but not ulcerative colitis, and this was unrelated to the degree of inflammation[66]. Reduced levels of somatostatin have been seen in IBD[67], but these reflect both neuronal and enteroendocrine cell pools of the peptide, and so are hard to interpret. Catecholamine-containing nerves are apparently increased in ulcerative colitis[68,69], but tissue catecholamine levels were in one study unaffected[68] and in another increased[70]. Finally, there is a preliminary report of an up-regulation of nitric oxide synthase in neurons of the submucous and myenteric plexuses in Crohn's disease[71].

INFLAMMATORY CELLS AS TARGETS FOR THE ENTERIC AND AUTONOMIC NERVOUS SYSTEMS

Mast cells and nerves are found in association in villi of the small intestine[72,73]. Stead et al. have shown that in rats infected with a nematode there is remodeling of nerve fibers in the villi associated with changes in the mast cell density of the tissue[74]. This implies a structural and presumably functional nerve–mast cell relationship in the bowel, which is supported by studies described above that demonstrate the importance of mast cells in nerve-mediated secretory events. The role of mast cells in models of IBD such as TNBS-treated animals is less clear, and their relationships with nerves have yet to be examined. Since the submucosa is an important interface of nerves, mast cells and blood vessels, all of which may play a role in neurogenic inflammation, the relationships of these structures in this region in inflammation deserve examination. In a recent ultrastructural study in patients with IBD, Dvorak *et al.* demonstrated that nerve–mast cell associations were significantly increased (as were mast cells) in ulcerative colitis compared to Crohn's disease or control tissues[75]. However, this study showed that the distances between nerves and mast cells were greater than those described in other animal or human studies[72,73]. This does not imply that they were not linked functionally, and further examination of this issue is required

Other cells – such as macrophages, plasma cells and eosinophils – are probably also involved in neurally mediated responses and are also associated with nerves. Macrophages are present in the ENS and eosinophils, and plasma cells have been shown to be innervated in human and animal GI tract[76–78].

Another cell type of relevance to inflammation is the lymphocyte. The GI tract is a rich source of lymphocytes, and indeed plays a vital role in exposure to antigens and in lymphocyte recirculation[79,80]. Ottaway was the first to show a structural and functional link between the VIP innervation and lymphocyte function[81]. Substance P also affects lymphocyte function, and can increase lymphocyte trafficking through peripheral lymph nodes. In preliminary experiments we have demonstrated that substance P and CGRP can increase trafficking through the GI tract[82]. In this context it is interesting to note that capsaicin-treated rats have been shown to respond less vigorously to an antigenic challenge, and substance P can reverse this effect[83,84]. Taken together these findings suggest that neuropeptides may prime cells of the immune system to respond to a challenge, such as an inflammatory stimulus, and hence they are able to modulate the functional capacity of the immune system in a given situation.

MODULATION OF INFLAMMATION USING NEUROACTIVE COMPOUNDS

Can nerves initiate or maintain the inflammatory state once it has been initiated? This is an important question, since it could lead to novel therapeutic strategies for the management of IBD. Recent evidence in humans and animals broadly supports the idea of a nervous involvement in the inflammatory process. In 1985, the α_2-adrenergic agonist clonidine was used clinically in the treatment of ulcerative colitis[85]. Though the results of this study looked promising, others have reported less successful results[86,87] and the side-effects of this compound probably preclude its wide use as an agent. Another compound of interest is nicotine. Treatment of ulcerative colitis patients with nicotine gum or transdermal nicotine patches was found to be effective in some patients[88,89]. As with the clonidine studies, the site of action of nicotine has not been determined. Given the enormous number of actions of nicotine centrally and peripherally it is unclear to what extent a peripheral neuromodulatory action might be a factor in its effects.

Another class of drugs which have been reported to be beneficial are local anesthetics. Björck *et al.* have reported that topical lidocaine improves the histological and clinical appearance of proctitis and proctosigmoiditis[90,91]. To follow up on this we performed a controlled study of the effects of lidocaine in TNBS-induced colitis in rats, in which we confirmed and extended these findings[92]. In particular we observed that pretreatment of rats with lidocaine substantially reduced the severity of colitis, and treatment after the initiation of inflammation was also effective in reducing disease severity. Though it is clear that local anesthetics can have actions other than to block conduction of nervous impulses, this mechanism is an appealing one to consider for future studies.

SUMMARY

The role of the ENS in intestinal inflammation has been established. At this stage more questions remain than have been answered as to how it is involved, and to what extent alterations in structure or neuronal phenotype contribute to the pathogenesis of IBD. Many of the functional disturbances observed in IBD are likely due to an alteration in the ENS, either structurally through disruptions of nerve–target relationships or by modifications of neurotransmitters or their receptors. Careful studies investigating the effects of intestinal inflammation on the ENS at the cellular and molecular level are required to achieve a complete understanding of these complex diseases. Finally, it appears that the ENS might be a potential therapeutic target in IBD, and that neuroactive drugs that act locally could represent useful agents in the management of this disease.

Acknowledgements

This work was supported by grants from the Medical Research Council of Canada and the Crohn's and Colitis Foundation of Canada. Keith Sharkey is an Alberta Heritage Foundation for Medical Research (AHFMR) Scholar, and Edward Parr is a recipient of an AHFMR studentship.

References

1. Storsteen KA, Kernohan JW, Bargen JA. The myenteric plexus in chronic ulcerative colitis. Surg Gynecol Obstet. 1953;97:335–43.
2. Davis DR, Dockerty MB, Mayo CW. The myenteric plexus in regional enteritis: A study of the number of ganglion cells in the ileum in 24 cases. Surg Gynecol Obstet. 1955;101:208–16.

3. Shakiroff BGP, Hinton JW. Denervation of the pelvic colon for ulcerative colitis. Surg Forum. 1950;1:134–9.
4. Thorek P. Vagotomy for idiopathic ulcerative colitis and regional enteritis. Results in 21 cases. JAMA. 1951;145:140–6.
5. Dennis C, Eddy FD, Frykman HM, McCarthy HM, Westover D. The response to vagotomy in idiopathic ulcerative colitis and regional enteritis. Ann Surg. 1948;128:479–96.
6. Lindgren S, Stewenius J, Sjölund K, Lilja B, Sudkvist G. Autonomic vagal nerve dysfuntion in patients with ulcerative colitis. Scand J Gastroenterol. 1993;28:638–42.
7. Lindgren S, Lilja B, Rosen I, Sundkvist G. Disturbed autonomic nerve function in patients with Crohn's disease. Scand J Gastroenterol. 1991;26:361–6.
8. Furness JB, Costa M. The enteric nervous system. Edinburgh: Churchill Livingstone; 1987.
9. Dockray GJ, Sharkey KA. Neurochemistry of visceral afferent neurones. In: Cervero F, Morrison JFB, editors. Progress in brain research, Vol. 67: Visceral sensation. Amsterdam: Elsevier; 1986:133–48.
10. Holzer P. Capsaicin: cellular targets, mechanisms of action, and selectivity for thin sensory neurons. Pharmacol Rev. 1991;43:143–201.
11. Maggi CA. Capsaicin-sensitive nerves in the gastrointestinal tract. Arch Int Pharmacodyn. 1990;303:157–66.
12. Sharkey KA. Substance P and calcitonin gene-related peptide (CGRP) in gastrointestinal inflammation. Ann NY Acad Sci. 1992;664:425–42.
13. Chahl LA, Szolcsanyi J, Lembeck F, editors. Antidromic vasodilatation and neurogenic inflammation. Budapest: Akademiai Kiado; 1984.
14. Costa M, Furness JB, Gibbins IL. Chemical coding of enteric neurons. Prog Brain Res. 1986;68:217–40.
15. Bornstein JC, Furness JB. Enteric neurons and their chemical coding. In: Holle GE, Wood JD, editors. Advances in the innervation of the gastrointestinal tract. Amsterdam: Excerpta Medica; 1992:101–14.
16. Costa M, Brookes S, Waterman S, Mayo R. Enteric neuronal circuitry and transmitters controlling intestinal motor function. In: Holle GE, Wood JD, editors. Advances in the innervation of the gastrointestinal tract. Amsterdam: Excerpta Medica; 1992:115–24.
17. Bornstein JC, Furness JB. Correlated electrophysiological and histochemical studies of submucous neurons and their contribution to understanding enteric neural circuits. J Auton Nerv Syst. 1988;25:1–13.
18. Sharkey KA, Coggins PJ, Tetzlaff W, Zwiers H, Bisby MA, Davison JS. Distribution of growth-association protein, B-50 (GAP-43) in the mammalian enteric nervous system. Neuroscience. 1990;38:13–20.
19. Parr EJ, Sharkey KA. The use of constitutive nuclear oncoproteins to count neurons in the enteric nervous system of the guinea-pig. Cell Tissue Res. 1994;277:325–31.
20. Parr EJ, Gibson AW, Sharkey KA. C-myc antigens in the mammalian enteric nervous system. Neuroscience. 1994;58:807–16.
21. Payan DG. Neuropeptides and inflammation: the role of substance P. Annu Rev Med. 1989;40:341–52.
22. Miller MJS, Sadowska-Krowicka H, Jeng AY et al. Substance P levels in experimental ileitis in guinea pigs: effects of misoprostol. Am J Physiol. 1993;265:G321–30.
23. Palmer JM, Greenwood B. Regional content of enteric substance P and vasoactive intestinal peptide during intestinal inflammation in the parasitized ferret. Neuropeptides. 1993;25:95–103.
24. Eysselein VE, Reinshagen M, Cominelli F et al. Calcitonin gene-related peptide and substance P decrease in the rabbit colon during colitis. A time study. Gastroenterology. 1991;101:1211–19.
25. Swain MG, Agro A, Blennerhassett P, Stanisz A, Collins SM. Increased levels of substance P in the myenteric plexus of trichinella-infected rats. Gastroenterology. 1992;102:1913–19.
26. Hurst SM, Stanisz AM, Sharkey KA, Collins SM. Interleukin 1β-induced increase in substance P in rat myenteric plexus. Gastroenterology. 1993;105:1754–60.
27. Sharkey KA, Ihns Y. The effects of experimental ileitis on vasoactive intestinal polypeptide (VIP)-immunoreactivity in the guinea pig. Gastroenterology. 1993;104:A780 (abstr.).
28. Kishimoto S, Kobayashi H, Shimizu S et al. Changes of colonic vasoactive intestinal peptide and cholinergic activity in rats with chemical colitis. Dig Dis Sci. 1992;37:1729–37.

29. Schulte-Bockholt A, Fink JG, Otterson MF, Telford GL, Hopp K, Koch TR. Gene expression of VIP in sigmoid colon from chronic ulcerative colitis (CUC). Gastroenterology. 1993;104:A578 (abstr.).
30. Eysselein VE, Reinshagen M, Patel A, Davis W, Nast C, Sternini C. Calcitonin gene-related peptide in inflammatory bowel disease and experimentally induced colitis. Ann NY Acad Sci. 1992;657:319–27.
31. Evangelista S, Meli A. Influence of capsaicin-sensitive fibres on experimentally-induced colitis in rats. J Pharm Pharmacol. 1989;41:574–5.
32. Karmeli F, Eliakim R, Rachmilewitz D. Capsaicin pretreatment augments mucosal damage in acetic acid colitis indicating the role of capsaicin sensitive afferent neurons in maintaining colonic mucosal integrity. Gastroenterology. 1993;104:A833 (abstr.).
33. Domek MJ, Blackman E, Vidrich A, Kao J, Baker M, Leung FW. Capsaicin pretreatment increases severity of dextran sulfate sodium (DSS)-induced colonic damage in rats. Gastroenterology. 1993;104:A71 (abstr.).
34. Crowe SE, Sestini P, Perdue MH. Allergic reactions of rat jejunal mucosa. Ion transport responses to luminal antigen and inflammatory mediators. Gastroenterology. 1990;99:74–82.
35. MacNaughton WK, Leach KE, Prud'homme-Lalonde L, Ho W, Sharkey KA. Ionizing radiation reduces neurally evoked electrolyte transport in rat ileum through a mast cell-dependent mechanism. Gastroenterology. 1994;106:324–35.
36. LaMont JT. Mucus: the front line of intestinal mucosal defense. Ann NY Acad Sci. 1992;664:190–201.
37. Moore BA, Sharkey KA, Mantle M. Neural mediation of cholera toxin-induced mucin secretion in the rat small intestine. Am J Physiol. 1993;265:G1050–6.
38. Laporte JL, Dauge-Geffroy MC, Chariot J, Roze C, Potet F. [Sensory fibers sensitive to capsaicin can modulate secretion of the duodenal mucus. A morphometric study in rats]. Gastroenterol Clin Biol. 1993;17:535–41.
39. Martinolle JP, Moré J, Dubech N, Garcia-Villar R. Inverse regulation of α- and β-adrenoceptors during trinitrobenzenesulfonic acid (TNB)-induced inflammation in guinea-pig small intestine. Life Sci. 1993;52:1499–508.
40. Collins SM, Blennerhassett PA, Blennerhassett MG, Vermillion DL. Impaired acetylcholine release from the myenteric plexus of Trichinella-infected rats. Am J Physiol. 1989;257:G898–903.
41. Swain MG, Blennerhassett PA, Collins SM. Impaired sympathetic nerve function in the inflamed rat intestine. Gastroenterology. 1991;100:675–82.
42. Collins SM, Hurst SM, Main C et al. Effect of inflammation of enteric nerves: Cytokine-induced changes in neurotransmitter content and release. Ann NY Acad Sci. 1992;664:415–24.
43. Palmer JM. Immunomodulation of electrical and synaptic behavior of myenteric neurons of guinea pig small intestine during infection with Trichinella spiralis. In: Collins SM, Snape WJ, editors. Effects of immune cells and inflammation on smooth muscle and enteric nerves. Boca Raton: CRC Press; 1990:181–95.
44. Wood JD. Histamine signals in enteric neuroimmune interactions. Ann NY Acad Sci. 1992;664:275–83.
45. Frieling T. Different types of stimuli evoke spike discharge in submucous neurons of the large intestine driving cyclical chloride secretion. In: Holle GE, Wood JD, editors. Advances in the innervation of the gastrointestinal tract. Amsterdam: Excerpta Medica; 1992:425–31.
46. Gabella G. On the plasticity of form and structure of enteric ganglia. J Auton Nerv Syst. 1990;30:S59–66.
47. Poncino A, Geuna S, Scherini E, Giacobini Robecchi MG, Filogamo G. DNA synthesis experimentally induced in neurons: tetraploidy or hyperdiploidy? Int J Dev Neurosci. 1990;8:621–3.
48. Siemers PT, Dobbins WO. The Meissner plexus in Crohn's disease of the colon. Surg Gynecol Obstet. 1974;138:39–42.
49. Reynolds BA, Weiss S. Generation of neurons and astrocytes from isolated cells of the adult mammalian central nervous system. Science. 1992;255:1707–10.
50. Dvorak AM, Osage JE, Monahan RA, Dickersin GR. Crohn's disease: transmission electron microscopic studies. III. Target tissues. Proliferation of and injury to smooth muscle and

the autonomic nervous system. Hum Pathol. 1980;11:620–34.

51. Steinhoff MM, Kodner IJ, DeShryver Kecskemeti K. Axonal degeneration/necrosis: a possible ultrastructural marker for Crohn's disease. Mod Pathol. 1988;1:182–7.

52. Dvorak AM, Onderdonk AB, McLeod RS et al. Axonal necrosis of enteric autonomic nerves in continent ileal pouches: possible implications for pathogenesis of Crohn's disease. Ann Surg. 1993;217:260–71.

53. Geboes K, Rutgeerts P, Ectors N et al. Major histocompatibility class II expression on the small intestinal nervous system in Crohn's disease. Gastroenterology. 1992;103:439–47.

54. Strobach RS, Ross AH, Markin RS, Zetterman RK, Linder J. Neural patterns in inflammatory bowel disease: an immunohistochemical survey. Mod Pathol. 1990;3:488–93.

55. O'Morain C, Bishop AE, McGregor GP et al. Vasoactive intestinal peptide concentrations and immunocytochemical studies in rectal biopsies from patients with inflammatory bowel disease. Gut. 1984;25:57–61.

56. Bishop AE, Polak JM, Bryant MG, Bloom SR, Hamilton S. Abnormalities of vasoactive intestinal polypeptide-containing nerves in Crohn's disease. Gastroenterology. 1980;79:853–60.

57. Sjolund K, Schaffalitzky de Muckadell OB, Fahrenkrug J, Hakanson R, Peterson BG, Sundler F. Peptide-containing nerve fibres in the gut wall in Crohn's disease. Gut. 1983;24:724–33.

58. Mazumdar S, Das KM. Immunocytochemical localization of vasoactive intestinal peptide and substance P in the colon from normal subjects and patients with inflammatory bowel disease. Am J Gastroenterol. 1992;87:176–81.

59. Koch TR, Carney JA, Go VLW, Szurszewski JH. Altered inhibitory innervation of circular smooth muscle in Crohn's colitis. Association with decreased vasoactive intestinal polypeptide levels. Gastroenterology. 1990;98:1437–44.

60. Kubota Y, Petras RE, Ottaway CA, Tubbs RR, Farmer RG, Fiocchi C. Colonic vasoactive intestinal peptide nerves in inflammatory bowel disease. Gastroenterology. 1992;102:1242–51.

61. Koch TR, Carney JA, Go VLW. Distribution and quantitation of gut neuropeptides in normal intestine and inflammatory bowel diseases. Dig Dis Sci. 1987;32:369–76.

62. Duffy LC, Zielezny MA, Riepenhoff Talty M et al. Vasoactive intestinal peptide as a laboratory supplement to clinical activity index in inflammatory bowel disease. Dig Dis Sci. 1989;34:1528–35.

63. Goldin E, Karmeli F, Selinger Z, Rachmilewitz D. Colonic substance P levels are increased in ulcerative colitis and decreased in chronic severe constipation. Dig Dis Sci. 1989;34:754–7.

64. Bernstein CN, Robert ME, Eysselein VE. Rectal substance P concentrations are increased in ulcerative colitis but not in Crohn's disease. Am J Gastroenterol. 1993;88:908–13.

65. Mantyh PW, Catton MD, Boehmer CG et al. Receptors for sensory neuropeptides in human inflammatory diseases: Implications for the effector role of sensory neurons. Peptides. 1989;10:627–45.

66. Watanabe T, Kubota Y, Sawada T, Muto T. Distribution and quantification of somatostatin in inflammatory disease. Dis Colon Rectum. 1992;35:488–94.

67. Koch TR, Carney JA, Morris VA, Go VLW. Somatostatin in the idiopathic inflammatory bowel diseases. Dis Colon Rectum. 1988;31:198–203.

68. Koch TR, Cave DR, Ford H, Kirsner J. Histofluorescent and radioenzymatic analysis of colonic catecholamines in man. J Auton Nerv Syst. 1984;11:383–91.

69. Kyösola K, Penttilä O, Salaspuro M. Rectal mucosal adrenergic innervation and enterochromaffin cells in ulcerative colitis and irritable colon. Scand J Gastroenterol. 1977;12:363–7.

70. Penttilä O, Kyösola K, Klinge E, Ahonen A, Tallqvist G. Studies of rectal mucosal catecholamines in ulcerative colitis. Ann Clin Res. 1975;7:32–6.

71. Geboes K, Mebis J, Rutgeerts P, Ectors N, Vantrappen G. Demonstration of nitric oxide positive neurons in Crohn's disease. Gastroenterology. 1993;104:A705 (abstr.).

72. Stead RH, Tomioka M, Quinonez G, Simon GT, Felten SY, Bienenstock J. Intestinal mucosal mast cells in normal and nematode-infected rat intestines are in intimate contact with peptidergic nerves. Proc Natl Acad Sci USA. 1987;84:2975–9.

73. Stead RH, Dixon MF, Bramwell NH, Riddell RH, Bienenstock J. Mast cells are closely apposed to nerves in the human gastrointestinal mucosa. Gastroenterology. 1989;97:575–

85.

74. Stead RH. Nerve remodeling during intestinal inflammation. Ann NY Acad Sci. 1992;664:443–55.
75. Dvorak AM, McLeod RS, Onderdonk AB et al. Human gut mucosal mast cells: Ultrastructural observations and anatomic variation in mast cell-nerve associations in vivo. Int Arch Allergy Appl Immunol. 1992;98:158–68.
76. Mikkelsen HB, Rumessen JJ. Characterization of macrophage-like cells in the external layers of human small and large intestine. Cell Tissue Res. 1992;270:273–9.
77. Dvorak AM. Ultrastructure of human gastrointestinal system. Interactions among mast cells, eosinophils, nerves and muscle in human disease. In: Collins SM, Snape WJ, editors. Effects of immune cells and inflammation on smooth muscle and enteric nerves. Boca Raton: CRC Press; 1990:139–66.
78. Arizono N, Matsuda S, Hattori T, Kojima Y, Maeda T, Galli SJ. Anatomical variation in mast cell nerve associations in the rat small intestine, heart, lung, and skin. Similarities of distances between neural processes and mast cells, eosinophils, or plasma cells in the jejunal lamina propria. Lab Invest. 1990;62:626–34.
79. Weihe E, Nohr D, Michel S et al. Molecular anatomy of the neuro-immune connection. Int J Neurosci. 1991;59:1–23.
80. Ottaway CA. Neuroimmunomodulation in the intestinal mucosa. Gastroenterol Clin N Am. 1991;20:511–29.
81. Ottaway CA. Vasoactive intestinal peptide as a modulator of lymphocyte and immune function. Ann NY Acad Sci. 1988;527:486–500.
82. Sharkey KA, Kirk DR, Graham TL. Substance P and CGRP modify lymphocyte output from the mesenteric lymphatic duct of the rat. Gastroenterology. 1992;102:A757 (abstr.).
83. Nilsson G, Ahlstedt S. Altered lymphocyte proliferation of immunized rats after neurological manipulation with capsaicin. Int J Immunopharmacol. 1988;10:747–51.
84. Helme RD, Eglezos A, Dandie GW, Andrews PV, Boyd RL. The effect of substance P on the regional lymph node antibody response to antigenic stimulation in capsaicin-pretreated rats. J Immunol. 1987;139:3470–3.
85. Lechin F, van der Dijs B, Insausti CL et al. Treatment of ulcerative colitis with clonidine. J Clin Pharmacol. 1985;25:255–62.
86. Sutherland LR. Clonidine in the treatment of ulcerative colitis. Can J Gastroenterol. 1988;2(Suppl. A):53–56A.
87. Melander M, Almer S, Strom M. Clonidine in ulcerative colitis and proctitis. J Intern Med. 1993;233:93–94 (letter).
88. Lashner BA, Hanauer SB, Silverstein MD. Testing nicotine gum for ulcerative colitis patients. Experience with single-patient trials. Dig Dis Sci. 1990;35:827–32.
89. Pullan RD, Ganesh S, Mani V et al. Transdermal nicotine treatment for ulcerative colitis: a controlled trial. Gastroenterology. 1993;104:A765 (abstr.).
90. Björck S, Dahlström A, Ahlman H. Topical treatment of ulcerative proctitis with lidocaine. Scand J Gastroenterol. 1989;24:1061–72.
91. Björck S, Dahlström A, Johansson L, Ahlman H. Treatment of the mucosa with local anesthetics in ulcerative colitis. Agents Actions. 1992;35(Suppl.):C60–72.
92. McCafferty D-M, Sharkey KA, Wallace JL. Beneficial effects of local or systemic lidocaine in experimental colitis. Am J Physiol. 1994;266:G560–G567.

16
The role of smooth muscle in intestinal inflammation

S. M. COLLINS, I. KHAN, B. VALLANCE and C. HOGABOAM

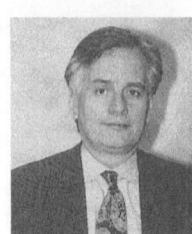

S. M. COLLINS

CHANGES IN SMOOTH MUSCLE CONTRACTION

Regional differences in muscle responses to inflammation

The observation that active ulcerative colitis is accompanied by a reduction in motor activity in the distal colon[1-3] suggests that the contractility of colonic smooth muscle may be impaired as a result of inflammation. this has been confirmed in an *in-vitro* study of human colonic circular muscle in which contraction induced by either bethanechol or KCl was significantly reduced in comparison to muscle obtained from patients without inflammatory bowel disease (IBD)[4], suggesting that the underlying mechanism is located at the postreceptor level in the excitation–contraction coupling of the muscle cell. Similar observations have been made in animal models of colitis[5]. In our study[5], a similar decrease in colonic smooth muscle contractility was observed in colitis induced by chemical injury (acetic acid or trinitrobenzene sulfonic acid, TNB), as well as infection (*Trichinella spiralis*). These results also illustrate that inflammation-induced changes in smooth muscle are nonspecific in that they do not appear to be influenced by the manner in which colitis is induced.

There are no reports of small bowel motility in Crohn's disease patients upon which to speculate about the nature of any underlying change in muscle contraction. However, an *in-vitro* study from this laboratory demonstrated that both circular and longitudinal muscles from the inflamed ileum of patients with Crohn's disease exhibited increased contractility when compared to muscle from patients without IBD[6]. The increased contractility occurred following stimulation with either carbamylcholine or histamine, suggesting that the underlying mechanism was not exclusively at the receptor level, although differences in the dose–response relationships between control and inflamed tissues suggested that some alterations in the ligand-recognition properties of receptors may contribute to the observed changes.

Taken in conjunction with the results obtained in the inflamed human colon, the results imply that the nature of inflammation-induced changes in intestinal muscle is region-specific. This is supported by results from animal studies in which inflammation induced in either the small intestine or colon by the same stimulus (*T. spiralis*) resulted in a similar profile of altered contractility; there was increased tension development by muscle from the inflamed small intestine[7] and a reduction in tension development by muscle from the inflamed colon[5].

Mechanisms underlying altered muscle contraction in the inflamed intestine

Information regarding the mechanisms underlying altered smooth muscle function in the inflamed intestine is primarily derived from studies on animal models of acute intestinal inflammation. It should be emphasized that these models are not of IBD *per se*, but are paradigms for testing the impact of inflammation on tissue function and exploring underlying mechanisms. This laboratory has focused its efforts on primary nematode infection of rodents, since these models have been in long-standing use for the study of immuno-physiological interactions in the gut[8], and an extensive literature exists regarding the immunological responses of the rodent host to nematode infection.

In keeping with the postulate that the mechanisms underlying changes in smooth muscle contractility in the inflamed intestine are, for the most part, receptor-independent is the finding of suppressed sodium pump activity in muscle from the inflamed jejunum of *T. spiralis*-infected rats[9]. In that study we showed that ouabain-sensitive rubidium-86 uptake by longitudinal muscle was reduced by > 80% compared to control, and that this was accompanied by a corresponding decrease in the activity of PNPPase (p-nitrophenyl-phosphatase), an enzyme marker of sodium-pump activity. The molecular mechanism underlying this change was also explored, and suppression of sodium pump activity likely occurs at the level of gene transcription of the α-1 isoform of the sodium pump protein[10]. Since this pump is electrogenic, its suppression during inflammation would therefore lead to hyper-excitability of the muscle, since membrane potential would be reduced to a level closer to the threshold for contraction. However, it is plausible that the increased contractility of muscle in the inflamed gut is multifactorial, because others have shown in this model that there is an increase in the contractile protein content of muscle[11].

Trophic changes in muscle from the inflamed intestine

In Crohn's disease strictures there is profound thickening of both the muscularis mucosae and propria and muscle cell proliferation[12,13]. Furthermore, there are preliminary data suggesting that intestinal muscle cells from IBD patients exhibit altered growth patterns compared to controls[14]. The mechanisms underlying the hyperplasia of smooth muscle in the inflamed intestine remain to be determined, but studies in animal models indicate that both hyperplasia and hypertrophy of the muscularis externa occur during intestinal inflammation[15]. Subsequent studies have indicated that these trophic changes are determined by different mediators potentially involved in the inflammatory response (see below). For example, interleukin-1β (IL-1β) and platelet-derived growth factor have calcium-dependent mitogenic effects on human[16] and rodent intestinal smooth muscle growth *in vitro*. Furthermore, in a similar system we have preliminary data suggesting that the constitutive release of nitric oxide modulates intestinal smooth muscle proliferation. Studies are ongoing to explore the relative impact of proinflammatory and anti-inflammatory substances to intestinal smooth muscle proliferation.

The inflammatory basis for altered muscle contraction and growth

Changes in muscle contraction are absent from corticosteroid-treated, nematode-infected rats in whom the inflammatory response has been suppressed[17]. In addition, the changes are absent from congenitally athymic rats following *T. spiralis* infection[18]. Moreover, the changes in muscle contraction are restored following successful reconstitution of T lymphocyte function prior to infection[18]. These findings, taken in conjunction with the demonstration of T cell infiltration of the muscle layer within the first 48 h of infection[19] support the hypothesis that the increased contraction of smooth muscle from the inflamed intestine of *T. spiralis*-infected rats is T lymphocyte-dependent. Similar observations have been made in nematode-infected mice[20]. In addition, it is well known that certain inbred mouse strains develop a greater or more effective immune responsiveness to nematode infections than other strains[21-23]. Our preliminary studies using inbred mice indicate that changes in muscle contractility may also be genetically determined, and that there is a positive correlation between the increased contractility of muscle and the ability of the animal to expel the parasite from the gut. This correlation is potentially important as the process of worm expulsion is also T lymphocyte-dependent and a series of studies have indicated that CD4+ T helper cells are likely responsible (for review see ref. 24). This has prompted our ongoing investigation of the role of CD4+ cell subpopulations and their cytokine products as mediators of the observed changes in muscle contraction.

Space prohibits an exhaustive review of factors which affect intestinal smooth muscle growth, but suffice it to say that the phenomenon of intestinal smooth muscle proliferation during inflammation is mediated by immune cells and the mediators they produce. For example, the hyperplasia of intestinal muscle in the *T. spiralis*-infected rat is T lymphocyte-dependent[25]. Whether this reflects a direct or indirect interaction between lymphocytes and muscle cells is currently being investigated. Furthermore, during TNB colitis in rats, another model of intestinal inflammation characterized by profound smooth muscle hyperplasia, the presence of proliferating smooth muscle cells in the external muscle layers was abolished by oral administration of a nitric oxide synthase inhibitor[26]. Although its source(s) in the muscle layer is currently speculative, nitric oxide also appears to play a role in smooth muscle hyperplasia during intestinal inflammation. Studies are ongoing into other potential immune mechanisms of regulation of smooth muscle growth during inflammation.

MUSCLE CELLS AS ACTIVE PARTICIPANTS IN INTESTINAL INFLAMMATION

Collagen production by intestinal muscle cells

Several observations prompt consideration of an active role by muscle in the inflammatory process in the gut. In IBD, ultrastructural studies have shown changes in muscle suggestive of active protein synthesis[27]. In addition, some muscle cells are surrounded by collagen, and it is known that human intestinal smooth muscle cells in culture synthesize and secrete collagen types I, III and V[28]. Transforming growth factor beta (TGF-β) stimulates collagen synthesis by muscle cells[29] and preliminary studies from this laboratory indicate that TGF-β-induced stimulation of collagen synthesis by muscle cells involves the influx of extracellular Ca^{2+} through verapamil-sensitive channels.

Collagen synthesis by muscle is not only clinically important in the context of stricture formation, but illustrates two important concepts. The first is that muscle cells engage in noncontractile activities that contribute to the inflammatory process, and the second is that muscle cells are receptive to immune modulation, as illustrated by their responsiveness to the cytokine TGF-β. Further examples of these concepts will be discussed below.

Cytokine production by muscle cells

A previous study by Kao *et al.* showed that inflammatory mediator production in the gut is not restricted to cells of the mucosa and lamina propria; these authors showed that there was exaggerated production of prostaglandin E_2 (PGE_2) in the muscularis externa of the colon, inflamed following the administration of formalin and immune complexes to rabbits[30]. In the absence of a discernible inflammatory cell infiltrate in the musclaris externa, the production of PGE_2 was attributed to muscle cells, which have been known for some time to produce prostaglandins.

Recent work has extended this observation to address cytokine production by muscle cells. Although the concept of cytokine production by cells other than those of bone marrow origin is not new, the application of this to intestinal muscle is novel. Two observations in the nematode-infected rat have prompted this investigation. First, we have observed ultrastructural changes in muscle cells of the inflamed rat jejunum that are similar to those observed in muscle from patients with IBD. These include enhancement of the Golgi apparatus and prominence of the rough endoplasmic reticulum suggestive of active protein synthesis. Second, we have found evidence of cytokine gene expression and protein production in the muscularis externa of the inflamed jejunum following *T. spiralis* infection in rats[31]. Specifically, we have shown that there is constitutive expression of interleukin-1β (IL-1β) mRNA and protein in the muscularis externa, and that this increases within 12 h of infection. The increased expression of IL-1β is followed by the expression of other cytokines, including IL-6 and tumor necrosis factor alpha (TNF-α). These observations prompted an evaluation of the ability of intestinal muscle cells to express cytokine genes and secrete cytokine proteins. Since the expression of IL-1β was enhanced earliest in the muscularis externa, we suspected that this cytokine might be the stimulus for the induction of other cytokine genes in smooth muscle. Our results to date provide clear evidence that muscle cells express cytokine genes and secrete the corresponding proteins. First, IL-1β induces its own gene expression in muscle cells, and this is accompanied by protein production[32]. Second, IL-1β also induces IL-6 gene expression, and this is also accompanied by protein secretion[33]. Ongoing studies are evaluating the ability of muscle cells to produce other cytokines including TNF-α and TGF-β.

MHC II expression on smooth muscle cells

We have already demonstrated lymphocytic infiltration of the muscularis externa in the intestine of *T. spiralis*-infected rats, and we have also shown the expression of MHC II in this tissue during infection[19]; the precise location of the MHC II complexes has yet to be determined. Similar observations have been made in *T. spiralis*-infected mice; in addition to MHC II expression we have also documented the expression of the adhesion molecule ICAM-1 in the muscularis externa of infected mice[34]. The functional significance of these findings remains to be determined. Parallel studies using cultured muscle cells isolated from the mouse intestine have shown that MHC II and ICAM-1 expression can be induced following exposure to interferon gamma (IFN-γ) and the IFN-γ effect was potentiated by TNF-α or IL-β[34]. These findings raise the possibility that muscle may contribute to immune activation via MHC II-linked antigen presentation, and this speculation is based upon the observation that antigen presentation has been demonstrated in a variety of cell types including human myoblasts[35] and vascular smooth muscle[36]. It is possible that increased intestinal permeability, as well as changes in vascular permeability in the gut wall during nematode infection, permit access of luminal as well as parasite antigens to the muscularis externa[37]. Cytokines released by lymphocytes that infiltrate the muscle layer may induce MHC II and ICAM-1 expression by muscle cells. If this is accompanied by antigen processing and presentation, together with the elaboration of co-stimulatory factors such as IL-1β, lymphocyte activation may occur followed by clonal selection of the T cell population. Current research is evaluating whether smooth muscle cells are capable of activating lymphocyte via antigen presentation.

Clinical significance

The implications of inflammation-induced changes in smooth muscle contractility and growth are obvious in the context of symptom generation in intestinal inflammatory conditions including IBD. The clinical consequence of a more active role for muscle cells in immune activation are perhaps more subtle, but are nevertheless worthy of consideration. For example, IBD in remission is often accompanied by symptoms suggestive of irritable bowel syndrome[38] and persistent functional abnormalities in the bowel[1,39]. These abnormalities persist in the face of a normal appearance of the overlying mucosa. It is possible that the mucosal injury and inflammation that characterizes active IBD induces changes in the muscularis externa which persist following resolution of the mucosal changes; recent data from animal studies support this hypothesis[40]. These persistent changes in the neuromuscular layers could be maintained through the elaboration of cytokines and other mediators by muscle cells. This scenario requires that cytokines are able to alter the physiology of neuromuscular tissues, and evidence in this regard has already been obtained[41,42].

Acknowledgements

This work was supported by a grant from the Medical Research Council (MRC) of Canada to S.M.C. Dr C. M. Hogaboam is a recipient of an MRC Fellowship.

References

1. Rao SSC, Read NW, Brown C, Bruce C, Holdsworth CD. Studies on the mechanism of bowel disturbance in ulcerative colitis. Gastroenterology. 1987;93:934–40.
2. Kern FJ, Almy TP, Abbot FK, Bogdonoff MD. Motility of the distal colon in nonspecific ulcerative colitis. Gastroenterology. 1951;19:492–503.
3. Snape WJ, Matarazzo SA, Cohen S. Abnormal gastrocolonic response in patients with ulcerative colitis. Gut. 1980;21:392–6.
4. Snape WJ, Williams R, Hyman PE. Defect in colonic muscle contraction in patients with ulcerative colitis. Am J Physiol. 1991;261:G987–91.
5. Grossi L, McHugh K, Collins SM. On the specificity of altered muscle function in experimental colitis in rats. Gastroenterology. 1993;104:1049–56.
6. Vermillion DL, Huizinga JD, Ridell RH, Collins SM. Altered small intestinal smooth muscle function in Crohn's disease. Gastroenterology. 1993;104:1692–700.
7. Vermillion DL, Collins SM. Increased responsiveness of jejunal longitudinal muscle in *Trichinella*-infected rats. Am J Physiol. 1988;254:G124–9.

8. Russell DA, Castro GA. Physiology of the gastrointestinal tract in the parasitized host. In: Johnson LR, editor. Physiology of the gastrointestinal tract, 2nd edn. New York: Raven Press; 1987:1749–80.
9. Muller MJ, Huizinga JD, Collins SM. Altered smooth muscle contraction and sodium pump activity in the inflamed rat intestine. Am J Physiol. 1989;257:G570–7.
10. Khan I, Collins SM. Altered sodium pump gene expression in the inflamed intestine of the nematode-infected rat. Am J Physiol. 1993;264:G1160–8.
11. Bowers RL, Castro GA, Lai M, Harari Y, Weisbrodt NW. Actin mRNA expression in intestinal smooth muscle of rats infected with *Trichinella spiralis*. Gastroenterology. 1990;99:1236 (abstr.).
12. Graham MF, Diegelmann RF, Elson CO *et al.* Collagen content and types in the intestinal strictures of Crohn's disease. Gastroenterology. 1988;94:257–65.
13. Dvorak AM, Connell AB, Dickersin GR. Crohn's disease, a scanning electron microscopic study. Hum Pathol. 1979;10:165–77.
14. Shah M, Willey A, Graham MP. Inflammatory bowel disease induces changes in the *in vitro* phenotype of human intestinal muscle cells. Gastroenterology. 1993;104:779 (abstr.).
15. Blennerhassett MG, Vignjevic P, Vermillion DL, Collins SM. Inflammation causes hyperplasia and hypertrophy in smooth muscle of rat small intestine. Am J Physiol. 1992;262: G1041–6.
16. Scheinfeld BA, Collins SM, Blennerhassett MG. Verapamil inhibits interleukin-1β-mediated hyperplasia of human intestinal smooth muscle. Gastroenterology. 1994;106:A768.
17. Marzio L, Blennerhassett P, Chiverton S, Vermillion DL, Langer J, Collins SM. Altered smooth muscle function in worm-free gut regions of *Trichinella*-infected rats. Am J Physiol. 1990;259:G306–13.
18. Vermillion DL, Ernst PB, Collins SM. T-lymphocyte modulation of intestinal muscle function in the *Trichinella*-infected rat. Gastroenterology. 1991;101:31–8.
19. Dzwonkowski P, Stead RH, Blennerhassett MG, Collins SM. Induction of class II major histocompatibility complex (MHCII) in enteric smooth muscle. Gastroenterology. 1991;100:A577 (abstr.).
20. Vallance BA, Blennerhassett PA, Collins SM. T lymphocyte dependence of persistent intestinal muscle function post infection by *Trichinella spiralis* in the mouse. Gastroenterology. 1994;106:A1054.
21. Else KJ, Hultner L, Grencis RK. Cellular immune responses to the murine nematode parasite *Trichuris muris*. II. Differential induction of Th-cell subsets in resistant versus susceptible mice. Immunology. 1992;75:232–7.
22. Else KJ, Grencis RK. Cellular immune responses to the murine nematode parasite *Trichuris muris*. I. Differential cytokine production during acute or chronic infection. Immunology. 1991;72:508–13.
23. Zhu DH, Bell RG. IL-2 production, IL-2 receptor expression, and IL-2 responsiveness of spleen and mesenteric lymph node cells from inbred mice infected with *Trichinella spiralis*. J Immunol. 1989;142:3262–7.
24. Wakelin D. Allergic inflammation as a hypothesis for the expulsion of worms from tissues. Parasitol Today. 1993;9:115–16.
25. Blennerhassett G, Vignjevic P, Vermillion DL, Ernst PB, Collins SM. Intestinal inflammation induces T-lymphocyte-dependent hyperplasia of jejunal smooth muscle. Gastroenterology. 1990;98:A328 (abstr.).
26. Hogaboam CM, Jacobson K, Collins SM, Blennerhassett MG. The selective beneficial effects of nitric oxide inhibition in experimental colitis. Gastroenterology. 1994;106:A700.
27. Dvorak AM, Osage JE, Monahan RA, Dickersin GR. Crohn's disease: transmission electron microscopic studies. III. Target tissues. Proliferation of and injury to smooth muscle and the autonomic nervous system. Hum Pathol. 1980;11:620–34.
28. Graham MF, Drucker DE, Diegelmann RF, Elson CO. Collagen synthesis by human intestinal smooth muscle cells in culture. Gastroenterology. 1987;92:400–5.
29. Graham MF, Bryson GR, Diegelmann RF. Transforming growth factor beta 1 selectively augments collagen synthesis by human intestinal smooth muscle cells. Gastroenterology. 1990;99:447–53.
30. Kao HW, Zipser RD. Exaggerated prostaglandin production by colonic smooth muscle in rabbit colitis. Dig Dis Sci. 1988;33:697–704.

31. Khan I, Blennerhassett P, Gauldie J, Collins SM. Cytokine mRNA profile in smooth muscle from the inflamed intestine of the nematode-infected rat. Gastroenterology. 1992;102:A645 (abstract).

32. Khan I, Kataeva G, Blennerhassett MG, Collins SM. Auto-induction of interleukin-1β gene expression in enteric smooth muscle cells. Gastroenterology. 1993;104:A534 (abstr.).

33. Khan I, Collins SM. Interleukin-1β induces the expression of interleukin-6 in intestinal smooth muscle cells. Gastroenterology. 1994;106:A710.

34. Hogaboam CM, Hewlett B, Stead RH, Snider DP, Collins SM. Cytokine-induced class II major histocompatibility antigen and intracellular adhesion molecular expression on murine intestinal smooth muscle cells. Gastroenterology. 1994;106:A700.

35. Goebels N, Michaelis D, Wekerle H, Hohfeld R. Human myoblasts as antigen presenting cells. J Immunol. 1992;149:661–7.

36. Hart MN, Waldschmidt MM, Hanley-Hyde JH, Moore SA, Kemp JD, Schelper RL. Brain microvascular smooth muscle expresses Class II antigens. J Immunol. 1987;138:2960–3.

37. Blennerhassett MG, Catallo D. Dexamethasone blocks vascular leakage, but not endothelial activation, in smooth muscle of inflamed rat jejunum. Gastroenterology. 1993;104:A670 (abstr.).

38. Isgar B, Harman M, Kaye MD, Whorwell PJ. Symptoms of irritable bowel syndrome in ulcerative colitis in remission. Gut. 1983;24:190–2.

39. Rao SSC, Read NW, Stobart JAH, Haynes WG, Benjamin S, Holdsworth CD. Anorectal contractility under basal conditions and during rectal infusion of saline in ulcerative colitis. Gut. 1988;29:769–77.

40. Vallance BA, Blennerhassett PA, Collins SM. Murine trichinosis: a model of post-infective smooth muscle dysfunction. Gastroenterology. 1994;106:A584.

41. Beasley D, Cohen RA, Levinsky NG. Interleukin-1 inhibits contraction of vascular smooth muscle. J Clin Invest. 1989;83:331–5.

42. Collins SM, Hurst SM, Main C et al. Effect of inflammation of enteric nerves. Cytokine-induced changes in neurotransmitter content and release. Ann NY Acad Sci. 1992;664:415–24.

17
Brain–gut interactions in IBD: mechanisms of anorexia in animal models of experimental colitis

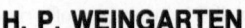

H. P. WEINGARTEN

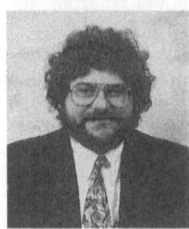

INTRODUCTION

The perspective motivating the present research originates from the assertion that a complete understanding of the symptomatology and etiology of inflammatory bowel disease (IBD) cannot be derived from investigations of one organ, the bowel, in isolation. Rather, it is acknowledged that physiological processes within the bowel are influenced constantly by signals from other organs, primarily the brain, via neural and hormonal communication routes (Fig. 1). On the efferent side, disturbances in brain–gut communication may precipitate or maintain inflammation in the bowel, especially in situations related to stress[1]. On the afferent side, altered communication between gut and brain must underlie the behavioral symptomatology associated with IBD. This chapter focuses on one of these symptoms – the reduction of eating (anorexia) and weight loss associated with IBD, particularly Crohn's disease and ulcerative colitis.

It is estimated that anywhere from 22%[2] to 70%[3] of Crohn's patients exhibit weight loss, a reduction of caloric intake being one of the major causes. Anorexia is manifest especially during acute exacerbations of IBD and, in children, the inadequate nutrition is a major contributor to growth deficiencies[4,5]. The weight loss in adult Crohn's patients is so severe that this clinical group is often used as a weight loss control for studies of anorexia nervosa[6]. Although the malnutrition of the IBD patient is associated with

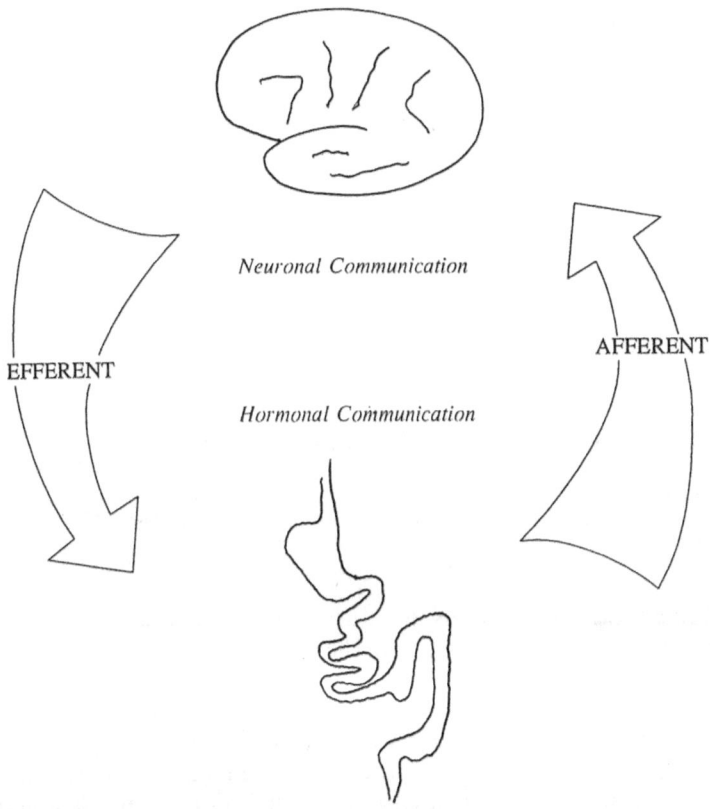

Neuronal Communication

EFFERENT

AFFERENT

Hormonal Communication

Fig. 1 Schematic representation of bidirectional communication between gut and brain

increased morbidity, and amelioration of the nutritional deficiencies is associated with a more positive prognosis[3,7,8] the mechanisms by which inflammation of the gastrointestinal tract result in anorexia are unknown. Since the brain is the organ ultimately responsible for the direction of behavior, treatment of IBD-associated anorexia and weight loss must involve an understanding of how signals from the inflamed gut are communicated to the brain, and identification of the processes that are turned on in the brain upon receipt of these signals to suppress food intake.

THE PHENOMENON: ANOREXIA FOLLOWING COLON INFLAMMATION

The initial step in our research strategy was to identify preparations in which the relationship between gut inflammation and anorexia could be productively examined. First, we characterized changes in food intake and body weight in several parasite animal models of gastrointestinal inflammation (*Trichinella spiralis* and *Nippostrongylus brasiliensis*). Although

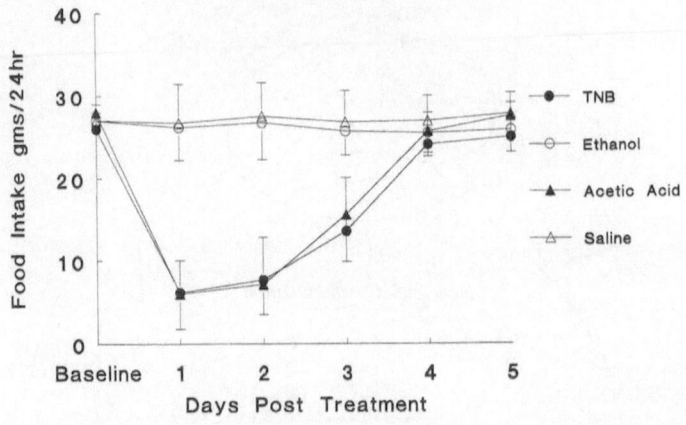

Fig. 2 Profile of anorexia following colon inflammation in the rat. Data shown are levels of 24-h food intakes in baseline period and for 5 days after treatment with TNB in ethanol ($n = 50$), 50% ethanol vehicle ($n = 58$), 4% acetic acid ($n = 25$) or saline vehicle ($n = 27$). Data are group means $\pm$ SEM. (Reprinted from *American Journal of Physiology* 264: R873, 1993, with permission)

we replicated the observations of others[9] of a reduced food intake in nematode-infected rats associated with the period of intestinal inflammation, we found the results variable. More importantly, in these models the site of infection is the proximal small intestine where the parasites invade the epithelium and cause substantial structural damage. Since the proximal duodenum is a site of potential importance in the regulation of feeding[10], it is difficult to distinguish a direct effect of the infection on intestinal feeding systems from that resulting from the host's inflammatory response. Thus, we next concentrated on models of colitis, since the distal colon is far removed from the site of putative satiety signals and because colitis is more congruous with the distribution of human IBD.

We established that two – trinitrobenzene sulfonic acid (TNB[11]) and acetic acid[12] – animal models of experimental colitis were associated with virtually identical, robust and highly reproducible suppressions of food intake and body weight (Fig. 2). Daily caloric intake was reduced by approximately 80%, 70% and 50% on the first 3 days after the induction of colitis. Food intake normalized by the fourth post-treatment day. The anorexia was associated with a significant weight loss that outlasted the period of food intake suppression[13].

Especially because of the large, and early-onset, inhibition of food intake, it is tempting to suggest that the unwillingness of the colitic animals to eat results simply from the trauma or malaise resulting from the procedures used to induce the inflammation. However, several experiments demonstrate convincingly that neither trauma nor malaise resulting from the colitis-inducing treatments are adequate explanations for the anorexia of these animals[13-15]. For example:

1. Although the anorexia is fully manifest when rats are maintained on

liquid diets, TNB-treated animals demonstrate no reduction of water intake, indicating that they have the behavioral capacity to perform the behaviors necessary to ingest food and that the anorexia is specific to nutrient.

2. TNB-treated rats manifest the complete profile of anorexia when maintained on a low-residue elemental diet, even though the potential malaise associated with the passage of fecal material over the inflamed segment is not a factor under these feeding conditions.

3. Computerized meal pattern analysis reveals that the anorexia of treated animals results *specifically* from a reduced meal size; TNB-treated animals do not decrease the number of meals initiated during the period of anorexia. This finding demonstrates that the anorexia does not result from a failure to initiate eating, but rather from the elaboration of an exaggerated satiety signal once food has entered the gut.

4. TNB-treated rats show no anorexia in sham-feeding preparations, where the ingested food does not accumulate in the gut. This result indicates that TNB-treated rats have normal appetite and motivation to eat, and that the exaggerated satiety signal that terminates meals prematurely in these animals requires gastric distension or stimulation of postgastric tissues.

5. TNB-treated rats show no elevations of plasma oxytocin, a biological marker of treatments that suppress eating via gastrointestinal malaise.

The results from the TNB and acetic acid colitis models demonstrate a specific, reliable and robust suppression of eating associated with colon inflammation independent of the stimulus used to initiate the inflammatory response. These studies characterize the phenomenology of colitis-associated anorexia and validate the use of these animal models for the further investigation of the relationship between gut inflammation and eating. In subsequent experiments we sought to answer two fundamental questions regarding the mechanisms of anorexia following colon inflammation:

1. What is the nature of the biological signal that causes the suppression of eating following colon inflammation?

2. How do the anorexigenic signals from the inflamed colon communicate with the brain?

NATURE OF THE ANOREXIGENIC SIGNAL

The temporal relationship between the anorexia and the inflammation in the TNB model indicated that the suppression of food intake was associated with the acute phase of inflammation. In addition, we had confirmed early on that the degree of anorexia correlated significantly with the degree of tissue inflammation as indexed by myeloperoxidase (MPO) (Fig. 3). Thus, we concentrated our search for the anorexigenic signals on biological responses associated with the early parts of the inflammatory cascade. First, we defined whether the suppression of eating depended on the production of cyclooxygenase or lipoxygenase metabolites of arachidonic acid[13]. Leuko-

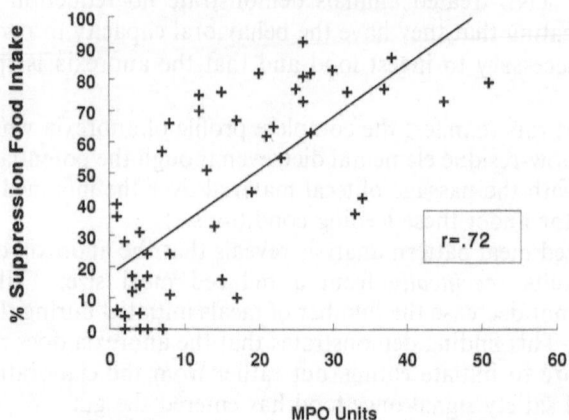

Fig. 3 Correlation between MPO levels in colon on day 5 and magnitude of anorexia. The degree of anorexia was calculated as the average percentage suppression of 24-h food intake on the first 2 days after TNB treatment compared to baseline intake

Table 1

Treatment	Effect on MPO activity	Effect on tissue levels	Effect on anorexia
MK 886	0	↓ LTB$_4$	0
Indomethacin	0	↓ PGE$_2$	50% reversal

triene synthesis was inhibited by repeated intrarectal infusion (10 mg/kg per infusion) of the 5'-lipoxygenase inhibitor, MK 886. Prostaglandin synthesis was inhibited by repeated intraperitoneal injection (5 mg/kg per injection) of the cyclooxygenase inhibitor indomethacin. The results are summarized in Table 1.

The doses of MK 886 and indomethacin we selected had no effect on the degree of colon inflammation induced by the TNB treatment during the period under examination (5 days post-TNB treatment), as indexed by the fact that neither treatment changed the degree of MPO activity in colon compared to TNB-treated rats receiving control treatments. This ensured that any influence of MK 886 and indomethacin on anorexia could be attributed to effects of inflammatory mediators themselves, and not on the degree of tissue inflammation *per se*. In addition, the ability of MK 886 and indomethacin to reduce colon levels of LTB$_4$ and PGE$_4$ in TNB-treated animals to normal levels demonstrated the biological efficacy of the treatments. The critical observation, however, is that only the inhibition of prostaglandin synthesis significantly reversed the anorexia following TNB treatment; leukotriene synthesis inhibition was without effect.

We then evaluated the involvement of the acute phase cytokine, IL-1, in TNB-induced anorexia. Several sets of data implicate IL-1 in the anorexia following colon inflammation. First, food intake is suppressed in the first 24 h following colon inflammation and colon levels of IL-1 are already

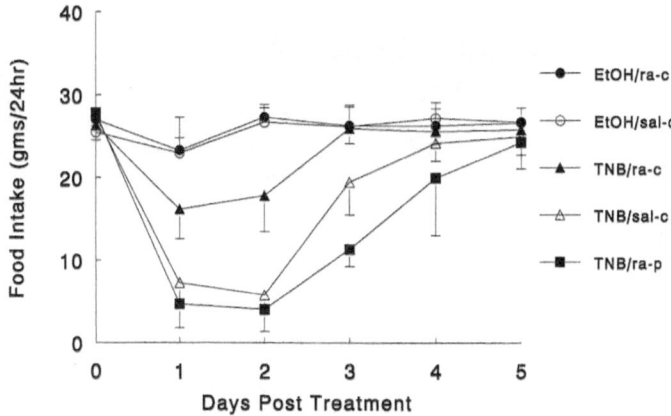

Fig. 4 Twenty-four-hour food intakes before treatment (day 0) and for 5 days after treatment with TNB + i.c.v. rhIL1ra (▲), TNB + i.c.v. saline (△), TNB + s.c. rhIL1ra (■), ethanol + i.c.v. rhIL1ra (●), or ethanol + i.c.v. saline (○). Data are group means ± 1 SEM. (Reprinted from *American Journal of Physiology* 266: R1661, 1994, with permission)

markedly elevated on the first day following TNB administration[16]. Second, acute injection of IL-1 suppresses eating[17–19] and chronic administration of IL-1 peripherally results in a profile of anorexia nearly identical to that produced by TNB treatment[20,21]. Third, both TNB-induced[13] and IL-1-induced[18,22] inhibition of eating are attenuated by inhibition of cyclo-oxygenase products of arachidonic acid metabolism.

To evaluate the role of IL-1 we used osmotic minipumps to deliver 24 µg/h recombinant human IL-1 receptor antagonist (rhIL1ra)[23] chronically into either the periphery (subcutaneously) or the brain (intracerebroventricularly). Infusion of rhIL1ra directly into the brain resulted in a significant reversal of the anorexia and weight loss associated with TNB treatment; peripheral infusion at this dose was without effect[24] (see Fig. 4). These results indicate the necessity of central IL-1 receptors in the expression of the anorexia associated with acute experimental colitis. The suggestion that the cytokine expression in the brain, and not in the periphery, is more intimately associated with the anorexia following gut inflammation is consistent with a similar conclusion derived from studies evaluating the relative importance of peripheral and central tumor necrosis factor in the anorexia and cachexia associated with cancer[25].

COMMUNICATION OF THE ANOREXIGENIC SIGNAL FROM PERIPHERY TO BRAIN

Whatever the exact nature of the anorexigenic signal produced by the inflamed segment, it is obvious that this message must be communicated to the brain in order to affect eating. This reality forces consideration of the mechanisms by which the anorexigenic signal is transmitted to the central nervous system. The possibilities are outlined in Fig. 5.

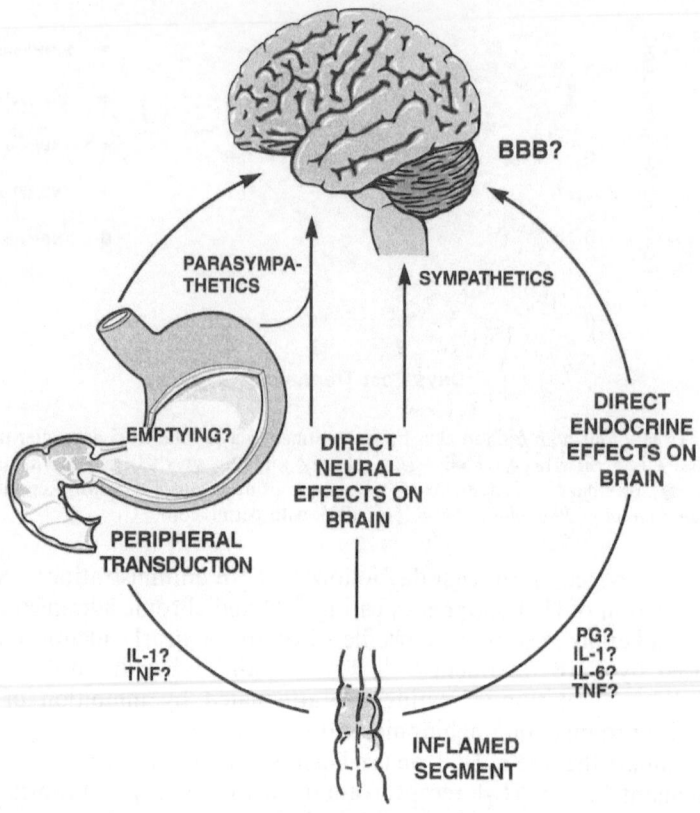

Fig. 5 Schematic representation of the possible mechanisms by which anorexigenic signals from the inflamed segment may be communicated to the brain. (Abbreviations: BBB = blood–brain barrier; IL-1 = interleukin-1; IL-6 = interleukin-6; PG = prostaglandin; TNF = tumor necrosis factor)

Inflammation of the colon is associated with production of high levels of acute-phase cytokines, such as IL-1 and TNF, both of which suppress eating when injected peripherally[17,26]. We have also demonstrated that TNB treatment results in a significant increase in serum IL-6 for at least 3 days following treatment (Weingarten and Gauldie, unpublished). It is possible that these peripherally released cytokines represent anorexigenic signals that are transmitted to the brain in a classic endocrine manner. This hypothesis requires that peripheral cytokines have access to brain via either transport mechanisms in the blood–brain barrier[27] or circumventricular organs with porous or absent blood–brain barriers[28]. Alternatively, it may be that the anorexigenic signal communicates with the brain indirectly requiring one, or several, transductions in the periphery of the signal from the inflamed segment before it is received by brain. This indirect signalling is analogous to the way in which the gut peptide cholecystokinin (CCK) signals satiety[29]; CCK released by cells in the proximal duodenum affect neural or smooth

Table 2

Treatment	Effect on MPO	Effect on anorexia
Vagotomy (VGx)	↑	0
Area postrema ablation (APx)	↑	0
APx + nucleus solitary tract ablation	↑	0

muscle elements in the pylorus and, thus, alter vagal afferent traffic to a pattern that signals satiety. This possibility is reinforced by the observations that inflammatory mediators[30] and TNB-induced colitis both result in a delayed rate of gastric emptying[14].

As a preliminary examination of the route by which the colitis-produced anorexigenic signals reach the brain, we examined the effects of total subdiaphragmatic vagotomy, selective area postrema ablations and combined area postrema/nucleus of the solitary tract ablations on the profile of anorexia in the TNB colitis model[31]. The results are summarized in Table 2.

Consistent with a previous report that produced peripheral vagal deafferentation by capsaicin[32], both peripheral (subdiaphragmatic) vagotomy and central (APx + nucleus solitary tract ablation) vagotomy increased the inflammatory response to intrarectal TNB. However, none of these treatments affected the magnitude or time-course of the TNB-induced suppression of food intake. These results indicate that:

1. The expression of anorexia following colon inflammation is not mediated by vagal afferent activity, nor does it require the entry of an anorexigenic signal into the brain via the area postrema.
2. Although gastric emptying is delayed in association with colon inflammation, this disturbance is not necessary for the expression of the anorexia.
3. Although CCK may be involved in the eating-suppressive effects of IL-1[33], CCK is not a necessary mediator of TNB-induced anorexia.

SUMMARY AND CHALLENGES FOR FUTURE RESEARCH

The specific biological signals that mediate the anorexic effects of gastrointestinal inflammation remain to be elucidated. Although it is clear that inflammation of the gut leads to the elaboration of multiple inflammatory mediators and cytokines in the periphery, it appears that it is cytokine expression in the central nervous system that is critical to the anorexia associated with colitis. There is now ample evidence that immune signals that suppress food intake activate cytokine expression in brain (e.g. ref. 34). Understanding how the inflammation-related signals in the periphery are communicated to the central nervous system and activate cytokine production in the brain remains an enormous challenge. This problem is nearly identical to an analogous and persisting problem in the understanding of the etiology of fever[35]. Elucidation of these gut–brain communication mechanisms is essential to the development of appropriate and efficacious treatments for the eating and weight disturbances associated with IBD.

It is also recognized that IBD is a chronic condition characterized by recurring relapses and acute exacerbations of the disease following periods of apparent remission. The studies presented to date, that focus on the properties and mechanisms of anorexia upon the initial inflammatory episode, are preliminary, but necessary, to the study of the mechanisms of chronic reductions of eating and weight that characterize IBD. The successful application of the current research to IBD will require extension of these investigations into models that appropriately mimic the recurring and relapsing nature of human IBD.

Acknowledgements

All of the research described in this paper was conducted as part of an ongoing collaboration with Dr S. M. Collins of the McMaster University Department of Medicine (Division of Gastroenterology), and was funded by operating grants from the Medical Research Council of Canada. Some of the experiments described in this paper constitute portions of a dissertation submitted by Kevin McHugh to the Faculty of Graduate Studies in partial fulfillment of the requirements for the PhD degree. We thank Dawn Elston and Bernadetta Michalski for excellent technical assistance with these studies.

References

1. McHugh K, Weingarten HP, Khan I, Riddell R, Collins SM. Stress-induced exacerbation of experimental colitis in the rat. Gastroenterology. 1993;104:A1051.
2. Farmer RG, Hawk WA, Turnbull RB Jr. Clinical patterns in Crohn's disease: a statistical study of 615 cases. Gastroenterology. 1975;68:627–35.
3. Silk DBA, Payne-James J. Inflammatory bowel disease: nutritional implications and treatment. Proc Nutr Soc. 1989;48:355–61.
4. Clark ML. Role of nutrition in inflammatory bowel disease: an overview. Gut. 1986;27: 72–5.
5. Kirschner BS. Nutritional consequences of inflammatory bowel disease on growth. J Am Coll Nutr. 1988;7:301–8.
6. McCallum RW, Grill BB, Lange R, Plansky A, Galss EE, Greenfeld DG. Definition of a gastric emptying abnormality in patients with anorexia nervosa. Dig Dis Sci. 1985;30: 713–22.
7. Greenberg GR, Flemming CR, Jeejeebhoy IH, Rosenberg IH, Sales D, Tremaine WJ. Controlled trial of bowel rest and nutritional support in the management of Crohn's disease. Gut. 1988;29:1309–15.
8. Heatley RV. Assessing the nutritional state in inflammatory bowel disease. Gut. 1986;27: 61–6.
9. Castro GA, Copeland EM, Dudricks SJ, Johnson LR. Enteral and parenteral feeding to evaluate malabsorption in intestinal parasitism. Am J Trop Med Hyg. 1979;28:500–7.
10. Smith GP, Gibbs J. Postprandial satiety. In: Sprague JM, Epstein AN, editors. Progress in psychobiology and physiological psychology. NY: Academic Press; 1979:179–242.
11. Morris GP, Beck PL, Herridge MS, Depew WT, Szewczuk MR, Wallace JL. Hapten-induced model of chronic inflammation and ulceration in the rat colon. Gastroenterology. 1989;96:795–803.
12. MacPherson BR, Pfeiffer CJ. Experimental procedures of diffuse colitis in rats. Digestion. 1978;17:135–54.
13. McHugh K, Weingarten HP, Keenan C, Wallace JL, Collins SM. On the suppression of food intake in experimental models of colitis in the rat. Am J Physiol. 1993;264:R871–6.
14. McHugh K, Castonguay TW, Collins SM, Weingarten HP. Characterization of suppression

of food intake following acute colon inflammation in the rat. Am J Physiol. 1993;265: R1001–5.

15. Hansell E, Collins SM, Verbalis JG, Stricker EM, Weingarten HP. Plasma oxytocin levels are not elevated during colitis-induced anorexia in rats. 11th International Conference on the Physiology of Food and Fluid Intake. Oxford, England. 1993.

16. Rachmileiwtz D, Simon PL, Schwartz LW, Griswold DE, Fondacaro JD, Wasserman MA. Inflammatory mediators of experimental colitis in rats. Gastroenterology. 1989;97:326–37.

17. Dinarello C. Interleukin-1 and interleukin-1 antagonism. Blood. 1991;77:1627–52.

18. Hellerstein MK, Meydani SN, Meydani M, Wu K, Dinarello C. Interleukin-1-induced anorexia in the rat. J Clin Invest. 1989;84:228–35.

19. Plata-Salaman CR, French-Mullen JMH. Intracerebroventricular administration of a specific IL-1 receptor antagonist blocks food and water intake suppression induced by interleukin-1B. Physiol Behav. 1992;51:1277–9.

20. Mrosovsky N, Molony LA, Conn CA, Kluger MJ. Anorexia effects of interleukin-1 in the rat. Am J Physiol. 1989;257:R1315–21.

21. Otterness IG, Seymour PA, Golden HW, Reynolds JA, Daumy GO. The effects of continuous administration of murine interleukin-1 in the rat. Physiol Behav. 988;43:797–804.

22. Uehara A, Ishikawa Y, Okumura T et al. Indomethacin blocks the anorexic action of interleukin-1. Eur J Pharmacol. 1989;170:257–60.

23. Eisenberg SP, Evans RJ, Arend WP et al. Primary structure and functional expression from complementary DNA of a human interleukin-1 receptor antagonist. Nature (Lond.). 1990;343:341–6.

24. McHugh K, Collins SM, Weingarten HP. Central interleukin-1 receptors contribute to suppression of feeding after acute colitis in the rat. Am J Physiol. 1994;266:R1659–63.

25. Tracey KJ, Morgello S, Koplin B et al. Metabolic effects of cachectin/tumor necrosis factor are modified by site of production. J Clin Invest. 1990;86:2014–24.

26. Plata-Salaman CR. Immunomodulators and feeding regulation: a humoral link between the immune and nervous systems. Br Behav Immun. 1989;3:193–213.

27. Banks WA, Kastin AJ. Blood to brain transport of interleukin links the immune and central nervous systems. Life Sci. 1991;48:117–21.

28. Rothwell NJ. Functions and mechanisms of interleukin-1 in the brain. Trends Physiol Sci. 1991;12:430–5.

29. Smith GP, Jerome C, Norgren R. Afferent axons in the abdominal vagus mediate satiety of cholecystokinin in rats. Am J Physiol. 1985;261:R64–9.

30. Robert A, Olafsson AS, Lancaster C, Zhang WR. Interleukin-1 is cytoprotective, anti-secretory, stimulates PGE-2 synthesis by the stomach and retards gastric emptying. Life Sci. 1991;48:123–34.

31. Weingarten HP, Ladenheim EE, Emond M, Collins SM. Neither subdiaphragmatic vagotomy nor area postrema lesions block anorexia following colon inflammation in the rat. Soc Neurosci Abstr. 19: no 240.10.

32. Evangelista S, Meli A. Influence of capsaicin-sensitive fibres on experimentally-induced colitis in rats. J Pharm Pharmacol. 1989;41:574–5.

33. Daun JM, McCarthy DO. The role of cholecystokinin in interleukin-1-induced anorexia. Physiol Behav. 1993;54:237–41.

34. Ban E, Haour F, Lenstra R. Brain interleukin 1 gene expression induced by peripheral lipopolysaccharide administration. Cytokine. 1992;4:48–54.

35. Blatteis CM. Neuromodulative actions of cytokines. Yale J Biol Med. 1990;63:133–46.

PART 2:
TRENDS IN IBD THERAPY
1994

Section VI
Critical appraisal of clinical trials

18
How to critically appraise a clinical trial

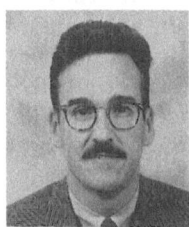

L. R. SUTHERLAND

INTRODUCTION

The prescription of medications is a daily activity for most physicians. The act of prescribing incorporates a number of factors including issues related to effectiveness, appropriate use, comparability with other medications, adverse events and cost. The answers to most of these issues can be found within the body of the available medical literature. But therein lies a dilemma. Clinicians wish to base their therapeutic decisions on scientific data but are often overwhelmed by the number of case reports, open series and other therapeutic trials that are published each year.

For example, a search within Medline for 1992 identified 3285 citations for the therapy of gastrointestinal disease. The majority of the publications, however, were isolated case reports, preliminary studies of groups of patients all of whom received the same medication ('open series') or reviews. It is doubtful that any of these reports would modify practice patterns. Such references should be skimmed and considered as perhaps previews as to how therapy may change in the future. However, the history of medicine, including gastroenterology, is littered with reports of medications and interventions which appeared promising in small open series but failed the more rigorous methodology of the clinical trial.

Returning to the 3285 citations, simply restricting the search to randomized trials will reduce the number of papers to 227. That is still a large number of papers to review, but a task that can be managed and enhanced by the application of a few simple rules[1].

This review will outline strategies which should allow clinicians to develop a personal screening plan to reduce the number of papers that have to be carefully reviewed. A second goal is to assist in identifying those publications which could potentially alter the pattern of prescribing medications.

THE ABSTRACT

Is the trial double-blind, randomized and controlled?

Although the natural history of the development of an indication for a particular medication includes an 'open-label' study or 'open series' in which all patients receive the medication, the impact of such a study on clinical practice should be minimal. Harold Conn categorized such studies as 'honest efforts'. They should alert the clinician to the possibility that drug X may be of benefit for a particular disease. However, the results are likely to be greatly biased towards efficacy for the drug, and the sample size is generally small. Following the publication of such a case series, several additional clinical trials should be performed before the medication can be recommended for a particular disease or indication.

The first step to critical appraisal is to scan the title and abstract for three key words: randomized, controlled, double-blind. The inclusion of these words or phrases in the abstract or key word section should alert the clinican to the possibility that this report might actually alter the way in which he or she practices medicine. Blinding of both patient and investigator, the use of a control substance (either placebo or other active medication) and randomization to prevent entry bias should produce a trial of reasonable quality. These techniques are fundamental to reducing the inherent bias, which is the clinical assumption that the new medication will be superior to the conventional therapy, present in any trial. If the abstract confirms the inclusion of these key phrases, the reader should move on to the Methods section.

THE METHODS SECTION

This is one of the most important sections of the paper, but is often skipped by the reader. This practice is often encouraged by the publisher or editor who, in a few journals, prints this section in the smallest type!

Randomization

As Meinert has suggested[2], the process of randomization provides part of the basis for statistical analysis, but from a practical point of view its major effect is to increase the chances of a bias-free treatment assignment. Randomization implies that each patient has an equal chance to receive either treatment. Physicians may often have a bias towards one or another therapy, and may influence the trial results by assigning their patients to one or another treatment preferentially. The ideal strategy is for patients to be assigned by sealed envelopes based on random-number generation. In the case of a multicenter trial the system may be centralized. Schemes which rely on birth dates, hospital identification numbers or days of the month are susceptible to bias. Using a sealed envelope is not foolproof. There are several stories of investigators pulling envelopes until they found the therapeutic assignment they were looking for! A log which reports patient assignment by entry number and entry date provides a check against such interference.

The control

The control is the medication or intervention to which the newer therapy is being compared. Studies which do not include a control intervention do not have the same credibility as those that do. Within the context of the pharmaceutical sphere the control will either be a placebo or another active medication. The control should be identical in appearance to the active medication. An added 'plus' is if the placebo tastes the same. Study participants have been known to compare notes with each other, or to take their medications to pharmacists, chemists, etc. for analysis in order to break the code.

In many cases, particularly when two active medications are being compared, it is not possible to construct identical capsules. The appropriate adjustment in this case is to conduct a 'double-dummy' trial in which placebos, identical to both active medications, are prepared and the patients are assigned to either active medication and the placebo of the alternative therapy. The failure to use such a technique will cast a shadow over a study. For example, in one of the few comparison studies of two 5-ASA preparations for maintenance of remission in ulcerative colitis, a double-dummy technique was not used[3].

In a recent report of the use of 5-ASA for prevention of postoperative recurrence of Crohn's disease, although patients were randomized, they were randomized to either treatment or no medication[4], rather than a placebo. Although the authors dealt with the issue in their discussion, and felt that they had demonstrated no ill-effect from the lack of a placebo, the study would have been enhanced by the use of one.

Blinding

Blinding is another essential element required in order to have confidence in the study results. The term usually implies that both the patient and the physician are blinded to the treatment assignment. The term 'triple blind' refers to blinding of the statistician doing the analysis to the drug assignment.

Blinding is easiest to perform if two medications are being compared (see above, the control). It is more difficult if two different interventions are being compared. For example, how would one blind a study comparing TPN with corticosteroid therapy? A variety of strategies could be utilized. One possibility would be to define the outcome by objective criteria (change in hemoglobin, albumin, etc.), which would be analyzed by individuals unaware of the assignments. More subjective evaluations could be performed by individuals blinded to the assignment who might, for example, evaluate the participants using a telephone interview.

Other Issues

How do the patients in this study compare with the patients in your own practice? A study of high quality will inform the reader as to the number of patients that had to be assessed in order to arrive at the study population. Minor points to note in the Methods section include acquisition dates (starting and stopping) and the use of a reject log. It is not uncommon to screen two to three times the number of patients required to arrive at the patient population. Was a log of screened patients kept? How do the excluded patients differ from those who were included? This information will assist the reader in relating the study population to his or her own practice.

How many patients dropped out of the study? This will give an impression as to the side-effect profile. If the medication is poorly tolerated a greater proportion of patients will drop out. This rule does not apply as well in placebo controlled trials, where a higher rate of dropout can be expected. Patients who are doing poorly are assumed to be on placebo and are withdrawn.

Awareness of these points will help the reader to determine how relevant the study population is to their own practice. For example, if the study took several years to recruit a small number of patients, or most of the patients approached declined, then the study population may not be representative of the total patient population.

Compliance should be assessed preferably by biological tests (serum or urine analysis) but pill counts are better than nothing.

STATISTICAL METHODS

Most clinicians skip over the Statistical Methods section and regard it as a lot of mumbo-jumbo or a black box. To a certain extent the clinician has to rely on the abilities of the journal reviewers and editors to be sure that the appropriate statistical techniques were utilized. There are, however, a certain number of questions that physicians should ask each time they review a clinical trial.

First, was an intention-to-treat compared to a per-protocol analysis utilized? In the intention-to-treat analysis all patients who took even one tablet are included in the analysis. The per-protocol analysis is confined to patients who have complied with all aspects of the protocol. An intention-to-treat analysis is more conservative, tends to give results that are less biased towards showing efficacy and may reflect what happens in the real world. In contrast, the per-protocol analysis provides information related to what to expect in the group of patients who tolerate the medication and who are compliant.

Second, it is worthwhile checking to see if any mention is made regarding a sample size calculation. The sample size calculation is particularly important if a 'negative' trial is reported. In certain cases the conclusion that drug A is equivalent to drug B or placebo may be a function of low statistical power to detect a difference, related to an insufficient number of study subjects. Many of the early trials for the therapy of Crohn's disease which did not demonstrate efficacy are flawed because of small sample size[5]. It was not until the 1980s, when trials involving hundreds of patients were performed, that the possible beneficial effects of 5-ASA could be identified. Broadly speaking, studies which utilize small patient groups can detect only very large differences in outcome. The larger the study sample, the smaller the difference in efficacy that can be detected. If there is no mention of such issues in either the Methods or Discussion section, this may indicate a poorly designed study.

Third, do the investigators report their major results with 95% confidence intervals? Confidence intervals provide the clinician with the range of possible results if the experiment was repeated, using the same number of patients, 95 out of 100 times. The values are sensitive to the number of patients enrolled in the trial. If the intervals include unity or a range of positive and negative values, the results are not statistically significant. Although most clinicians focus on the p value to help them evaluate the results of a study, consideration of confidence intervals is often more helpful, and may explain inconsistent results.

Finally, presentation of the data in the form of a life table will often clarify response rates to various medications.

RESULTS

How was the randomization assessed?

There should be an attempt to determine if the treatment groups are comparable in terms of basic demographic characteristics and disease variables. An acceptable Results section includes the comparison of the treatment groups to determine if the randomization was successful.

Readers should not be distracted by concerns related to statistical significance compared to clinical significance. Consider a modest difference in effect between two medications which is statistically significant. The effect may be clinically important if the disease is serious or lethal, but may not be clinically important if the disease is not life-threatening. Whether or not the p value is 0.05, 0.01 or 0.001 does not determine clinical significance.

Subgroup analysis, if not part of the original study design, should be considered as pointing the directions for future research rather than as definitive findings. Adverse events should be detailed, and the timing of significant endpoints should be readily apparent to the reader.

Table 1 Simple checklist for reviewing clinical trials

Method of randomization	Pharmacy or random numbers
Blinded	Placebo identical in appearance and taste, double-dummy technique if not possible to give both medications in identical capsules
Entry criteria	Clearly stated. List of patients screened provided
Patient population	Results account for each patient; i.e. completed, eliminated, adverse reactions
Statistics	Intent-to-treat analysis. Sample size calculation or reference to consideration of α or β error. Confidence intervals. Life table analysis
Compliance	Tested by pill count or biological equivalent

CONCLUSIONS

Given the incredible growth of the medical literature and the responsibility that we as physicians have to remain current, strategies are necessary to focus attention on reports that might alter clinical practice. Critically appraising the literature should assist in mastering the continued growing information available on which to base decisions for therapeutics. A simple checklist (Table 1) may assist.

Clinicians and health-care agencies wish to base their decisions regarding therapeutics on objective evidence gained through the execution of clinical trials. Just as with most things in life, not all trials are equal in terms of quality or reliability. Decisions regarding therapeutics should be based only on properly executed trials of high quality. It is not necessary to be a biostatistician or clinical trials expert in order to critically appraise the trial literature. A few simple concepts will assist in reviewing any report of a therapeutic intervention.

References

1. Department of Clinical Epidemiology and Biostatistics, McMaster University Health Sciences Centre. How to read medical journals: V. To distinguish useful from useless or even harmful therapy. CMAJ. 1981;124:1156–62.
2. Meinert CL. Clinical trials design conduct, and analysis. Oxford: Oxford University Press; 1986.
3. Courtney MG, Nunes DP, Bergin CF et al. Randomised comparison of olsalazine and mesalazine in prevention of relapses in ulcerative colitis. Lancet. 1992;339:1279–81.
4. Caprilli R, Andreoli A, Capurso L et al. Oral mesalazine (5-aminosalicylic acid: Asacol) for the prevention of post-operative recurrence of Crohn's disease. Aliment Pharmacol Ther. 1994;8:35–43.
5. Sutherland LR. Editorial: 5-aminosalicylates for prevention of recurrence in patients with Crohn's disease: Time for a reappraisal? J Clin Gastroenterol. 1991;13:5–7.

19
Finding the right index for IBD

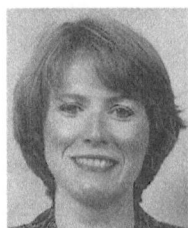

E. J. IRVINE

INTRODUCTION

A broad library of health status instruments has been developed and applied to assess the impact of inflammatory bowel disease (IBD) or its treatment upon patients' lives. These instruments include conventional disease activity indices and health-related quality-of-life instruments which are complementary in the appraisal of IBD[1]. The focus of this discussion will be to review the clinical disease activity indices and their limitations, and to propose guidelines which may assist in selecting an index for a particular situation.

APPLICATIONS OF CLINICAL DISEASE ACTIVITY INDICES

Many disease activity instruments have been generated to permit assessment of the efficacy of new therapies or to predict the clinical course of disease for individuals or groups of patients. The model index for determining therapeutic efficacy will differ considerably from an index to predict long-term outcome.

Consider an activity index to assess drug treatment in active disease. The possible primary outcomes of such a study[2] would include the proportion of patients 'in remission' ('improved', 'unchanged' or 'worsened') at the end of the trial. Other less important outcomes might be the 'mean' or 'median' change in index score or median 'time to improvement'. Similarly, if assessing a drug for prevention of relapse, the analogous outcomes would be the proportion of patients who remain 'in remission', the 'mean change in disease activity score' in the population study groups and the 'median time to

Table 1 The ideal activity index

1 Simple to administer (acceptable to physicians and patients)
2 Quantitative (numerical value)
3 Composite:
subjective symptoms
objective features
signs, endoscopy, histology
blood, urine, tissue parameters of inflammation
4 Valid (able to measure clinical disease activity)
5 Reliable (limited measurement error or observer bias)
6 Responsive (able to reflect important clinical change)
7 Relate to the study question, population and intervention being evaluated

worsening' in each treatment group[2].

In contrast, the outcomes of interest in natural history studies are features such as mortality rate, rate of disease complications or disease-related surgeries, hospitalizations, extension of disease, or rate of drug resistance. Conventional activity indices are generally poor predictors of clinical course. Useful predictive features must be present early in the natural history, are usually discrete categorical parameters and should remain stable with time. A few examples are site or extent of disease, number of prior surgeries and prior resistance to corticosteroids. Predictive traits can be used in clinical trials to define homogeneous study populations (eligibility criteria), prerandomization stratification variables or in *post-hoc* analyses to generate new hypotheses. The remainder of the discussion will focus on activity rather than predictive indices.

THE IDEAL CLINICAL ACTIVITY INDEX

To be able to clearly define study outcomes in clinical trials a newly developed activity index should be adequately assessed for the psychometric properties of validity (ability to reflect clinical activity and intestinal inflammation), reliability (high precision and limited measurement error) and ability to detect a clinically important change in health state (for review, see ref. 3). Only then is there a good chance that it will reflect the clinical state at each assessment, give consistent results when no change in clinical status has occurred and be sensitive to important changes during the study.

The ideal index should be simple to administer, quantitative, evaluating subjective symptoms, physical findings (radiologic or endoscopic attributes) and laboratory (blood, urine, stool or tissue) markers of inflammation. When possible it should be applied in a fashion that relates to the specific research question, the qualities of study population (e.g. patients with perianal Crohn's disease, fibrostenotic symptoms, etc.), and the expected actions or mechanisms of the drug or intervention under evaluation. Many 'activity indices' have been developed and applied in Crohn's disease and ulcerative colitis but few fulfill all of these requirements (Table 1).

AVAILABLE INDICES AND THEIR LIMITATIONS

Indices of disease activity available for ulcerative colitis and Crohn's disease (reviewed in refs 1, 4 and 5) are rarely used in daily practise since clinicians perform a quick assessment of 'global' activity based on a few criteria. During clinical trials, however, objective reproducible criteria are necessary to ensure that there is standardization among many clinicians or centers involving large groups of patients.

One of the first activity indices devised was the Truelove and Witts classification of mild, severe and fulminant ulcerative colitis, which was used to assess the efficacy of cortisone in patients with active ulcerative colitis[6]. This semiquantitative index has no clear definition of what constitutes a moderate exacerbation. This complicates the classification of patients with some but not all features in a single category, and also leads to difficulty in defining improvement or worsening except when patients are in complete remission with absence of all features of active disease.

An improvement upon some of these shortcomings was observed when the St Marks' index for extensive ulcerative colitis furnished 11 different features, including symptoms of bowel function, physical findings of temperature, abdominal tenderness and sigmoidoscopic appearance grading each item from 0 to 3 with a quantitative score range of 0–22[7]. However, many of the features of this index are not pertinent for patients with distal proctocolitis, since few of these patients experience constitutional symptoms, abdominal tenderness or impaired daily activities. This resulted in the development of a relevant index[8] which assessed rectal bleeding, stool frequency, sigmoidoscopic appearance and global physician assessment, giving a score range of 0–12.

These and other indices were developed using the technique of 'face validation' in which clinicians identified the items and response scales based on intuition and experience. Although improvement could be defined by changes in category or score, clear definitions of remission, improvement and worsening were not given before application.

A review of a series of recent trials in patients with proctosigmoiditis revealed substantial variability in the subjective symptoms chosen for assessment. Many but not all evaluated stool frequency and consistency and rectal bleeding, but none evaluated fecal incontinence or straining. A larger proportion of recent studies have evaluated sigmoidoscopic appearance, as described by Baron et al., which grades activity on a four-point scale from 0 – inactive to 3 – severely active. This scale was evaluated for interobserver variation when it was first defined[9]. Morphologic grading of inflammation has also been standardized and minor adaptations of the grades used by Riley et al.[10] appear in much of the recent ulcerative colitis literature. Because of the heterogeneity of features of Crohn's disease, neither endoscopic nor histologic assessments have been as consistently useful in determining activity.

The Crohn's disease activity index (CDAI)[11,12], probably the most familiar index used in North America, was developed using 'construct validation' techniques in which 18 candidate items were evaluated in 112 patients at 187 visits. Multiple regression analysis was used to identify the eight features

Table 2 Properties of a predictive index for IBD

1 Easily recognizable clinical or laboratory parameter
2 Categorical data (discrete categories, usually not numerical)
3 Objective feature (not subjective)
4 Feature which is relatively constant with time
5 Discriminates between groups of patients

which best predicted the physician's global assessment of very well, fair, poor or very poor. The scores of the final eight items of disease activity are variably weighted to yield a score range from 0 to about 700. Active disease is considered greater than 150 and severe disease greater than 450. The full validation of this score was performed during the National Cooperative Crohn's Disease Study[13].

Major criticisms of the CDAI (reviewed in refs 1, 3 and 5) were the need to keep a 7-day diary of subjective symptoms, the interobserver variation in index calculation and the substantial weighting given the subjective symptoms. The only laboratory indicator, the hematocrit, may be influenced by non-disease problems, and active perianal disease or obesity will give a falsely low activity score, while prior surgery and frequent stools will yield an overly high one. These problems resulted in the development of the Simple Index[14], which reduced the number of features from eight to five, eliminated the weighting coefficients and the need for patients to keep a diary (score range 0–29). The Dutch Activity Index[15], which also attempted to address the criticisms of the CDAI, consists of nine items identified by stepwise regression and construct validation techniques. However, this index is heavily influenced by the serum albumin and confounded by nutritional state, disease extent and duration of exacerbation. Despite the drawbacks of these indices, they have each been applied successfully in clinical trials and shown therapeutic benefits such as obtaining a good rate of remission with prednisone or sulfasalazine[13], a more rapid response if these two drugs were combined[16] and that Pentasa 4 g/day provides greater therapeutic gain than 1 g/day[17].

In the past decade a large number of indices has been developed for Crohn's disease with the differences occurring in the subjective symptoms, objective findings and laboratory markers assessed[3,5]. Several studies have shown variable correlation of these activity scores with one another in the same or similar groups of patients[18]. Not surprisingly, 'No single index of disease activity or severity in either Crohn's disease or ulcerative colitis has achieved universal acceptance' (J. Singleton, personal communication, 1994).

Obstacles to standardizing disease activity or comparing results among trials of IBD relate to differences between Crohn's disease and ulcerative colitis, the heterogeneity of each disease, the characteristics of the particular study population, the therapy being tested, the investigators' preferences for which index to apply and the attributes of the index itself. We are now beginning to see new indices being developed for specific populations such as the pediatric population, because of the problems of growth and maturation which are poorly assessed by the adult indices[19]. Similarly, the author has developed and validated an index specifically for assessment of activity of

Table 3 Selecting an index for a particular study

Take into account the following parameters:
1   Disease characteristics
2   Study population characteristics
3   Intervention being tested
4   Investigators' preference or comfort
5   Index attributes

perianal Crohn's disease[20].

Laboratory blood, urine and tissue markers are increasingly being assessed in clinical trials[3,5], and these are not necessarily incorporated into the composite indices. The potential advantages of these biochemical markers, acute-phase reactants, cytokines, adhesion molecules, etc., are that they may more precisely reflect the tissue inflammation, they are often automated and thus more easily assessed in a blinded fashion. Nevertheless, like clinical indices, they must be tested for validity, measurement error and responsiveness to change in clinical state. As with endoscopy and histology in Crohn's disease, it is possible to observe improvements in symptoms with residual perturbation of inflammatory parameters.

SELECTING THE INDEX

No single index can satisfy the needs of all trials. Nevertheless, the clinical symptoms, objective findings and laboratory measurements may be selected independently based on the study objectives and target population. Thus, a trial testing a new drug for perianal disease would require application of an index reflecting severity of subjective perianal problems[20], objective assessment of the anatomical disease using endoscopy or ultrasound[21] and a laboratory evaluation such as the serum haptoglobin[5] which may reflect the degree of inflammation.

Definitions of remission, improvement, absence of change or worsening, the important outcome events in any clinical trial, must be defined by the investigators based on the study objectives and expected mechanism of treatment. Although available disease activity indices have been adequate for previous trials, as patient populations are stratified more homogeneously, and different therapeutic interventions are tested, more refined 'indices' and health status instruments will be needed to assess subpopulations of patients. Endoscopic indices for Crohn's disease need to be simplified and made more user-friendly. As newer imaging techniques are refined, so too will new endoscopic or imaging indices be developed. Laboratory indices should be determined by both the disease parameters and the presumed mechanism of drug action. Finally, it should be emphasized that, to assess the full spectrum of outcomes in clinical trials, health-related quality of life and adverse effects of treatment should be included.

References

1. Garrett JW, Drossman DA. Health status in IBD: biological and behavioural considerations. Gastroenterology. 1990;99:90–6.
2. Irvine EJ. Assessing outcome in randomized clinical trials: inflammatory bowel disease. Can J Gastroenterol. 1993;7:561–7.
3. Irvine EJ, Feagan B, Rochon J et al. Quality of life: a valid and reliable measure of therapeutic efficacy in the treatment of inflammatory bowel disease. Gastroenterology. 1994;106:287–96.
4. Hodgson HJF, Mazean MA. Assessment of drug therapy in IBD. Aliment Pharmacol Ther. 1991;5:555–84.
5. Kjeldsen J, Schaffalitzky de Muckadell OB. Assessment of disease severity and activity in inflammatory bowel disease. Scand J Gastroenterol. 1993;28:1–9.
6. Truelove SC, Witts LJ. Cortisone in ulcerative colitis: final report on a therapeutic trial. Br Med J. 1955;2:1041–4.
7. Powell-Tuck J, Brown RL, Lennard-Jones JE. A comparison of oral prednisone given as single or multiple daily doses for active proctocolitis. Scand J Gastroenterol. 1978;13:833–7.
8. Sutherland LR, Martin F, Greer S et al. 5-Aminosalicylic acid enema in the treatment of distal ulcerative colitis, proctosigmoiditis and proctitis. Gastroenterology. 1987;92:1894–8.
9. Baron JH, Connell AM, Lennard-Jones JE. Variation between observers in describing mucosal appearances in procto colitis. Br Med J. 1964;1:89–92.
10. Riley SA, Mani V, Goodman MJ, Herd ME, Dutt S, Turnberg LA. Comparison of delayed release 5-aminosalicylic acid (mesalazine) and sulphasalazine in the treatment of mild to moderate ulcerative colitis relapse. Gut. 1988;29:669–74.
11. Best WR, Becktel JM, Singleton JW, Kern R. Development of a Crohn's disease activity index. Gastroenterology. 1976;70:439–44.
12. Best WR, Becktel JM, Singleton JW. Rederived values of the eight coefficients of the Crohn's disease activity index (CDAI). Gastroenterology. 1979;77:843–6.
13. Summers RM, Switz DM, Sessions JT et al. National Cooperative Crohn's Disease Study: Results of drug treatment. Gastroenterology. 1979;77:847–69.
14. Harvey RF, Bradshaw JM. A simple index of Crohn's disease activity. Lancet. 1980;1:514–15.
15. Van Hees PAM, Van Elteren PH, Van Lier HJJ, Van Tongeren JHM. An index of inflammatory activity in patients with Crohn's disease. Gut. 1980;21:279–86.
16. Rijk MC, Van Hogezand RA, Van Lier HJJ, Van Tongeren JHM. Sulphasalazine and prednisone compared with sulphasalazine for treating active Crohn's disease. Ann Intern Med. 1991;114:445–50.
17. Singleton JW, Hanauer SB, Gitnick GL et al. Mesalamine capsules for the treatment of active Crohn's disease. Results of a 16 week trial. Gastroenterology. 1993;104:1293–301.
18. Reed JF, Faust LA. An analysis of Crohn's disease activity indices from a registry of patients in eastern Pennsylvania. Can J Gastroenterol. 1991;5:199–208.
19. Hyams JS, Ferry GD, Mandel FS et al. Development and validation of a pediatric Crohn's disease activity index. J Pediatr Gastroenterol Nutr. 1991;12:439–47.
20. Irvine EJ, Stoskopf B, Donnelly M. A disease activity index for patients with perianal Crohn's disease (CD). Gastroenterology. 1990;98:A177 (abstr.).
21. Tio TL, Mulder CIJ, Wiijers OB et al. Endosonography of perianal and pericolorectal fistula and or abscess in Crohn's disease. Gastrointest Endosc. 1994;4:331–6.

20
Special problems associated with surgical trials in IBD

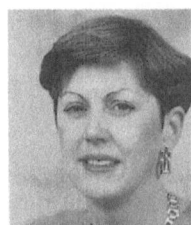

R. S. McLEOD

INTRODUCTION

Decisions about the effectiveness of a treatment may be made based on careful observations. This may be appropriate if the condition is universally fatal or has a high mortality rate and the treatment effect is large. In these situations the value of the treatment is self-evident, and it is unlikely that other factors are responsible for the difference in outcome. However, in modern surgical practice these situations are uncommon. More often, technological developments or surgical interventions lead to small improvements in survival, symptoms or quality of life, and it is necessary to control for extraneous factors to be certain that the observed difference is indeed due to the treatment.

It is accepted that the randomized controlled trial is the best trial design to determine treatment effectiveness. There are several attributes of the randomized controlled trial which minimize the risk of random error and systematic (bias) error, and thus minimize the risk of making an incorrect conclusion about treatment effectiveness. Firstly, subjects are randomly allocated to two groups: a treatment group in which the new treatment is tested and a control group in which standard therapy or placebo is administered. Secondly, the interventions and follow-up are standardized and performed prospectively. Thus, hopefully both groups are similar in all respects except for the single factor being studied. Not only does this guard against differences in factors known to be important, but it also ensures that there are not differences due to other factors which have not yet been

Table 1 Methodological issues of concern
in surgical trials

1	Placebo effect of surgery
2	Blinding
3	Standardization of the procedure
4	Timing of the trial
5	Obsolete procedure

identified.

Although the randomized controlled trial has been accepted by physicians, there is a relative paucity of randomized controlled trials published in the surgical literature. In a review of three surgical journals, *British Journal of Surgery, Diseases of the Colon and Rectum*, and *Surgery*, only 6% of all clinical articles published in these journals in 1980 were randomized controlled trials[1]. Only 16% of articles were comparative studies. Unfortunately, the proportion of randomized controlled trials published in these journals in 1990 was unchanged.

The reason for the lack of randomized controlled trials does not appear to be due to the lack of controversy regarding surgical procedures. In the surgical management of inflammatory bowel disease there is controversy regarding the necessity of a mucosectomy and a defunctioning ileostomy in performing a pelvic pouch procedure. The role of strictureplasty in the management of Crohn's disease is unresolved. The relative merits of surgical and medical treatments have been debated. For instance, do patients with limited terminal ileal Crohn's disease do better with early surgery or medical therapy?

In this chapter, problems precluding or hindering the performance of randomized controlled trials testing surgical therapies will be categorized and discussed under two general headings: methodological issues and feasibility issues.

METHODOLOGICAL ISSUES

The methodological issues that must be addressed by an investigator studying a surgical procedure are similar to those encountered by the investigator testing a medical therapy. However, because of the nature of surgery, these issues may present more of a problem to the surgical investigator. These issues are listed in Table 1. While they make the performance of a trial more difficult, none of them precludes the performance of a randomized controlled trial.

Placebo effect of surgery

Any intervention may have a placebo effect, and it is for this reason that placebo medication is administered to the control group in medical trials. While this is possible in a trial assessing medical therapy, it is usually not feasible or ethical to perform a sham operation when testing a surgical procedure. It appears, also, that the placebo effect of surgery may be greater than with medication. For example, Diamont reported on a series of 18 patients in which 13 had ligation of their internal mammary artery for coronary artery disease and five had a sham operation[2]. All of the latter group reported subjective improvement in their symptoms.

The placebo effect may be difficult to overcome, especially in situations where patient assessment is the important outcome. An example of such a situation might be a trial comparing surgery to medical management in Crohn's disease, where quality of life is the primary outcome. In this situation the patient's assessment of quality of life may be altered by his or her having had a surgical procedure. In situations where outcome is measured with 'hard' outcomes (e.g. development of a cancer, death) or where outcome is assessed by a blinded observer, the placebo effect is less of a concern.

Blinding

The issue of blinding is of importance because of the issue of the placebo effect of surgery. Blinding of the patient and investigators may be difficult, if not impossible, if a surgical therapy is being compared to a medical therapy. It is less difficult if two surgical therapies are being compared, although even in this situation the scars or the side-effects of the two procedures may differ, so the patient is aware of the procedure performed.

Blinding is critical in the assessment of the procedure. If not, there may be a bias in favor of one of the treatment arms. In some situations, even though the patient and investigator are unblinded, it may be possible to have the outcome assessed by a blinded assessor. In situations where the primary outcome is a change in symptoms or quality of life as assessed by the patient, it may be possible to measure a 'hard' outcome in addition, and if it correlates with the patient's assessment then there is less concern about the possibility of bias due to a placebo effect. An example might be to correlate the endoscopic appearance with the patient's symptoms in patients with recurrent Crohn's disease.

Standardization of the procedure

Standardization of the procedure is difficult, since surgeons may vary in their experience with, and their ability to perform, a surgical procedure; there may be individual differences in performing the procedure; and finally, there may be technical modifications as the procedure evolves. There are strategies, however, to ensure that critical aspects of the procedure are standardized. These include ensuring that all surgeons agree on the performance of these aspects of the procedure, providing teaching sessions and obtaining documentation that the procedure has been performed satisfactorily (for example, resection margins may be assessed to ensure that they are free of macroscopic evidence of Crohn's disease). Finally, one can limit the number of surgeons participating in the trial. The decision to do so may vary depending on the complexity of the surgical procedure and the concern about the generalizability of the results, since limiting the number of surgeons may decrease the generalizability.

Timing of the trial

Chalmers has argued that the first patient in whom a procedure is performed should be randomized[3]. Most surgeons would argue, however, that there is a learning curve in any procedure, and that modifications to the technique are made frequently at its inception. By including these early patients one would bias the results against the new procedure. On the other hand, it may be difficult to initiate a trial when the procedure is widely accepted by both the patient and surgical community.

Obsolete procedure

There are concerns that, given the time necessary to accrue patients and complete a trial, the results of the trial may not be relevant because modifications may have been made to the procedure, or other procedures may have been developed in the interim. This argument, however, is equally pertinent to medical trials, where there may be more information available on the optimal dosage, or new drugs may have become available since the start of the trial.

FEASIBILITY ISSUES

While methodological issues may challenge the investigator, feasibility issues may preclude the performance of a randomized controlled trial. These issues inclue: uncommon condition, patient preferences and surgeon preferences.

Uncommon condition

The prevalence of inflammatory bowel disease, including both ulcerative colitis and Crohn's disease, in North America is approximately 50 cases per 100000 population[4]. Although a large proportion of these patients may require surgery at some time, there may be relatively few patients who fit the entry criteria for a particular trial given the various sites, severity and manifestations of the disease. For instance, trials assessing surgery for perianal disease, segmental colitis and gastroduodenal Crohn's disease would be difficult to perform because of the relative rarity of these sites of disease. Similarly, the indications for strictureplasty are relatively uncommon.

Patient preferences

Patient preferences may preclude the performance of a randomized controlled trial. In a medical trial, patients who are randomized to one treatment arm have the possibility of being offered the effective treatment at the conclusion of the trial. Thus, they may benefit directly from the results of the trial. For example, following a trial assessing maintenance therapy for either Crohn's disease or ulcerative colitis, patients may be eligible to receive the more efficacious treatment. Surgical procedures, however, are usually permanent. Thus, there is little chance of the patient receiving the more effective treatment at the conclusion of the trial and thus benefiting from the results of the treatment. As a result, patients may be reluctant to enter a trial, particularly if the treatments are viewed as being unequal. For example, if a trial were performed to compare recurrence rates following total proctocolectomy or colectomy and ileorectal anastomosis in Crohn's disease, the patient would be left with a permanent ileostomy if he or she were randomized to the total proctocolectomy group regardless of the results of the trial. In such situations, if there is genuine equipoise about the effectiveness of the two treatments, it is likely that patients will have a preference for one treatment or the other, and refuse randomization. However, there are trials which have compared surgery to a medical therapy (EC–IC bypass procedure)[5] and surgical procedures of differing magnitude (lumpectomy versus mastectomy for breast cancer)[6]. Thus, more research is required to determine whether patient preferences do indeed preclude the performance of randomized controlled trials, and what factors affect their decision-making. Physicians' opinions on the reasons for patients not participating in trials may not necessarily reflect patients' opinions.

Surgeon preferences

Perhaps one of the major reasons for the lack of surgical trials is the greater acceptance on the part of surgeons of results from case reports and series. There is little incentive for surgeons to do randomized controlled trials, and perhaps some disincentives. Unlike medications, surgical procedures are not regulated by a regulatory agency such as the Health Protection Branch (HPB) in Canada or the Federal Drug Administration (FDA) in the USA. Surgeons can proceed with performing a new operation with little constraint even from their hospital or local ethics committee. On the other hand, if a trial is initiated, then the surgeon must seek approval from the ethics committee and consent from the patient. A good example of the lack of regulation has been the explosion of laparoscopic techniques in general surgery without any substantive trials having been performed. Economic disincentives may also make participation in trials unattractive. In the case of laparoscopic cholecystectomy, surgeons who failed to perform this procedure suddenly began noticing the effects on their practices. Many surgeons felt it necessary to begin performing this procedure even though the results and complications were not fully evaluated. Another disincentive is the lack of funding for surgical trials. Because of the HPB and FDA regulations, which require investigation of drugs prior to their release, industry is interested in providing funding to perform medical trials. These sources are generally not available for funding surgical trials, and funding must come from other sources. Finally, the lack of professional acclaim for clinical as opposed to laboratory research for academic surgeons may be another factor.

CONCLUSIONS

Should more randomized controlled trials be performed to test surgical therapies in inflammatory bowel disease? The answer is unequivocally 'yes'. However, these trials must address important clinically relevant questions, have appropriate outcome measures and be methodologically sound. In most instances this will mean multicenter trials. There must be commitment on the part of surgeons, and adequate funding must be available. Finally there are some situations where randomized controlled trials cannot be performed and, in these situations, trial designs which are less rigorous than the randomized controlled trial, but more rigorous than the case series, may need to be adopted.

References

1. Solomon MJ, McLeod RS. Clinical studies in surgical journals – have we improved? Dis Colon Rectum. 1993;36:43–8.
2. Dimond EG, Kittle CF, Crockett JE. Evaluation of internal mammary artery ligation and sham procedure in angina pectoris. Circulation. 1958;18:712–13.
3. Chalmers TC. Randomization of the first patient. Med Clin Am. 1975;59:1035.
4. Donaldson RM. Crohn's disease. In: Sleisenger MH, Fordtran JS, editors. Gastrointestinal disease: pathophysiology, diagnosis, management. Philadelphia: Saunders; 1983:1088.
5. The EC/IC Bypass Study Group: Failure of extracranial–intracranial arterial bypass to reduce the risk of ischemic stroke: results of an international randomized trial. N Engl J Med. 1985;313:1191–200.
6. Fisher B et al. Eight year results of a RCT comparing total mastectomy and lumpectomy with or without irradiation in the treatment of breast cancer. N Engl J Med. 1989;320:822.

21
Trends in IBD therapy: a meta-analytic approach

G. W. WHITING, J. LAU, B. KUPELNICK and T. C. CHALMERS

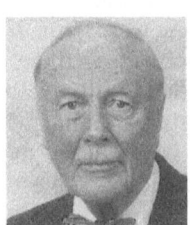

T. C. CHALMERS

INTRODUCTION

Meta-analysis is more than a statistical technique for pooling data from multiple primary research reports. Instead it is a wholly new and precise discipline for gathering and transferring the results of primary research projects in a valid and understandable format so that they can be applied to patient care by physicians and those who set medical policy.

Crohn's disease is a perfect example of the serious problem physicians and health-care policy-makers face when they try to keep up with the potential impact of medical research on medical practice. In a disease of unknown etiology, one with acute and chronic manifestations, there is bound to be an increasing explosion of important clinical trials. Publication of review articles written by the clinical experts has been the classical way of keeping everybody informed. That route has been found increasingly to be flawed because of the appearance of evidence of lack of thorough literature searches, and of bias in the selection and interpretation of published trials in many fields. There is no reason to think that Crohn's disease would be any different. In contrast to meta-analysis, the writer of reviews and textbook chapters does not present all of the evidence on which opinions and recommendations are based.

The purpose of this chapter is to illustrate the application of all aspects of the technique of meta-analysis to the pharmacologic treatment of acute attacks of Crohn's disease, a common clinical problem requiring frequent updates of therapeutic advances.

CRITERIA FOR A GOOD META-ANALYSIS

If meta-analyses are to be reliable conduits of original medical information they must be reliably performed. Calling something a meta-analysis or *structured* review calls into play certain methodological rules which, if neglected, could and should lead to rejection by editors or peer reviewers of the whole effort. This protection of the reader works only if there is a reasonable agreement about the characteristics of an acceptable meta-analysis. The search for the original data must be as complete as possible, bias must be minimized by blinding papers before decisions are made by the investigators, and all steps must be carried out in duplicate to minimize errors. These initial steps are illustrated schematically in Fig. 1. Once a subject has been selected, references are sought in review articles and recent randomized controlled trials (RCT). MeSH terms and key words for a Medline search are gleaned from a recovery of the first articles in Medline. However, it has been demonstrated at least six times[1] that a Medline search for clinical trials recovers only about 50% of the articles found by other means. Most of the clinical trials found elsewhere are actually in Medline when an author search is carried out, so the defect lies in subject cataloguing.

The conscientious clinical investigator will also have been perusing *Current Contents* each week for inflammatory disease trials. As in other diseases there are also special publications of bibliographies and abstracts, in this case, *Trends in Inflammatory Bowel Disease Therapy*, published in June 1993 by Interfalk, Canada.

Once a number of candidate papers have been logged in, a preliminary screening is carried out and the review articles and uncontrolled trials rejected. A matrix of comparisons (see below) is then constructed, and a decision made about which meta-analyses to undertake. The selected papers are then 'differentially photocopied' – by that is meant the process by which a technician blots out before photocopying all information relative to the sources, dates, and results of each trial. The former are left blank and the latter are disguised as A and B, or X and Y. One copy of this blinded paper is placed in the master file with the original and one copy is given to each investigator, along with an unaltered copy to be consulted when all of the questions that could be answered from the blinded copy are answered. Pertinent data are extracted by each investigator, and quality questionnaires are filled out using only the Methods and Results sections[2]. A consensus conference is then held to iron out the differences, which typically occur 15–20% of the time. There are occasional exceptions to the above process, as when a few papers are well known to all and others are added late, but an attempt is made to do each study properly. Because those familiar with the field will easily recognize a few papers, an attempt is made in each instance to have as one of the investigators a methodologist or student, in addition to the expert in the field.

After the consensus conference tables of results are constructed in a standard format and the statistical analyses carried out by more than one method.

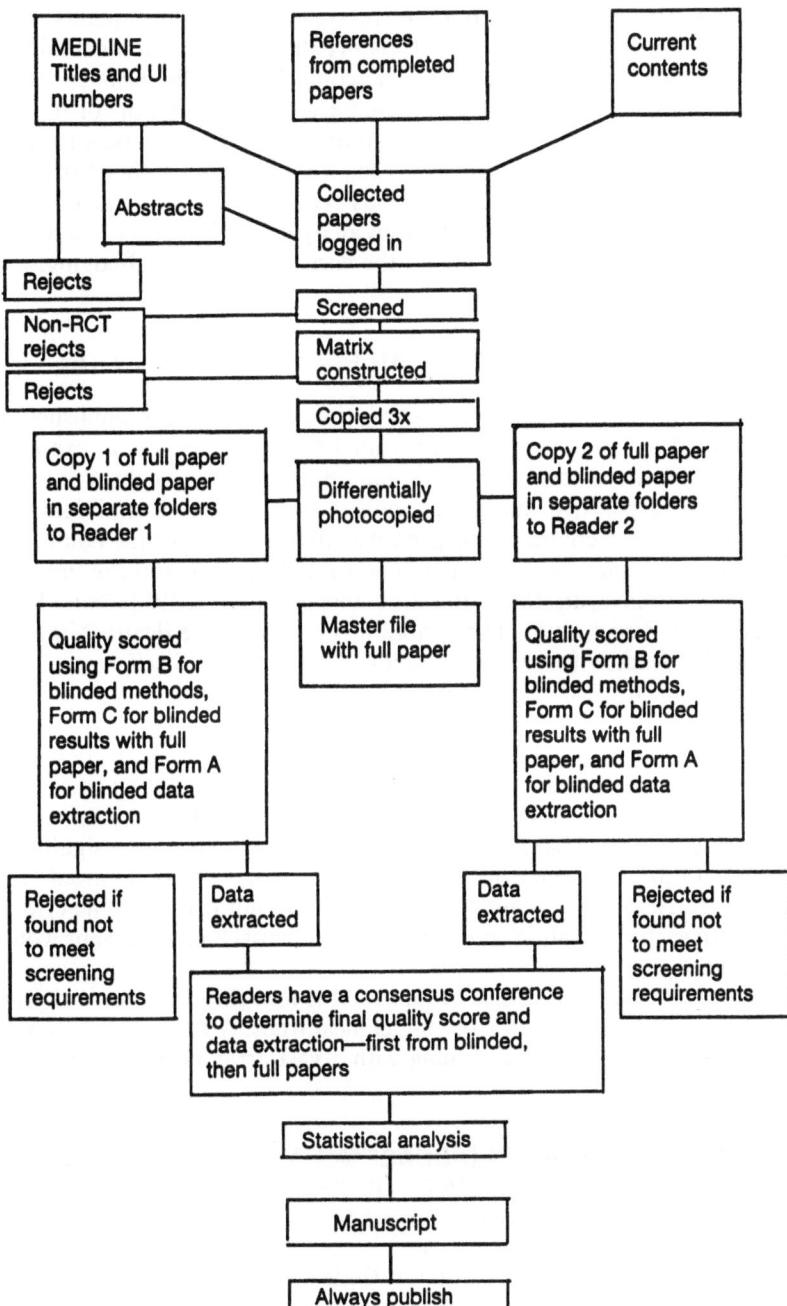

Fig. 1 Diagram of a meta-analytic process designed to ensure that all relevant published articles are included, that bias is minimized by blinding information that might influence selection of papers and extraction of data, and that errors are minimized by duplicate performance

Unfortunately there is no quantitative system for scoring quality as a reflection of the fact that bias might distort the results, so the confidence intervals are not weighted by the quality scores. Instead the included RCTs are listed in order of descending quality score, so the investigators or readers can do their own sensitivity analyses by omitting the worst papers to see if the results are inordinately influenced by the worst research. Other sensitivity analyses can then be carried out, such as removing studies with outlying treatments or unusual patients. Subgroup analyses can be carried out at this stage, but with great caution to avoid the accusation of data-dredging.

CUMULATIVE META-ANALYSIS, AN EXCITING INNOVATION

If a new meta-analysis is performed every time a new study is published or found, critical new information is presented to the reader. As an example, the left-hand chart on Fig. 2 shows a standard format meta-analysis of RCTs comparing perioperative antibiotics with a placebo or no antibiotics in patients undergoing colorectal surgery, usually for cancer of the colon, but also of interest to surgeons removing inflamed bowels. The dots are the odds ratio, under 1.0 favoring the antibiotics, and the lines the 95% confidence intervals around each ratio. The endpoint is perioperative death. Although most of the studies favor the antibiotics, none is in itself statistically significant. The trials also reported the postoperative infection rates, and here the control rates were higher and the differences more often significant. However, by the time 200 patients had been randomized, in 1971, the differences were statistically significant and, although fluctuating some with regard to degree, the confidence intervals never crossed the unity line in the ensuing 20 years. The final illustrative Z and p values were highly significant ($2p = 0.0016$) in 1987 when the last study in this series was reported. The term 'illustrative p' value is used because we have not corrected the critical p value with each calculation, as some strict frequentist biostatisticians would have us do.

Cumulative meta-analysis has brought to the fore the importance of prior clinical trials in planning and stopping clinical trials. A Bayesian approach[3] seems more appropriate when dealing with a vast array of published RCTs.

TREATMENT OF CROHN'S DISEASE AS AN EXAMPLE OF THE NEED TO FIND EFFICIENT WAYS OF DEALING WITH THE GLUT OF PUBLISHED AND UNPUBLISHED RCTs

Three years ago we developed for the *Online Journal of Current Clinical Trials* a matrical approach to the large number of available clinical trials of drugs and diet for the treatment of acute attacks of Crohn's disease[4]. The different drugs and diets considered by the authors of each RCT to be the experimental approach were placed in the rows, and the control treatments of each RCT were the columns. Into the appropriate cells were placed each study identified by the number of patients randomized and a code for the

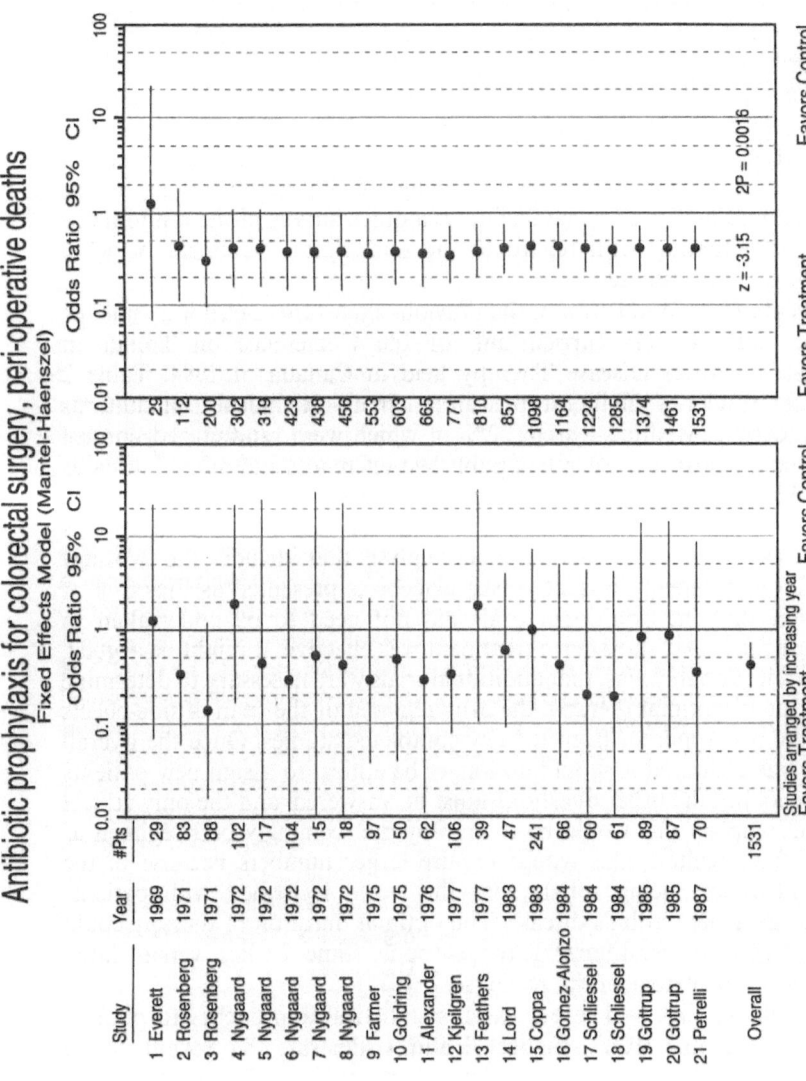

Fig. 2 An example of the meta-analytic approaches to randomized control trials of the efficacy of perioperative antibiotics in reducing the operative death rates from surgery for cancer of the colon. The standard chart on the left reveals none of the individual trials to be statistically significant, and the cumulative meta-analysis on the right reveals statistical significance to have been achieved by 1975. In this case heterogeneity is not significant, so that the random- and fixed-effects models give the same answer

outcome chosen by the authors as the principal one (Table 1). This process enabled the author and reader to keep close track of the papers appearing in each cell, so that the need for a meta-analysis can be determined. For instance, a pooling of the trials of an immunosuppressant drug summarized in cell A1 was clearly indicated and was carried out[4]. The success rate of the combined different immunosuppressant drugs in short-term studies of varying duration was significantly better than a placebo. The cells A2 and A4 would bear watching, and A3 and A5 appear to be statistically significant, but could be checked with a meta-analysis. The cells under the columns B to E are comparisons of one active treatment with another and, because of a lower failure rate among the controls, will require many more studies before meta-analysis is indicated. The diet studies are going to require individual analysis because most are studying different modifications. So use of the proposed matrical format facilitates a quick survey of the randomized control trial situation with regard to the nonsurgical treatment of acute attacks of Crohn's disease.

Four years after completion of the previous literature search it is time for a repeat, and one was carried out for the Conference on Trends in Inflammatory Bowel Disease Therapy held in Canada in 1994. Table 2 presents the results of the literature search. Ninety-six clinical trial citations were found by a Medline search, 22% of which were randomized control trials of acute treatments. Search of published references and other databases revealed 11 more RCTs, an additional one-third.

A matrix of the RCTs published from January 1990 to March 1994 is presented as Table 3. An updated meta-analysis that includes the two new trials of an immunosuppressant versus placebo is presented as Figs 3-6. It is apparent that the additional trials did not need to be undertaken to establish the fact that short-term treatment was effective. It might be argued, and indeed it probably was, that additional trials were necessary to determine the duration of optimal therapy, the drug regimen or the span of side-effects which were not apparent from the few completed studies. Once the overall question was answered it should no longer be ethical to assign new patients to a placebo; but the other questions must be answered, and the only ethical way to accomplish this would be to employ the seemingly best regimen as the control thereafter. This would require larger numbers because of the smaller differences being sought, but the world is loaded with patients diagnosed as acute Crohn's disease. The optimal duration of therapy could be determined by randomizing the stopping time earlier versus later, depending on the extent of the response.

The graphs in Figs 3-6 reveal various statistical approaches to pooling the data in the nine RCTs. Figures 3 and 4 illustrate the advantages of employing both the fixed- and random-effects models. The results of the trials are heterogeneous ($p < 0.01$), and the cumulative meta-analyses best illustrate the differences resulting from widening the confidence intervals with the random-effects model. The reduction in the odds ratios is statistically significant (confidence intervals no longer crossing one) from 1980 on in the fixed-effects model and only after 1989 in the random-effects model. In Fig. 5 the random-effects model units are different, absolute percentage change,

Table 1 Therapy comparison matrix of RCT of therapy for acute attacks of Crohn's disease

Experimental therapy	Comparison therapy					
	Placebo	Sulfasalazine	Steroids	Diet	Other	Totals
Immunosuppression	26?* 72++ 42+ 12+ 15+ 42++ 134?		3?		37++ 36?	10
T-cell stimulants	33+ 9? 19? 21?					4
Sulfasalazine	26++ 54++				42− 23?	4
5-ASA	12? 67+	30+ 23?				4
Antibiotics	20+ 100++ 52++ 7?				72+ 52?	6
Steroids	47++ 38++ 85++	38+			38+	5
Diet	36++		6+ 7+ 9?	19? 10++ 36? 16? 28+ 20++		10
Combination	56++ 20+ 163++		163−	21++	72++	6
Other	55? 18? 29? 199+ 21+ 16? 18?		80++ 22?			9
Totals	33	3	7	7	8	58

The rows are the experimental therapies, the columns the control therapies, and the cells list each pertinent study, giving the total number of patients and symbols for outcome as follows: ++, statistically significant in favor of the experimental therapy; +, trend in favor of the experimental; ?, no clinically interesting difference; −, trend in favor of the control therapy; −−, statistically significant in favour of the control therapy

Data are from Fig. 1 of ref. 4.

Table 2 Results of a Medline search for citations related to the treatment of Crohn's disease between January 1990 and April 1994

Type of study	Number of citations
Review articles	22
Randomized control trials	
Acute treatment	21 (11)
Maintaining remission	12
Total	33
Non-randomized and uncontrolled	7
Meta-analysis of RCT	1
Total clinical trial citations	96

RCT of acute treatment are expanded by 11 additional ones culled from the reference lists of recent publications

References to the 32 randomized control trials in the matrix of new trials listed by cell in the matrix

Matrix cell
D5. Riordan AM, Hunter JO, Cowan RE *et al.* Treatment of active Crohn's disease by exclusion diet: East Anglian multicentre controlled trial. Lancet. 1993;342:1131–4.
C6. Gorard DA, Hunt B, Payne-James JJ *et al.* Initial response and subsequent course of Crohn's disease treated with elemental diet or prednisolone. Gut. 1993;34:1198–202.
C6. Gonazlez-Huix F, de Leon R, Fernandez-Banares F *et al.* Polymeric enteral diets as primary treatment of active Crohn's disease: a prospective steroid controlled trial. Gut. 1993;34:778–82.
A5. Singleton JW, Hanauer SB, Gitnick GL *et al.* Mesalamine capsules for the treatment of active Crohn's disease: results of a 16-week trial. Pentasa Crohn's Disease Study Group. Gastroenterology. 1993;104:1293–301.
C5. Landi B, Anh TN, Cortot A *et al.* Endoscopic monitoring of Crohn's disease treatment: a prospective, randomized clinical trial. The Groupe d'Etudes Therapeutiques des Affections Inflammatoires Digestives. Gastroenterology. 1992;102:1647–53.
C6. Sanderson IR, Udeen S, Davies PS, Savage MO, Walker-Smith JA. Remission induced by an elemental diet in small bowel Crohn's disease. Arch Dis Child. 1987;61:123–7.
A4. Sutherland L, Singleton J, Sessions J *et al.* Double blind, placebo controlled trial of metronidazole in Crohn's disease. Gut. 1991;32:1071–5.
B4. Ursing B, Alm T, Barany F *et al.* A comparative study of metronidazole and sulfasalazine for active Crohn's disease: the cooperative Crohn's disease study in Sweden. II. Result. Gastroenterology. 1982;83:550–62.
D6. Harries AD, Jones LA, Danis V *et al.* Controlled trial of supplemented oral nutrition in Crohn's disease. Lancet. 1983;1:887–90.
D6. Park RH, Galloway A, Danesh BJ, Russell RI. Double blind trial comparing elemental and polymeric diet as primary treatment for active Crohn's disease. Gut. 1989;30:A1453–4 (abstr.).
A1. Brynskov J, Freund L, Rasmussen SN *et al.* A placebo-controlled, double-blind, randomized trial of cyclosporine therapy in active chronic Crohn's disease. N Engl J Med. 1989;321:845–50.
A5. Bergman L, Krause U. Postoperative treatment with corticosteroids and salazosulphapyridine (Salazopyrin) after radical resection for Crohn's disease. Scand J Gastroenterol. 1976;11:651–66.
A8. Brillanti S, Biasco G, Azzaroni D *et al.* Pentasa versus sulphasalazine tablets in the treatment of active Crohn's ileocolitis. Scand J Gastroenterol Suppl. 1989;158:129–30.
D6. Greenberg GR, Fleming CR, Jeejeebhoy KN, Rosenberg IH, Sales D, Tremaine WJ. Controlled trial of bowel rest and nutritional support in the management of Crohn's disease. Gut. 1988;29:1309–15.

continued

Table 2 *continued*

A3. Rasmussen SN, Lauritsen K, Tage-Jensen U *et al.* 5-Aminosalicylic acid in the treatment of Crohn's disease. A 16-week double-blind, placebo-controlled, multicentre study with Pentasa. Scand J Gastroenterol. 1987;22:877–83.

A1. Arora S, Katkov WN, Cooley J *et al.* A double-blind, randomized, placebo-controlled trial of methotrexate in Crohn's disease. Gastroenterology. 1992;102:A591 (abstr.).

D6. Giaffer MH, North G, Holdsworth CD. Controlled trial of polymeric versus elemental diet in treatment of active Crohn's disease. Lancet. 1990;335:816–19.

E5. Saverymuttu S, Hodgson HJ, Chadwick VS. Controlled trial comparing prednisolone with an elemental diet plus non-absorbable antibiotics in active Crohn's disease. Gut. 1985;26:994–8.

C6. Hunt JB, Payne-James JJ, Palmer KR *et al.* A randomised controlled trial of elemental diet and prednisolone as primary therapy in acute exacerbations of Crohn's disease. Gastroenterology. 1989;96:A224 (abstr.).

A2. Van Hees PA, Van Lier HJ, Van Elteren PH *et al.* Effect of sulphasalazine in patients with active Crohn's disease: a controlled double-blind study. Gut. 1981;22:404–9.

D5. O'Morain C, Segal AW, Levi AJ. Elemental diet as primary treatment of acute Crohn's disease: a controlled trial. Br Med J. 1984;288:1859–62.

A3. Griffiths A, Koletzko S, Sylvester F, Marcon M, Sherman P. Slow-release 5-aminosalicylic acid therapy in children with small intestinal Crohn's disease. J Pediatr Gastroenterol Nutr. 1993;17:186–92.

D6. Raouf AH, Hildrey V, Daniel J *et al.* Enteral feeding as sole treatment for Crohn's disease: controlled trial of whole protein v amino acid based feed and a case study of dietary challenge. Gut. 1991;32:702–7.

D6. Rigaud D, Cosnes J, Le Quintrec Y *et al.* Controlled trial comparing two types of enteral nutrition in treatment of active Crohn's disease: elemental versus polymeric diet. Gut. 1991;32:1492–7.

B9. Rijk MC, van Hogezand RA, van Lier HJ, van Tongeren JH. Sulphasalazine and prednisone compared with sulphasalazine for treating active Crohn disease. A double-blind, randomized, multicenter trial. Ann Intern Med. 1991;114:445–50.

C7. Ewe K, Press AG, Singe CC *et al.* Azathioprine combined with prednisolone or monotherapy with prednisolone in active Crohn's disease. Gastroenterology. 1993;105:367–72.

E6. Lochs H, Steinardt HJ, Klaus-Wentz B *et al.* Comparison of enteral nutrition and drug treatment in active Crohn's disease. Results of the European Cooperative Crohn's Disease Study. IV. Gastroenterology. 1991;101:881–8.

C6. Thomas AG, Taylor F, Miller V. Dietary intake and nutritional treatment in childhood Crohn's disease. J Pediatr Gastroenterol Nutr. 1993;17:75–81.

C6, D7, C7. Lindor KD, Fleming CR, Burnes JU, Nelson JK, Ilstrup DM. A randomized prospective trial comparing a defined formula diet, corticosteroids, and a defined formula diet plus corticosteroids in active Crohn's disease. Mayo Clin Proc. 1992;67:328–33.

C7. Afdhal NH, Long A, Lennon J, Crowe J, O'Donoghue DP. Controlled trial of antimycobacterial therapy in Crohn's disease. Clofazimine versus placebo. Dig Dis Sci. 1991;36:449–53.

C5. Brignola C, De Simone G, Iannone P *et al.* Influence of steroid treatment's duration in patients with active Crohn's disease. Agents Actions. 1992 (Spec No): C90–2.

C3. Jenss H, Hartmann F, Scholmerich J, German ASA-Study Group. 5-Aminosalicylic acid versus methylprednisolone in the tretment of active Crohn's disease — first results of double blind clinial trial. Scand J Gastroenterol. Suppl. 1989;158:136.

and the varying control rates of failure are also shown. For Fig. 6 the order of the trials was changed from ascending year to descending control rate to illustrate something we have found almost universally in meta-analyses, a direct correlation between response rate and the rate of events in the control group (J. Cappelleri, J. Lau, C. H. Schmid and T. C. Chalmers, manuscript in preparation).

The above procedures will be new and somewhat disturbing to both gastroenterologists and biostatisticians, and considerable thought and dialog

Table 3 Matrix of randomized control trials of treatment of acute attacks of Crohn's disease published from January 1990 through March 1994

Experimental therapy*	Comparison therapy				
	A Placebo	B Sulfasalazine	C Steroids	D Diet	E Other
1 Immunosuppression	71++ 28+				
2 Sulfasalazine	26++				
3 5-ASA	14++ 67+		55 − −		
4 Metronidazole	56++	78?			
5 Steroids	310++ 84?		96? 54+	78++ 21?	37?
6 Diet			32? 42? 29? 15? 24? 19?	14 − − 30++ 51? 28+ 24? 30?	107 − −
7 Combination therapy			49+ 18+ 42++	17+	
8 Mesalazine (Pentasa)		34?			
9 Sulfasalazine + prednisone		60+			

*Numbers plotted are comparisons, not individual papers, due to some papers comparing more than two treatments
Cells contrain number of patients in each RCT and results of major endpoint chosen by author: ++, statistically significant favoring experimental therapy; +, trend towards experimental; ?, no clinically meaningful difference; −, trend favoring the control treatment; − −, statistically significant favoring the control therapy

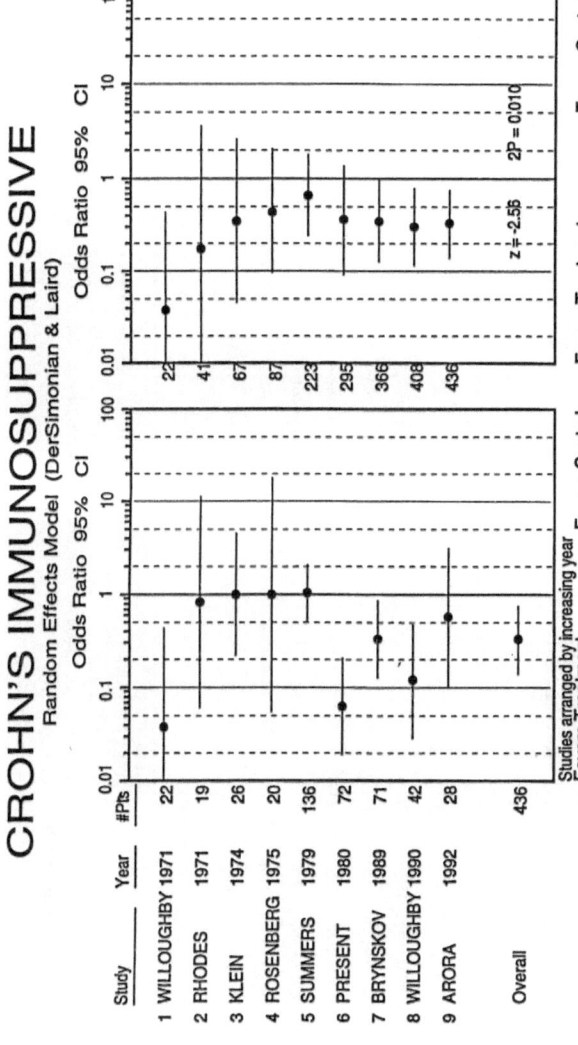

Fig. 3 Nine randomized control trials of immunosuppressive therapy versus placebo for acute attacks of Crohn's disease. Results expressed as odds ratio, experimental treatment better with odds ratio less than 1. Random-effects model. Studies ordered by year of publication, standard on left and cumulative on right

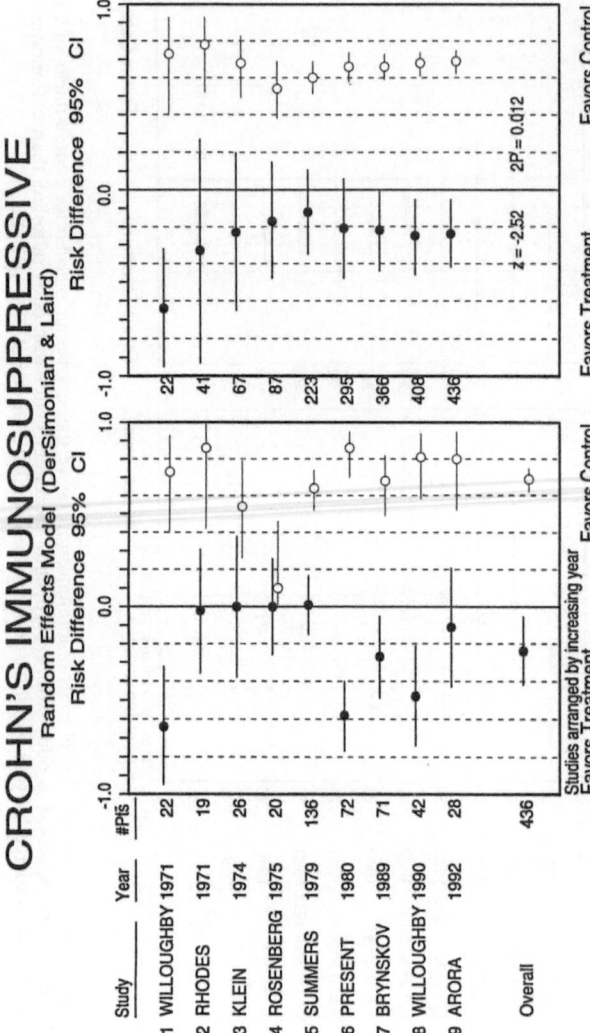

Fig. 4 Same as in Fig. 3, but results are expressed as absolute percentage difference. Open circles are rate of failure in placebo-treated groups

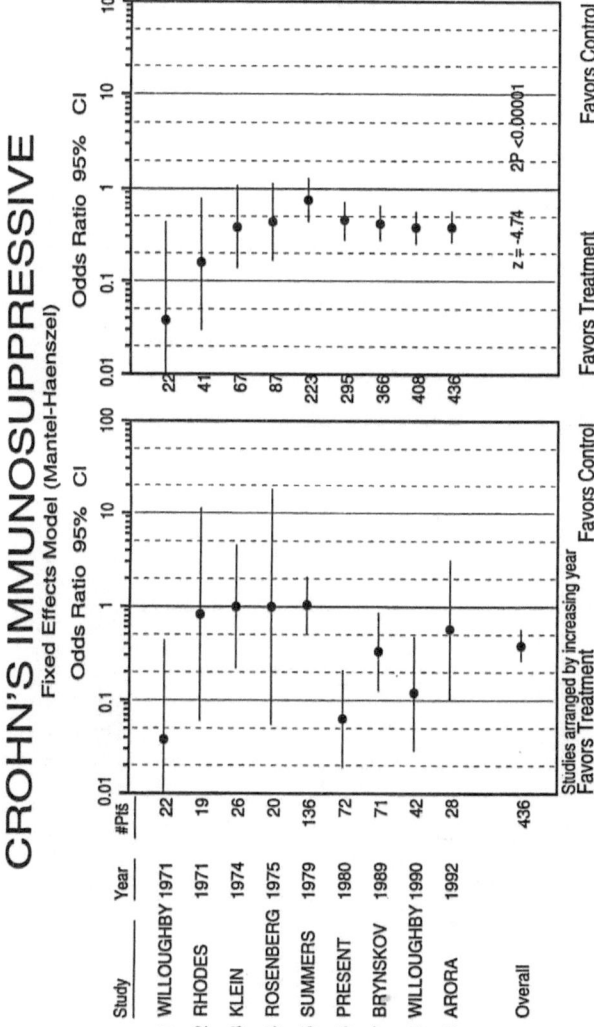

Fig. 5 Same as in Fig. 3, but analyses by fixed-effects model. Note on right that significance at the $p = 0.05$ level is achieved by 1980 instead of in 1989 as in the random-effects model

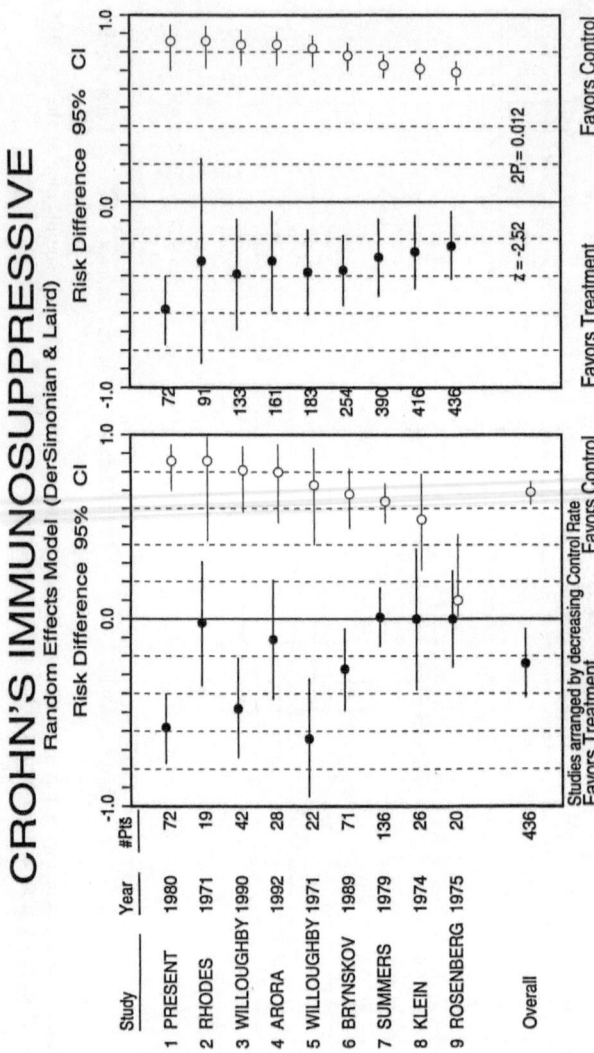

Fig. 6 Same as in Fig. 4, but studies are arranged according to the rate of failure in the control group, in descending order

are indicated. However, such are the consequences of the very large number of trials of the treatment of Crohn's disease. The situation would actually be more acute were clinicians to randomize the 'first patient'[6-8], as they should, as long as the optimal treatment of the acute disease has not been discovered. That is not likely to occur unless the exact etiology is known, and a large number of patients will have presented themselves for treatment before that happens.

Acknowledgements

This work was supported in part by a grant from the Agency for Health Care Policy and Research, R01HS07782.

References

1. Chalmers TC, Lau J. Meta-analytic stimulus for changes in clinical trials. Stat Meth Med Res. 1993;2:161–72.
2. Chalmers TC, Smith Jr H, Blackburn B et al. A method for assessing the quality of a randomized control trial. Contr Clin Trials. 1981;2:31–49.
3. Lewis RJ, Wears RL. An introduction to the Bayesian analysis of clinical trials. Ann Emerg Med. 1993;22:8:1328–35.
4. Morris RD, Lau J, Arena NJ, Nardine FE, Chalmers TC. A clinical trials database as a research tool in health care. Online J Curr Clin Trials (serial online). 1992;1992(Doc. No. 14).
5. Chalmers TC. When should randomization begin? [Letter]. Lancet. 1968;1:858.
6. Chalmers TC. Randomization of the first patient. Med Clin N Am. 1975;59:1035–8.
7. Chalmers TC. The need for early randomization in the development of new drugs for AIDS. J AIDS. 1990;3(Suppl. 2):S10–15.
8. Chalmers TC. Randomize the first patient! N Engl J Med. 1977;296:107.

Section VII
Basic science: genetics, markers and models

22
New IBD markers: definition of disease heterogeneity

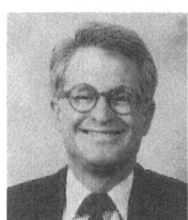

S. R. TARGAN

INTRODUCTION

The objective of this chapter is to relate recent findings that support the use of molecular and cellular techniques to define subsets of patients with inflammatory bowel disease (IBD). An example of the potential of using these methods to define disease subgroups by genetic and subclinical markers is an 'aggressive' form of rheumatoid arthritis, which recently has been shown to express a specific HLA-DR4 allele[1]. This subgroup of patients with rheumatoid arthritis is defined clinically by a progressively active course that is resistant to standard therapy, including corticosteroids. Such patients do, however, respond very well to treatment with the immune suppressant, methotrexate. Those patients with the HLA-DR4 allele are now placed immediately on methotrexate. Thus, this description of a subgroup of patients has led to a completely altered treatment protocol, and is the first instance where a genetic marker is being used to define a subset of patients for treatment with a selected therapy in an immunologically mediated disease. In ulcerative colitis and Crohn's disease, subsets of patients may also be defined by genetic and subclinical markers that reflect specific types of mucosal inflammation, and each type may represent a unique opportunity for individualized treatment approaches.

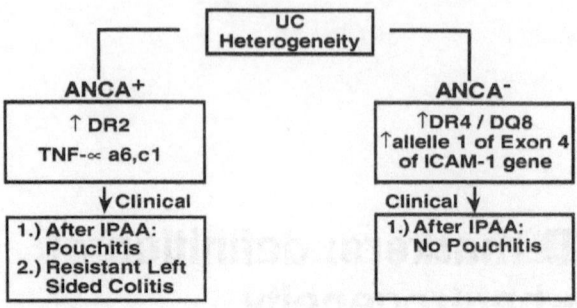

Fig. 1

GENETIC AND SUBCLINICAL CHARACTERIZATION OF PATIENTS WITH IBD

HLA and ANCA

As with other immunologic diseases, subgroups of patients with IBD have a varied clinical presentation, and this has led to investigations to determine whether this variation may actually represent a set of diseases that display a similar clinical picture. The differences may be based on heterogeneous genetic backgrounds. Genetic heterogeneity was first shown in two diseases: (a) type I diabetes and type II diabetes have different genetic profiles[2]; (b) juvenile rheumatoid arthritis of a particular clinical phenotype has different HLA associations from the other types[3].

In recent years a series of observations has suggested that within each type of IBD (particularly within ulcerative colitis but also currently emerging in Crohn's disease) there are heterogeneous clinical phenotypes. The following is a discussion of ulcerative colitis as an example of a genetically heterogeneous syndrome. These concepts are schematized in Fig. 1.

Genetic and subclinical markers have been associated with ulcerative colitis. Particularly informative has been the finding that in ulcerative colitis there has been an increased association of HLA-DR2 and a decreased association with HLA-DR4. Furthermore, the population can be divided into those patients who express anti-neutrophil cytoplasmic antibodies (ANCA) and those who do not. HLA associations differ based on the presence or absence of ANCA[4]. HLA-DR2 is associated only with patients expressing ANCA, while HLA-DR4 is associated with the ulcerative colitis population *not* expressing ANCA. Presence or absence of ANCA appears to breed true in families, i.e. unaffected family members of ulcerative colitis probands with ANCA also have ANCA; the converse is also true[5]. These initial findings suggest a correlation between ANCA and the so-called 'familial ulcerative colitis' which may differ from the 'spontaneous' ulcerative colitis that appears to arise in the absence of a family association.

A genetic/subclinical characterization has been made recently in patients with familial colon cancer, separating this population from those patients with spontaneous colon cancer. The initial gene associations were made with pedigrees of familial cancer. Subsequent studies will define the relationships of these gene alterations when spontaneous cancers arise in the general population.

ICAM1 and exon 5

Initial data suggested that the serum marker ANCA may differentiate patients with two distinct types of colitis. Subsequent studies demonstrated additional genetic associations further describing the populations with and without ANCA. The adhesion molecule termed ICAM1 is a critical structure located on many cell types and is very important for regulating the immune response. The gene structure for that particular molecule is now known, and polymorphisms within that gene have also been described[6]. It is now apparent that a different allele of the ICAM1 molecule in a particular part of the gene termed 'exon 5' is differentially associated within the ulcerative colitis population. There is an increased association of exon 4 with ulcerative colitis patients who do *not* express ANCA, but this increase is not noted in those who do. Thus, a second genetic association becomes apparent upon dividing the ulcerative colitis population by ANCA. These genes are associated with the regulation of inflammation, and the findings suggest that there may be a different type of mucosal inflammatory process among those patients that have ANCA circulating in their serum compared to those who do not[7,8]

Subgroups defined at the mucosal level

The presence of ANCA antibodies in the serum of patients with ulcerative colitis potentially is a marker of an underlying selective immune regulatory abnormality manifested by a specific type of inflammation that may differ from inflammation in patients without this marker. This hypothesis was generated from the findings of several recent studies which have shown differential familial, genetic and clinical associations between ulcerative colitis patients expressing ANCA and those who do not[4-6]. These findings support the thesis that ANCA is a marker that defines the mucosal inflammatory process of ulcerative colitis patients as different from the inflammation of patients who do not produce ANCA. If ANCA is a marker for a disease-related immune response process, it is assumed that there are B cells within the colonic mucosa that produce these antibodies. Studies have shown that ANCA secreting B-cell clones are present in only 60–70% of both involved and uninvolved mucosa of ulcerative colitis patients. This percentage parallels that found for the presence of ANCA in the serum of ulcerative colitis patients, suggesting that the presence or absence of serum ANCA is reflective of the mucosal B-cell ANCA production. More importantly, this finding implicates these clones in a disease-specific mucosal immune response in ANCA-expressing ulcerative colitis patients which differs from the mucosal response of ulcerative colitis patients not expressing ANCA. It is likely that the B-cell clones which produce ANCA are involved in an ulcerative colitis-related immune response rather than the ANCA antibodies playing a direct role in the disease pathogenesis. Therefore, the presence or absence of ANCA-producing B cells may reflect a different mucosal inflammatory response occurring among the different groups of patients, and suggests that there could be distinct types of clinical disease which can be differentiated based on ANCA.

Subgroups defined by clinical parameters

An example of a subgroup defined initially by clinical parameters comprises those patients with very severe disease that undergo an ileal pouch–anal anastomosis and subsequently develop inflammation in those pouches. Investigations were performed to determine their genetic and subclinical marker profiles and distinctions were found. The great majority of patients in this group express ANCA. By contrast those patients that have a similar operation but do not develop pouchitis do not express ANCA[9,10]. This study was the first investigation following a clinical observation. The investigation yielded corroborative and provocative results further emphasizing the heterogeneity among the population of patients diagnosed with 'ulcerative colitis'.

To date the diagnosis of ulcerative colitis, and the description of subpopulations, has been made purely on an anatomical basis, i.e. proctitis, left-sided colitis and pancolitis, or relative to their clinical presentation of mild, moderate and severe. However, the population has not been divided by 'type of inflammation', which may now be possible by separation of the populations along the lines of the markers defined above. Type of inflammation may be characterized by the responsiveness of the patient to a particular medication as part of the natural history of the disease process. As has been shown in the example of rheumatoid arthritis, these markers may determine how 'aggressive' the process is, and how 'responsive' it is to standard or 'progressive' courses of medication. It is now incumbent upon clinical researchers and physicians to begin to characterize and stratify ulcerative colitis and Crohn's disease on the basis of the aggressiveness of inflammation and the extent of disease by molecular and cellular technology, in conjunction with the natural clinical course, and response to therapy.

An attempt was made to utilize the markers currently available to define an additional clinical group differentiated by ANCA. In conjunction with the Mayo Clinic we investigated the incidence of ANCA in treatment-resistant, left-sided colitis who were resistant to the standard treatments including oral and intravenous corticosteroids. Ninety percent of patients with 'resistant' left-sided disease had ANCA, which is a substantially higher figure than the overall group of ulcerative colitis patients, of which 60% express ANCA[11].

A similar picture is now emerging in Crohn's disease. Although ANCA is present at low levels in only a small group of Crohn's patients (15–20%) it marks for a different gene association than those Crohn's patients that have ANCA-free serum[12].

In summary, building on our early findings dividing subgroups of patients with IBD, and ulcerative colitis in particular, we now have three 'levels' of differentiation; (a) genetic and subclinical markers; (b) mucosal cell profile; and (c) clinical distinctions. It is likely that further markers will be found from this same base, and these concepts are being applied to other disease processes contemporaneously.

THE PRESENT AND FUTURE OF TREATMENT BASED ON DEFINITION OF DISEASE HETEROGENEITY

It is very important that when new trials of medications are initiated, and when retrospective analyses of patient populations are undertaken, efforts are made so that markers may be properly associated with those patients. Excellent examples of such redefined patient populations in 1994 include those patients with ulcerative colitis and Crohn's disease who are resistant to corticosteroids, thus requiring immunosuppressive agents such as 6-mercaptopurine and methotrexate, or cyclosporine. Further definition could be obtained by determining response and nonresponse to the various immunosuppressive agents. As in rheumatoid arthritis, these groupings would then 'mark' these patients so that they may be treated with appropriate modality at the presentation of their disease, and not 5 years later when we have discovered that they are resistant.

Subgrouping of patients by genetic and molecular markers is the wave of the future, and our thinking about these diseases should be altered and patient populations stratified by these more modern concepts. Using the criteria described above, varying mucosal inflammatory processes associated with a specific treatment response profile can improve the amount of time taken to find the best therapeutic options for the well-defined patient.

References

1. Weyand CM, Hikok K, Conn DL, Goronzy JJ. The influence of HLA-DRB1 genes on disease severity in rheumatoid arthritis. Ann Intern Med. 1992;117:801–6.
2. Pociot F, Briant L, Jongeneel CV et al. Association of tumor necrosis factor (TNF) and class II major histocompatibility complex alleles with the secretion of TNF-α and TNF-β by human mononuclear cells: a possible link to insulin-dependent diabetes. Eur J Immunol. 1993;23:224–31.
3. Nepom B, Nepom G, Schaller J et al. Characterization of specific HLA DR4-associated histocompatibility markers in patients with juvenile rheumatoid arthritis. J Clin Invest. 1984;74:287–91.
4. Yang H-Y, Rotter JI, Toyoda H et al. Ulcerative colitis: a genetically heterogeneous disorder defined by genetic (HLA class II) and subclinical (anti-neutrophil cytoplasmic antibodies (ANCA)) markers. J Clin Invest. 1993;92:1080–4.
5. Shanahan F, Duerr R, Landers C et al. Neutrophil autoantibodies in ulcerative colitis. A family study with evidence for genetic heterogeneity. Gastroenterology. 1992;103:456–61.
6. Yang H, Vora D, Targan S, Toyoda H, Beaudet A, Rotter JI. Genetic heterogeneity within UC and Crohn's disease defined by anti-neutrophil cytoplasmic antibodies (ANCAs) and intercellular adhesion molecule-1 (ICAM-1) polymorphisms. Gastroenterology. 1994 (In press) (abstr.).
7. Targan SR, Landers C, Vidrich A, MacDermott RP. Perinuclear antineutrophil cytoplasmic

antibodies (p-ANCA) are spontaneously produced by B-cells from involved and uninvolved mucosa of ulcerative colitis (UC) patients (Submitted).

8. Targan SR, Landers C, Vidrich A, MacDermott RP. Perinuclear antineutrophil cytoplasmic antibodies (p-ANCA) are spontaneously produced by B-cells from involved and uninvolved mucosa of ulcerative colitis (UC) patients. Gastroenterology. 1994 (In press) (abstr.).

9. Sandborn WJ, Tremaine WJ, Batts K, Pemberton JH, Phillips SF. Definition of pouchitis following ileal pouch anal anastomosis (IPAA): a pouchitis disease activity index. Gastroenterology. 1993;104:A774.

10. Vecchi M, Gionchetti P, Bianchi MB et al. p-ANCA reactivity in ulcerative colitis patients with and without pouchitis after proctocolectomy. Gastroenterology. 1993;104:A796.

11. Sandborn WJ, Landers CJ, Steiner BL, Tremaine WJ, Targan SR. The prevalence of antineutrophil cytoplasmic antibody (ANCA) is unexpectedly high in patients with treatment-resistant, left-sided ulcerative colitis (UC). Gastroenterology. 1994 (In press) (abstr.).

12. Yang H-Y, Vora D, Targan S, Toyoda H, Beaudet A, Rotter J. Association of intercellular adhesion molecule-1 (ICAM-1) polymorphisms with subsets of inflammatory bowel disease (IBD) stratified by antineutrophil cytoplasmic antibodies (ANCA) (Submitted).

23
Lessons in IBD pathogenesis from new animal models of spontaneous colitis

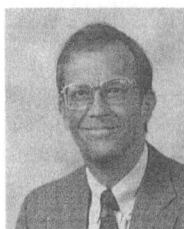

R. B. SARTOR

INTRODUCTION

Until recently, most experimental models of intestinal inflammation have been induced in laboratory animals by exposure to a variety of toxins of questionable environmental relevance[1,2] (Table 1). The exception to this rule is the cottontop tamarin, which spontaneously develops colitis and adenocarcinoma of the colon. However, this New World marmoset is on the endangered species list and is not widely available. Existing animal models have provided very important insights into soluble mediators involved in acute and, in some cases, chronic intestinal inflammation. However, the acute injury response to toxins is of limited value to understanding basic immunoregulatory defects relevant to the pathogenesis of idiopathic chronic inflammatory bowel disease in humans.

Significant improvements in traditional animal models have been made

Table 1 Established animal models of intestinal inflammation

Mucosal	Intermediate	Transmural
Cottontop tamarin	Acetic acid (rat)	Trinitrobenzene sulfonic acid (rat, mouse)
Carrageenan (guinea pig)		
Dextran sulfate sodium (mouse)		Peptidoglycan-polysaccharide (rat)
Immune complex (rabbit)		Indomethacin (rat, dog)

Table 2 New rodent models of spontaneous intestinal inflammation

Spontaneous mutation	Genetically engineered	Reconstituted
C_3H HeJ Bir mouse	HLA-B_{27}/$\beta 2\mu$ transgenic rat	CD45RBhi → SCID mouse
	IL-2 deleted mouse	
	IL-10 deleted mouse	
	$\alpha\beta$ TCR deleted mouse	
	TGF-β_1 deleted mouse	

by exploring the differential genetic susceptibility of inbred rat strains to bacterial cell wall polymers[1,3]. Inbred Lewis rats develop a biphasic, spontaneously relapsing granulomatous enterocolitis with associated fibrosis, arthritis, granulomatous hepatitis, anemia and leukocytosis after intramural injection of peptidoglycan–polysaccharide (PG-PS) polymers. The chronic phase of PG-PS-induced enterocolitis is T lymphocyte-mediated and persists for at least 6 months. In contrast, Fischer F344 rats (MHC-matched with Lewis) and Buffalo rats develop only transient intestinal injury and no extraintestinal inflammation. Although the PG-PS model has several unique features, intramural injection of PG-PS at the time of laparotomy is a tedious and nonphysiologic means of inducing experimental and intestinal inflammation.

Recent advances in molecular biologic techniques have made it practical to overexpress or delete genes of interest in rodents as well as in viruses, bacteria, yeast and cultured cells. Overexpression (transgenic) and deletion (knockout, KO) of specific HLA, cytokine and T cell receptor genes in rodents have provided important and sometimes surprising models of spontaneous colitis (Table 2). These new models, in combination with a spontaneous mutation in C_3H/HeJ mice, restoration of T cell subsets to immunocompromised mice, and induction of intestinal inflammation by PG-PS, indomethacin and trinitrobenzene-sulfonic acid (TNB-SA) in inbred rodent strains have provided novel insights into mechanisms of chronic intestinal and systemic inflammation.

This chapter describes clinical, histologic and immunologic features of these animal models, concentrating on the newer, genetically engineered rodents which spontaneously develop chronic intestinal inflammation. These new rodent models provide the tools to dissect the basic mechanisms of chronic intestinal and systemic inflammation and provide relevant insights into the pathogenesis of inflammatory bowel disease.

C₃H/HeJ BIR SUBSTRAIN MOUSE

In 1992 Birkenmeier and colleagues[4] at Jackson Laboratories and the University of Alabama described a heritable form of colitis in mice. Over the past 10 years it became apparent that individual C_3H/HeJ mice episodically developed diarrhea and perianal ulceration with no demonstrable pathogens. Selective breeding of mice exhibiting diarrhea established a pedigree in which there is a 50% incidence of spontaneous colitis. There is a male predominance (67% incidence in males, 31% in females) and seasonal variation (winter > summer). The time-course of inflammation is biphasic. The most reproducible inflammation develops at 3–5 weeks of age with spontaneous resolution in most mice. Some mice exhibit chronic inflammation. It is unclear whether the chronic phase is a result of failure to resolve the acute inflammation or spontaneous reactivation of chronic inflammation. Clinical manifestations of inflammation include occasional diarrhea, hemoccult positive stools and perianal ulceration. Inflammation is routinely found in the cecum near the ileocecal valve, but can involve the left colon. Histologic characteristics include focal linear ulcers with infiltration of mononuclear cells and neutrophils. Extraintestinal manifestations other than perianal ulceration have not yet been reported.

The mechanism(s) of spontaneous colitis in the C_3H/HeJ Bir substrain mouse have not yet been determined. Presumably the propensity to develop inflammation is the result of the spontaneous mutation of a specific gene. Attempts to identify this gene are in progress and, if successful, will provide important clues to direct investigations of specific gene mutations in IBD patients. The C_3H/HeJ parent strain is interesting in its own right by virtue of being resistant to bacterial lipopolysaccharide (LPS or endotoxin). Like the parent strain, macrophages from C_3H/HeJ Bir mice fail to produce IL-1 or TNF-α in response to *in-vitro* LPS stimulation[5].

HLA-B$_{27}$ TRANSGENIC RATS

HLA-B$_{27}/\beta_2$ microglobulin ($\beta2\mu$) transgenic rodents were developed to determine if experimental *in-vivo* expression of this class I MHC molecule would drive a systemic inflammatory response which resembles the human HLA-B27 syndrome. HLA-B$_{27}/\beta_2\mu$ transgenic mice fail to exhibit clinical evidence of spontaneous inflammation, but are more susceptible to experimental infection with *Yersinia*[6]. However, transgenic rats which expressed high copy numbers of the human HLA-B$_{27}/\beta_2\mu$ gene develop a systemic syndrome of polyarthritis, dermatitis, hair loss, nail changes, myocarditis, epididymitis, progressive wasting, gastritis and colitis[7]. Surprisingly, diarrhea usually precedes other manifestations and is clinically evident in 50% of transgenic rats by 10 weeks of age and in almost 100% by 20 weeks of age[8]. The chronic diarrhea is not grossly bloody, and is associated with intermittent perianal ulceration (R.B. Sartor, unpublished observations). The colon is grossly thickened and granular, but has no discrete ulceration, nodularity, or strictures. Histologically there is an infiltration by mononuclear cells into the lamina propria, with occasional crypt abscesses in severe cases. Inflammation is confined to the mucosa in almost all rats. Crypts are hyperplastic with reactive atypia and goblet cell depletion. The majority of rats exhibit focal areas of gastric inflammation in the lamina propria and submucosa with a proliferation of mucus-neck cells and grandular ectasia. In the joints, neutrophils accumulate in the joint space; the synomium is hyperplastic, infiltrated with mononuclear cells, and pannus erodes the bone.

Several studies have been performed to determine the mechanisms of progressive intestinal and systemic inflammation in this model. The susceptibility to inflammatory disease correlates with the level of human HLA-$B_{27}/\beta_2\mu$ expression on lymphoid cells[8]. Eighty percent of hemizygous transgenic rats in two lines which express greater than 50 copies of recombinant HLA-$B_{27}/\beta_2\mu$/cell develop clinically evident colitis and systemic disease by 10–16 weeks of age. Rats from lines expressing low copy numbers of B_{27} fail to develop inflammation even in the homozygous state, whereas homozygous but not heterozygous offspring of mid-level line developed clinical disease. Interestingly, there is no apparent difference in frequency or onset of colitis or systemic inflammation in Lewis or Fischer rat lines which express equivalent copy numbers of the transgene. The lack of clinically apparent spontaneous inflammation in transgenic *mice* expressing high copy numbers of the same construct is difficult to explain.

Clinical disease can be transferred by bone marrow cells from HLA-B_{27}-positive donors to irradiated B_{27}-negative recipients[9]. Disease can also be transferred by fetal liver cells, but not by mature lymph node or spleen cells, indicating that repopulation of the recipient by B_{27}-positive progenitor cells is necessary for disease initiation and that donor cells do not need to be derived from rats with active inflammation. Moreover, disease remitted in B_{27}-positive, irradiated recipients following engraftment with B_{27}-negative cells. These studies demonstrate the colitis is mediated by immunocytes, and that HLA-B_{27} expression by nonimmune cells (epithelial, endothelial, etc.) is neither sufficient nor necessary for colitis induction.

Preliminary studies demonstrate a fundamental role of ubiquitous conventional flora in the pathogenesis of HLA-B_{27} associated colitis and arthritis[10] (R.B. Sartor, unpublished results). HLA-$B_{27}/\beta_2\mu$ transgenic rats raised in a sterile (germ-free) environment fail to develop clinically apparent diarrhea or arthritis and no elevation of colonic myeloperoxidase or IL-1, in contrast to rats housed under conventional conditions with no demonstrable bacterial pathogens. In our preliminary studies the incidence of arthritis in HLA-B_{27} transgenic rats repopulated with specific pathogen-free bacterial flora is less than that in those raised in a conventional rodent facility. Despite the absence of colitis and arthritis, germ-free transgenic rats develop hair loss, dermatitis and epididymitis to the same degree as conventional B_{27}-positive rats.

IL-2 KNOCKOUT MICE

IL-2 is a key immunoregulatory cytokine produced by activated TH_1 lymphocytes whose principal activities are to stimulate proliferation and activation of effector and regulatory lymphocytes[11]. Mice homozygous for the mutated IL-2 gene (IL-2 $-/-$) develop normally for 3–4 weeks, but then exhibit a progressive wasting syndrome[12]. Approximately 50% of mice died by 9 weeks of age with evidence of splenomegaly, lymphadenopathy and severe hemolytic anemia. Surviving mice develop chronic diarrhea, episodic bloody stools and rectal prolapse, which becomes clinically evident between 6 and 15 weeks of age. Progressive disease results in death by 10–25 weeks of age. These mice develop pancolitis, with the left colon affected to a greater degree, but no evidence of small intestinal inflammation. The inflamed colon is thickened with crypt hyperplasia but inflammation is confined to the mucosa. The mucosa is ulcerated, crypt abscesses are present, the lamina propria is infiltrated by mononuclear cells and neutrophils. In advanced stages, epithelial dysplasia is noted. Amyloidosis develops in the liver, spleen and kidney.

Immunopathogenesis of colitis in this model has been explored by immunohistochemical staining. The number of T and B cells within the lamina propria dramatically increased in colitic mice with T lymphocytes, up to 100 times higher than controls. In the late stages of disease, colonic B cells are reduced. T lymphocytes in inflamed colons are activated, as indicated by the CD_{44} (activated memory T cells) and CD_{69} (early T cell activation) markers. T cells within inflammatory foci have increased proliferation rates. Lamina propria IgG_1 and IgA secreting cells are dramatically increased and serum IgA is elevated to 16–64 times control values. Anticolon antibodies are increased until late stages of inflammation, but are part of a generalized autoantibody response.

Bacterial and viral pathogens were not detected, and there was no evidence of horizontal disease transmission in normal littermates. However, normal luminal bacteria were implicated by no clinical or histologic evidence of colitis in three IL-2-deficient mice followed for 5 months. Knockout mice raised under specific pathogen-free conditions develop no clinical signs of colitis, but had evidence of mild histologic and immunologic abnormalities by 17–20 weeks of age.

IL-10-DEFICIENT MICE

IL-10, a product of TH_2 lymphocytes, is believed to have predominantly immunosuppressive activity by virtue of its ability to down-regulate macrophage, natural killer cells and lymphocyte activation and cytokine production[11]. IL-10-deficient mice spontaneously develop chronic inflammation of their entire intestinal tract, with the most severe inflammation noted in the duodenum, proximal jejunum and right colon[13]. These mice develop a progressive wasting syndrome with anemia, which begins by 3–4 weeks of age, and results in a mortality of 30% by 5–6 weeks. Male and female mice are equally affected. The proximal small bowel is markedly thickened due to mucosal and crypt hyperplasia. The crypt architecture is deranged and dysplastic with a decrease in Peyer's patches. Superficial erosions are present with exudate. Away from ulcerated areas the lamina propria is infiltrated by mononuclear cells, neutrophils and occasional multinucleated giant cells. Inflammation diminishes in the distal small bowel, with an atrophy of the ileal mucosa. Colonic lesions are predominantly atrophic. Liver histology is normal but the bone marrow demonstrates an increased myeloid/erythroid ratio.

The majority of plasma cells in the inflamed intestine produced IgA or IgG_1 and expression of MHC class II molecules was increased on small intestinal and colonic epithelial cells. Serum IgG_1 and IgA levels were increased in the IL-10 $-/-$ mice. The antibody response to immunization

Table 3 Pathogenesis of colitis in $\alpha\beta$ TCR-deficient mice

Strain	CD4 + $\alpha\beta$ T cells	B cells	Colitis
Wild-type	+	+	No
TCR δ KO	+	+	No
Nude	–	+	No
RAG-1 KO	–	–	No
TCR α KO	–	+	Yes
TCR β KO	–	+	Yes
TCR $\beta \times \delta$ KO	–	+	Yes
Class II MHC KO	–	+	Yes

with a T cell-dependent antigen was no different in IL-10 deleted and control mice. However, *in vivo Nippostrongylus* infection stimulated a TH_1 ($\uparrow$ IFN-γ) lymphokine response in IL-10 $-/-$ mice in contrast to the usual TH_2 (IL-4, IL-5) response in controls. Interestingly, spleen cells from the knockout mice produced 20-fold more IL-6 and TNF-α than normal mice following LPS stimulation. These results suggest that deficient production of IL-10, which suppresses activation and cytokine synthesis by macrophages, natural killer cells and T cells, could lead to chronic stimulation by luminal bacterial components. This hypothesis is supported by the observation that IL-10-deficient mice reared under specific pathogen-free conditions have only isolated left-sided colitis with no histologic evidence of small intestinal inflammation.

$\alpha\beta$ T CELL RECEPTOR-DEFICIENT MICE

The T cell receptor (TCR) is a heterodimer composed of either $\alpha + \beta$ or $\gamma + \delta$ subunits. Antigen binding to the TCR complex in conjunction with accessory ligand binding and costimulatory cytokines is required for antigen-specific activation of T lymphocytes. Mutation of various components of the TCR has been elegantly studied by Monbaerts et al.[14]. Deletion of the α or β chains of the TCR in mice induces a spontaneous colitis with onset by 3–4 months of age and mortality by 6–12 months. Mice develop nonbloody diarrhea, weight loss and rectal prolapse due to a pancolitis, left > right-sided. The colon is quite thickened due to massive crypt hyperplasia, goblet cell depletion, acute and chronic inflammation of the lamina propria and crypt abscesses. Macroscopic mucosal ulcerations and rectal bleeding are not seen. The small intestine is grossly and histologically normal, but mesenteric lymph nodes are enlarged and focal hepatic inflammatory cell infiltrates are present in some mice.

The authors examined multiple deletion constructs to investigate mechanisms of immunodeficiency leading to colitis in this model (Table 3). The common denominator in mice which developed colitis is the absence of $\alpha\beta$ T lymphocytes and the presence of functional B cells. An important clue is the lack of colitis in mice with mutated recombination-activating genes (RAG-1) and in SCID mice, which are totally deficient in mature T and B lymphocytes. These results suggest that spontaneous colitis in this model is the result of lack of appropriate $\alpha\beta$ T cell-mediated suppression of B cells. Analysis of the $\alpha\beta$ TCR mutation in several inbred mouse strains demonstrated that the 129/Sv and C_3H/He genetic backgrounds were permissive and Balb/c was more resistant.

LYMPHOCYTES SUBSET RECONSTITUTED IMMUNODEFICIENT MICE

The severe combined immunodeficient (SCID) mouse and nude rat can be populated with immunocytes without rejection, which permits the *in-vitro* study of the activity of various T cell subpopulations. Based on studies by Powrie and colleagues[15] in nude rats, several groups have described colitis resulting from injection of T lymphoycyte subsets divided on the basis of density of binding of the monoclonal antibody CD45RB into SCID mice[16,17]. CD45RB[hi] lymphocytes have been shown to secrete profiles of TH_1 lymphokines, whereas CD45 low cells secrete TH_2 lymphokines. Injection of unfractionated cells or combined CD45RB[hi] and low subsets caused no disease. However, injection of only CD45RB[hi] lymphocytes induced chronic wasting beginning 10–30 days after reconstitution and a 30% mortality rate at 12 weeks. Intestinal inflammation is predominantly in the colon (left > right) but was mild in the small intestine. Histologic examination of the small intestine reveals focal mononuclear infiltrates in the lamina propria. Colon inflammation is characterized by focal ulceration, chronically thickened mucosa with crypt hyperplasia and a mononuclear cell infiltrate of the lamina propria with occasional neutrophils and transmural inflammation. Mild periportal infiltrates are seen in the liver.

IFN-γ-mRNA tissue concentrations were substantially higher than normal values in SCID mice reconstituted with CD45RB[hi] cells, but IL-10 levels were not increased[17]. IL-4 levels were undetectable in all mice and TNF-α was elevated in reconstituted mice with and without colitis. These results indicate that CD45[lo] lymphocytes can suppress intestinal inflammation, which is mediated by the reciprocal CD45[hi] population and suggest that a dysregulation between TH_1 and TH_2 lymphokine production may contribute to chronic intestinal inflammation. These studies graphically illustrate the essential role of competent immunosuppressive cells in homeostasis of the intestinal mucosa.

TGF-β_1-DEFICIENT MICE

Transforming growth factor β (TGF-β) is a macrophage product which has pleiotrophic immunologic activities including monocyte chemotaxis and stimulation of collagen synthesis by intestinal smooth muscle cells and fibroblasts[11]. An important immunoregulatory activity of this molecule is suppression of lymphocyte proliferation. TGF-β_1 knockout mice have increased *in-utero* mortality, but appear to develop normally until weaning (3 weeks of age), when they develop a wasting syndrome and systemic inflammation consisting of myocarditis, bronchoalveolar inflammation, pancreatitis, and dermatitis[18,19]. One of the two reported TGF-β_1-deficient lines develops diarrhea and has an as yet incompletely described colitis[18]. The

Table 4 Immunologic mechanisms of spontaneous colitis in genetically engineered rodents

Defective T cell suppression: CD45RB^{hi} → SCID, $\alpha\beta$TCR$-/-$, TGF-β1$-/-$
↑ TH$_1$/TH$_2$ lymphokines: IL-10$-/-$, ? CD45RB^{hi} → SCID
↑ B cell response: IL-2$-/-$, $\alpha\beta$TCR$-/-$

mechanisms of chronic systemic inflammation and colitis in this model remain obscure, but may be related to defective suppression of lymphocytes. Of interest, many of the organs involved are colonized by ubiquitous bacteria.

SUMMARY AND CONCLUSIONS

Chronic intestinal inflammation which develops in response to spontaneous gene mutations, targeted deletion or overexpression of specific genes or selective manipulation of lymphocyte subsets can provide important insights into mechanisms of intestinal inflammation[20]. Several broad immunologic mechanisms which mediate spontaneous colitis are listed in Table 4. The similarities of chronic intestinal inflammation in these models to idiopathic ulcerative colitis and Crohn's disease suggest that similar mechanisms may be active in human IBD.

A theme common to many of these models is that intestinal inflammation develops as a result of defective immunosuppression. The models of TGF-β_1 knockout, $\alpha\beta$ TCR deletion and CD45RB^{hi} reconstitution of SCID mice clearly demonstrate the consequences of ineffective T lymphocyte suppression, and suggest that T cell suppression is critical to normal mucosal homeostasis. The disordered balance between TH$_1$ and TH$_2$ lymphokine profiles in IL-10 knockout and CD45RB^{hi} → SCID mice further document the importance of effective immunoregulation by lymphocytes. How these animal studies relate to the proposed TH$_1$ profile of Crohn's disease and TH$_2$ for ulcerative colitis remains to be determined, but it is of interest that IL-10 $-/-$ and reconstituted SCID mice have small intestinal inflammation and TH$_1$ lymphokine profiles. The TCR deletion studies and IL-2 knockout mice strongly suggest that, in the absence of regulatory T cells, uncontrolled B lymphocyte activation is capable of mediating mucosal damage.

A second concept is that specific gene mutations can cause spontaneous intestinal inflammation, and that clinically and histologically similar lesions can arise from different immunoregulatory defects. These observations illustrate the limited repertoire of mechanisms of tissue injury, suggest that a variety of immunoregulatory defects may induce human IBD and imply that there may be multiple etiologies for these disorders. Moreover, the etiologic heterogeneity among ulcerative colitis and Crohn's disease patients may be responsible for clinical subsets of patients with predictable patterns of disease, complications and response to medications.

A third concept is that host genetic susceptibility determines the aggressiveness, chronicity and complications of intestinal inflammation. The effect of genetic susceptibility is illustrated by the C$_3$H/HeJ Bir mouse and differential responses to experimental intestinal inflammation in Lewis vs Fischer rats in the PG-PS and indomethacin models[3,21] and C$_3$H/He or 129/Sv vs Balb/c mice in the $\alpha\beta$ TCR knockout model[14]. Identification of genetic mechanisms of defective immunoregulation in susceptible rodents could direct the search for genetic susceptibility factors in IBD patients.

Fourthly, transfer studies in the HLA-B27/$\beta_2\mu$ transgenic rats demonstrate that bone marrow-derived cells can mediate chronic intestinal and systemic inflammation. The inflammatory response of these cells is genetically programmed, since progenitor cells can be derived from fetuses which do not exhibit evidence of intestinal or systemic inflammation. Moreover, display of HLA-B27 on host epithelial cells is not sufficient for induction of disease. This observation suggests that increased expression of MHC molecules during experimental or idiopathic inflammation is a consequence of the inflammatory reaction and not necessary for chronic intestinal inflammation. Resolution of spontaneous intestinal inflammation in HLA-B_{27}+ rats after irradiation and successful bone marrow engraftment from nontransgenic rats raises the possibility of therapeutic bone marrow transplantation in IBD patients.

Finally, attenuation of spontaneous intestinal inflammation in IL-2- and IL-10-deficient mice raised in a pathogen-free environment and lack of evidence of colitis in IL-2 knockout mice and HLA-B_{27}/$\beta2\mu$ mice living in germ-free (sterile) conditions dramatically illustrates the critical pathogenetic role of ubiquitous luminal bacterial constituents. These results parallel those observed in indomethacin-induced enterocolitis where Lewis rats conventionalized with specific pathogen-free flora develop chronic mild small bowel ulcers but germ-free littermates have no evidence of chronic inflammation[22]. Because microbiologic conditions vary between rodent facilities, direct comparisons of the clinical features of each of these spontaneous colitis models must be made under similar conditions, optimally using animals colonized with the same flora. It is unknown whether spontaneous colitis develops as the result of luminal bacteria invading tissues of immunocompromised hosts (IL-2, and TCR knockout mice), a hyperactive response to bacterial components (LPS, PG-PS) in rodents which lack effective immunosuppressor cytokines (IL-10, TGF-β knockout mice) or an exaggerated antibody response to ubiquitous bacterial antigens (IL-2, TCR knockout models and CD45^{hi} → SCID mice).

These genetically engineered rodent models have only recently been described, so their usefulness has been only superficially exploited. Similar types of spontaneous intestinal inflammation will almost certainly be discovered as new knockout and transgenic rodents are generated to study other immunoregulatory molecules. Application of sophisticated molecular and immunologic techniques, and further genetic manipulation by selective crossbreeding with well-characterized mouse strains, should generate important insights and new enthusiasm to explore mechanisms of chronic intestinal inflammation.

Acknowledgements

This work was supported by USPHS grants DK 40249, DK 47700 and DK 34987 and the Crohn's and Colitis Foundation of America. The author gratefully acknowledges the expert secretarial assistance of Robert Tuttle and Shirley Willard.

References

1. Sartor RB. Animal models of intestinal inflammation: relevance to IBD. In: MacDermott RP, Stenson W, editors. Inflammatory bowel disease. New York: Elsevier; 1991:337–54.
2. Stenson WF. Animal models of inflammatory bowel disease. In: Targan SR, editor. Inflammatory bowel disease from bench to bedside. Baltimore: Williams & Wilkins; 1994:180–92.
3. McCall RD, Haskill S, Zimmerman E et al. Tissue IL-1 and IL-1 receptor antagonist expression in enterocolitis in resistant and susceptible rats. Gastroenterology. 1994;106: 960–72.
4. Birkenmeier EH, Stundberg JP, Elson CO. A heritable form of colitis in mice. Gastroenterology. 1992;102:A596.
5. McCabe RP, Mills T, Ridwan B, et al. Immunologic reactivity of C_3H/HeJ mice with spontaneous colitis. Gastroenterology. 1993;104:A656.
6. Nickerson CI, Luthra HS, David CS. Role of enterobacteria and HLA-B27 in spondyloarthropathics: studies with transgenic mice. Ann Rheum Dis. 1990;49:426–33.
7. Hammer RE, Maika SD, Richardson JA, Tang J, Taurog JD. Spontaneous inflammatory disease in transgenic rats expressing HLA-B27 and human $\beta_2\mu$: an animal model of HLA-B27-associated human disorders. Cell. 1990;63:1099–112.
8. Taurog JD, Maika S,D Simmons WA, Breban M, Hammer RE. Susceptibility to inflammatory disease in HLA-B27 transgenic rat lines correlates with the level of B27 expression. J Immunol. 1993;150:4186.
9. Breban M, Hammer RE, Richardson JA, Taurog JD. Transfer of the inflammatory disease of HLA-B37 transgenic rats by bone marrow engraftment. J Exp Med. 1993;178:1607–16.
10. Taurog JD, Hammer RE, Balish E et al. Effect of the germfree state on the inflammatory disease of HLA-B27 transgenic rats: a split result. Arthritis Rheum. 1993;36:S46.
11. Sartor RB. Viewpoints on digestive diseases. Cytokines in intestinal inflammation: pathophysiological and clinical considerations. Gastroenterology. 1994;106:533–9.
12. Sadlack B, Merg H, Schorle H et al. Ulcerative colitis-like disease in mice with a disrupted interleukin-2 gene. Cell. 1993;75:253–61.
13. Kuhn R, Lohler J, Rennick D, Rajowsky K, Muller W. Interleukin-10-deficient mice develop chronic enterocolitis. Cell. 1993;75:263–79.
14. Mombaerts P, Mizoguchi E, Grusby M et al. Spontaneous development of inflammatory bowel disease in T cell receptor mutant mice. Cell. 1993;75:275–82.
15. Powrie F, Mason D. Ox-22^{high} CD4+ T cells induce wasting disease with multiple organ pathology: Prevention by the Ox-22^{low} subset. J Exp Med. 1990;172:1701–8.
16. Morrisey PJ, Charrier K, Braddy S, Liggitt D, Watson JD. CD4+ T cells that express high levels of CD45RB induce wasting disease when transferred into cogenic severe combined immunodeficient mice. Disease development is prevented by cotransfer of purified CD4+ T cells. J Exp Med. 1993;178:237–44.
17. Powrie F, Leach MW, Mauze S, Caddle LB, Coffman RL. Phenotypically distinct subsets of CD4+ T cells induce or protect from chronic intestinal inflammation in C. B-17 SCID mice. Int Immunol. 1993;5:1461–71.
18. Kulkarni AB, Huh CG, Becker D et al. Transforming growth factor $\beta1$ null mutation in mice causes excessive inflammatory response and early death. Proc Natl Acad Sci. 1993;90:770–4.
19. Shull MM, Ormsby I, Kier AB et al. Targeted disruption of the mouse transforming growth factor-$\beta1$ gene results in multifocal inflammatory disease. Nature. 1992;359:693–9.
20. Strober W, Ehrhardt RO. Chronic intestinal inflammation: an unexpected outcome in cytokine or T cell receptor mutant mice. Cell. 1993;75:203–5.
21. Sartor RB, Bender DE, Holt LC. Susceptibility of inbred rat strains to intestinal and extraintestinal inflammation induced by indomethacin. Gastroenterology. 1992;102:A690.
22. Sartor RB, Bender DE, Grenther T, Holt LC. Absolute requirement for ubiquitous luminal bacteria in the pathogenesis of chronic intestinal inflammation. Gastroenterology. 1994 (In press).

24
Potential human models of IBD

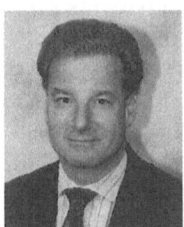

S. B. HANAUER

INTRODUCTION

The absence of an animal model that correlates with the course of either ulcerative colitis or Crohn's disease has impeded basic research to define the etiopathogenesis of inflammatory bowel disease (IBD) and clinical research involving potential therapeutic agents. Basic progress in animal (primarily mouse) genetic typing accompanied by both 'knockout' and 'transgenic' techniques may eventually identify genetic predispositions that will apply to the human IBD. Meanwhile, continued clinical research in IBD has elucidated many aspects of the immune and inflammatory cascades contributing to the pathogenesis of ulcerative colitis and Crohn's disease which may translate into a better understanding of the clinical manifestations and course, and may promise eventual therapeutic improvements. Concurrently, new serologic markers (e.g. ANCA) and genetic phenotyping (e.g. HLA-DR2) offer potential correlates to clinical subgroups that may clarify aspects of the heterogeneity within IBD. The diversity amongst patients and evolving epidemiology of IBD as ethnic populations assume Western diets and culture (including smoking) suggest that an eventual reclassification of IBD is likely. We need to continue to consider these possibilities in search of subsets of human models of IBD. Meanwhile, there are a number of potential models that can be utilized to study the pathogenesis, natural history and therapies.

RISK FACTORS

Several risk factors for the development of IBD may be considered models in predisposed individuals to distinguish the susceptibility towards environmental exposure/injury. Thus far the family history of IBD presents the most available means of evaluating potential candidates for developing disease. Linkage studies are under way which may eventually identify patients 'at risk', as may serologic studies (e.g. pANCA). Unfortunately, there is no facile means of assessing preclinical disease; therefore the natural history of relatives with identified markers such as HLA-DR2 or pANCA should be observed, especially in the 'multiplex' families. These individuals also afford the potential of measuring other potential 'preclinical' markers or response parameters. For instance, intestinal permeability has been utilized with variable results in active and quiescent IBD and as a marker for preclinical relapse[1]. The original finding of increased permeability in family members of patients with Crohn's disease has not been verified[2]; however, the concept of permeability as a potential marker should not be abandoned. Further, provocative permeability testing using NSAID may increase the sensitivity of permeability studies[3]. The influence of cigarette smoking on permeability in relatives of IBD patients could also be explored, especially in relatives of patients with ulcerative colitis who may have an increased risk of developing clinical disease if they stopped smoking. It would also be of great interest to evaluate family members documented to have increased permeability with additional studies such as leukocyte scans or even ileocolonoscopy to rule out preclinical mucosal/histologic disease.

PRECLINICAL MARKERS

Preclinical markers of IBD may also be identified in patients with recognized predisposing diseases such as HLA-B27-associated spondyloarthritis. Patients with ankylosing spondylitis have a high incidence of associated ileitis with endoscopic and histologic features that are indistinguishable from Crohn's disease[4]. Additional studies of mucosal immune function in these individuals should provide insight into both initiating (or predisposing) and amplifying factors[5]. Few natural history studies have been performed in this subgroup of patients.

NSAID-induced small bowel and colonic damage has recently been observed to mimic many of the mucosal (and potentially clinical) features of IBD[6]. This affords the opportunity to evaluate both a risk factor for IBD in susceptible individuals (e.g. relatives) but also the normal reparative mechanisms that may be absent or deficient (including eicosanoids, cytokines and growth factors).

MODELS

Alternative *acute models* of idiopathic IBD include enterocolitides of known etiology such as infectious, ischemic or radiation-induced mucosal damage where there is the potential to measure regulatory immune, inflammatory events and tissue repair in healthy individuals, IBD patients and relatives.

Potential models of IBD exist even within the disease course. In ulcerative colitis there are two excellent models to assess mucosal events: the margin of disease and pouchitis. The margin between active inflammation and 'normal' mucosa has been inadequately studied. More often, patients with distal colitis are included with pancolitics when mediators or histology are examined. The disease margin is a prototype for defining mucosal abnormalities in the same individual with an identical genetic disposition. Local immune, inflammatory and regenerative features need to be studied in the patients. Likewise, pouchitis offers another example of an aberrant tissue response to (presumably) similar environmental exposures in patients with ulcerative colitis and familial polyposis. Genetic dispositions can be compared between these groups but, even within ulcerative colitis patients, the natural history of pouchitis beginning with the diverted or naive pouch followed by bacterial proliferation and the defined risk for subclinical and clinical disease, as well as the potential for healing with antibiotic therapy, offer the opportunity to study patients in a sequential fashion[7]. It appears that risk factors may also, predictably, be applied to patients prior to the formation of an ileal pouch, such as the presence of extraintestinal manifestations or pANCA.

Potential models for the study of Crohn's disease also exist within the disease spectrum and clinical course. The aphthous ulcer occurs in healthy individuals and patients with NSAID exposure, and as isolated findings as a presumed 'primary' lesion or event in Crohn's disease. Further exploration of the immunoinflammatory and mediator events in and around these Crohn's, infectious or NSAID-induced lesions offer additional insight into pathogenic differences. Two additional models of Crohn's disease include the anastomotic site and fecal diversion. The predisposition for Crohn's disease to recur at the proximal to the anastomotic margin affords the potential to sequentially monitor mucosal events, and has recently been the focus of several interventional studies to prophylax or alter both endoscopic and clinical disease. Similarly, diversion of the fecal stream in Crohn's disease offers an alternative model to study the inflammatory process[8].

A number of newly described colitides also need to be examined as models for IBD as additional epidemiologic, clinical, histopathologic, immune and associated factors are explored. The recent recognition of collagenous, microscopic diversion and HIV-associated enterocolitis affords the opportunity to examine potential similarities and differences with the classic IBD syndromes[9].

In the examination and evaluation of these and other potential human models of IBD it is important *not* to be limited to current paradigms of etiopathogenesis[10]. We must be humbled by the recent example of *H. pylori* in peptic ulcer disease. When confronted with the current dogma seeking an immunologic 'truth' as a predisposing cause of IBD, we should remain open to alternative hypotheses including dysfunctional epithelium, alternative microorganisms (including viral vasculitis and epithelial bacteria), and molecular mimicry or autoimmunity, and use these concepts for hypothesis-testing rather than exceptions to our current conceived formulations on etiopathogenesis.

References

1. Hollander D. The intestinal permeability barrier: a hypothesis as to its regulation and involvement in Crohn's disease. Scand J Gastroenterol. 1992;27:721–6.
2. Munkholm P, Langholz E, Hollander D et al. Intestinal permeability in patients with Crohn's disease and ulcerative colitis and their first degree relatives. Gut. 1994;35:68–72.
3. Pironi L, Miglioli M, Ruggeri E et al. Effect of non-steroidal anti-inflammatory drugs (NSAID) on intestinal permeability in first degree relatives of patients with Crohn's disease. Gastroenterology. 1992;102:A679.
4. Mielants H, Veys EM, Goemaere S, Cuvelier C, DeVos M. A prospective study of patients with spondyloarthropathy with special reference to HLA-B27 and to gut histology. J Rheumatol. 1993;20:1353–8.
5. Cuvelier CA, DeWever N, Mielants H, DeVos M, Veys EM, Roels H. Expression of T cell receptors alpha beta and gamma delta in the ileal mucosa of patients with Crohn's disease and with spondylarthropathy. Clin Exp Immunol. 1992;90:275–9.
6. Bjarnason I, Hayllar J, MacPherson AJ, Russell AS. Side effects of nonsteroidal anti-inflammatory drugs on the small and large intestine in humans. Gastroenterology. 1993;104:1832–47.
7. Luukkonen P, Jarvinen H, Tanskanen M, Kahri A. Pouchitis – recurrence of the inflammatory bowel disease? Gut. 1994;35:243–6.
8. Winslet MC, Allan A, Poxon V, Youngs D, Keighley MRB. Faecal diversion for Crohn's colitis: a model to study the role of the faecal stream in the inflammatory process. Gut. 1994;35:236–42.
9. Kingsmore SF, Kingsmore DB, Hall BD, Wilson JAP, Gottfried MR, Allen NB. Cooccurrence of collagenous colitis with seronegative spondylarthropathy: Report of a case and literature review. J Rheumatol. 1994;20:2153–7.
10. Kuhn TS. The structure of scientific revolutions. Chicago, IL: University of Chicago Press; 1962.

Section VIII
Basic science: pathogenesis

25
New concepts of pathogenesis in IBD

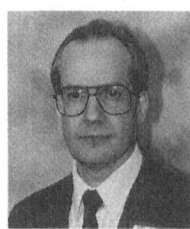

C. FIOCCHI

INTRODUCTION

Inflammatory bowel disease (IBD) still remains an enigma and there is no real understanding of its etiology and pathogenesis. In spite of this, efforts directed at uncovering predisposing factors, identifying specific etiologic agents, creating new animal models, investigating immunologic abnormalities, and developing novel and more effective forms of therapy continue to expand. Until the cause and mechanism(s) of IBD are clearly understood there remain many implicated factors, as demonstrated by the variety of topics presented in the chapters of this book. To a large extent this reflects limitations in knowledge, even though there is general agreement that both Crohn's disease (CD) and ulcerative colitis (UC) are intricate multifactorial entities. In the face of this discouraging complexity an in-depth discussion of IBD pathogenesis can be quite extensive and diffuse. This laborious approach has already been taken, and comprehensive reviews are available[1,2]. This chapter will instead focus on selected and recent developments, particularly those having an impact on the pathophysiology of IBD.

PREDISPOSING FACTORS

Epidemiology

Epidemiological studies of IBD patients and their families have been carried out for a long time. The outcome of such studies has generated two essential pieces of information: the presence of a worldwide trend for an increased incidence of IBD (CD in particular), and the now well-established notion of an enhanced susceptibility to UC and CD among family members. Except for these important findings the large number of population studies performed so far has not contributed much more to the critical question of whether IBD is predominantly a genetic disorder or is environmentally conditioned. A simple way of addressing this controversy is to put forward a classical multifactorial model, where many genes and multiple environmental influences determine the individual risk for developing IBD[3]. In reality, unless new clinical, familial or population clues surface, there is little chance that traditional epidemiology will contribute something new to IBD pathogenesis[4].

IMMUNOGENETICS

While classical epidemiology is practically at a standstill, significant progress is being made in the related field of immunogenetics. Following on previous observations of an enhanced frequency of certain HLA-DR haplotypes in selected and homogeneous populations[5], new data have been gathered to support the possibility of distinct associations of HLA class II genes with IBD. Toyoda *et al.* have recently reported a positive association of UC with the HLA-DR2 allele, and of CD with the HLA-DR1/DQw5 alleles[6]. This endorses the long-held concept that the two forms of IBD are distinct, and provides additional evidence for disease susceptibility and possible genetic heterogeneity. The latter concept is further strengthened by the observation that subgrouping of UC patients is possible when the HLA class II genes are analyzed in association with subclinical markers, such as antineutrophil cytoplasmic antiody (ANCA): ANCA-positive patients have an increased frequency of HLA-DR2 compared to ANCA-negative controls, whereas ANCA-negative patients have an increased frequency of HLA-DR4 as compared to ANCA-positive patients[7].

Susceptibility markers

Detection of autoantibodies is a common finding in patients affected by chronic disorders with immune or inflammatory manifestations. The same is true for IBD, where an association with numerous immune-related conditions has long been recognized. In addition to serum antibodies against gut epithelial antigens[8], the presence of a novel type of perinuclear ANCA (pANCA) has been reported[9]. When antibody titers in the serum of patients with UC are compared to those of subjects with other colitides they are significantly higher, leading to the suggestion that they represent a marker of this form of IBD[10]. Furthermore, an increased pANCA prevalence was also found among healthy relatives in UC-affected families, making this autoantibody a potential marker of genetic susceptibility[11]. Subsequent studies have generally supported these interesting observations, although the presence of additional autoantibodies in sera of UC patients has also been recently confirmed and associated with a generalized activation of the immune system in IBD[12].

INFECTIOUS AGENTS

Bacteria

The possibility that either form of IBD has a specific bacterial etiology has been considered since CD and UC were recognized as distinct clinical entities. Over the years, interest in searching for unique microorganisms has been wavering, but has never been abandoned. The approach taken to identifying new organisms has changed and become more sophisticated, but the quantity or quality of the results fall below what could be expected from more refined methodologies. Mimicking classical studies with serum antibodies, examination of immune cells from the general circulation or active IBD lesions has shown an augmented reactivity to a variety of bacterial antigens, but unique and selective responses have yet to be discovered[13,14]. The recent emphasis on a possible mycobacterial etiology of CD has spurred much interest and raised many hopes, but evidence that patients' peripheral or mucosal mononuclear cells mount a specific response against mycobacterial antigens is still missing[15]. Reactivity of circulating T lymphocytes to the 65 kDa heat-shock protein of mycobacterial origin is often detected, but this may simply reflect a nonspecific response shared by many chronic inflammatory and autoimmune disorders[16]. Clustering of CD in families is a well-described phenomenon, and this has been proposed as evidence for exposure of various family members to infectious microorganisms, but this is indirect and circumstantial at best[17].

Viruses

The most recent development in the area of causative microorganisms has been the demonstration that intestinal tissue of CD patients harbors persistent measles virus[18]. The virus is located in endothelial cells that are part of granulomas presumably leading to a vasculitis responsible not only for bowel inflammation but also the characteristic skip lesions of CD[19]. This is a novel, exciting and intriguing hypothesis that deserves to be pursued.

ANIMAL MODELS

After decades of limited and occasional interest the field of experimental colitis is experiencing a true explosion. In the past few years a substantial number of models in mice, rats, rabbits and immunodeficient animals have been developed and extensively tested (Table 1). The subject has recently been reviewed in detail[20], and it has been suggested that the sensible

Table 1 Animal models of IBD

Exogenous induction		Endogenous induction	
Irritants	Ethanol, acetic acid	Spontaneous	Cotton top tamarin, C3H/HeJ mouse
Drugs	Nonsteroidal anti-inflammatory drugs, indomethacin	Clonal deletion	Cyclosporin A
Immunologic	Immune complexes, trinitrobenzene sulfonic acid	T-cell reconstruction	$CD45RB^{high}$ CD4+ T cells in severe combined immunodeficiency mice
Bacterial products	Peptidoglycan-polysaccharide	Transgenic	HLA-B27
Feeding	Dextran sulfate	Gene targeting	IL-2, IL-10, T-cell receptor 'knockout' mice
Nitric oxide-related	Peroxynitrite		
Surgery	Ileopouchitis		

utilization of selected models can significantly contribute to understanding the pathogenesis of human IBD[21].

Exogenous induction

Among the models induced by the administration of exogenous agents one of the most informative is that where a chronic colitis is initiated in rats by injecting the bowel wall with peptidoglycan-polysaccharide, a component of the cell membrane of certain bacteria[22]. Particularly attractive features of this model are the induction by naturally occurring substances that may be present in the gut lumen, the formation of granulomas, the accompanying systemic manifestations, and in particular the chronicity of inflammation that recurs in a biphasic fashion, suggesting a primary immune sensitization followed by a secondary response. This is a particularly attractive model also because of the observation that the rat strain has a major impact on the severity of colitis, suggesting an important contribution by genetic factors as proposed for humans[23]. Another recently described model is one in which colitis appears in mice that have ingested dextran sulfate. An initial insult to the epithelial layer is followed by a secondary and chronic inflammatory infiltrate in the lamina propria[24]. With the discovery of nitric oxide (NO) as a potential mediator of intestinal injury, new models centered on the production of NO in the intestinal wall have been very recently reported, although its exact role may vary from model to model[25,26]. Finally, the development of a model mimicking ileopouchitis in Lewis rats submitted to bowel reconstruction has been reported in preliminary form[27].

Endogenous induction

In theory a colitis model that does not require the administration of a foreign substance might be a better model of IBD. Unfortunately the few spontaneous models, such as the South American cotton top tamarin or the C3H/HeJ mouse, have practical limitations. The newest way to create IBD models is by manipulation of the immune system. A cyclosporin A-induced autoimmune disease in mature T cell-deprived mice shows striking inflammatory lesions in the colon leaving the small bowel intact[28]. This model reinforces the idea of how important autoimmune events are in the pathogenesis of IBD. A wasting syndrome associated with colonic inflammatory cell infiltration is induced in immunodeficient (SCID) mice reconstituted with purified CD45RB^{high}CD4+ T cells, indicating that specific subsets of T helper cells may be critically important to bowel damage[29,30].

At present the most original models are those obtained by engineering the animal's genetic make-up. In addition to the spontaneous bowel inflammation appearing in rats transfected with the human HLA-B27 allele[31], colitis or enterocolitis have been reported in mice undergoing gene-targeted disruption of the interleukin (IL)-2, IL-10, or T cell receptor genes[32-34]. As discussed by Strober and Ehrhardt, these 'knockout' animals suggest that chronic intestinal inflammation may arise from vastly different immune abnormalities, point to T cells as primary culprits for inducing mucosal inflammation, and stress how unique the intestine must be as a specific target of injury, considering that these animals lack the same gene products systemically[35]. To this effect there is intriguing evidence that these animals do not develop colitis in a germ-free environment, but only if they harbor a normal lumenal content. If this is confirmed, the long-held suspicion that the interaction of enteric antigens with the local immune system is a *sine-qua-non* condition to develop IBD may be finally proved.

IMMUNOLOGIC FACTORS

Humoral immunity

The possibility that immune phenomena could be implicated in the pathogenesis of IBD was initially considered after the original demonstration that sera from UC patients could crossreact with colonic epithelial cells. From that pioneer observation demonstrating the existence of anticolon antibodies in IBD, a large number of studies have confirmed the presence of abnormalities in the production, type and class distribution of systemic and mucosal immunoglobulins[36]. Of particular interest are the changes in IgG distribution observed in the serum and mucosa of UC patients, where the predominance of IgG1 and the reduction of IgG2 subclasses is found in both patients and monozygotic twins, suggesting at least a partial genetic contribution to those abnormalities[37]. More interesting than the simple concentration or distribution of antibodies in UC or CD is the question of whether some of them are true autoantibodies, which would support a possible autoimmune nature of IBD[38].

Autoantibodies

Once considered the hallmark of autoimmune disease, the mere presence of self-reactive immunoglobulins no longer implies sickness, but rather a phenomenon associated with aging, or an epiphenomenon not relevant to tissue damage, as seems to be the case for pANCA. However, if high titers of antibodies are consistently present, and antibodies are located in and specifically react with an affected organ or tissue, then the possibility that they are responsible for immune-mediated injury should be seriously considered. As in many other conditions with immunologic features, autoreactive antibodies have been described in IBD, but few have withstood the test of time and careful control studies. At present only one putative autoantigen has been well characterized and shown to be reproducibly associated with high levels of specific autoantibodies. In a series of studies Das and collaborators have identified a tissue-bound IgG that is eluted only from the colon of UC patients. After identifying a 40 kDa protein reactive with such IgG, a monoclonal antibody developed against this protein localized the antigen to the colon, skin and biliary epithelium[39]. This striking distribution matches perfectly with the localization of UC and the most common sites of the extraintestinal manifestations of this disease, lending further support to the notion that 40 kDa could be the target of a true autoreactive response. Later the same investigators demonstrated that deposits of IgG1 and activated complement colocalize with the 40 kDa protein in UC colon, suggesting a possible mechanism of tissue destruction[40]. Further developments include the preliminary characterization of the autoantigen as a P40 protein belonging to the tropomyosin family, a group of common structural proteins, and the detection of antibodies reactive to tropomyosin in 95% of sera from patients with UC[41]. Finally, most sera of patients with primary sclerosing cholangitis can block the binding of the monoclonal antibody in an inhibition assay using sections of bile ducts or gallbladder[42]. This indicates that patients with primary sclerosing cholangitis have circulating antibodies able to bind to an epitope of the peptide shared by biliary and colonic epithelium, further strengthening the possibility of autoimmunity in UC pathogenesis. In spite of this series of elegant studies it still remains to be conclusively established whether a tropomyosin is the primary target of an immune response in UC, and whether antibodies directed against it have real pathogenic potential.

Cellular immunity

Investigation of the type, distribution and function of the immune cells in the systemic circulation and intestine of IBD patients has been a major focus of attention for many years. For well over a decade this attention has gradually shifted from the peripheral circulation to the gut mucosa. Initially, only classical immune cells, such as T and B lymphocytes, were examined, until it became evident that other types of local cells exhibited similar properties and secreted the same products as those of mononuclear cells. Thus, the idea that cell-mediated immunity in the normal and diseased mucosa is solely mediated by 'immune' cells is no longer acceptable, and a whole new set of 'nonimmune' cells must be taken into account, substantially enhancing the complexity of assessing IBD immunopathophysiology.

Epithelial cells

One of the best examples of 'nonimmune' cells playing a role in IBD is that of epithelial cells. These are known to express HLA class II antigens on the cell surface, a condition indispensable for antigen presentation and accessory cell function. In the inflamed intestine expression of class II antigens is enhanced, suggesting an involvement of epithelial cells in the local immune response. Mostly based on the work of Mayer and collaborators, it is now accepted that these cells regulate intestinal immunity in health and disease. The most prominent observations were the ability of epithelial cells to present antigens, and the abnormality of this function in IBD, where helper T cells rather than suppressor cells are preferentially activated by CD or UC epithelial cells[43]. This could be a mechanism for expanding or perpetuating an undesirable and excessive immune reactivity in the gut. Other investigators have extended these observations, showing evidence that drugs beneficial to IBD patients can down-regulate HLA-DR antigens on epithelial cells[44,45].

Intraepithelial lymphocytes and lamina propria mononuclear cells

The intestinal mucosa is populated by a rich and extremely varied number of cells[46]. Knowledge of the population of intraepithelial lymphocytes (IEL) in IBD is still rather limited, but a few interesting observations have been made. As in the normal intestine, the majority of IEL display a dominant CD3+CD8+ phenotype, but the proportion bearing the $\gamma\delta$ T cell receptor (TCR$\gamma\delta$+) is decreased in CD and even more remarkably in UC[47,48]. The normal population of human IEL tends to display a restricted set of Vβ usage for its T cell receptor (TCR) suggesting oligoclonality[49], and this may also occur in IBD[50].

In the lamina propria T cells are second in number only to plasma cells attesting to their fundamental importance in local regulatory and effector functions. There is strong evidence that T cells play a major role in the morphological changes associated with tissue damage. In-situ activation of lamina propria T cells results in injury to the mucosa, and there is a quantitative relationship between the number of T cells and the degree of tissue destruction[51]. T lymphocytes have been evaluated extensively in control and IBD intestine, but no consistent shift of CD4+ or CD8+ subsets have been found. However, as in the intraepithelial compartment, the number carrying the TCR$\gamma\delta$ is decreased[47]. Obviously during a pathologic reaction many factors contribute to the final outcome of local immune response, but even in the normal mucosa there is evidence that the activation pathways most commonly used by local cells differ from those of circulating cells, a phenomenon which may depend on the unique make-up of the mucosal microenvironment[52]. Whether the IBD microenvironment is fundamentally different from that of the normal gut is being assessed. A possibility being currently investigated is that endogenous or exogenous superantigens may be present and induce the activation of specific types of mucosal T cells. Evidence supporting this possibility exists[53], but a firm link to selective usage of a restricted set of Vβ regions in IBD mucosa is still lacking[54,55], even though some preliminary reports suggest this possibility[56]. Nevertheless, IBD may still be similar to other autoimmune conditions associated with depletion or overrepresentation of certain T cells with a unique TCR Vβ region utilization[57], and this needs to be explored in detail.

Other immune cells continue to receive little attention, but this should not be interpreted as a sign that they are not important to IBD pathogenesis. Rather, this reflects technical problems in isolating or working with such cells that are often few in number. A general impression is that all of them tend to be activated and release bioactive mediators[58,59].

Mesenchymal cells

Once considered simple structural cells, fibroblasts and muscle cells are now recognized as metabolically active and biologically important players in overall gut homeostasis. Both cell types have shed the image of 'nonimmune' bystanders, and must be included in the realm of immunologically active cells. Although morphologically similar, mesenchymal cells from different parts of the body have unique functional characteristics, as demonstrated for colonic fibroblasts in regard to their capacity to produce collagen in comparison with skin fibroblasts[60]. During inflammation, especially when chronic, e.g. IBD, gut mesenchymal cells change both phenotypically as well as functionally[61,62], a phenomenon likely to be dependent on the inflammatory reaction in their proximity. In spite of these changes being secondary, this does not diminish their importance. In fact, pathologic findings typical of UC or CD, such as shortening of the bowel and stricture formation, are due to the effect of excessive collagen deposition and muscle cells hyperplasia. Recent data demonstrate the enhanced collagen production by fibroblasts in tissue culture, by immunohistochemistry and in-situ hybridization. Furthermore, the spectrum of functional responses and modulatory activity of mesenchymal cells is certainly broader than originally thought, in view of the capacity of these cells for proliferating in response to and generating mRNA for a variety of proinflammatory cytokines, including IL-1, IL-6 and tumor necrosis factor α (TNF-α)[63].

Cell adhesion molecules

With the expanding number of mucosal cell types that actively participate in the IBD reaction, and the multiple interactions occurring among them, it seems logical to assume that some mechanisms must be in place to allow or facilitate such intricate interplay. The obvious candidates for this complex and important function are adhesion molecules, a large group of cell surface proteins that allow contact, physical attachment and biological interaction between two or more cell types[64]. The role of adhesion molecules becomes even more important in inflammation, and they can be pivotal to the outcome of any inflammatory response given their ability to control cell-to-cell contact, as well as the entry and exit of inflammatory cells from tissues[65]. Evidence that adhesion molecules have an important role in IBD pathogenesis is accumulating. Although expression of the leukocyte adhesion molecules CD11/CD18 is not increased in circulating cells[66], an entirely different situation exists in actively inflamed gut. The percentage of tissue macrophages expressing LFA-1 (leukocyte function-associated antigen-1, CD11a) is strikingly increased in both UC and CD mucosa, and correlates with severity of inflammation[67]. High levels of ELAM-1 (endothelial leukocyte adhesion molecule-1) but not VAM-1 (vascular cell adhesion molecule-1) are detected in actively inflamed areas of CD or UC[68,69], in addition to an increase of ICAM-1 (intracellular adhesion molecule-1) and E- and P-selectins in venules, and VLA-4 (very late activation antigen-4) on mononuclear cells[70]. The enhanced expression of several adhesion molecules can be functionally translated into an abnormal function of peripheral and intestinal mononuclear cells in IBD: blood cells show an enhanced tendency to form granulomas in vitro[71], and lamina propria lymphocytes lose selectivity in their interaction with high endothelial venules (HEV)[72]. Finally, considering how important adhesion molecules are in controlling the number and type of cells in inflammatory infiltrates, it is conceivable that blockade of adhesion molecule expression may result in modulation of inflammation itself. Preliminary evidence supporting this possibility has been recently reported in the cotton top tamarin, where the administration of anti-VLA-4 monoclonal antibody results in significant attenuation of acute colitis[73].

Soluble mediators

Among the numerous components of the immune and inflammatory reaction of IBD none has received so much attention as soluble mediators. This is a broad term that includes any molecule produced by activated cells and released in the immediate vicinity, such as eicosanoids, growth factors and cytokines. The unparalleled interest in cytokines is explained by their extremely broad and potent activity on almost every aspect of pathophysiology in development, immunity and inflammation, and their potential for providing unprecedented insights into mechanisms of disease and novel therapeutic approaches[74].

Lipid mediators

The enhanced production of eicosanoids (prostanoids and leukotrienes) in IBD mucosa was one of the first findings demonstrating that inflammatory cells secrete bioactive substances at the level of the diseased mucosa, and for the first time implicated soluble mediators in the pathogenesis of UC and CD. This concept has become well established, and until recently inflammatory cells were considered to be solely responsible for the enhanced production of prostaglandins, thromboxanes and leukotrienes. This concept has changed rather dramatically in the past few years with the demonstration that other cell types also play an active role in local eicosanoid metabolism. The most novel finding is clear proof that epithelial cells are involved in this process, and produce lipid mediators even under normal circumstances. At active sites of inflammation these cells produce significantly increased amounts of platelet-activating factor and 12-lipoxygenase[75,76]. These are important observations because they expand the number of cells involved in inflammation, and in particular broaden the spectrum of activities of epithelial cells in the local immune response.

Cytokines

The field of intestinal cytokines in normal and abnormal mucosal immunity is experiencing a true explosion of interest and knowledge. Unfortunately this positive trend is complicated in IBD by conflicting reports on the levels of cytokines in the serum, culture supernatants or intestinal tissues of CD and UC patients. This confusing situation is due, at least in part, to the use of vastly different methodological approaches (stimulated vs unstimulated conditions, bioassays vs immunoassays, mRNA assessment by immunoblotting or polymerase chain reaction (PCR), etc.), and different patient populations (adult vs pediatric, acute vs chronic, on vs off medication, etc.). Several excellent and comprehensive reviews are available to the reader interested in an in-depth evaluation of this subject[77-80]. For the sake of space, and keeping in mind the scope of this chapter, discussion will be limited to the most recent and salient developments.

Of the several immunoregulatory cytokines (IL-2, IL-4, IL-5, IL-10 and interferon-γ – IFN-γ) IL-2 probably has a direct role in the pathogenesis of CD. In spite of contradictory results on its levels under various experimental conditions, patients with CD receiving treatment with high doses of this cytokine for cancer immunotherapy experience symptomatic exacerbations[81]. In contrast, patients with active disease that develop AIDS and loss of IL-2-producing CD4+ T cells enter remission[82]. The genes for IL-2 and its receptor (IL-2R) are usually expressed at a higher degree in CD than UC[83,84], and so are its products, including the soluble form of the IL-2R whose circulating levels roughly reflect the severity of immune activation in CD but not UC mucosa[85].

The production of the so-called proinflammatory cytokines (IL-1, IL-6, IL-8 and TNF-α) is almost invariably increased, although results from different investigators are not always uniform. All agree that the production of IL-1 in IBD tissue is markedly and consistently elevated during active disease. Much of the interest related to this potent proinflammatory substance is now centered on its antagonist, the IL-1 receptor antagonist (IL-1ra), a natural protein that blocks the receptor for IL-1 without triggering an inflammatory response[86]. Two points deserve special attention: more than the levels of IL-1 itself, the most important factor in determining how much inflammatory activity will ensue may actually depend on the relative concentration of IL-1ra and IL-1, or the IL-1ra/IL-1 ratio. Evidence indicates that a mucosal imbalance between these two molecules is present in IBD, and this may lead to chronic inflammation[87]; in addition, genetic polymorphism for the allelic frequencies of IL-1ra may be another factor predisposing to UC or a more severe form of it[88].

The production, cellular source and overall role of TNF-α in IBD continues to be quite controversial, but except for one group of studies, this cytokine does not appear to be produced in exceedingly large amounts as predicated by the severity of inflammation in CD or UC, or other forms of gut injury[89,90]. The potent proinflammatory mediator IL-8, which is primarily a chemotactic agent for neutrophils, is also receiving attention in IBD. Gut tissue actively involved in UC or CD contains extremely elevated levels of this chemokine, even though in the peripheral blood circulating antibodies to IL-8 are found only in UC[91-93]. A novel and interesting aspect of IL-8 is its apparent production by gut epithelial cells, reinforcing the idea that these cells are indeed involved in gut inflammation[94].

Growth factors

Growth factors represent a large group of peptides produced by multiple cell types, and they affect the growth and differentiation of epithelial cells. There is strong evidence that these peptides are involved in various stages of the IBD process[80]. Some of them, such as insulin growth factor-I (IGF-I) have been implicated in the pathogenesis of experimental colitis and hepatitis in rats[95], indicating that growth factors are broadly involved in any inflammatory response of the gastrointestinal tract. The expression of some of these factors, such as trefoil peptides associated with gut ulceration, and the angiogenic peptide basic fibroblast growth factor (bFGF), is enhanced in IBD[96,97]. Growth factors in general, and transforming growth factor $\beta 1$ (TGF-$\beta 1$), in particular, are likely to be involved in the healing process accompanying intestinal inflammation, a function which can be co-modulated by other growth factors such as transforming growth factor-α (TGF-α), and epidermal growth factor (EGF) and cytokines (IL-1β and IFN-γ)[98,99].

Neuropeptides

The existence of a 'brain–gut axis' has long been suspected, but until recently this concept was based more on intuition and clinical impression rather than concrete scientific evidence. With the demonstration of how rich the enteric nervous system is, and how intimate is the relationship between nerve fibers and immune cells, the basis for supporting the brain–gut axis gained considerable strength[100]. In addition, well-defined physical and biochemical pathways linking the stress response to the regulation of inflammatory diseases have been established[101], providing additional backing for the clinical observation that stress can induce a clinical flare-up in IBD patients. Evidence is now unquestionable that the enteric nervous system has a definitive role in regulating the function of humoral as well as cellular gut immunity. This function is mediated through the secretion of a large number of neuropeptides, or 'cytokine equivalents' for the nervous cells. These are located in close physical proximity to T and B cells, macrophages, mast cells, etc., and during inflammation nerve cells surprisingly express HLA-DR antigens to an extent correlating to that of epithelial cells[102]. Thus, the role of enteric nerves and their interaction with local immunocytes is much more extensive and important than previously noted. For instance, a recent report shows how vasoactive intestinal peptide (VIP) markedly up-regulates IgA and down-regulates IgG production by human colonic lamina propria mononuclear cells in vitro[103]. The function of VIP and other neural substances is likely to be much more extensive, and future work will define the impact of enteric neuropeptides on mucosal immunity.

Oxygen metabolites

Reactive oxygen metabolites (ROM) do not fit the same definition of soluble mediators used for the above substances, since they do not circulate, and their existence is transient. Nevertheless, they represent another type of secretory product of activated inflammatory cells[104], being highly cytotoxic to a variety of cells in vitro and in vivo. There is abundant evidence that large amounts of ROM are produced in IBD by various types of mucosal cell[105,106]. In addition to the gut, circulating monocytes from IBD patients can release ROM, a phenomenon that can be triggered by bacterial products[107]. Oxygen metabolites have been proposed as possible final pathways of injury for many of the immune and nonimmune events occurring in the inflamed bowel of humans and animals[108,109]. This concept is supported by studies showing beneficial effects of oxygen radical scavengers in IBD[110].

MISCELLANEOUS FACTORS

A feature common to many complex and chronic conditions is the proposed multifactorial origin, where the cumulative effect of several factors results in the triggering or modulation of the disease. Perhaps no better example of this exists than IBD, since a number of observations have been made in regard to various factors or conditions for which there is limited scientific evidence or logical explanation.

Smoking

The initial studies describing the effect of smoking on the clinical course of CD or UC were received with skepticism. However, when reports from various centers started accumulating it became impossible to dismiss data showing a beneficial effect of smoking in UC and a detrimental effect in CD[111,112]. This opposite dichotomy is exceedingly puzzling, but the findings are so consistent and reproducible that the effect of smoking may actually reflect some event fundamentally linked to the etiopathogenesis of both forms of IBD[113]. The mechanism by which smoking may modulate the clinical manifestations of IBD is just as perplexing and enigmatic, and not surprisingly nicotine has been blamed, in spite of the fact that there is no obvious evidence implicating this alkaloid. In spite of this, a study recently published shows that the addition of transdermal nicotine to conventional treatment significantly improves symptoms in UC patients[114].

Intestinal permeability

The finding of an increased intestinal permeability in Crohn's disease patients is not surprising, but the suggested existence of a similar defect in healthy relatives has raised substantial interest as a potential predisposing factor. This observation has attracted considerable attention, but results have been controversial, some reports reinforcing and others denying the existence of altered intestinal permeability in unaffected relatives of CD subjects[115-117]. In one study, increased permeability was detected even in the lungs of CD patients[117]. The key question in regard to these curious observations is whether a permeability defect is a primary etiologic factor or is secondary to intestinal inflammation[118]. This is no easy question to address, but careful studies have identified at least a subset of healthy relatives with high permeability in the absence of obvious clinical evidence of disease[119]. The arduous aspect of this problem is how to precisely define 'absence of disease', since very early defects of epithelial structure and function can probably be so subtle as to be undetectable by routine methods and thus go unnoticed. Until better methods to evaluate permeability or define normality of absorptive mechanisms are developed, the answer to the question of increased intestinal permeability in CD is likely to remain elusive.

SUMMARY AND CONCLUSIONS

The ultimate goal of fully understanding the pathogenesis of IBD is that of helping patients by developing scientifically based, truly efficacious treatments that have high specificity and are free of side-effects. Although not quite at hand, realizing this goal appears feasible based on the rapidly accumulating knowledge on the various immunopathogenic components of IBD. Many of the new therapies now undergoing clinical trials are based on this approach[120]. The strongest emphasis is in creating new interventions based on an understanding of inflammatory mediators[121], and this has resulted in therapies varying from administering injections of IL-1ra to simple dietary manipulations[122]. The drugs that clinicians and patients alike have relied upon for years are taking on new names and appearances, but it remains to be proven that this has really improved their effectiveness in addition to the cost[123]. A new series of immunosuppressive drugs is being tested, but most of them suffer from the same disadvantages of the old ones, i.e. toxicity, side-effects and lack of specificity[124]. Finally, not all that is new and better must carry the luster and respect of the laboratory bench. Clinical observation is still a centerpiece of medical care, and can still be used to improve or change therapy. A good example of this is the use of short-chain fatty acid or butyrate enemas for UC, apparently with promising results[125,126]. Solid scientific evidence for a long-held 'energy-deficient state' in UC is still limited[127], but common sense and intuition may go a long way.

References

1. Fiocchi C. Pathophysiology: facts, hopes and implications for treatment. In: Scholmerich J, Kruis W, Goebell H, Hohenberger W, Gross V, editors. Inflammatory bowel disease: pathophysiology as basis of treatment. Lancaster: Kluwer; 1993:257–79.
2. Shanahan F. Pathogenesis of ulcerative colitis. Lancet. 1993;342:407–11.
3. Sofaer J. Crohn's disease: the genetic contribution. Gut. 1993;34:869–71.
4. Lashner BA, Kirsner JB. The epidemiology of inflammatory bowel disease: are we learning anything new? Gastroenterology. 1992;103:696–8.
5. Asakura H, Tsuchiya M, Aiso S et al. Association of the human lymphocyte-DR2 antigen with Japanese ulcerative colitis. Gastroenterology. 1982;82:413–18.
6. Toyoda H, Wang S-J, Yang H-J et al. Distinct associations of HLA class II genes with inflammatory bowel disease. Gastroenterology. 1993;104:741–8.
7. Yang H, Rotter JI, Toyoda H et al. Ulcerative colitis: a genetically heterogeneous disorder defined by genetic (HLA class II) and subclinical (antineutrophil cytoplasmic antibodies) markers. J Clin Invest. 1993;92:1080–4.
8. Fiocchi C, Roche JK, Michener WM. High prevalence of antibodies to intestinal epithelial antigens in patients with inflammatory bowel disease and their relatives. Ann Intern Med. 1989;110:786–94.
9. Saxon A, Shanahan F, Landers C, Ganz T, Targan S. A distinct subset of anti-neutrophil cytoplasmic antibodies is associated with inflammatory bowel disease. J Allergy Clin

Immunol. 1990;86:202–10.

10. Duerr RH, Targan SR, Landers CJ, Sutherland LR, Shanahan F. Anti-neutrophil cytoplasmic antibodies in ulcerative colitis. Comparison with other colitides/diarrheal diseases. Gastroenterology. 1991;100:1590–6.

11. Shanahan F, Duerr RH, Rotter JI et al. Neutrophil autoantibodies in ulcerative colitis: familial aggregation and genetic heterogeneity. Gastroenterology. 1992;103:456–61.

12. Dalekos GN, Manoussakis MN, Goussia AC, Tsianos EV, Moutsopoulos HM. Soluble interleukin-2 receptors, antineutrophil cytoplasmic antibodies, and other autoantibodies in patients with ulcerative colitis. Gut. 1993;34:658–64.

13. Fiocchi C, Battisto JR, Farmer RG. Studies on isolated gut mucosal lymphocytes in inflammatory bowel disease. Detection of activated T cells and enhanced proliferation to *Staphylococcus aureus* and lipopolysaccharides. Dig Dis Sci. 1981;26:728–36.

14. Pirzer U, Schonhaar A, Fleischer B, Hermann E, Buschenfelde K-HM. Reactivity of infiltration T lymphocytes with microbial antigens in Crohn's disease. Lancet. 1991;338:1238–9.

15. Ibbotson JP, Lowes JR, Chahal H et al. Mucosal cell-mediated immunity to mycobacterial, enterobacterial and other microbial antigens in inflammatory bowel disease. Clin Exp Immunol. 1992;87:224–30.

16. Szewczuk MR, Depew WT. Evidence for T lymphocyte reactivity to the 65 kilodalton heat shock protein of mycobacterium in active Crohn's disease. Clin Invest Med. 1992;15:494–505.

17. Kruiningen HJV, Colombel JF, Cartun RW et al. An in-depth study of Crohn's disease in two French families. Gastroenterology. 1993;104:351–60.

18. Wakefield AJ, Pittilo RM, Sim R et al. Evidence of persistent measles virus infection in Crohn's disease. J Med Virol. 1993;39:345–53.

19. Wakefield AJ, Sawyerr AM, Hudson M, Dhillon AP, Pounder RE. Smoking, the oral contraceptive pill, and Crohn's disease. Dig Dis Sci. 1991;36:1147–50.

20. Stenson WF. Animal models of inflammatory bowel disease. In Targan SR, Shanahan F, editors. Inflammatory bowel disease. From bench to bedside. Baltimore: Williams & Wilkins; 1994:180–92.

21. Fiocchi C. Cytokines and animal models: a combined path to inflammatory bowel disease pathogenesis. Gastroenterology. 1993;104:1202–19.

22. Yamada T, Sartor RB, Marshall S, Specian RD, Grisham MB. Mucosal injury and inflammation in a model of chronic granulomatous colitis in rats. Gastroenterology. 1993;104:759–71.

23. McCall RD, Haskill S, Zimmermann EM, Lund PK, Thompson CR, Sartor RB. Tissue interleukin-1 and interleukin-1 receptor antagonist expression in enterocolitis in resistant and susceptible rats. Gastroenterology. 1994;106:960–72.

24. Cooper HS, Murthy SNS, Shah RS, Sedergran DJ. Clinicopathologic study of dextran sulfate sodium experimental murine colitis. Lab Invest. 1993;69:238–49.

25. Caplan MS, Hedlund E, Hill N, MacKendrick W. The role of endogenous nitric oxide and platelet-activating factor in hypoxia-induced intestinal injury in rats. Gastroenterology. 1994;106:346–52.

26. Rachmilewitz D, Stamler JS, Karmeli F et al. Peroxynitrite-induced rat colitis – a new model of colonic inflammation. Gastroenterology. 1994;105:1681–8.

27. Lacey SR, Lichtman S. Development of an animal model for ileoanal pouchitis. J Pediatr Surg. 1993;28:574–5.

28. Bucy RP, Xu XY, Li J, Huang GQ. Cyclosporin A-induced autoimmune disease in mice. J Immunol. 1993;154:1039–50.

29. Powrie F, Leach MW, Mauze S, Cadde LB, Coffman RL. Phenotypically distinct subsets of CD4+ T cells induce or protect from chronic intestinal inflammation in C. B-17 scid mice. Int Immunol. 1993;5:1461–71.

30. Morrisy PJ, Charrier K, Braddy S, Liggit D, Watson JD. CD4+ T cells that express high levels of CD45RB induce wasting disease when transferred into congenic severe combined immunodeficient mice. Disease development is prevented by cotransfer of purified CD4+ T cells. J Exp Med. 1993;178:237–44.

31. Hammer RE, Maika SD, Richardson JA, Tang J-P, Taurog JD. Spontaneous inflammatory disease in transgenic rats expressing HLA-B27 and human b2m: an animal model of HLA-

B27-associated human disorders. Cell. 1990;63:1099–112.

32. Sadlack B, Mertz H, Schorle H, Schimpl A, Feller AC, Horak I. Ulcerative colitis-like disease in mice with a disrupted interleukin-2 gene. Cell. 1993;75:253–61.

33. Kuhn R, Lohler J, Rennick D, Rajewsky K, Muller W. Interleukin-10-deficient mice develop chronic enterocolitis. Cell. 1993;75:263–74.

34. Mombaerts P, Mizoguchi E, Grusby MG, Glimcher LH, Bhan AK, Tonegawa S. Spontaneous development of inflammatory bowel disease in T cell receptor mutant mice. Cell. 1993;75:275–82.

35. Strober W, Ehrhardt RO. Chronic intestinal inflammation: an unexpected outcome in cytokine or T cell receptor mutant mice. Cell. 1993;75:203–5.

36. Brandtzaeg P, Halstensen TS, Kett K. Immunopathology of inflammatory bowel disease. In: MacDermott RP, Stenson WF, editors. Inflammatory bowel disease. New York: Elsevier; 1992:95–136.

37. Helgeland L, Tysk C, Jarnerot G et al. IgG subclass distribution in serum and rectal mucosa of monozygotic twins with or without inflammatory bowel disease. Gut. 1992;33:1358–64.

38. Snook J. Are the inflammatory bowel diseases autoimmune disorders? Gut. 1990;31:961–3.

39. Das KM, Vecchi M, Sakamaki S. A shared and unique epitope(s) on human colon, skin, and biliary epithelium detected by a monoclonal antibody. Gastroenterology. 1990;98:464–9.

40. Halstensen TS, Das KM, Brandtzaeg P. Epithelial deposits of immunoglobulin G1 and activated complement colocalise with the M_r 40 kD putative autoantigen in ulcerative colitis. Gut. 1993;34:650–7.

41. Das KM, Dasgupta A, Mandal A, Geng X. Autoimmunity to cytoskeletal protein tropomyosin. J Immunol. 1993;150:2487–93.

42. Mandal A, Dasgupta A, Jeffers L et al. Autoantibodies in sclerosing cholangitis against a shared peptide in biliary and colon epithelium. Gastroenterology. 1994;106:185–92.

43. Mayer L, Eisenhardt D. Lack of induction of suppressor T cells by intestinal epithelial cells from patients with inflammatory bowel disease. J Clin Invest. 1990;86:1255–60.

44. Hoang P, Crotty B, Dalton HR, Jewell DP. Epithelial cells bearing class II molecules stimulate allogeneic human colonic intraepithelial lymphocytes. Gut. 1992;33:1089–93.

45. Crotty B, Hoang P, Dalton HR, Jewell DP. Salicylates used in inflammatory bowel disease and colchicine impair interferon-γ induced HLA-DR expression. Gut. 1992;33:59–64.

46. Fiocchi C. Mucosal cellular immunity. In: Targan SR, Shanahan F, editors. Immunology and immunopathology of the liver and gastrointestinal tract. New York: Igaku-Shoin; 1990:107–38.

47. Fukushima K, Masuda T, Ohtani H et al. Immunohistochemical characterization, distribution, and ultrastructure of lymphocytes bearing T-cell receptor γδ in inflammatory bowel disease. Gastroenterology. 1991;101:670–8.

48. Hoang P, Senju M, Lowes JR, Jewell DP. Phenotypic characterization of isolated intraepithelial lymphocytes in patients with ulcerative colitis and normal controls. Dig Dis Sci. 1992;37:1725–8.

49. VanKerckhove C, Russell GJ, Deusch K et al. Oligoclonality of human intestinal intraepithelial T cells. J Exp Med. 1992;175:57–63.

50. Landau SB, Balk SP, Yang L, Burke SK, Blumberg RS. T-cell receptor (TCR) γ variable region utilization is altered in ulcerative colitis. Gastroenterology. 1992;102:A650.

51. Lionetti P, Breese E, Braegger CP, Murch SH, Taylor J, MacDonald TT. T-cell activation can induce either mucosal destruction or adaptation in cultured human fetal small intestine. Gastroenterology. 1993;105:373–81.

52. Qiao L, Schurmann G, Autschbach F, Wallich R, Meuer SC. Human intestinal mucosa alters T-cell reactivities. Gastroenterology. 1993;105:814–19.

53. Aisenberg J, Ebert EC, Mayer L. T-cell activation in human intestinal mucosa: the role of superantigens. Gastroenterology. 1993;105:1421–30.

54. Posnett DN, Schmelkin I, Burton DA, August A, McGrath H, Mayer LF. T cell antigen receptor V gene usage. Increases in Vβ8+ T cells in Crohn's disease. J Clin Invest. 1990;85:1770–6.

55. Spencer J, Choy MY, MacDonald TT. T cell receptor Vβ expression by mucosal T cells. J Clin Pathol. 1991;44:915–18.

56. Duchmann R, Strober W, Fiocchi C, James SP. TCR Vβ2 gene expression is selective in control but not in IBD lamina propria lymphocytes. Gastroenterology. 1992;102:617.

57. Paliard X, West SG, Lafferty JA et al. Evidence for the effects of a superantigen in rheumatoid arthritis. Science. 1991;253:325–9.

58. Sperber K, Ogata S, Sylvester C et al. A novel human macrophage-derived intestinal mucin secretagogue: implications for the pathogenesis of inflammatory bowel disease. Gastroenterology. 1993;104:1302–9.

59. Fox CC, Lichtenstein LM, Roche JK. Intestinal mast cell responses in idiopathic inflammatory bowel disease. Dig Dis Sci. 1993;38:1105–12.

60. Martens MFWC, Huyben CMLC, Hendriks T. Collagen synthesis in fibroblasts from human colon: regulatory aspects and differences with skin fibroblasts. Gut. 1992;33:1664–70.

61. Lee EY, Stesnson WF, DeChryver-Kecskemeti K. Thickening of muscularis mucosae in Crohn's disease. Mod Pathol. 1991;4:87–90.

62. Vermillion DL, Huizinga JD, Riddell RH, Collins SM. Altered small intestinal smooth muscle function in Crohn's disease. Gastroenterology. 1993;104:1692–9.

63. Strong SA, Klein JS, West GA, Fiocchi C. Activation of intestinal mesenchymal cells by IL1β induces inflammatory cytokine and procollagen gene expression. Gastroenterology. 1993;104:A784.

64. Springer TA. Adhesion receptors of the immune system. Nature. 1990;346:425–34.

65. Cronstein BC, Weissmann G. The adhesion molecules of inflammation. Arthritis Rheum. 1993;36:147–57.

66. Greenfield SM, Hamblin A, Punchard NA, Thompson RPH. Expression of adhesion molecules on circulating leucocytes in patients with inflammatory bowel disease. Clin Sci. 1992;83:221–6.

67. Malizia G, Calabrese A, Cottone M et al. Expression of leukocyte adhesion molecules by mucosal mononuclear phagocytes in inflammatory bowel disease. Gastroenterology. 1991;100:150–9.

68. Koizumi M, King N, Lobb R, Benjamin C, Podolsky DK. Expression of vascular adhesion molecules in inflammatory bowel disease. Gastroenterology. 1992;103:840–7.

69. Ohtani H, Nakamura S, Watanabe Y et al. Light and electron microscopic immunolocalization of endothelial leucocyte adhesion molecules-1 in inflammatory bowel disease. Virchows Arch A Pathol Anat. 1992;420:403–9.

70. Nakamura S, Ohtani H, Watanabe Y et al. In situ expression of the cell adhesion molecules in inflammatory bowel disease. Lab Invest. 1993;69:77–85.

71. Mishra L, Mishra BB, Harris M, Bayless TM, Muchmore AV. In-vitro cell aggregation and cell adhesion molecules in Crohn's disease. Gastroenterology. 1993;104:772–9.

72. Salmi M, Granfors K, MacDermott RP, Jalkanen S. Aberrant binding of lamina propria lymphocytes to vascular endothelium in inflammatory bowel disease. Gastroenterology. 1994;106:596–605.

73. Podolsky DK, Lobb R, King N et al. Attenuation of colitis in the cotton-top tamarin by anti-alpha 4 integrin monoclonal antibody. J Clin Invest. 1993;92:372–80.

74. Oppenheim JJ, Neta R, Pathophysiological roles of cytokines in development, immunity, and inflammation. FASEB J. 1994;8:158–62.

75. Ferraris L, Karmeli F, Eliakim R, Klein J, Fiocchi C, Rachmilewitz D. Intestinal epithelial cells contribute to the enhanced generation of platelet activating factor in ulcerative colitis. Gut. 1993;34:665–8.

76. Shannon VR, Stenson WF, Holtzman MJ. Induction of epithelial arachidonate 12-lipoxygenase at active sites of inflammatory bowel disease. Am J Physiol. 1993;264:G104–11.

77. Fiocchi C. Cytokines. In: MacDermott RP, Stenson W, editors. Inflammatory bowel disease. New York: Elsevier; 1992:137–62.

78. Fiocchi C. Cytokines. In: Targan SR, Shanahan F, editors. Inflammatory bowel disease. From bench to bedside. Baltimore: Williams & Wilkins; 1994:106–22.

79. Sartor RB. Cytokines in intestinal inflammation: pathophysiological and clinical considerations. Gastroenterology. 1994;106:533–9.

80. Podolsky DK, Fiocchi C. Cytokines and growth factors in inflammatory bowel disease. In: Kirsner JB, Shorter RG, editors. Inflammatory bowel disease. Lea & Febiger; 1995 (In

press).

81. Sparano JA, Brandt LJ, Dutcher JP, DuBois JS, Atkins MB. Symptomatic exacerbation of Crohn disease after treatment with high-dose interleukin-2. Ann Intern Med. 1993;118:617–18.

82. James SP. Remission of Crohn's disease after human immunodeficiency virus infection. Gastroenterology. 1988;95:1667–9.

83. Matsuura T, West GA, Klein JS et al. Immune activation gene products are resistant to IL4 inhibitory activity in Crohn's disease (CD). Gastroenterology. 1993;194:A739.

84. Mullin GE, Lazenby AJ, Harris ML, Bayless TM, James SP. Increased interleukin-2 messenger RNA in the intestinal mucosal lesions of Crohn's disease but not ulcerative colitis. Gastroenterology. 1992;102:1620–7.

85. Matsuura T, West GA, Klein JS, Ferraris L, Fiocchi C. Soluble interleukin 2, CD8 and CD4 receptors in inflammatory bowel disease. A comparative study of peripheral blood and intestinal mucosal levels. Gastroenterology. 1992;102:2006–14.

86. Arend WP. Interleukin-1 receptor antagonism. J Clin Invest. 1991;88:1445–51.

87. Casini-Raggi V, Kam L, Jin Y, Fiocchi C, Pizarro TT, Cominelli F. Mucosal imbalance of interleukin-1 and interleukin-1 receptor antagonist in inflammatory bowel disease: a potential mechanism of chronic intestinal inflammation. 1994 (Submitted).

88. Mansfield JC, Holden H, Tarlow JK et al. Novel genetic association between ulcerative colitis and the anti-inflammatory cytokine interleukin-1 receptor antagonist. Gastroenterology. 1994;106:637–42.

89. Hymas JS, Treem WR, Eddy E, Wyzga N, Moore RE. Tumor necrosis factor-α is not elevated in children with inflammatory bowel disease. J Pediatr Gastroenterol Nutr. 1991;12:233–6.

90. Tan X, Hsueh W, Gonazles-Crussi F. Cellular localization of tumor necrosis factor (TNF-)-α transcripts in normal bowel and in necrotizing enterocolitis. Am J Pathol. 1993;142:1858–65.

91. Izzo RS, Witkon K, Chen AI, Hadjiyane C, Weinstein MI, Pellecchia C. Interleukin-8 and neutrophil markers in colonic mucosa from patients with ulcerative colitis. Am J Gastroenterol. 1992;87:1447–52.

92. Izzo RS, Witkon K, Chen AI, Hadjiyane C, Weinstein MI, Pellecchia C. Neutrophil-activating peptide (interleukin-8) in colonic mucosa from patients with Crohn's disease. Scand J Gastroenterol. 1993;28:269–300.

93. Mahida YR, Ceska M, Effenberger F, Kurlak L, Lindley I, Hawkey CJ. Enhanced synthesis of neutrophil-activating peptide-I/interleukin-8 in active ulcerative colitis. Clin Sci. 1992;82:273–5.

94. Eckmann L, Jung HC, Schurer-Maly C, Panja A, Morzycka-Wroblewska E, Kagnoff MF. Differential cytokine expression by human intestinal epithelial cell lines: regulated expression of interleukin 8. Gastroenterology. 1994;105:1689–97.

95. Zimmermann EM, Sartor RB, McCall RD, Pardo M, Bender D, Lund PK. Insulin growth factor I and interleukin 1β messenger RNA in a rat model of granulomatous enterocolitis and hepatitis. Gastroenterology. 1993;105:399–409.

96. Wright NA, Poulsom R, Stamp G et al. Trefoil peptide gene expression in gastrointestinal epithelial cells in inflammatory bowel disease. Gastroenterology. 1993;194:12–20.

97. Ohtani H, Nakamura S, Watanabe Y, Mizoi T, Saku T, Nagura H. Immunocytochemical localization of basic fibroblast growth factor in carcinomas and inflammatory lesions of the human digestive tract. Lab Invest. 1993;68:520–7.

98. Ciacci C, Lind SE, Podolsky DK. Transforming growth factor β regulation of migration in wounded rat intestinal epithelial monolayers. Gastroenterology. 1993;105:93–101.

99. Dignass AU, Podolsky DK. Cytokine modulation of intestinal epithelial cell restitution: central role of transforming growth factor β. Gastroenterology. 1993;105:1323–32.

100. Goetzel EJ, Sreedharan SP. Mediators of communication and adaptation in the neuroendocrine and immune systems. FASEB J. 1992;6:2646–52.

101. Sternberg EM, Chrousos GP, Wilder RL, Gold PW. The stress response and the regulation of inflammatory disease. Ann Intern Med. 1992;117:854–66.

102. Geboes K, Rutgeerts P, Ectors N et al. Major histocompatibility class II expression on the small intestinal nervous system in Crohn's disease. Gastroenterology. 1992;103:439–47.

103. Boirivant M, Fais S, Annibale B, Agostini D, Fave GD, Pallone F. Vasoactive intestinal polypeptide modulates the in vitro immunoglobulin A production by intestinal lamina propria lymphocytes. Gastroenterology. 1994;106:576–82.

104. Lloyd AR, Oppenheim JJ. Poly's lament: the neglected role of the polymorphonuclear neutrophil in the afferent limb of the immune response. Immunol Today. 1992;13.

105. Simmonds NJ, Rampton DS. Inflammatory bowel disease – a radical view. Gut. 1993;34:865–8.

106. Oshitani N, Kitano A, Okabe H, Nakamura S, Matsumoto T, Kobayashi K. Location of superoxide anion generation in human colonic mucosa obtained by biopsy. Gut. 1993;34:936–8.

107. Baldassano RN, Schreiber S, Johnston RB, Fu RD, Muraki T, MacDermott RP. Crohn's disease monocytes are primed for accentuated release of toxic oxygen metabolites. Gastroenterology. 1993;105:60–6.

108. Bilotta J, Waye JD. Hydrogen peroxide enteritis: the 'Snow White' sign. Gastrointest Endosc. 1989;35:428–30.

109. Tamai H, Levin S, Gaginella TS. Induction of colitis in rats by 2'-2'-azobis (2-amidinopropane) dihydrochloride. Inflammation. 1992;16:69–81.

110. Williams JP. Phagocytes, toxic oxygen metabolites and inflammatory bowel disease: implications for treatment. Ann R Coll Surg Engl. 1990;72:253–62.

111. Rudra T, Motley RJ, Rhodes J. Does smoking improve colitis? Scand J Gastroenterol. 1989;170(Suppl.):61–3.

112. Cottone M, Rosselli M, Orlando A et al. Smoking habits and recurrence of Crohn's disease. Gastroenterology. 1994;106:643–8.

113. Rhodes T, Thomas GAO. Smoking: good or bad for inflammatory bowel disease? Gastroenterology. 1994;106:807–10.

114. Pullman RD, Rhodes J, Ganesh S et al. Transdermal nicotine for active ulcerative colitis. N Engl J Med. 1994;330:811–15.

115. Katz KD, Hollander D, Vadheim CM et al. Intestinal permeability in patients with Crohn's disease and their healthy relatives. Gastroenterology. 1989;97:927–31.

116. Teahon K, Smethurst P, Levi AJ, Menzies IS, Bjarnason I. Intestinal permeability in patients with Crohn's disease and their first degree relatives. Gut. 1992;33:320–3.

117. Adenis A, Colombel J-F, Lecouffe P et al. Increased pulmonary and intestinal permeability in Crohn's disease. Gut. 1992;33:678–82.

118. Hollander D. Permeability in Crohn's disease: altered barrier function in healthy relatives? Gastroenterology. 1993;1993:1848–73.

119. May GR, Sutherland LR, Meddings JB. Is small intestinal permeability really increased in relatives of patients with Crohn's disease? Gastroenterology. 1993;104:1627–32.

120. Jewell DP, Campieri M, Jarnerot G, Modigliani R, Rask-Madsen J. New therapeutic modalities for inflammatory bowel disease. Gastroenterol Int. 1993;6:1–12.

121. Hawkey CJ, Mahida YR, Hawthorne AB. Therapeutic interventions in gastrointestinal disease based on an understanding of inflammatory mediators. Agents Actions. 1992 (Special Conference Issue):C22–5.

122. Stenson WF, Cort D, Rodgers J et al. Dietary supplementation with fish oil in ulcerative colitis. Ann Intern Med. 1992;116:609–14.

123. Sutherland LR, May GR, Shaffer EA. Sulfasalazine revisited: a meta-analysis of 5-aminosalycylic acid in the treatment of ulcerative colitis. Ann Intern Med. 1993;118:540–9.

124. Sandborn WJ, Tremaine WJ. Cyclosporine treatment of inflammatory bowel disease. Mayo Clin Proc. 1992;67:981–90.

125. Scheppach W, Sommer H, Kirchner T et al. Effect of butyrate enemas on the colonic mucosa in distal ulcerative colitis. Gastroenterology. 1992;103:51–6.

126. Breuer RI, Buto SK, Christ ML et al. Rectal irrigation with short-chain fatty acids for distal ulcerative colitis. Dig Dis Sci. 1991;36:185–7.

127. Roediger WEW. The colonic epithelium in ulcerative colitis: an energy-deficiency disease? Lancet. 1980;2:712–15.

26
The gut–brain axis in IBD: an investigator's perspective

S. M. COLLINS, H. P. WEINGARTEN and K. McHUGH

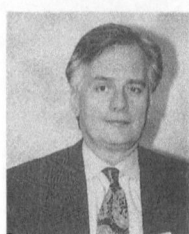

S. M. COLLINS

INTRODUCTION

The gut–brain axis is a neurohumoral bidirectional communication network that integrates behavior and intestinal function. Brain-to-gut communication is evident in many demonstrations of central nervous system (CNS) control of intestinal physiology, including motility and acid secretion. This may be relevant to the pathogenesis of functional bowel disease and stress-induced peptic ulceration. Gut-to-brain communication is reflected in studies on feeding behavior which have identified satiety signals originating from the upper and lower gut to influence appetitive behavior. With growing acceptance of neuroimmune interactions it is possible to extrapolate our knowledge of brain–gut interactions to increase our understanding of the pathophysiology of inflammatory bowel disease (IBD).

INFLAMMATION AND FEEDING BEHAVIOR

Weight loss and growth retardation in children with IBD[1] is multifactorial and likely reflects impaired nutrient absorption, increased metabolic demands and decreased food intake (anorexia)[2]. Weight loss may be so severe that Crohn's disease patients have been used as a body weight control in studies of anorexia nervosa[3]. However, the mechanisms whereby inflammation produces anorexia are unknown, but may reflect perturbation of satiety signals that originate in the gut[4] or the effects of inflammatory mediators on feeding control centers in the brain.

In recent studies we have investigated food intake in rats with colitis induced by trinitrobenzene (TNB) sulfonic acid[5]. Intrarectal administration of TNB resulted in a significant increase in myeloperoxidase (MPO) activity in the colon during the first 5 days, and this was accompanied by a substantial decrease in feeding that was maximum during the first 48 h and was reversible after 4 days. Changes in food intake were accompanied by a significant decrease in body weight. The suppression of feeding was independent of the manner in which colitis was induced, as a similar response was observed in rats with colitis induced by acetic acid. Anorexia also occurred regardless of whether nutrient was presented solid or liquid, and was also evident with the ingestion of an elemental diet[6]. Since neither water intake nor sham feeding was suppressed, it is unlikely that the reduction in feeding reflects a general malaise phenomenon. Moreover, meal pattern analysis revealed that rats exhibited a normal frequency of meal initiation, but simply consumed less at each meal; this pattern is not consistent with a general malaise effect[7].

Subsequent study revealed that the anorexia is sensitive to cyclooxygenase inhibitors[6] as well as an interleukin-1 (IL-1) receptor antagonist delivered either into the peritoneal cavity or, more effectively, into the CNS[8]. Since several actions of IL-1 are prostaglandin-mediated, these results suggest that IL-1 plays a pivotal role in mediating the anorexia associated with TNB colitis. Ongoing studies are examining the contributions of IL-6 and tumor necrosis factor alpha (TNF-α) to the anorexia observed in this model.

These observations illustrate that inflammation induces gut-to-brain signaling resulting in the expression of anorexia in a model of experimental colitis.

STRESS AND IBD

The impact of stress on organic disease has been examined in several organ systems, such as the cardiovascular system, and in the context of disease processes such as neoplasia and type I diabetes[9]. However in the case of IBD the contribution of stress remains controversial. Earlier investigators entertained the idea that some physiological consequences of stress, such as sustained intestinal muscle spasm, might actually cause mucosal inflammation that could not be attributed to ischemia[10]. While stress is not generally considered to be a causal factor in the pathogenesis of IBD, there are some studies that support the notion that stress may exacerbate IBD. There are two lines of evidence in this regard: first, some have demonstrated a temporal association between stressful life events and exacerbations of IBD[11,12], although this has not been confirmed by other studies[13,14]; second, lifestyle adjustments, including stress management, have been reported to improve the course of IBD, resulting in fewer exacerbations[15].

Research conducted in the past decade has demonstrated the biological plausibility of a relationship between stressful stimuli and immune function in experimental animals[16,17] and humans[18]. A dominant theme of this research concerns the interplay between neuropeptides, hormones and cytokines (for review see ref. 19). Cytokines such as IL-1 and TNF-α share certain physiological properties with the stress-associated hormone corticotrophin-releasing factor (CRF)[20] and are co-produced in the hypothalamus and released in response to stress[21]. In addition to contributing to the stress response, cytokine production by immunocytes may be modulated as a result of the stress response. For example, stress alters IL-2 gene expression and protein production by T lymphocytes and leukocytes in experimental animals and humans[17,18]. Of importance in this regard is the existence of neuropeptide receptors on immune cells, including those in the gut (for review see refs 22 and 23), and it should be noted that the expression of these receptors is, in turn, susceptible to the effects of stress[24]. Conversely, it has been shown that cytokines may profoundly influence neurotransmitter content and release in nerves, including those in the enteric nervous system[25]. These findings provide the basis for the existence of dynamic bidirectional interactions between the immune system and both the central and enteric nervous systems. As cytokines, such as IL-1, play an important role in the initiation, maintenance and control of intestinal inflmmatory processes[26–28], it is not unreasonable to anticipate that stress might alter intestinal inflammatory conditions by influencing cytokine profiles.

Preliminary data from our laboratory provide evidence in support of the hypothesis that there is a causal relationship between stress and the exacerbation of intestinal inflammation[29]. In these studies, acute colitis was induced in rats by intrarectal administration of TNB, and the animals were allowed to recover for 6 weeks before being subjected to mild restraint stress. The stress *per se* did not induce inflammation in those rats without colitis, and caused a significant increase in inflammatory activity, as relected by the activity of MPO in the colon, in those rats with previous colitis. Interestingly, the stress-induced reactivation of colitis was accompanied by a reduction in the expression of IL-1β mRNA in the colon. We speculate that IL-1 plays a protective role at this late stage of colitis[26], and that the expression of the cytokine in the gut was down-regulated by corticosteroids released as part of the stress response.

These data provide evidence in favour of a causal link between stress and intestinal inflammation, and prompt further exploration of the relationship between stress and IBD activity in humans.

THE RELATIONSHIP OF IBD AND IRRITABLE BOWEL SYNDROME (IBS)

There has been debate over the existence of a special relationship between IBD and IBS[30]. The observations upon which a relationship is suspected are as follows. Patients in remission from IBD often complain of symptoms suggestive of an irritable bowel[31]. This could reflect the coexistence of IBD with a highly prevalent disorder. Alternatively, it could represent the fact that inflammation in the gut leads to irritability of the gut. This notion is derived from the fact, which is now well established, that active mucosal inflammation causes changes in neuromuscular function not only at the site of inflammation[32,33] but also at non-inflamed remote sites[34,35]. Our data also indicate that changes in nerve and muscle function persist after the mucosal inflammation has subsided, as reflected by a normal level of activity of MPO activity and normal histology[36,37]. These persistent changes in tissue function may correspond to changes in sensory-motor function observed in experimental animals and humans following inflammatory episodes. MacPherson and Pfeiffer showed that colitis induced in cats caused colonic motor changes that persisted long after changes in mucosal inflammation had subsided[38]. Similar observations were made by Sethi and Sarna in dogs with pancolitis induced by acetic acid[39,40]. In patients with a previous history of *Salmonella* enteritis, others have shown that there is persistent IBS-like symptomatology and evidence of changes in rectal sensitivity and motor responsiveness[41]. These findings are similar to those obtained in IBD patients in histologically proven remission[42,43]. Taken in conjunction with the animal studies and the study on *Salmonella* patients post-*Salmonella* infection, this author concludes that mucosal inflammation results in persistent neuromotor dysfunction, and thus a basis for ongoing symptoms, once the inflammatory changes have subsided.

Based on recent studies from this laboratory one may speculate that the following sequence of events occurs. Mucosal injury and subsequent inflammation leads to changes in function of the deeper neuromuscular tissues. In addition to changing physiological function in these tissues, the inflammatory process leads to a phenotypic shift in the neuromuscular tissues such that they are able to express genes for cytokines[44]. The locally produced cytokines are therefore in a position to maintain the altered physiological function of these tissues. The underlying assumption is that the inflammatory process in the mucosa is subject to tighter control, and is more rapidly down-regulated, whereas the changes in the deeper neuromuscular tissues lack the presence of an equivalent control mechanism, thereby permitting changes to persist through autostimulation[44].

Thus, the emerging hypothesis is that IBD produces IBS by virtue of the inflammatory response to involve the neuromuscular tissues to the extent that they maintain a state of dysfuntion that persists after resolution of the mucosal inflammation.

References

1. Kirschner BS. Nutritional consequences of inflammatory bowel disease on growth. J Am Coll Nutr. 1988;7:301–8.
2. Gee MI, Grace MGA, Wensel R, Sherbaniuk R, Thompson ABR. Nutritional status of gastroenterology outpatients: comparison of inflammatory bowel disease with functional disorders. J Am Diet Assoc. 1985;85:1466–74.
3. McCallum R, Grill BB, Lange R, Planky A, Glass EE, Greenfeld DG. Definition of a gastric emptying abnormality in patients with anorexia nervosa. Dig Dis Sci. 1985;30:713–22.
4. Conover KL, Weingarten HP, Collins SM. A procedure for within-trial repeated measurement of gastric emptying in the rat. Physiol Behav. 1987;39:303–8.
5. Morris GP, Beck PL, Herridge MS, Depew WT, Szewczuk MR, Wallace JL. Hapten-induced model of chronic inflammation and ulceration in the rat colon. Gastroenterology. 1989;96:795–803.

6. McHugh KJ, Weingarten HP, Keenan C, Wallace J, Collins SM. On the suppression of food intake in experimental colitis in the rat. Am J Physiol. 1993;264:R871–6.
7. McHugh K, Weingarten HP, Collins SM. The role of delayed gastric emptying in anorexia induced by intestinal inflammation in the rat. Soc Neurosci. 1991;17:493(abstr.).
8. McHugh K, Weingarten HP, Collins SM. Anorexia in experimental colitis is mediated by interleukin-1 at both a peripheral and central level. Gastroenterology. 1993;104: A1051(abstr.).
9. Vialettes B, Ozanon JP, Kaplansky S et al. Stress antecedents and immune status in recently diagnosed type I (insulin dependent) diabetes mellitus. Diabet Metab. 1989;15:45–50.
10. Lium R. Etiology of ulcerative colitis. II. Effects of induced muscular spasm on colonic explants in dogs with comment on relation of muscular spasm to ulcerative colitis. Arch Intern Med. 1939;63:210–25.
11. Garrett VD, Brantley PJ, Jones GN, McKnight GT. The relation between daily stress and Crohn's disease. J Behav Med. 1991;14:87–96.
12. Duffy LC, Zielezny MA, Marshall JR et al. Lag time between stress events and risk of recurrent episodes of inflammatory bowel disease. Epidemiology. 1991;2:141–5.
13. Duffy LC, Zielezny MA, Marshall JR et al. Relevance of major stress events as an indicator of disease activity prevalence in inflammatory bowel disease. Behav Med. 1991;17:101–10.
14. North CS, Alpers DH, Helzer JE, Spitznagel EL, Clouse RE. Do life events or depression exacerbate inflammatory bowel disease? Ann Intern Med. 1991;114:381–6.
15. Milne B, Joachim G, Niedhardt J. A stress management programme for inflammatory bowel disease patients. J Adv Nurs. 1986;11:561–7.
16. Halper JP, Miller AH, Trestman RL, Santucci AC, Lackner C, Stein M. Biochemical mechanisms of stress-induced impairment of rat T cell mitogenesis. J Neuroimmunol. 1991;32:241–7.
17. Batuman OA, Sajewski D, Ottenweller JE, Pitman DL, Natelson BH. Effects of repeated stress on T cell numbers and function in rats. Brain Behav Immun. 1990;4:105–17.
18. Glaser R, Kennedy S, Lafuse WP et al. Psychological stress-induced modulation of interleukin 2 receptor gene expression and interleukin 2 production in peripheral blood leukocytes. Arch Gen Psychiatry. 1990;47:707–12.
19. Eskay RL, Grino M, Chen HT. Interleukins, signal transduction, and the immune system-mediated stress response. Adv Exp Med Biol. 1990;274:331–43.
20. Biandi M, Sacerdote P, Locatelli L, Mantegazza P, Panerai AE. Corticotropin releasing hormone, interleukin-1 alpha, and tumor necrosis factor-alpha share characteristics of stress mediators. Brain Res. 1991;546:139–42.
21. Minami M, Kuraishi Y, Yamaguchi T, Nakai S, Hirai Y, Satoh M. Immobilization stress induces interleukin-1 beta mRNA in the rat hypothalamus. Neurosci Lett. 1991;123:254–6.
22. Shanahan F, Anton P. Neuroendocrine modulation of the immune system: possible implications for inflammatory bowel disease. Dig Dis Sci. 1988;33:41–9S.
23. Ottaway CA. Neuroimmunomodulation in the intestinal mucosa. Gastroenterol Clin N Am. 1991;20:511–29.
24. Wiik P, Opstad PK, Knardahl S, Byum A. Receptors for vasoactive intestinal peptide (VIP) on human mononuclear leucocytes are upregulated during prolonged strain and energy deficiency. Peptides. 1988;9:181–6.
25. Hurst S, Collins SM. Interleukin-1 beta modulation of norepinephrine release from rat myenteric nerves. Am J Physiol. 1993;264:G30–5.
26. Cominelli F, Nast CC, Llerena R, Dinarello CA, Zipser RD. Interleukin 1 suppresses inflammation in rabbit colitis. Mediation by endogenous prostaglandins. J Clin Invest. 1990;85:582–6.
27. Cominelli F, Nast CC, Dinarello CA, Gentilini P, Zipser RD. Regulation of eicosanoid production in rabbit colon by interleukin-1. Gastroenteroloy. 1989;97:1400–5.
28. Cominelli F, Nast CC, Clark BD et al. Interleukin 1 (IL-1) gene expression, synthesis, and effect of specific IL-1 receptor blockade in rabbit immune complex colitis. J Clin Invest. 1990;86:972–80.
29. McHugh K, Weingarten HP, Khan I, Riddell R, Collins SM. Stress-induced exacerbation of experimental colitis in the rat. Gastroenterology. 1993;104:A1051(abstr.).
30. Bayless TM, Harris ML. Inflammatory bowel disease and irritable bowel syndrome. Med Clin N Am. 1990;74:21–8.

31. Isgar B, Harman M, Kaye MD, Whorwell PJ. Symptoms of irritable bowel syndrome in ulcerative colitis in remission. Gut. 1983;24:190–2.
32. Swain MG, Agro A, Blennerhassett P, Stanisz A, Collins SM. Increased levels of substance P in the myenteric plexus of *Trichinella*-infected rats. Gastroenterology. 1992;102:1913–19.
33. Vermillion DL, Collins SM. Increased responsiveness of jejunal longitudinal muscle in *Trichinella*-infected rats. Am J Physiol (Gastrointest Liver Physiol.). 1988;254:G124–9.
34. Marzio L, Blennerhassett P, Chiverton S, Vermillion DL, Langer J, Collins SM. Altered smooth muscle function in worm-free gut regions of *Trichinella*-infected rats. Am J Physiol. 1990;259:G306–13.
35. Jacobson K, McHugh K, Collins SM. Distal colitis causes changes in enteric nerve function at distant non-inflamed sites in the gut. Gastroenterology. 1993;104:717(abstr.).
36. Collins SM, Blennerhassett PA, Blennerhassett MG, Vermillion DL. Impaired acetylcholine release from the myenteric plexus of *Trichinella*-infected rats. Am J Physiol. 1989;257:G898–903.
37. Vallance BA, Blennerhassett PA, Collins SM. Murine trichinosis: a model of post-infective smooth muscle dysfunction. Gastroenterology. 1994;106:A582.
38. MacPherson BR, Shearin NL, Pfeiffer CJ. Experimental diffuse colitis in cats: observations on motor activity. J Surg Res. 1978;25:42–9.
39. Sethi AK, Sarna SK. Colonic motor response to a meal in acute colitis. Gastroenterology. 1991;101:1537–46.
40. Sethi AK, Sarna SK. Colonic motility in acute colitis in conscious dogs. Gastroenterology. 1991;100:954–63.
41. Bergin AJ, Donnelly TC, McKendrick MW, Read NW. Changes in anorectal function in persistent bowel disturbance following salmonella gastroenteritis. Eur J Gastroenterol Hepatol. 1993;5:617–20.
42. Rao SSC, Read NW, Brown C, Bruce C, Holdsworth CD. Studies on the mechanism of bowel disturbance in ulcerative colitis. Gastroenterology. 1987;93:934–40.
43. Rao SSC, Read NW, Stobart JAH, Haynes WG, Benjamin S, Holdsworth CD. Anorectal contractility under basal conditions and during rectal infusion of saline in ulcerative colitis. Gut. 1988;29:769–77.
44. Khan I, Kataeva G, Blennerhassett MG, Collins SM. Auto-induction of interleukin-1β gene expression in enteric smooth muscle cells. Gastroenterology. 1993;104:A534.

27
Gut–brain interactions in IBD: a clinician's perspective

T. M. BAYLESS

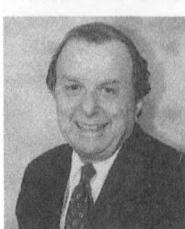

RELATIONSHIP OF STRESS AND IBD

While most physicians, and some patients, consider psychosocial factors as important in aggravating the symptoms of already existing IBD, most of the information is based on varied anecdotal observations and bolstered by a few recent scientific studies. However, a belief in an association between the mind and IBD is tempered by a tendency for patients and some physicians to view psychosocial and stress-related issues with speculation, bias and some stigmatization. On the positive side, patients with proctitis who have experienced recrudescence of mucosal friability and rectal bleeding within a day of a severe life stress provide a dramatic example of such 'hard-to-dismiss' anecdotes. While psychosocial factors may not initiate inflammation in IBD, it is possible that they lead to alterations in the immune response and thereby alter disease activity. Thus, impulses started in the brain may act as aggravating factors for already-established bowel inflammation, rather than as primary causative factors.

Physicians have varying opinions about the research linking psychological stress with IBD. Mitchell and Drossman surveyed 1000 members of the American Gastroenterological Association (including 530 in clinical practice and 330 in academic practice plus 110 trainees). They found that, in general, the physicians agreed that psychosocial factors contributed to clinical exacerbation of symptoms, especially in ulcerative colitis. However, these clinicians did not feel that such factors were involved in the etiology of IBD. Older physicians were more convinced, based on their clinical experience, of the role of psychosocial factors in exacerbating IBD than were younger physicians, who relied more heavily on their prior education. The majority of those surveyed did not believe there was any personality style characteristic of IBD patients, nor did they feel that the psychosocial impact on patients with IBD was any different from that observed with other chronic illnesses such as arthritis or diabetes mellitus[1].

KNOWN MIND–GUT PHYSIOLOGIC INTERACTIONS

Specific physiologic 'reflexes' or gut responses to a meal are well documented. These easily stimulated mind/gastrointestinal (GI) tract reactions include: salivation, gastric secretion, gastric motility and colonic motility. Some are mediated via the enteric nervous system (or 'small brain')[2].

It is now acceptable to state that intestinal inflammation has many neurohormonally influenced effects on the GI tract, such as the secretory diarrhea of IBD and the intestinal cramping experienced by so many patients with colitis. The 'physiologic' responses that occur in health would still be expected to occur in the IBD patient and, in addition, to perhaps be accentuated by inflammation and its multiple effects on gut function.

EFFECTS OF STRESS ON THE GI TRACT

Many of the physiologic events that occur in health, and may be aggravated by intestinal inflammation, can also be effected by various psychic stimuli such as fear, anger or 'stress'. The salivation and increased gastric secretion and gastric motility that occur when one thinks of a delicious meal is well documented by physiologists. Changes in intestinal and colonic motility to various stressful stimuli were well demonstrated by Wolfe and Wolf and by Almy and colleagues[3]. Few would deny that emotional distress will produce changes in bowel function in many individuals and produce abdominal discomfort in some[4].

Some of the symptoms described by patients with IBD probably relate to changes in motility and in awareness of painful sensations. These motility changes and pain may, at times, be independent of disease activity.

MECHANISMS FOR STRESS/GUT FUNCTION RELATIONSHIP

Stress and gut physiology are presumably related through the highly innervated nerve plexi and neuroendocrine links to the enteric nervous system ('the small brain') and its spinal and autonomic connections to the central nervous system[2,5]. Thus psychologic or environmental stimuli are able, by their neural–hormonal connections, to have an effect on motility and on visceral perception. The mind/gut system is further modulated by various neurotransmitters, including VIP, TRH, 5-HT, CCK, substance P and the enkephalins.

ANIMAL RESEARCH ON STRESS AND MUCOSAL CHANGES

A number of studies in animals support the presence of an association between stress and changes in mucosal morphology and, indirectly, with gastrointestinal disease. Acute gastric erosions were produced in rats by physical restraint, prolonged swimming or premature weaning[3]. Monkeys placed in a conditioned anxiety situation or restrained in chairs developed gastroduodenitis. Two had chronic colitis[6]. Interestingly, colitis led to the death of four gibbons after the death of their mate. This was considered a major disruption in the social environment by the authors[7,8]. The studies of the cottontop tamarin by Wood et al show that they remain well in the wild, but when they are caged, with a disruption of their social order, most develop an ulcerating colitis[9].

HUMAN RESEARCH ON PSYCHOSOCIAL FACTORS AND SYMPTOMS

Clinical and epidemiologic studies have suggested a relationship between psychosocial stress and symptom onset or exacerbation[3]. Social structure is characterized as a 'permissive' factor in susceptibility to disease. Persons who experience social disorganization are more susceptible to various medical conditions. The first cases of ulcerative colitis described in Bedouin Arabs occurred in individuals who were moved from their traditional nomadic life to 'modern' living in government housing.

EFFECTS OF STRESS ON PATIENTS WITH IBD

Time-lag studies have indicated that stress, especially major life events, precedes illness aggravation in patients with IBD, but that this is not disease-specific. The symptoms studied, pain and diarrhea, were more likely to be physiologic responses to acute stress, rather than reflections of increased disease activity.

North, Alpers and their colleagues in St Louis studied the effects of major life events and mood on bowel symptoms and pain in 32 patients with IBD, but could find no association with symptoms 1–2 months later. However, they did note an association between depressive symptoms and the severity of symptoms[10]. A strong relationship between major life events, especially health-related events, and symptom exacerbation (including pain, bowel dysfunction and bleeding) was found in a study from Hamilton, Ontario. Duffy, Marshall and their colleagues found that patients with a history of major life events at the outset of the study had a significantly greater risk of active disease than those without such a history[11]. The latter report was able to show a relationship between stress and GI symptoms because they focused on acute responses to stress rather than on events that had occurred months earlier. By focusing on daily stressors, other investigators found a significant association between acute daily stress and bowel symptoms over a 4-week period, in 10 patients with Crohn's disease[12].

The few careful studies of a relationship between psychosocial factors and symptoms in patients with IBD can be summarized. First, epidemiologic and clinical observations have, in the past, suggested an association between stress and illness exacerbation; this is general and not unique to IBD. Secondly, recent studies relating major life events with symptom exacerbation in patients with IBD have yielded somewhat conflicting results, but a positive association is suggested. Thirdly, the major stressors are not unique to IBD and include illness or death in the family, separation or divorce, other major losses or interpersonal conflict. Lastly, daily stressors seem to be associated with exacerbation of symptoms in patients with IBD, as well as with other illnesses.

CONCURRENT PSYCHOLOGICAL ASSOCIATIONS WITH IBD

Studies of unselected populations indicated that the psychological profiles of patients with IBD are similar to normal subjects, although with wide variation. Patients with IBD have slightly higher frequencies of psychiatric diagnoses and slightly greater psychological distress (most often related to anxiety and depression) than normal controls, but this is at a level comparable to patients with other chronic illnesses. Patients with IBD clearly have fewer psychological problems than patients coming to physicians with the irritable bowel syndrome (IBS). Patients with Crohn's disease have more psychological disturbances than patients with ulcerative colitis, and the degree of psychological distress correlates directly with the severity and chronicity of disease (which is usually greater with Crohn's disease). These findings suggest that psychological disturbances are a component of illness in general, rather than being etiologic or specific for IBD.

MODULATION OF IMMUNE REGULATION BY STRESS

Current scientific research supports the prospect that environmental factors influence disease susceptibility through the central nervous system. Stress is associated with alterations in both humoral and cellular immune mechanisms in humans and in experimental animals. While psychosocial factors may not initiate inflammation in IBD, it is possible that they lead to alterations in the immune response and thereby alter disease activity.

The effects of psychosocial stressors on the immune system are probably mediated through bidirectional, interconnected pathways between the brain, the enteric nervous system, the neuroendocrine axis and the immune system.

There is increasing evidence that alterations of enteric nervous system function may be important in the pathogenesis of IBD. Substance P appears to be a mediator of neurogenic inflammation in the GI tract, the skin and the respiratory tract. Interleukin-1 has effects on intestinal epithelial ion secretion which contribute to the diarrhea of IBD. VIP also stimulates intestinal secretion and is a known mediator of diarrhea. VIP-containing neurones and rectal mucosal VIP levels are increased in patients with Crohn's disease.

271

COEXISTENCE OF IBS AND IBD IN THE SAME PATIENT

IBS is quite a common combination of symptoms that accounts for one-third to one-half of all patients seen in many digestive disease clinics and practices. There is unanimity of opinion as to the sensitivity of patients with IBS to acute and chronic stress.

Since 10–13% of the general population have a tendency to IBS, it is to be expected that this same percentage of IBD patients would have both conditions: IBD and IBS. Because IBS is much more common than IBD it is not surprising that many patients with IBD were initially told that they had IBS. Conversely, when a patient who truly had IBS later develops IBD the physician usually forgets the pre-existing IBS, but the patient assumes she or he had IBD all along. The negative influence of this type of assumption on the physician–patient relationship is not measurable, but is certainly possible to imagine[13].

Whether some of the stress-related symptoms described in some patients with IBD are due, even in part, to a coexisting IBS is not known. Definitive methods of identifying the gut motor responses of IBS would be needed for a definitive answer to this question.

EXAMPLES OF CLINICALLY RELEVANT PATHOPHYSIOLOGY

Some examples of clinically relevant alterations in pathophysiology include *acute proctosigmoiditis* being associated with an increase in IBS symptoms in the spastic and inflamed left colon. Because of spasm in the sigmoid colon, often accentuated by a large or fatty meal, the patient experiences distension of the descending colon and pain in the left upper quadrant. The patient and the physician may incorrectly interpret this 'splenic flexure syndrome' as an extension of the still distally located inflammation.

Pain and diarrhea based on distension of an irritable left colon after *ileocolonic resection* results from excessive distension of the left colon by the larger stool volume following loss of absorptive surface of the ileum and right colon. Again, the patient (and even the doctor) may think that the Crohn's disease has suddenly appeared in the descending colon, which was normal by colonoscopy just before surgery. Patients with IBS are also more symptomatic, with small amounts of unabsorbed carbohydrates, such as fructose, sorbitol and lactose.

Patients with severe IBS also have an irritable small bowel, especially when it is formed into a closed reservoir as an *ileoanal pouch*, and they have at least eight to 10 bowel movements per day because of the spasticity and small capacity of the ileoanal pouch. The stomach to pouch transit time may also be quite rapid. Explaining the coexistence of IBD and IBS to the patient is often quite helpful to the patient and to the doctor. Avoiding this operation in a patient with severe IBS as well as ulcerative colitis is an even greater service to all concerned.

Although the thesis of coexistence of IBS and IBD is a simple one, it is rarely mentioned in the literature. I have found this concept very helpful in evaluating and advising 'complicated' or 'difficult' patients with IBD[13]. Functional gastrointestinal disease probably coexists with other 'organic' illnesses, such as peptic ulcer and reflux esophagitis. The astute physician will be alert to these overlapping diagnoses.

As a final thought, one hopes and assumes that scientific explanations of these mind–gut interactions will be forthcoming.

References

1. Mitchell CM, Drossman DA. Survey of the AGA membership relating to patients with functional gastrointestinal disorders. Gastroenterology. 1987;92:1282–4.
2. Wood JD. Enteric neuroimmune interactions. In: Walker WA, Harmatz PR, Wershil BK, editors. Immunophysiology of the gut. New York: Academic Press; 1993.
3. Drossman DA. Psychosocial considerations in gastroenterology. In: Sleisenger MH, Fordtran JS, Cello JP, Feldman M, editors. Gastrointestinal disease: pathophysiology, diagnosis, management. Philadelphia: Saunders; 1993:3–17.
4. Drossman DA, Sandler RS, McKee DC, Lovitz AJ. Bowel patterns among subjects not seeking health care. Use of a questionnaire to identify a population with bowel dysfunction. Gastroenterology. 1982;83:529–34.
5. Mayer EA, Raybould HE. Role of visceral afferent mechanisms in functional bowel disorders. Gastroenterology. 1990;99:1688–704.
6. Porter RW, Brady JV, Conrad D, Mason JW, Calambos R, Rioch D. Some experimental observations on gastrointestinal lesions in behaviorally conditioned monkeys. Psychosom Med. 1958;20:379–94.
7. Stout C, Snyder RL. Ulcerative colitis-like lesions in Siamang gibbons. Gastroenterology. 1969;57:256–60.
8. Engel GL. Psychological factors in ulcerative colitis in man and gibbon. Gastroenterology. 1969;57:362–4.
9. Drossman DA. Is the cotton-topped tamarin a model for behavioral research? Dig Dis Sci. 1985;30:24–7S.
10. North CS, Alpers DH, Helzer JE, Spitznagel EL, Clouse RE. Do life events or depression exacerbate inflammatory bowel disease? Ann Intern Med. 1991;114:381–6.
11. Duffy LC, Zielezny MA, Marshall JR et al. Relevance of major stress events as an indicator of disease activity prevalence in inflammatory bowel disease. Behav Med. 1991;17:101–10.
12. Garrett VD, Brantly PJ, Jones GN, McKnight GT. The relation between daily stress and Crohn's disease. J Behav Med. 1991;14:87.
13. Bayless TM. Coexistent irritable bowel syndrome and inflammatory bowel disease. In: Bayless TM, editor. Current management of inflammatory bowel disease. Toronto: Decker; 1989:59–62.

Section IX
Surgical issues in IBD

28
Cancer risk in IBD

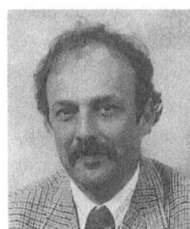

A. EKBOM

An association between cancer in different sites and inflammatory bowel disease has been reported in many studies starting in the 1920s[1]. Associations between every conceivable site and type have been proposed. There are, however, very few population-based studies of a size sufficiently large to give reliable risk estimates. In most instances the relationship between inflammatory bowel disease and different malignancies has emanated from either small case series or follow-up studies of patient groups where the selection bias is a concern, and which most authors have not taken into consideration. It is also worth pointing out that somewhere between 20% and 30% of any population in the westernized world will be diagnosed with some sort of cancer during their lifetime. Thus, in order to ensure reliable risk estimates, there is a need for a control population. Such studies also have to be performed outside referral centers where selection bias can be operating.

In a population-based study of 3121 patients with ulcerative colitis and 1655 patients with Crohn's disease[2] we were able to confirm an overall increased risk for cancer both among patients with ulcerative colitis, 202 observed cases of cancer compared to 142.1 expected (standardized incidence ratio (SIR) = 1.6, 95% confidence interval (CI) 1.4–1.8) and in Crohn's disease 58 observed cases compared to 47.1 expected (SIR = 1.2, 95% CI 0.9–1.6).

Surveillance bias could be a concern in a cohort of patients with regular contacts with the health-care system. However, the standardized mortality ratio (SMR) was also increased for malignant diseases. In the case of ulcerative colitis (SMR = 1.3, 95% CI 1.1–1.6) and for Crohn's disease (SMR = 1.1, 95% CI 0.7–1.6). After excluding colorectal cancer the relative risk for cancer was close to 1.0 for both ulcerative colitis (SIR = 1.0, 95% CI 0.9–1.2) and Crohn's disease (SIR = 1.1, 95% CI 0.8–1.5). The risk estimate was almost the same when we analyzed the standardized mortality ratio for ulcerative colitis (SMR = 1.0, 95% CI 0.7–1.5) and for Crohn's disease (SMR = 0.9, 95% CI 0.8–1.3). Colorectal cancer therefore seems to be the major cause of the increased morbidity and mortality in malignancies in patients with inflammatory bowel disease.

There was a tendency toward an increased risk for cancer of the bile ducts among patients with extensive colitis (SIR = 1.9, 95% CI 1.7–4.0) which is consistent with other studies[3,4] and for cancer of the small intestine among patients with Crohn's disease (SIR = 3.4, 95% CI 0.1–18.6) also previously reported[5,6]. The risk estimate in the study from the Uppsala Health Care Region is, however, lower than previously reported. One feasible explanation for this is that a combination of Crohn's disease and a bypassed intestine seems to carry the highest risk[5]. This procedure is very rarely used in Sweden, or Israel where similar results have been reported[7]. There was also an increased number of malignancies of the connective tissues (sarcomas) for both ulcerative colitis (SIR = 4.0, 95% CI 1.0–10.2) and Crohn's disease (SIR = 2.5, 95% CI 0.1–13.9), an association also previously reported[8]. There was a decreased risk of cancer of the respiratory tract among patients with ulcerative colitis (SIR = 0.5, 95% CI 0.2–1.0), giving further credence to non-smoking status as a risk factor for ulcerative colitis[9]. Surprisingly, we could not find any increased risk for cancer of the respiratory tracts among cases with Crohn's disease (SIR = 0.8, 95% CI 0.2–0.4), thus casting some doubts on smoking as a risk factor for Crohn's disease. Finally, we also found, in accordance with previous studies from New York[10] and Cleveland[3], a statistically significant decreased risk of breast cancer among patients with extensive colitis (SIR = 0.4, 95% CI 0.1–1.0), although the underlying reason for this still remains unknown.

The risk of colorectal cancer among patients with Crohn's disease varies greatly in different studies, with risk estimates between 2.5 and 20.0[6,11–13]. In the study from the Uppsala Health Care Region, Sweden[13], we found an overall increased risk of 2.5 for patients with Crohn's disease (95% CI 1.3–4.3) with no differences among females and males. However, in patients where the disease was confined to terminal ileum at the time of diagnosis the risk for colorectal cancer did not differ from that of the background population. On the other hand, patients with any colonic involvement at the time of diagosis had a substantially increased risk (SIR = 5.6, 95% CI 2.1–12.2). Age at diagnosis also seemed to affect the risk estimates substantially. Those with any colonic involvement and diagnosed before the age of 30 entailed a SIR of 20.9 (95% CI 6.8–48.7) compared to SIR = 2.2 (95% CI 0.6–5.7) among those diagnosed after the age of 30. This is consistent with the results from the study from the Mayo Clinic[11], where an overall risk of 20.0 was found as 80% of the patients in that study had colonic involvement at the time of diagnosis.

As for Crohn's disease the risk estimates given in different studies of the risk for colorectal cancer in patients with ulcerative colitis vary substantially. However, with the exception of two Danish studies[14,15] an increased risk has been found in all other studies[3,4,16-27]. The cumulative incidence 25–35 years after diagnosis ranges from 8%[6] to 43%[18], and standardized incidence ratios between 2[26] and 30[25] have been reported. In a multivariate analysis in the study from the Uppsala Health Care Region[16] age at diagnosis was found to be an independent factor for an increased risk for colorectal cancer. Low age (less than 15 years) entailed a cumulative incidence 35 years after diagnosis of 40%, which is very close to that reported from the Mayo Clinic[18], a study also confined to patients less than 15 years of age at time of diagnosis. Moreover, further follow-up of patients in the Uppsala study has revealed that 50% of all patients with pancolitis diagnosed before the age of 15 will be diagnosed with a colorectal cancer before the age of 50. These findings suggest that a prophylactic proctocolectomy in this patient group might be an appropriate alternative compared to close surveillance, in order to reduce the mortality in colorectal cancer, which is the main reason for the reduced long-time relative survival in patients with ulcerative colitis[28].

It has been proposed that a patient with ulcerative colitis is at maximum risk for development of colorectal cancer about the age of 50 regardless of the age at onset or duration of disease[22]. In the study from the Uppsala Health Care Region, Sweden[16], we were unable to confirm that hypothesis. We found a consistently higher relative risk than for the normal population persisting among patients even after the age of 70, which seems to refute that hypothesis.

Extent of disease at time of diagnosis is also an independent risk factor for colorectal cancer[16]. Patients with proctitis did not differ significantly in the risk for colorectal cancer from the background population (SIR = 1.7, 95% CI 0.8–3.2) even after analyzing rectal cancer as a single entity. These findings imply that it is not the inflammation as such, but some additional exposure is needed for a malignant transformation in this patient group. There is an increased risk of colorectal cancer among patients with left-sided colitis at diagnosis confirmed in some studies[21,27]. In the analysis of the results from the Uppsala Health Care Region, Sweden, this increased risk was also found, although the risk estimate was substantially lower (SIR = 2.8, 95% CI 1.6–4.4) compared to patients with pancolitis at diagnosis (SIR = 14.8, 95% CI 11.4–188.4). Moreover, the latency period seems to be 10–15 years longer compared to pancolitis before a patient with left-sided colitis is at an increased risk of colorectal cancer (Fig. 1). If this increased risk is due to patients initially diagnosed as left-sided colitis, in which the disease subsequently has progressed to pancolitis, or if the risk is present among patients with their disease confined to the left colon remains, however, unknown.

In one[14] of the studies where no association could be found between ulcerative colitis and colorectal cancer it was probably due to the short follow-up, 10 or fewer years after diagnosis. In the other[15], however, the follow-up was substantially longer, although the authors analyzed left-sided colitis and pancolitis as one entity which could at least partly explain the lack of any association found. However, the authors suggest an alternative explanation that modern treatment strategies using pharmacologic com-

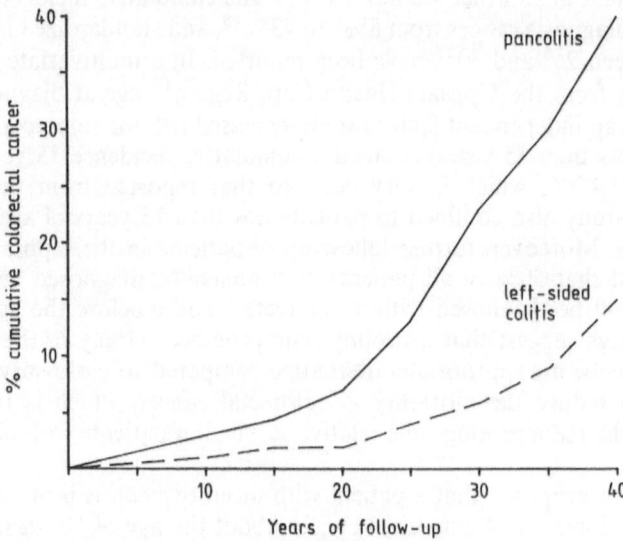

Fig. 1 Cumulative incidence of colorectal cancer for patients with pancolitis and left-sided colitis at diagnosis. The solid line shows those in whom pancolitis was diagnosed and the dashed line those who were given the diagnosis of left-sided colitis

pounds such as sulfasalazine could be one feasible reason for the lack of any increased risk of colorectal cancer in their patient group. The same observation was also made in a study from the UK[29] of colonoscopic surveillance among patients with ulcerative colitis, where the authors wrote: 'A review of the notes of our cancer patients suggests that virtually none of them were taking disease suppressive drugs, such as slazopyrin, regularly or at all'. Moreover, a similar mechanism has also been proposed in Israel in the 1980s[30]. In order to study whether additional risk factors or protective agents could be identified for colorectal cancer among patients with ulcerative colitis we recently conducted a case–control study[31]. Cases were found by a renewed follow-up of the previous study[16]. We could identify 102 patients who had been diagnosed with colorectal cancer after a previous diagnosis of ulcerative colitis. Two controls were identified for each case and were matched for sex, extent of disease at time of diagnosis and calendar year of the diagnosis of ulcerative colitis. Moreover, the controls had to be alive without colorectal cancer with an intact or partly intact colon at the time of diagnosis of colorectal cancer of the case. Six controls were excluded due to a proctocolectomy done prior to the diagnosis of the colorectal cancer in the case, thus leaving 196 controls. After retrieving the charts from cases and controls in a uniform manner we analyzed, among other things, to what extent pharmacotherapy and disease activity had any impact on the risk for colorectal cancer.

Disease activity entailed a protective effect when we compared those with more than one exacerbation on the average per year to those with less than one. Those with the higher disease activity had a decreased risk (RR = 0.70,

95% CI 0.44–1.14). Pharmacologic therapy, especially sulfasalazine, entailed an even higher protective effect. In a comparison between those who had completed at least one 3-month course of sulfasalazine medication and those who never had completed a 3-month course we found a highly significant protective effect (RR = 0.34, 95% CI 0.19–0.62). The risk estimates for both disease activity and pharmacologic therapy, sulfasalazine, prevailed and was only marginally changed in a multivariate analysis with mutual adjustment for the two factors. The results thus confirm the observations made in Denmark, the UK and Israel. One feasible explanation is, of course, the intervention of prostaglandin synthesis by salicylate compounds which could inhibit various stages of the carcinogenic process[32], a parallel to the reduced risk of sporadic colorectal cancer in aspirin users[33].

CONCLUSION

Colorectal cancer in patients with ulcerative colitis is the only malignancy which has any impact on the morbidity and mortality in cancer in patients with inflammatory bowel disease. This increased risk can be reduced through pharmacologic therapy.

References

1. Bargen JA. Chronic ulcerative colitis associated with malignant disease. Arch Surg. 1928;17:561–76.
2. Ekbom A, Helmick C, Zack M, Adami HO. Extracolonic malignancies in inflammatory bowel disease. Cancer. 1991;67:2015–19.
3. Mir-Madjlessi SH, Farmer RG, Easly KA, Beck GJ. Colorectal cancer and extra-colonic malignancies in ulcerative colitis. Cancer. 1986;58:1569–74.
4. Prior P, Gyde SN, Macartney JC, Thompson H, Waterhouse JAH, Allan RN. Cancer morbidity in ulcerative colitis. Gut. 1982;23:490–7.
5. Senay E, Sachar DB, Keohane M, Greenstein AJ. Small bowel carcinoma in Crohn's disease. Distinguishing features and risk factors. Cancer. 1989;63:360–3.
6. Greenstein AJ, Sachar DB, Smith H, Janowitz HD, Aufses AH. A comparison of cancer risk in Crohn's disease and ulcerative colitis. Cancer. 1981;48:2742–5.
7. Fireman Z, Grossman A, Lilos P et al. Intestinal cancer in patients with Crohn's disease. Scand J Gastroenterol. 1989;24:346–50.
8. Israel K, Nissenblatt M. Association of inflammatory bowel disease (IBD) with indolent soft-tissue sarcomas: report of two cases and review of literature. J Surg Oncol. 1986;32:125–30.
9. Lindberg E, Tysk C, Andersson K, Järnerot G. Smoking and inflammatory bowel disease: A case control study. Gut. 1988;29:352–7.
10. Greenstein J, Gennuso R, Sachar DB et al. Extraintestinal cancers in inflammatory bowel disease. Cancer. 1985;56:2914–21.
11. Weedon DD, Shorter RG, Ilstrup DM, Huizenga KA, Taylor WF. Crohn's disease and cancer. N Engl J Med. 1973;289:1099–102.
12. Gyde SN, Prior P, Macartney JC, Thompson H, Waterhouse JAH, Allan RN. Malignancy in Crohn's disease. Gut. 1980;21:1024–9.
13. Ekbom A, Helmick C, Zack M, Adami HO. Increased risk of large-bowel cancer in Crohn's disease with colonic involvement. Lancet. 1990;336:357–9.
14. Bonnevie O, Binder V, Anthonisen P, Riis P. The prognosis of ulcerative colitis. Scand J Gastroenterol. 1974;9:81–91.
15. Langholtz E, Munkholm P, Davidsen M, Binder V. Colorectal cancer risk and mortality

in patients with ulcerative colitis. Gastroenterology. 1992;103:1444–51.

16. Ekbom A, Helmick C, Zack M, Adami HO. Ulcerative colitis and colorectal cancer. A population-based study. N Engl J Med. 1990;323:1228–33.

17. Broström O, Löfberg R, Nordenvall B, Öst Å, Hellers G. The risk of colorectal cancer in ulcerative colitis: an epidemiologic study. Scand J Gastroenterol. 1987;22:1193–9.

18. Devroede GJ, Taylor WF, Saucer WG, Jackman RJ, Stickler GB. Cancer risk and life expectancy of children with ulcerative colitis. N Engl J Med. 1971;285:17–21.

19. Edwards FC, Truelove SC. The course and prognosis of ulcerative colitis. IV. Carcinoma of the colon. Gut. 1964;5:15–22.

20. Gilat T, Fireman Z, Grossman A et al. Colorectal cancer in patients with ulcerative colitis: a population study in central Israel. Gastroenterology. 1988;94:870–7.

21. Greenstein A, Sachar D, Smith H et al. Cancer in universal and left-sided ulcerative colitis: factors determining risk. Gastroenterology. 1979;77:290–4.

22. Gyde SN, Prior P, Allan RN et al. Colorectal cancer in ulcerative colitis: a cohort study of primary referrals from three centres. Gut. 1988;29:206–17.

23. Katzka I, Brody R, Morris E, Katz S. Assessment of colorectal cancer risk in patients with ulcerative colitis: experience from a private practice. Gastroenterology. 1983;85:22–9.

24. Kewenter J, Ahlman H, Hultén L. Cancer risk in extensive ulcerative colitis. Ann Surg. 1978;188:824–8.

25. Lennard-Jones ME, Morson BC, Ritchie JK, Williams CB. Cancer surveillance in ulcerative colitis: experience over 15 years. Lancet. 1983;2:149–53.

26. Maratka Z, Nedbal J, Kocianova J, Havelka J, Kudrmann J, Hendl J. Incidence of colorectal cancer in proctocolitis: a retrospective study of 959 cases over 40 years. Gut. 1985;26:43–9.

27. Samuelsson SM. Ulcerös colit och proctit. Uppsala: Department of Social Medicine. Thesis, University of Uppsala; 1976.

28. Ekbom A, Helmick CG, Zack M, Holmberg L, Adami HO. Survival and causes of death in patients with inflammatory bowel disease. A population-based study. Gastroenterology. 1992;103:954–60.

29. Lynch DAF, Lobo AJ, Sobala GM, Dixon MF, Axon ATR. Failure of colonoscopic surveillance in ulcerative colitis. Gut. 1993;34:1075–80.

30. Odes HS, Fraser D. Ulcerative colitis in Israel: epidemiology, morbidity and genetics. Public Health Rev. 1989/90;17:297–319.

31. Pinczowski D, Ekbom A, Baron J, Yuen J, Adami HO. Risk factors for colorectal cancer among patients with ulcerative colitis – a case–control study. Gastroenterology. 1994;107:117–20.

32. Marmett L. Aspirin and the potential role of prostaglandins in colon cancer. Cancer Res. 1992;52:5575–89.

33. Thun M, Namboodiri N, Heath CJ. Aspirin use and reduced risk of fatal colon cancer. N Engl J Med. 1991;325:1593–6.

29
Management of stomal complications

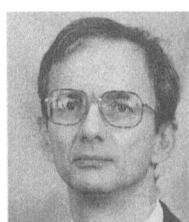

S. R. NORDGREN

INTRODUCTION

An intestinal stoma is of constant concern to anyone who has it. However, a well-constructed intestinal stoma can reduce the physical and psychological stress on its bearer. Creation of an intestinal stoma, be it temporary or permanent, therefore requires good judgement and surgical skill. However complicated or difficult the intra-abdominal part of the operation that necessitated the stoma has been, it is the quality and the function of the stoma that determines a significant part of the long-term quality of life. Problems related to the stoma must be specifically asked and searched for, as these kinds of problems are not always revealed spontaneously. In the following a short survey of stomal complications and their management will be reviewed and discussed.

THE TERMINAL ILEOSTOMY

A terminal ileostomy is the temporary or permanent result after proctocolectomy for patients mainly with ulcerative colitis (UC), Crohn's disease (CD) and familial polyposis (FAP). In UC and FAP it may be avoided by means of sphincter-saving reconstructive surgery. This is rarely so in CD.

A correctly sited, well-constructed and properly managed Brooke ileostomy[1] should, at least from a physical point of view, allow the patient to live an almost normal life. However, stomal complications do occur and frequently necessitate the need for revisional surgery.

Despite modern measures for skin protection and modern appliances

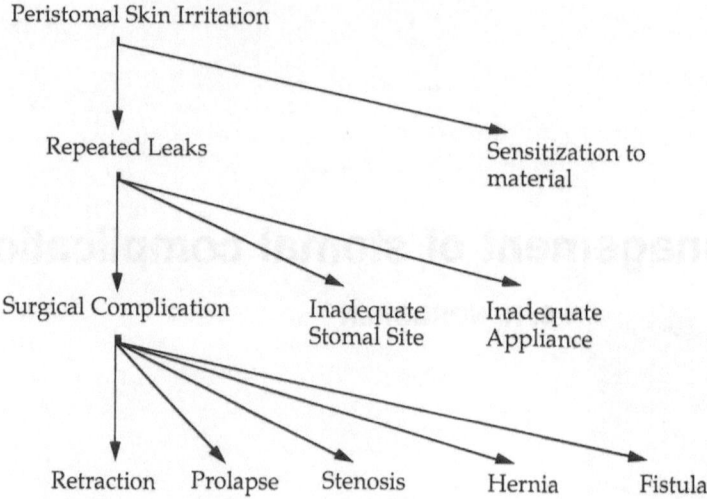

Fig. 1 Algorithm for assessment of ileostomy dysfunction

that are available today, peristomal skin irritation is the most common complication and most patients occasionally suffer from this inconvenience[2,3]. Whenever skin irritation develops, its cause should be carefully searched for, preferably in conjunction with an enterostomal therapist. An algorithm for the analysis of stomal complications is given in Fig. 1.

Peristomal irritation of the skin is most often a result of repeated exposure to stomal content, although sensitization to the appliance has to be ruled out. Repeated leakage may depend on imperfections in handling of the appliance or, more often, local conditions that make fitting of the appliance difficult. An inappropriately sited stoma, an abdominal scar or skinfold may be present, or the stoma may be subject to a surgical complication. To avoid the disability of stomal dysfunction it is important that surgically correctable problems are identified and surgical revision undertaken.

The surgical revision rate in a collected series of 2530 patients with UC, mainly based on questionnaires, was 19.3%[4-8]. The revision rate increases with time and interest spent in searching for stomal problems. According to our experience the cumulative risk of needing at least one revision after 10 years reached 0.75 in CD and 0.44 in UC (Fig. 2). The increased risk in CD compared to UC was verified by others[6,9] but not all[10]. The relative frequencies of various surgical complications appear in Table 1.

ILEOSTOMY COMPLICATIONS

Early ileostomy necrosis

Significant early edema of the postoperative ileostomy is common, and ischemia with sloughing of the mucosa occurs sometimes. Fortunately, early postoperative necrosis of the ileostomy is an uncommon complication. The

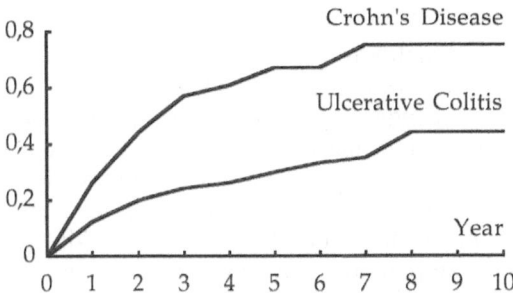

Fig. 2 Cumulative probability of need for the first ileostomy revision in patients with ulcerative colitis and Crohn's disease[8]

Table 1 Indications for ileostomy revision (collected series from 4, 8, 25)

	Total	Percentage
Retraction	87	35
Stenosis	74	30
Prolapse	25	10
Fistula	24	10
Miscellaneous	38	15

most common cause is a too narrow opening in the abdominal wall. However, in a patient with low cardiac output or mesenteric vascular occlusion it may be a part of total intestinal ischemia. We suggest that if there is any concern as to the viability of the ileostomy at its construction, the abdomen should not be closed until the stoma is matured satisfactorily.

Stenosis

Even when constructed according to modern principles ileostomy stenosis is still one of the most common long-term complications. Normally the ileal stoma should accept passage of the distal part of the fifth finger. However, a symptomatic stenosis does not occur until the stoma is quite narrow. This condition usually causes intermittent ileostomy discharge, pain at passage of undigested food material or even total stomal obstruction. The stenosis is almost invariably located at the skin level and the size of the skin opening can easily be gauged by the examining finger.

Stenosis is an unpredictable complication. After secondary healing of the mucocutaneous junction a stenosis is to be expected. In most patients it cannot be predicted and stenosis occurs regularly in some patients and not at all in others. Repeated instrumental dilatation does not prevent development of a stenosis, and may even worsen the condition. Treatment of a tight ileostomy stenosis involves excision of peristomal skin and re-establishment of the mucocutaneous junction. This operation may be done under local infiltration but general anesthesia is usually preferred by patients.

Prolapse

In patients with less ability to form peritoneal adhesions a sliding prolapse may occur on forceful straining, such as heavy lifting. A prolapse can also develop over time. Secondary inflammatory changes may occur, and a sliding prolapse becomes fixed. A fixed 'prolapse' may also be a stoma that was constructed too long. Surgical correction is necessary. Both the sliding and the fixed prolapse are repaired by excision of the stoma, close to the mucocutaneous junction to avoid enlargement of the skin opening, desussception of the stoma, amputation of its distal part, fixation to the abdominal aponeurosis and resuturing of the mucocutaneous junction.

Retraction

A retraction may be fixed or sliding. The pathophysiology behind sliding retraction is probably similar to that of a sliding prolapse. As stated above, a sliding stoma is frequently seen in patients that do not form peritoneal adhesions. Retraction of the stoma may also occur in patients who have put on weight. A retracted and flat stoma causes leakage of ileostomy fluid under the appliance with subsequent skin irritation.

Correction of stomal retraction involves peristomal incision and dissection of the small bowel all the way into the peritoneal cavity, so that sufficient length can be mobilized through the abdominal opening. The terminal bowel is carefully sutured to the abdominal parietes, the stoma everted and mucocutaneous sutures applied. If necessary, note that a 5 mm wide disk of skin can be nourished by small bowel perfusion, and re-establishment of the stoma can be done by suturing the peristomal disk of skin to the peristomal skin.

Speakman and co-workers[11] advocated the use of a linear stapler (TEA 55 or the S-GIA) to control sliding retraction. Anesthesia was not necessary. Their results appear less convincing, however, since a considerable number of postoperative problems occurred, such as stomal edema and bleeding. Three patients out of 10 developed abscess, ulcerations and sepsis.

Ulceration and fistula formation

According to our experience stomal ulcers and fistulas occur more frequently in patients with CD than in patients with UC, even when recurrent CD is excluded. The etiology of stomal fistulas varies, although a stomal ulcer or peristomal abscess is frequently involved in the pathogenesis. Recurrent CD should be excluded by endoscopy. If an abscess or cavity is found it should be drained before permanent repair.

When the fistulous tract involves subcutaneous tissue around the stoma it is probably safer to relocate the stoma and to leave the skin of the old stomal opening and the fistulous tract open to granulation and secondary healing[12]. If the fistula is distal to the skin level, as a perforation of the extra-abdominal ileal spout, a local procedure may be sufficient[2].

Ulcers or granulomas are most often observed on the caudal aspect of the ileostomy. A decubital ulcer from an appliance that is not properly cut or fixed should be suspected. The appliance should be assessed in collaboration with an enterostomal therapist. Secondary changes from long-standing ulcerations on the ileostomy may necessitate resection and construction of a new stoma.

Ileostomy hernia

Subcutaneous herniation at the site of an ileostomy is less common, particularly when compared to the incidence of colostomy hernia (see below). Herniation interferes greatly with ileostomy management, and is associated with sore skin and leakage. Moreover, subcutaneous kinking of the bowel in a hernia may cause episodes of obstruction.

Local revision may be successful but resiting the ileostomy, usually to the other side of the abdomen, may be required for satisfactory results. A snugly fitted belt may be a temporary solution.

Prestomal ileitis

Prestomal ileitis implies an inflammation of the prestomal mucosa. The principal symptoms are increased ileostomy discharge, watery consistency of the stools, pain in the peristomal area and sometimes blood in the stools. Extensive inflammation may cause peristomal abscess formation with fistulization to the peristomal skin. Intra-abdominal perforation may occur. Short segments of prestomal inflammation can be observed incidentally without any symptoms.

In the 'pre-Brooke era' inflammation of the prestomal ileum was most often seen as a result of stenosis of the stoma. The condition is difficult to distinguish from recurrent CD, and may not even occur except in CD[3].

Miscellaneous

Peristomal varicose veins are observed in patients with portal hypertension. Bleeding is the major problem, particularly when there is irritation to the peristomal skin. Bleeding may be profuse, and cross-stitch suture may be necessary for control. Measures to reduce the portal pressure should be considered. Cancer in the ileostomy has been observed in the extended follow-up of patients with ileostomy[13], and should be suspected when ulcers of the mucocutaneous junction are seen.

THE LOOP ILEOSTOMY

The loop ileostomy is a useful alternative to a defunctioning colostomy in elective colorectal surgery, or in an emergency operation when diversion of the fecal stream from the large bowel is required[14,15]. It is also useful for protection of an ileorectal anastomosis or an ileal reservoir. This stoma is normally supported by a short rod and sutured only to the skin, without sutures to the abdominal wall. When the supporting rod is removed, on day 7 postoperatively, granulation tissue keeps the stoma in place. Turning the ileal loop so that the active part of the stoma opens distally reduces the risk of skin irritation[15], an opinion not shared by all[14].

For the 6–10 weeks in which the loop ileostomy is normally required there are few problems with stability. If, for any reason, the loop ileostomy is retained beyond that period of time, sliding retraction or prolapse occurs. If this is the case closure of the ileostomy or conversion to a terminal end-ileostomy, with subcutaneous or intra-abdominal closure of the distal part, should be considered.

Complications necessitating surgical revision are rare. If a complication does occur, closure of the loop ileostomy should be considered, if possible. If not, it should be converted to a terminal ileostomy. Hospitalization for high ostomy output was reported by Wexner *et al.* in four out of 83 patients[14], and in 23 of 117 by Feinberg *et al.*[16]. Monitoring of urinary sodium excretion may be of help to predict which patients are at risk[17].

THE TRANSVERSE COLOSTOMY

The transverse colostomy is used for fecal diversion in left colonic obstruction or for protection of a colorectal anastomosis. Because of intercurrent medical problems in the group of patients at risk for a left colonic obstruction this stoma is often retained for the rest of the patient's life. From a functional point of view the transverse colostomy is a less favorable alternative for the patient. This stoma combines the problems of a colostomy (fecal odour) with the problems of an ileostomy (increased water loss and irritant action to the skin).

Furthermore, the stoma is usually inconveniently located immediately below the right costal margin where it interferes with clothing. Complications such as prolapse and peristomal hernia, are common.

Prolapse of the transverse colostomy, creating the typical 'ox-horn' appearance, is most frequently encountered when the stoma is retained for more than 2 months[18]. Adequate treatment is closure of the stoma, or conversion to an alternative enterostomy when possible.

We suggest that the transverse colostomy be avoided. Should it be necessary, a more convenient place for the stoma than the subcostal region should be tried, and construction of a terminal colostomy with primary eversion of the active, proximal limb and closure of the distal limb should be considered.

THE TERMINAL SIGMOID COLOSTOMY

The sigmoid colostomy is usually constructed in conjunction with an abdominoperineal resection for rectal cancer, or as a Hartmann procedure for complicated diverticulitis. Patients are often in their 60s or 70s, or even older. The operative procedure is often performed by young surgeons as an emergency procedure at a time of the day when full expertise is not at hand. Construction is often difficult due to obesity, a fat mesentery and multiple diverticula, and normal healing is frequently impaired. Due to the poor general condition of the patients postoperative rehabilitation is prolonged. Not infrequently, patients with a sigmoid colostomy are unable to manage the stoma on their own, which makes the colostomy a matter of concern for the family, relatives or home-care personnel.

Colostomy complications were investigated by Cubertafond et al.[19], based on a review of 4320 patients, including 1142 personal cases. Seventy-eight percent of the personal cases had a stoma of the left colon. The most common early complication was a peristomal infection with separation (10–25%). Late complications were seen in 7–56% of the patients. The most commonly seen late complications were hernia, prolapse and stenosis.

COMPLICATIONS OF THE SIGMOID COLOSTOMY

Early colostomy necrosis

Necrosis of the terminal part of the colon may occur due to faulty judgement of the adequacy of its blood supply. Normal perfusion may be reduced by compression through the stomal wound due to a fatty mesentery or inflammatory edema in the mesocolon. Should necrosis develop the level of viable bowel should be established by inspection or careful endoscopy. If ischemic changes extend down to the level of the aponeurosis early relaparotomy and reconstruction of the stoma should be considered, to avoid intraabdominal fecal leakage. An immediate reconstruction of a colostomy can be performed through the same opening and is definitely worthwhile, considering the long postoperative course of a necrotic stoma.

Separation at the mucocutaneous junction can normally be managed by conservative means. However, in secondary healing it should be noted that the risk of stenosis is proportional to the amount of secondary healing that occurs around the stoma. Secondary, or delayed, mucocutaneous suture is unsuccessful. We suggest that, also in the case of a colostomy, the abdominal wound should not be closed until the stoma is acceptable. Knowing that this violates the age-old wisdom of avoiding open bowel and open wounds, this violation is justified by the smooth healing of the colostomy.

Stenosis

Stenosis is largely a complication of the old technique when the colon was pulled through the abdominal opening and cut by cautery on the first postoperative day. This procedure, learnt by many active surgeons of today, invariably caused stenosis at the level of the skin. Digital or instrumental dilatation of a narrow colostomy is usually not helpful, and the trauma from dilatation may even accelerate the process. Refashioning of the colostomy, preferably under general anesthesia, is the method of choice. A circumferential incision is made around the stoma a few millimeters peripheral to the mucocutaneous junction. The colostomy is dissected from the skin, the ring of skin and underlying fibrous tissue is excised and the mucocutaneous junction re-established with interrupted monofilament sutures. This procedure becomes more complicated when a part of the subcutaneous bowel is damaged. A sufficient amount of bowel must be raised from the abdomen to allow a mucocutaneous suture without tension; if not, separation of the suture line with concomitant secondary healing with formation of granulations and new stenosis will inevitably occur.

Colostomy hernia

Herniation around a colostomy is so common that it is considered by some authors to be virtually inevitable[3]. Reported incidences vary between 1% and 50%[19,20]. All sizes, from small areas of bulging, noticed on straining, to grotesque enlargements of the abdominal wall with the colostomy on the top, occur. Colostomy hernia is particularly common when the colon has been brought out in the scar of a paramedian or iliac oblique incision. If a separate stab wound has been employed, hernias are usually smaller, although they still occur. Among measures presented to reduce the incidence of colostomy hernia are the extraperitoneal technique, meticulous suturing of the bowel to the peritoneum and bringing the colostomy through the rectus muscle instead of lateral to it.

Whittaker and Goligher studied the effect of an extraperitoneal technique for colostomy construction, in a nonrandomized study[21], and observed a reduced incidence of herniation, prolapse and retraction. However, the standard level of statistical significance was not reached, and the extraperitoneal technique has not been widely accepted.

Meticulous suturing of the bowel to the peritoneum has also been tried by Goligher[3] but this did not result in a lower incidence of hernia.

Bringing the stoma through the rectus abdominis muscle in order to reduce the incidence of hernia is controversial, but appears reasonable. It was effective in a retrospective study by Sjödahl et al.[22], and the technique is supported by us and others[23]. Bringing the terminal colon through a snugly fitting separate opening, and through the rectus muscle, is probably the best that can be done from a surgical–technical point of view to avoid colostomy herniation.

A well-fitted colostomy appliance with an attached belt is probably sufficient treatment for most small hernias that do occur.

Local repair of the abdominal wall without resiting of the colostomy is normally not effective, and is disappointingly often followed by recurrence of the hernia. Resiting of the colostomy is therefore the best radical treatment for this complication[20]. A method for local repair involving a synthetic mesh was recently described[24] when resiting was not appropriate.

Prolapse

Sliding prolapse or retraction of a colostomy is not the same serious problem as in a case of an ileostomy, because of the less irritant action of the bowel contents. However, prolapse of the stoma may lift off the appliance and cause leaks with unpleasant odour and staining of clothes.

It sometimes happens that the muscular coat of the bowel comes completely detached from the abdominal parieties, and a huge prolapse, measuring 15–20 cm, may occur. Patients in whom this complication is observed do not form adhesions between serosal layers. Radical treatment is amputation of the protruding part of the bowel with a new attempt to suturing the bowel to the abdominal parieties, followed by mucocutaneous suture.

Miscellaneous

Peristomal abscesses, sometimes with formation of fistulas may occur during healing of a stomal necrosis. A counter-incision further lateral and dorsal to the stoma may be necessary to achieve proper drainage. Laying open of the entire fistulous tract may be necessary to speed up granulation.

Recurrence of metastatic growths in the abdominal wall close to the stoma is uncommon in rectal cancer, but may occur in other malignancies. It should be remembered that the lesion that can be palpated in the stoma or through the skin only represents the top of an iceberg of metastatic tissue and local excision with refashioning of the stoma is only rarely possible. In this situation bringing forward a new part of the bowel as a stoma at another spot is probably the best way to help the patient.

CONCLUSION

The technical development of stomal appliances has reached a level where an enterostomy is compatible with an almost normal life. In the construction of an intestinal stoma extreme care should be taken to avoid all situations associated with risks for future stomal complications. Creation of a stoma is not a procedure for the inexperienced surgeon. It is our responsibility to extend efforts towards constructing a well-functioning enterostomy.

References

1. Brooke BN. The management of an ileostomy including its complications. Lancet. 1952;2:102–4.
2. Corman ML. Colon and rectal surgery, 3rd edn. Philadelphia: Lippincott; 1993.
3. Goligher JC. Surgery of the anus, rectum and colon, 5th edn. London: Baillière-Tindall.
4. Watts J, De Dombal F, Goligher J. Long term complications and prognosis following major surgery for ulcerative colitis. Br J Surg. 1966;53:1014–22.
5. Ritchie J. Ileostomy and excisional surgery for chronic inflammatory disease of the colon: a survey of one hospital region. Gut. 1971;12:528–40.
6. Roy P, Sauer W, Bearhs O, Farrow G. Experience with ileostomies. Am J Surg. 1970;119:77–86.

7. Morowitz D, Kirsner J. Ileostomy in ulcerative colitis. Am J Surg. 1981;141:370–5.
8. Carlstedt A, Fasth S, Hultén L, Nordgren S, Palselius I. Long-term ileostomy complications in patients with ulcerative colitis and Crohn's disease. Int J Colorect Dis. 1987;2:22–5.
9. Steinberg DM, Allan RN, Brooke BN, Cooke WWT, Alexander-Williams J. Sequelae of colectomy and ileostomy. Comparison between Crohn's colitis and ulcerative colitis. Gastroenterology. 1975;68:33–9.
10. Leong APK, Londono-Schimmer EE, Phillips MS. Life table analysis of stomal complications. Br J Surg. 1994 (In press).
11. Speakman CTM, Parker MC, Northover JMA. Outcome of stapled revision of retracted ileostomy. Br J Surg. 1991;78:935–6.
12. Greenstein A, Dicker ASM, Aufses A. Peri-ileostomy fistulae in Crohn's disease. Ann Surg. 1983;197:179–82.
13. Suarez V, Alexander-Williams J, O'Connor H, Campos A. Carcinoma developing in ileostomies after 25 or more years. Gastroenterology. 1988;95:205–8.
14. Wexner S, Taranow D, Johansen O et al. Loop ileostomy is a safe option for fecal diversion. Dis Colon Rectum. 1993;36:349–54.
15. Fasth S, Hultén L. Loop-ileostomy – a superior diverting stoma in colorectal surgery. World J Surg. 1984;8:401–7.
16. Feinberg S, McLeod R, Cohen Z. Complications of loop ileostomy. Am J Surg. 1987;153:102–7.
17. Svaninger G, Nordgren S, Palselius I, Fasth S, Hultén L. Sodium and potassium excretion in patients with ileostomies. Eur J Surg. 1991;157:601–5.
18. Wara P, Sørensen K, Berg V. Proximal fecal diversion: review of ten years experience. Dis Colon Rectum. 1981;24:114–19.
19. Cubertafond P, Gainant A, Barbier J, Coste G. Colostomies: indications et complications. Chirurgie. 1985;111:331–41.
20. Russel KP. Parastomal hernia. World J Surg. 1989;13:569–72.
21. Whittaker, Goligher JC. A comparison of the results of extraperitoneal and intraperitoneal techniques for construction of terminal iliac colostomies. Dis Colon Rectum. 1976;19:342–4.
22. Sjödahl R, Anderberg B, Bolin T. Parastomal hernia in relation to site of the abdominal stoma. Br J Surg. 1988;75:339–41.
23. Leslie D. The parastomal hernia. Surg Clin N Am. 1984;64:407–15.
24. Alexandre JH, Bouillot JL. Paracolostomal hernia: repair with use of a Dacron prosthesis. World J Surg. 1993;17:680–2.
25. Goldblatt M, Corman M, Haggit R. Ileostomy complications requiring revision: Lahey Clinic experience 1964–1973. Dis Colon Rectum. 1977;20:209.

30
Indications and contraindications to reconstructive surgery in ulcerative colitis

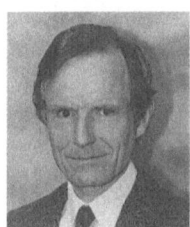

D. JOHNSTON

INTRODUCTION

Let us assume that the patient needs surgical treatment: either because of failure of medical treatment with steroids and/or azathioprine, or the occurrence of complications such as fulminating colitis, toxic dilatation, hemorrhage, perforation, or malignant or premalignant change. Thus patients who present for surgical treatment do not represent a homogeneous group: most are elective cases but a few are operated upon as emergencies, while a substantial minority require urgent operation. Some are young, some are old; some are relatively fit, others are debilitated and undernourished, while yet others may have serious associated disease of other organ systems. Hence strategies of treatment must take into account not only the extent and severity of the colitis, but the physical state of the patient, the degree of urgency of the operative procedure and finally the experience and training of the surgeon who operates.

Colitis in children tends to have a worse prognosis than colitis in adults; because with their long life expectancy there is a greater risk of carcinoma, while the debilitating effects of the disease process interfere with education and social relationships, and impair growth and sexual development. For these reasons surgical treatment is required in a greater proportion of children than of adults, and the decision to operate should not be delayed too long, lest the child be stunted and his or her education and social life devastated.

DIAGNOSIS

Infective causes of colitis must be excluded, leaving three main categories of disease, namely ulcerative colitis, Crohn's disease and colitis of an indeterminate nature. Crohn's disease should be excluded by normal clinical methods, supplemented by standard investigations such as colonoscopy with biopsies, air contrast barium enema and small bowel meal. A history of anal disease, patchy distribution of the disease in the colon and, of course, involvement of the small intestine, are all in favor of Crohn's disease. Reconstructive surgery is contraindicated in patients with Crohn's disease (see below) though the distinction between Crohn's disease and ulcerative colitis can on occasion be very difficult, and every large series of restorative proctocolectomies ostensibly for ulcerative colitis includes a few patients who eventually turn out to have Crohn's disease. In cases of particular diagnostic difficulty, when Crohn's disease is suspected but the small bowel seems to be completely normal on standard investigations, it may be prudent to remove the colon initially, leaving the rectum and establishing an ileostomy, so that an experienced pathologist may make a verdict on the large operative specimen rather than merely on biopsies. Whereas patients with Crohn's disease tend to fare badly after restorative proctocolectomy, patients with indeterminate colitis tend to do well. Hence the correct philosophy is to preserve the anal sphincter unless there is good evidence that the patient has Crohn's disease according to the opinion of an experienced pathologist.

CHOICE OF OPERATIVE PROCEDURE FOR ULCERATIVE COLITIS AND INDETERMINATE COLITIS

Until about 10 years ago the standard operation was panproctocolectomy and ileostomy. Today, however, the standard operative procedure is restorative proctocolectomy with a pelvic ileal reservoir anastomosed to the anal sphincter. A third possibility is colectomy with ileorectal anastomosis.

The point never to be forgotten is that the anal sphincter is nearly always healthy in patients with ulcerative colitis, though its mucosal lining may be inflamed in the upper third or so of the high-pressure zone. Since it is now accepted that a healthy anal sphincter is capable of providing excellent continence after removal of the entire rectum and colon, the burden of proof rests with those who would advocate ablation of the sphincter rather than with those who would preserve it. That is, in accord with the well-known principle, *primum non nocere*, the prevailing philosophy must be that the sphincter should be preserved, while more aggressive approaches which remove the sphincter should be regarded as unnecessary, unjustifiable and in future difficult to justify in law.

In the University Department of Surgery at Leeds General Infirmary we have made a systematic attempt to preserve the anal sphincter when operating for ulcerative colitis since 1977. Since 1980 we have performed very few primary panproctocolectomies with permanent ileostomy, though a few patients have ended up with a permanent stoma when the attempt at reconstruction to the anal sphincter has failed. Ileorectal anastomosis has not been used: there is no tradition of the use of this procedure in Leeds, because most patients who come to surgical treatment seem to have severe disease in the rectum and also because of the risk of cancer after ileorectal anastomosis. Thus the vast majority of patients have been treated by sphincter-saving restorative proctocolectomy, combined in most patients with a temporary defunctioning ileostomy.

Panproctocolectomy followed by the construction of a continent *Kock ileal reservoir* has not been used by us in the past 15 years. In our small series in the 1970s we were impressed by the complexity of the procedure and deterred by the eventual death of a nurse who succumbed to a series of postoperative complications. Patients with a conventional Brooke ileostomy, who have undergone panproctocolectomy, and who insist on being considered for the Kock pouch, should be referred to one or other of the few centers in the world where more than 50 such procedures have already been done.

PREOPERATIVE COUNSELLING

Before operation, much time needs to be spent with the patient by the physician, surgeon, stomatherapist and ideally, a patient who has already undergone the recommended operative procedure. The pros and cons of panproctocolectomy and ileostomy, ileorectal anastomosis and restorative proctocolectomy should be discussed fully, and the patient given ample time to reflect on what has been said and an opportunity to ask further questions at a subsequent meeting. Parents and relatives should be brought into these discussions as appropriate and, of course, this is particularly important in the case of children. As stated above, the bias nowadays should be towards preservation of the anal sphincter, and the advantages of restorative proctocolectomy in terms of preservation of continence, the avoidance of a stoma and of a perineal wound, and the better quality of life that may be expected, should be explained in detail. At the same time it is important not to paint too optimistic a picture. For example, it must be stated that, like any operative procedure, there is a slight risk to life itself (though the risk is less than that of continued colitis and the treatment thereof), that postoperative complications are quite common, that diarrhea and perianal excoriation tend to be troublesome for a few weeks after closure of the defunctioning ileostomy and that, in the long term, while the results are very good, they are by no means perfect, and in the end the procedure fails in 5–10% of patients, who then have to have a permanent ileostomy. The patient should be told that the *average* bowel frequency is four or five times during the day and perhaps once at night, but it is important to add that there is a considerable *range* of frequency of defecation, from twice to 10 times a day. This discouraging information should be tempered, however, by the added information that frequent bowel action, if it should occur, tends to be more under the patient's control, in the morning and after the evening meal, than is the bowel frequency of colitis, and also the urgent defecation that is one of the worst features of colitis is either absent or much improved after operation. The possibility of attacks of clinical pouchitis should be discussed. The need for a temporary defunctioning ileostomy should be explained and, of course, in patients who present in a debilitated state or as emergencies, the operation may have to be in three stages, beginning with simple colectomy, ileostomy and construction of a mucous fistula; the need for this type of approach should also be explained to the patient.

IS THE ANAL SPHINCTER ADEQUATE?

After surgical removal of the entire colon and rectum, the patient's continence and quality of life depend crucially on the anal sphincter. The adequacy of the sphincter for its task should therefore be evaluated carefully, by means of the history, examination and, if necessary, laboratory tests. The history is the most important method of evaluation. If a patient has severe colitis, with the frequency of defecation and urgency that that implies, yet remains continent, he or she will be continent after restorative proctocolectomy with a pelvic ileal reservoir. One should enquire carefully about common causes of sphincteric weakness, such as previous abscess or fistula, previous anal surgery or obstetric injury. Digital rectal examination will give further information about the strength of the sphincter and, if any doubt remains, anorectal function tests should be carried out to provide information on maximum resting anal pressure and maximum squeeze pressure. At the same time the opportunity is taken to evaluate the maximum tolerated volume (MTV) and compliance of the rectum, because if ileorectal anastomosis is contemplated it is important that the rectum should not be an unyielding fibrous tube, and the minimum MTV should be approximately 150 ml.

CONTRAINDICATIONS TO RESTORATIVE PROCTOCOLECTOMY

Inadequacy of the anal sphincter

This is a major contraindication. However, it must be borne in mind that debilitated patients who have been ill for a long time with ulcerative colitis tend to have low serum potassium levels, low serum albumin and weak muscles. In these circumstances removal of the colon and the establishment of an ileostomy may effect a remarkable improvement in the patient's general condition, and the anal sphincter may regain its normal power.

Diagnosis

The diagnosis should be one of ulcerative colitis or indeterminate colitis: Crohn's disease is a contraindication.

Previous small bowel resection

This should usually be regarded as a contraindication to reconstructive surgery, because anatomically it may then be difficult to construct an ileal reservoir and bring it down to the anal sphincter, while physiologically the effluent may be excessively profuse, liquid and corrosive.

Urgent or emergency operations

In toxic or debilitated patients these also represent a contraindication to reconstructive surgery. The correct policy then is to remove the entire colon, establish an end-ileostomy and bring out the upper end of the rectum as a mucous fistula. Reconstructive surgery can then be performed, when the patient is restored to good health.

Carcinoma

Carcinoma or severe dysplasia of the colon or rectum complicating colitis is often referred to as a contraindication to restorative surgery, but in practice is seldom a factor in the decision-making. It is, of course, vital to assess the colon and rectum properly, and to look for the presence of dysplasia and carcinoma. However, unless the carcinoma is located in the lower third of the rectum, there seems no good reason to rule out the possibility of reconstructive surgery, because nowadays most patients with rectal carcinoma are treated by sphincter-saving low anterior resection rather than abdominoperineal excision of the rectum. Again, if the patient is unlucky enough to have liver secondaries associated with colorectal carcinoma, the surgical approach should be as conservative as possible, so that the quality of life in the patient's remaining days should be as tolerable as possible. In view of the current lively debate about the desirability or otherwise of ablating the mucosal lining of the anal sphincter above the dentate line, it is particularly desirable that several biopsies should be taken from the anal transition zone and the mucosa immediately above it, because if moderate to severe epithelial dysplasia is present there, end-to-end pouch–anal anastomosis without mucosectomy is contraindicated, the correct procedure being either mucosal stripping with endo-anal pouch–anal anastomosis or, if the dysplasia is particularly severe and alarming, panproctocolectomy and ileostomy.

INDICATIONS AND CONTRAINDICATIONS FOR ILEORECTAL ANASTOMOSIS[1-4]

The main disadvantage of ileorectal anastomosis is that it does not cure the disease (either in the large bowel or in its extracolonic manifestations), and that it exposes the patient to a steadily increasing risk of developing rectal carcinoma. Despite annual sigmoidoscopic surveillance the onset of such a carcinoma is difficult to detect, because the rectal mucosa may be obscured by fluid feces and also because the entire rectal mucosa may be somewhat inflamed and abnormal-looking. Furthermore, the surveillance program itself is often faulty, and patients may default from follow-up. For reasons such as these the cancers that do develop tend to have a poor prognosis. The actual magnitude of the risk of cancer is much debated. It depends to some extent on how carefully patients have been selected for ileorectal anastomosis, on the duration of follow-up and on the assiduity with which the presence of cancer is sought. The incidences of cancer in the remaining rectum vary in different reports from 0% to over 20%, the average figure being about 5%. On follow-up of more than 20 years about 20% of patients will have developed cancer.

Ileorectal anastomosis is contraindicated if the rectum is severely affected by ulcerative colitis, and particularly if it is shrunken, fibrous and noncompliant or strictured. Obviously, if the rectum is the seat of carcinoma or severe dysplasia, it must be removed.

Nevertheless, despite the fact that colitis is usually at its most severe in the rectum, it would appear that a minority of patients with ulcerative colitis, perhaps 10–20% of all those who require surgical treatment, are suitable for colectomy with ileorectal anastomosis (IRA). The indications for IRA are that the anus should be healthy and the rectum should not be severely affected by disease. A short history of colitis is also desirable, because the risk of cancer should then be relatively low for at least 10 years after IRA. The procedure may also be indicated in elderly patients whose life expectancy is fairly short in any case, and in whom considerations of cancer risk are therefore less important than short-term considerations about quality of life. Paradoxically, however IRA is also worth considering in children, in whom life expectancy should be long and the risk of cancer therefore high. That is because IRA is a simpler operation than the pelvic pouch procedure, postoperative morbidity tends to be less and return to school quicker. In addition, provided the disease process is relatively mild in the rectum itself, the quality of life after IRA may be somewhat better than the quality of life after the pelvic pouch procedure, because bowel frequency may be more predictable and the risk of autonomic nerve damage in the pelvis is negligible. Therefore, in children and adolescents with colitis, it may be worth considering IRA for a period of 5–20 years, after which the rectum may be excised and an ileal pouch constructed with pouch–anal anastomosis. The major proviso, however, is that the parents must understand that there is a risk of cancer, and the need for regular sigmoidoscopic surveillance of the rectum must be clearly understood.

RESTORATIVE PROCTOCOLECTOMY WITH PELVIC ILEAL RESERVOIR[5–14]

This procedure is the operation of choice for most patients with ulcerative colitis. Worldwide experience over the past 15 years shows that it is very safe, with an operative mortality of less than 1%. Postoperative complications are still common, affecting approximately 40–50% of all patients. The most frequent complications are pelvic sepsis, with or without anastomotic dehiscence, small bowel obstruction, fistula to the vagina or elsewhere, and stricture at the pouch–anal anastomosis. Even in elective cases most surgeons still prefer to perform a temporary defunctioning ileostomy, which is closed 2–3 months later when the patient has recovered from the major operation. Nevertheless, several prospective trials in carefully selected patients in major centers have shown that one-stage restorative proctocolectomy yields good results, with an operative mortality and postoperative morbidity that are little different from the mortality and morbidity of the two-stage procedure. Our own experience in Leeds mirrors the results of these trials, but we would point out that when an ileostomy has been omitted, the septic complications, though no greater in *incidence*, are much more dangerous in *severity*. For example, in our own series of 50 one-stage procedures, three patients developed life-threatening peritonitis, and the need for emergency reoperation was greater than among 50 closely matched patients who underwent the two-stage procedure. For these reasons we would emphasize that the one-stage procedure must be used only in relatively 'fit' patients under strictly controlled conditions in specialized centers, that the technical aspects of the operation should be shown to be perfect (intact donuts, airtight suture lines) and that the surgeon who performs the operation should see the patient daily for 10 days after operation, and certainly not leave town. The very low operative mortality of the two-stage restorative proctocolectomy has been a shining achievement which should not be tarnished by ill-judged attempts to perform the operation in one stage in the majority of patients. Admittedly, such a policy will be successful in most patients, and it is unlikely that in any one center the operative mortality will rise statistically significantly, but our findings suggest that operative mortality is likely to be higher when the ileostomy is omitted, and we think it likely that a move to the one-stage procedure will increase operative mortality by 1–2%, an avoidable tragedy in the patients concerned. Furthermore, about 40% of the patients treated by restorative proctocolectomy are young women, and fecal leakage from the pelvic pouch or from the pouch–anal anastomosis is likely to give rise to pelvic peritonitis, which could endanger their prospects of having children. In either sex such leakage may lead to fibrosis and rigidity of the pelvic contents, which could impair anorectal function in the long term.

Restorative proctocolectomy in older patients

It used to be thought that sphincter-saving surgery was contraindicated in most patients over the age of 55 because their anal sphincters tended to be weaker than those of younger people, and the functional result tended to be worse. However, these views have had to be modified in recent years, because most major centers are now reporting good results in the older patients. Many of these patients have had colitis for many years, and their anal sphincters may have undergone 'work hypertrophy'. It is particularly important in the older patients to preserve the full power of the anal sphincter, and in our opinion this is best done by leaving the sphincter completely undisturbed. That is, mucosal stripping should be avoided and the pelvic reservoir should be stapled end-to-end to the top of the anal high-pressure zone, 1–2 cm above the dentate line.

END-TO-END POUCH–ANAL ANASTOMOSIS COMPARED WITH MUCOSECTOMY AND ENDO-ANAL ANASTOMOSIS

While there is general agreement that most patients should be treated by some form of reconstructive surgery, there is lively disagreement about the best method of performing the reconstruction, and some disagreement too about which pelvic reservoir should be used. At the Leeds General Infirmary we have employed the Fonkalsrud, J, S and W pouches in the past 15 years, and are currently conducting a prospective trial of large pouches versus small pouches and of the J, Utsunomiya pouch versus the W, Nicholls pouch. While our results with the quadruplicated W pouch are similar to those described by Nicholls, we have found, somewhat to our surprise, that a J pouch constructed from an equal length of ileum to that used in the W pouch yields similar results to those of the W reservoir.

END-TO-END OR MUCOSECTOMY PLUS ENDO-ANAL ANASTOMOSIS?

The method by which the pouch should be anastomosed to the anal sphincter is of great interest. The advocates of mucosectomy with endo-anal anastomosis at the dentate line stress the importance of ablating all inflammatory disease in the mucosa, even within the anal high-pressure zone, and claim to have achieved clinical results as good as those obtained when the entire sphincter is preserved. They also tend to emphasize the theoretical long-term danger of leaving some rectal-type mucosa in the upper anal canal. In contrast, we in Leeds, and others such as Martin in Cincinnati, were impressed by how the endo-anal procedure reduced resting pressure in the anal canal and how, in patients who sustained a particularly large fall in RAP, minor leakage of feces occurred, as the early writings from the Mayo Clinic made clear. The incidence of such leakage after mucosectomy and endo-anal anastomosis is about 50% in the first postoperative year, and tends to be worse at night.

Since the mid-1980s we have therefore preferred to leave the anal high-pressure zone intact, without stripping the mucosa above the dentate line, and have performed the reconstruction by the double-stapling technique. In our practice, at least, this has been associated with higher anal pressures, less leakage and better fine discrimination, such that the patients are more likely to be able to release gas or wind without having to go to sit on a toilet. There is also little doubt that avoidance of mucosectomy and hand-sewn endo-anal anastomosis renders the procedure technically more convenient. One technical difficulty associated with the end-to-end procedure, however, is the difficulty that the abdominal operator experiences in knowing exactly where to transect the bowel, and in certain cases, such as thick-set males with a narrow pelvis, it is expedient to mobilize the rectum and upper anus from the abdominal aspect and then to evert the anorectal stump, as in the Soave operation in children. From the perineal aspect the operator can then see exactly where to transect the bowel, about 1 cm above the dentate line, after which the closed anal stump is returned to its proper place and alimentary continuity restored by means of the circular stapling device.

It might be thought that preservation of a centimetre or two of mucosa above the dentate line might be associated with an increased incidence of fistulation to vagina or elsewhere, but this has not been our experience; nor have we found that patients so treated experienced greater urgency or frequency of defecation than those treated by endo-anal anastomosis. It should also be noted that the only cases of carcinoma so far reported after reconstructive surgery have been in patients who have undergone mucosal stripping, the performance of which does not guarantee that all at-risk mucosa has been removed.

Thus the argument continues, and the final verdict on the question of whether the anal mucosa should be stripped or not will depend on long-term clinical end-points, such as the respective incidences of carcinoma and the quality of life experienced by the patients after end-to-end or endo-anal pouch–anal anastomosis.

References

1. Kock NG, Myrvold HE, Nilsson LO, Philipson BM. Continent ileostomy. An account of 314 patients. Acta Chir Scand. 1981;147:67–72.
2. Jones PF, Gilroy Bevan P, Hawley PR. Ileostomy or ileorectal anastomosis for ulcerative colitis? Br Med J. 1978;1:1459–63.
3. Leijonmarck C-E, Lofberg R, Hellers G. Long-term results of ileorectal anastomosis in ulcerative colitis in Stockholm County. Dis Colon Rectum. 1990;33:195–200.
4. Watts JMcK, Hughes ESR. Ulcerative colitis and Crohn's disease: results after colectomy and ileorectal anastomosis. Br J Surg. 1977;64:77–83.
5. Cohen Z, McLeod RS, Stephen W, Stern HS, O'Connor B, Reznick R. Continuing evolution of the pelvic pouch procedure. Ann Surg. 1992;216:506–12.
6. Keighley MRB, Yoshioka K, Kmiot W. Prospective randomized trial to compare the stapled double lumen pouch and the sutured quadruple pouch for restorative proctocolectomy. Br J Surg. 1988;75:1008–11.
7. Kelly KA. Anal sphincter-saving operations for chronic ulcerative colitis. Am J Surg. 1992;163:5–11.
8. Nasmyth DG, Williams NS, Johnston D. Comparison of the function of triplicated and duplicated pelvic ileal reservoirs after mucosal proctectomy and ileoanal anastomosis for ulcerative colitis and adenomatous polyposis. Br J Surg. 1986;73:361–6.
9. Nasmyth DG, Godwin DGR, Dixon MF, Johnston D. Ileal ecology after pouch-anal anastomosis or ileostomy: a study of mucosal morphology, fecal bacteriology, fecal volatile fatty acids and their interrelationship. Gastroenterology. 1989;96:817–24.
10. Nicholls RJ, Pezim ME. Restorative proctocolectomy with ileal reservoir for ulcerative colitis and familial adenomatous polyposis: a comparison of 3 reservoir designs. Br J Surg. 1985;72:470–4.
11. Seow-Choen A, Tsunoda A, Nicholls RJ. Prospective randomized trial comparing anal function after hand sewn ileoanal anastomosis with mucosectomy versus stapled ileoanal anastomosis without mucosectomy in restorative proctocolectomy. Br J Surg. 1991;78:430–4.

12. Wexner SD, Jensen L, Rothenberger DA, Wong WD, Goldberg SM. Long term functional analysis of the ileoanal reservoir. Dis Colon Rectum. 1989;32:275–81.
13. Williams NS, Johnston D. The current status of mucosal proctectomy and ileo-anal anastomosis in the surgical treatment of ulcerative colitis and adenomatous polyposis. Br J Surg. 1985;72:159–68.
14. Johnston D, Holdsworth PJ, Nasmyth DG, Neal DE. Preservation of the entire anal canal in conservative proctocolectomy for ulcerative colitis. Br J Surg. 1987;74:940–4.

31
Pouchitis – what's new in etiology and management?

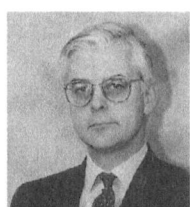

R. J. NICHOLLS

Pouchitis is a clinical condition associated with inflammation of the ileal reservoir. It was recognized first in continent ileostomies by Kock *et al.*[1] and subsequently in ileoanal ileal reservoirs by Handelsman *et al.*[2]. Histological changes in ileal reservoirs of a chronic inflammatory or atrophic type had been reported in both types of reconstruction by Philipson *et al.*[3] and Nicholls *et al*[4]. Subsequently it was appreciated that pouchitis occurs predominantly in ulcerative colitis and only rarely (if at all) in familial adenomatous polyposis. Various possible causes, including stasis, bacterial flora and biochemical factors (for example short-chain fatty acids or bile salts) have been studied. Various treatments from antibiotics, bile salts, short-chain fatty acids, xanthene oxidase inhibitors and conventional anti-inflammatory medication have been tried.

We are left with a somewhat confusing picture, due in part to ignorance concerning the etiopathology of inflammatory bowel disease, in part to a variable interpretation of diagnosis and in part to the possibility that acute inflammation may be due to various agents. The term 'pouchitis' implies inflammation; it cannot be diagnosed solely by the presence of symptoms or indeed by endoscopic appearances. There has to be histopathologic evidence of acute inflammation. Several studies have not used histopathology to make the diagnosis and, as a result, some patients deemed to have pouchitis may not have had this condition at all. There are various causes of frequency of defecation and other bowel symptoms that can be confused with pouchitis. These include physical factors, for example a small reservoir or emptying difficulties, intrinsic bowel motility, psychological factors, partial small-bowel obstruction and extramural inflammation. To diagnose pouchitis there must be inflammation present, and this is now generally accepted. There is a reasonable correlation between the severity of the histologic inflammation based on a semi-objective grading system and the symptoms[5].

HISTOPATHOLOGY OF THE RESERVOIR

Histopathologic examination of the ileal pouch mucosa shows several different abnormalities which may variably be represented and overlap with each other.

Chronic inflammation and villous atrophy

Almost all functioning pouches show some mucosal abnormality. These are common to patients with ulcerative colitis and familial adenomatous polyposis. They may vary in their severity but are qualitatively similar[6]. The changes are characterized by an increase in the presence of chronic inflammatory cells within the lamina propria. These include lymphocytes, plasma cells and sometimes eosinophils. In addition there is villous atrophy to a varying degree from individual to individual, and also within the same pouch. The degree of villous atrophy is associated with crypt hyperplasia.

These changes appear to occur early after restoration of the fecal stream[3,7,8]. They appear to be confined to the reservoir and only rarely extend into the proximal ileum[6]. The same authors have demonstrated more severe changes in the posterior than the anterior aspect of the lower part of the reservoir. Setti-Carraro et al.[9] in a study of 57 patients having four biopsies taken from the pouch at 5 cm intervals from distal to proximal, identified three groups of patients. These included group 1 ($n = 8$) in which none of the biopsies showed any acute inflammation, group 2 ($n = 25$) in which all biopsies showed acute inflammation and group 3 ($n = 26$) in which there was a gradient of decreasing inflammation from distal to proximal.

These changes may be the result of an alteration in milieu due to the presence of increased numbers of fecal bacteria compared with the normal ileostomy effluent. These may lead to changes in colonic intraluminal carbohydrate fermentation of dietary fiber with the increased production of short-chain fatty acids (SCFA) and changes in bile salt concentration and type. We do not yet know what the mucosal dynamics are in response to this alteration in microenvironment; nor do we know the factors responsible. Nasmyth et al.[10] have, however, presented data suggesting that the degree of villous atrophy is inversely related to the concentration of butyrate in the pouch feces. The degree of villous atrophy is also related to crypt cell turnover as determined immunohistochemically using the monoclonal antibody Ki-67[11]. A similar result was obtained by Martelli et al.[12], who demonstrated an increase in labeling index within the ileal mucosa in patients with ulcerative colitis after pouch construction. There was no change in patients with familial adenomatous polyposis.

COLONIC METAPLASIA

Histologically the presence of severe villous atrophy and crypt hyperplasia resembles colonic mucosa. When inflammation is present the picture looks like ulcerative colitis[11,13]. Studies have shown colonic-type mucin in ileal pouches irrespective of the original diagnosis. Using Alcian blue staining techniques and the monoclonal antibody PR3A5, which is thought to be specific for colon-type mucin, the presence of sulfated mucin has been demonstrated in ileal pouch mucosa[11,14]. A similar result as been reported using a $S_{35}-H_3$ glucosamine labeling technique[15].

These changes are, however, not complete. For example the pouch mucosa retains certain properties of small intestinal enterocytes with preservation of disaccharidase activity and the activity to absorb B_{12}, xylose and bile acids[14]. It is not known whether colonic metaplasia is a prerequisite for pouchitis[6].

'DIVERSION' CHANGES

In defunctioned pouches, that is before closure of the ileostomy, histologic abnormalities have been reported in a proportion of patients[16]. These include villous atrophy, chronic inflammation with eosinophil predominance and acute inflammation. The changes are not typical of ischemia or Crohn's disease and the authors speculated on the possibiity that they may represent a form of diversion ileitis analogous to that described in the rectum[17,18].

POUCHITIS

Pouchitis is characterized by the presence of acute inflammation. This is correlated with the severity of chronic inflammation[5,9,13,14]. The appearance is similar to ulcerative colitis in an active phase. Polymorphs appear to be located predominantly through the epithelium with crypt abscess formation; aggregates are seen in the lamina propria but are often focal. Ulceration is present. There may be evidence of colonic metaplasia but sometimes small intestinal sialomucins predominate[13]. Perhaps this is similar to the appearance of sialomucins in cases of acute ulcerative colitis[19]. In contrast with celiac disease, intra-epithelial lymphocyte counts in ileal pouches are low and do not increase in pouchitis[20].

Pouchitis is essentially confined to patients with ulcerative colitis. While case reports of its occurrence in familial adenomatosis have been reported, it is rare and histological confirmation is not always obtained. In 37 polyposis patients followed for a mean of 5 years there was not a single case[21].

The timing of these morphologic changes is unknown in detail. Some information is, however, available from a long-term histopathologic study of 60 patients with an original diagnosis of ulcerative colitis biopsied over a median period of 97 months (range 90–173 months). On the basis of histologic grade of the severity of acute and chronic inflammation the patients can be divided into three groups, A, B and C: in group A ($n = 27$) changes were minor with acute changes never seen; in group B ($n = 25$) chronic changes were more severe and there were transient episodes of acute inflammation; in group C ($n = 8$) severe chronic and severe acute inflammation were constantly present. Pouchitis never occurred in group A and was constantly present in group C. Patients were identified to their group within 6 months of closure of the ileostomy and remained in that group indefinitely. If these data are true, patients at risk of developing pouchitis can be identified on biopsy at an early stage in the postoperative course[9]. Verres et al.[22] have made similar observations. They have furthermore reported dysplasia to occur, albeit rarely but exclusively, in group C.

POSSIBLE EVOLUTION

On the basis of histopathologic observations a hypothetical sequence of events can be suggested. On construction of an ileal reservoir with defunctioning ileostomy, some cases will develop an inflammation in the mucosa associated with low intraluminal SCFA levels. This will be abolished with closure. The presence of feces containing bacterial counts similar to normal colonic feces then leads to chronic inflammation and villous atrophy. The degree of this will be variable according to the individual, but is less general in familial adenomatous polyposis than in ulcerative colitis. Stasis is always present to some degree in an ileal reservoir, whether a continent ileostomy or ileoanal construction.

As villous atrophy progresses, crypt hyperplasia occurs and mucin changes into colonic type. Colonic metaplasia can occur in both ulcerative colitis and familial adenomatous polyposis. It appears to be variable in its distribution and not complete, in that some small intestinal function is preserved.

Colonic metaplasia then renders the mucosa susceptible to the underlying pathologic process. With ulcerative colitis this results in inflammation, with familial adenomatous polyposis in the induction of adenoma formation.

POSSIBLE ETIOLOGICAL FACTORS

Bacteria

Bacterial counts in ileal reservoir feces are greater than in ileostomy effluent and approximate to those in normal feces. In addition there is a relative rise in the anaerobic count. The anaerobe to aerobe ratio in pouches is $100:1$ compared with about $4:1$ in ileostomy effluent[23]. These changes are likely to be due to stasis in the reservoir. In both Kock and ileoanal reservoirs stasis is present when compared with a constantly acting ileostomy. In both, total counts and increase in anaerobes have been reported[4,10,24,25].

While these changes may lead to mucosal alterations, for example chronic inflammation and villous atrophy, there is no evidence that stasis per se is responsible for pouchitis. A study assessing the efficiency of evacuation of the pouch has not shown any difference in patients with or without pouchitis[5,26]. Pouchitis is not related to the type of reservoir. Its incidence is no different in patients with S reservoirs needing catheterization compared with J reservoirs in which evacuation was not impeded[5]. Fleshman et al.[27] presented evidence that pouch inflammation was more likely in the presence of an ileoanal stricture, although pouchitis could still occur without it. Furthermore, there is no correlation between the number or species of bacteria or the presence or absence of pouchitis. No specific pathogenetic bacteria have been consistently found to be associated with pouchitis[25,26,28]. Onderdonk et al.[29] in an electron microscopic study of pouch mucosa combined with bacterial culture techniques, showed significantly greater total counts for aerobic bacteria associated with the mucosa in patients with pouchitis.

There is, however, much evidence (mostly anecdotal) that metronidazole improves pouch inflammation. The most objective evidence comes from a recent study employing indium-111-labelled granulocyte scanning in six patients with pouchitis[30]. This study showed a reduction in granulocyte migration to the pouch 1 month after metronidazole, associated with endoscopic and histologic improvement. In an interesting study, Dube and Huyen[31] identified 15 cases of pouchitis out of a total of 70 patients. Ten responded to metronidazole. Six patients, three responders and three non-responders, had gastric function studies. Fasting gastric pH was 1.3 or less in the former group and 4.2 or more in the latter. This suggests an effect of metronidazole on fecal flora. Metronidazole does not always work, however. In a double-blind crossover trial of 11 patients with chronic unremitting pouchitis there was only a slight diminution in the frequency of defecation and no significant change in histological grade or C-reactive protein[32].

METABOLIC EFFECTS OF ALTERED FECAL FLORA

Short-chain fatty acids (SCFA)

SCFA are produced by the fermentation by colonic bacteria of carbohydrate in dietary fiber. They are an important source of energy to the colonic epithelium and their lack may cause diversion colitis. Nasmyth et al.[10] reported higher SCFA concentrations in stool from ileal reservoirs than in normal ileostomy stool, and similar to normal feces. They also observed a relationship between butyrate concentrations and degree of villous atrophy: the higher the concentration, the lower the atrophy. This implied a protective influence of SCFA on limiting chronic changes. Clausen et al.[33] showed that SCFA concentrations were markedly lower in six patients with pouchitis compared with 28 without, with levels of 56.2 ± 13.3 mmol/l and 139.0 ± 8.5 mmol/l respectively. There was no change in the ratios of acetate to butyrate to propionate in either group. These authors produced evidence to indicate that this difference is due to lack of substrate rather than to the difference in the capacity of the flora to produce SCFA, since in-vitro production of SCFA of fecal homogenates in patients with pouchitis could be restored with the addition of saccharides. This suggested the possibility that pouchitis is due to a reduction of substrate available leading to low

SCFA. Wischmeyer et al.[34] demonstrated SCFA concentrations in stool of 11 pouchitis patients to be 25% of the level in 13 nonpouchitis patients. Further evidence indicating that SCFA may be important to influencing the state of the mucosa comes from a study of 14 patients in whom frequency of defecation was inversely related to the stool SCFA concentration[35]. Pouchitis did not respond to the installation of SCFA into the pouch by enema[36]. In contrast, some benefit was found in another study. Patients having had pouch operations for ulcerative colitis were recruited on the basis of a diagnosis of 'chronic pouchitis'. It is unclear whether this was confirmed histologically. Ten patients completed a trial of L-glutamine (1 g) given by suppository, and six had no recurrence of symptoms. Nine completed a trial of sodium butyrate (40 mmol) by suppository. Three had no recurrent symptoms. There is, however, no long-term follow up of this study, and no detailed statement of the criteria for improvement[37].

BILE SALTS

Hill and Owen[38] have reported high levels of deconjugated and secondary bile acids in the ileal reservoir compared with ileostomy effluent. Deconjugated bile acids can, through their detergent effect, damage membranes[39] and might therefore be a factor in pouchitis. The significant difference in total bile acid conjugates in six patients with pouchitis, 20 with ulcerative colitis without pouchitis and seven with familial adenomatous of 0.52 mg/g feces, 2.68 mg/g feces and 1.56 mg/g feces respectively requires further work for its corroboration[38]. Hulten[40] reported that cholestyramine was not helpful in pouchitis.

IMMUNE MECHANISM

The association of pouchitis with ulcerative colitis suggests a common etiopathogenesis. Clinically the conditions both show a natural history of exacerbations and remissions, either with resolution or with persisting chronic mucosal damage. Both are associated with an activity-related polyarthropathy. In pouchitis this is more likely to occur if it was present preoperatively[41]. Histologically there are close similarities, including the low numbers of intraepithelial lymphocytes, crypt abscesses and chronic cell infiltrate in the lamina propria. Increased IgG- and IgA-secreting plasma cells have been shown in the lamina propria in pouchitis in similar densities to those seen in ulcerative colitis[42]. Merrett et al.[43] studied biopsies from rectal mucosa and compared the finding with original colitic rectal mucosa in seven cases. Ig-containing cells were identified by immunohistochemistry. The total counts and profile of cells containing IgG, IgA, IgM and IgG1–4 were similar. De Silva et al.[11] have demonstrated increased numbers of RFD9 + macrophages in the mucosa, again a feature of noninfective inflammatory bowel disease. Gionchetti et al.[44] have confirmed this, and have shown them to be present in significantly higher proportions in pouchitis compared with nonpouchitis patients.

Mediators and inflammation have been shown to be increased in ileal pouches. Products of arachidonic acid metabolism (for example prostaglandin E2 and leukotriene B4) are present in mucosa and the lumen of ulcerative colitis[45]. In the pouch patients, Gertner et al.[46] have shown increased release of LTB4 in biopsies of patients with ulcerative colitis compared with polyposis. In addition, there was no difference in LTB4 released from biopsies taken from colitic pouches which were defunctioned compared to those which were functioning. Steroids which stabilize cell membranes, and aspirin which inhibits prostaglandin synthesis, may have what beneficial effect they do in pouchitis by a similar mechanism to that in ulcerative colitis. Chaussade et al.[47] have shown higher levels of platelet-activating factor (PAF) in the stool of pouch patients with pouchitis than those without. Overall density of cell immunoreactivity to tumor necrosis factor alpha (TNF-α) is increased in ulcerative colitis and Crohn's disease, and been confined to the lamina propria (mainly in subepithelial macrophages) in the flora[48]. In pouch mucosa TNF-α is also present, as determined by in situ hybridization of mRNA[49].

ISCHEMIA

Sakhuchi et al.[50], using laser doppler blood flow estimations, have suggested that ischemia may be a factor in pouchitis. Histopathologic examination of pouches has not shown changes typical of this pathology, however[51], and the intermittent relapsing and remitting nature of pouchitis is against ischemia.

Based on a possible ischemic etiology, allopurinol has been used in patients with acute ($n = 8$) and chronic ($n = 14$) pouchitis. It is important to note that the diagnosis was based on symptoms and not on histopathologic confirmation. In the former group, four responded and in the latter seven, but no data on long-term follow-up were given[52]. Further studies of appropriate placebos are required.

SUMMARY

Pouchitis is a man-made disease which appears clinically to resemble ulcerative colitis. It also appears to occur on a background of chronic inflammation, villous atrophy and colonic metaplasia. Histopathological confirmation of the diagnosis is essential. Patients at risk may be identified at an early stage after pouch construction by histopathological examination of a mucosal biopsy. Treatment using antibiotics, anti-inflammatory drugs, SCFA, xanthene oxydase inhibitors and cholestyramine is empirical. Like ulcerative colitis there is no specific cure. Further research studying the evolution of mucosal changes at a cellular and molecular level is the most likely way to increase understanding of the etiopathology and therefore the therapy.

References

1. Kock NG, Darle N, Hulton L, Kewenter J, Myrvold , Philipson B. Ileostomy. Curr Prob Surg. 1977;14:36–8.
2. Handelsman JC, Fishbein RH, Hoover HE, Smith GW, Haller JA. Endorectal pull-through operation in adults after colectomy and excision of rectal mucosa. Surgery. 1983;93:247–53.
3. Philipson B, Brandberg A, Jagenburg R, Kock NG, Lager I, Ahren C. Mucosal morphology, bacteriology and absorption in intra-abdominal ileostomy reservoir. Scand J Gastroenterol. 1975;10:145–53.
4. Nicholls RJ, Belleveau P, Neill M, Wilks M, Tabaqchali S. Restorative proctocolectomy with ileal reservoir: a patho-physiological assessment. Gut. 1981;22:462–8.
5. Moskowitz RL, Shepherd NA, Nicholls RJ. An assessment of inflammation in the reservoir after restorative proctocolectomy with ileo-anal ileal reservoir. Int J Colorectal Dis. 1986;1:167–74.
6. Shepherd NA, Healey CJ, Warren BF, Richman PI, Thomson WHF, Wilkinson SP. Distribution of mucosal pathology and an assessment of colonic phenotypic change in the pelvic ileal reservoir. Gut. 1993;34:101–5.
7. De Silva HJ, Millard PR, Prince C, Kettlewell M, Mortensen NJMcC, Jewell DP. Serial observations of the mucosal changes in ileoanal pouches. Gut. 1990;31:A1168–9.
8. Setti-Carraro P, Talbot IC, Nicholls RJ. The longitudinal distribution of endoscopic and histological changes in the ileal reservoir after restorative proctocolectomy. 1994 (Unpublished observations).
9. Setti-Carraro P, Talbot IC, Nicholls RJ. A long term appraisal of the histological appearances of the ileal reservoir mucosa after restorative proctocolectomy for ulcerative colitis. Gut. 1994 (In press).
10. Nasmyth DG, Godwin PGR, Dixon MF, Williams NS, Johnston D. Ileal ecology after pouch anal anastomosis or ileostomy. A study of mucosal morphology, fecal bacteriology, fecal volatile fatty acids and their interrelationship. Gastroenterology. 1989;96:817–24.
11. De Silva HJ, Gatter KC, Millard PR, Kettlewell M, Mortensen NJMcC, Jewell DB. Crypt cell proliferation and HLA-DR expression in pelvic ileal pouches. J Clin Pathol. 1990;43:824–49.
12. Martelli B, Talbot IC, Nicholls RJ. Changes in mucosal morphology and crypt cell turnover with construction of an ileoanal reservoir. 1994 (In press).
13. Shepherd NA, Jass JR, Duval I, Moskowitz RL, Nicholls RJ, Morson BC. Restorative proctocolectomy with ileal reservoir: pathological and histochemical study of mucosal biopsy specimens. J Clin Pathol. 1987;40:601–7.
14. De Silva HJ, Millard PR, Kettlewell M, Mortensen NJMcC, Jewell DP. Mucosal characteristics of pelvic ileal pouches. Gut. 1991;32:61–5.
15. Corfield AP, Warren BF, Bartolo DCC. Colonic metaplasia following restorative proctocolectomy monitored using a new metabolic labelling technique for mucin. J Pathol. 1990;160:170A.
16. Warren BF, Bartolo DCC, Collins CMP. Preclosure pouchitis – a new entity. J Pathol. 1990;160:170A.
17. Harig JM, Soergel KH, Komorowski RA, Wood CM. Treatment of diversion colitis with short chain fatty acid irrigation. N Engl J Med. 1989;320:23–38.
18. Editorial, Diversion colitis. Lancet. 1989;1:764.
19. Jass JR, England , Miller K. Value of mucin histochemistry in follow up surveillance of patients with long-standing ulcerative colitis. J Clin Pathol. 1986;39:393–8.
20. Shepherd NA. Pouchitis Workshop: The pathology of the ileal reservoir. Int J Colorectal Dis. 1989;4:206–8.
21. Madden MV, Neale KF, Nicholls RJ et al. Comparison of morbidity and function after colectomy with ileorectal anastomosis or restorative proctocolectomy for familial adenomatous polyposis. Br J Surg. 1991;78:789–92.
22. Veress B, Reinholt FP, Lindquist K, Liljeqvist L. Mucosal adaptation in the ileal reservoir after restorative proctocolectomy. A long term follow up study. Ann Chir. 1992;46:10–18.
23. Nasmyth DG, Williams NS. Pouch ecology. In: Nicholls RJ, Bartolo DCC, Mortensen NJMcC, editors. Restorative proctocolectomy. Oxford: Blackwell Scientific Publications;

1993:132–46.
24. Brandberg A, Kock NG, Philipson D. Bacterial flora in intraabdominal ileostomy reservoir. A study of 23 patients provided with 'continent ileostomy'. Gastroenterology. 1972;63:413–16.
25. Luukkonen P, Vultonen V, Sivonen A, Sipponen P, Jarveinen H. Faecal bacteriology and reservoir ileitis in patients operated on for ulcerative colitis. Dis Colon Rectum. 1988;31:864–7.
26. O'Connell PR, Rankin DR, Weiland LH, Kelly KA. Enteric bacteriology, absorption, morphology and emptying after ileal pouch–anal anastomosis. Br J Surg. 1986;73:909–14.
27. Fleshman JW, Cohen Z, McLeod RS, Stern H, Blair J. The ileal reservoir and ileoanal anastomosis procedure. Factors affecting technical and functional outcome. Dis Colon Rectum. 1988;31:10–16.
28. Hill MJ, Fernandez F. Pouch Workshop: Bacteriology I. Int J Colorectal Dis. 1989;4:217–19.
29. Onderdonk AB, Dvorak AM, Cisneos RL et al. Microbiologic assessment of tissue biopsy samples from ileal pouch patients. J Clin Microbiol. 1992;30:312–17.
30. Kmiot WA, Hesslewood SR, Smith N et al. Evaluation of the inflammatory infiltrate in pouchitis with IIIn-labelled granulocytes. Gastroenterology. 1993;104:981–8.
31. Dube S, Heyen F. Pouchitis and gastric hyposecretion: cause or effect? Int J Colorectal Dis. 1990;5:142–3.
32. Madden MV, McIntyre A, Nicholls RJ. Double blind cross over trial of Metronidazole in chronic unremitting pouchitis. Dig Dis Sci. 1994;39:1193–6.
33. Clausen MR, Trede M, Mortensen PB. Short chain fatty acids in pouch contacts from patients with and without pouchitis after ileal pouch–anal anastomosis. Gastroenterology. 1992;103:1144–53.
34. Wischmeyer P, Tremaine WJ, Haddad AC, Ambroze WL, Pemberton JH, Phillips SF. Fecal short chain fatty acids in patients with pouchitis after ileal pouch anal anastomosis. Gastroenterology. 1991;100:A848.
35. Ambroze WL, Pemberton JH, Phillips SF, Bell AM, Haddad AC. Fecal short chain fatty acid concentrations and effect on ileal pouch function. Dis Colon Rectum. 1993;36:235–9.
36. De Silva HJ, Ireland A, Kettlewell M, Mortensen NJMcC, Jewell DP. Short chain fatty acid irrigation in severe pouchitis (letter). N Engl J Med. 1989;321:1416–17.
37. Wischmeyer P, Pemberton JH, Phillips SF. Chronic pouchitis after ileal pouch–anal anastomosis: responses to butyrate and glutamine suppositories in a pilot study. Mayo Clin Proc. 1993;68:978–81.
38. Hill MJ, Owen RW. Pouch Workshop: Faecal bile acids in pouch and pouchitis patients. Int J Colorectal Dis. 1989;4:221–2.
39. Breuer NF, Rampton DS, Tammar A, Murphy GM, Dowling RH. Effect of colonic perfusion with sulfated and non-sulfated bile acids on mucosal structure and function in the rat. Gastroenterology. 1983;84:969–77.
40. Hulten L. Pouch Workshop: Pouchitis – incidence and characteristics in the continent ileostomy. Int J Colorectal Dis. 1989;4:208–10.
41. Lohmuller JL, Pemberton JH, Dozois RR, Ilstrup D, van Heerden J. Pouchitis and extraintestinal manifestations of inflammatory bowel disease after ileal pouch-anal anastomosis. Ann Surg. 1990;211:622–9.
42. Meuwissen SGM, Hoitsma H, Boot H, Seldenrijk CA. Pouchitis (pouch ileitis). Neth J Med. 1989;35:554–66.
43. Merrett MN, Gatter K, Heryet A, Jewell DP. Pattern of mucosal immunoglobulin (IG) producing cells is similar in ulcerative colitis and pouchitis. Gastroenterology. 1992;100:A935.
44. Gionchetti P, Campieri A, Belluzzi A et al. Macrophage subpopulations in pouchitis (letter). Gut. 1992;33:1008.
45. Lauritsen K, Larusen LS, Bukhave K, Rask-Madsen J. Inflammatory intermediaries in inflammatory bowel disease. Int J Colorectal Dis. 1989;4:75–90.
46. Gertner DJ, Madden MV, De Nucci G et al. Increased leukotriene B4 release from ileal pouch mucosa in ulcerative colitis compared with familial adenomatous polyposis. Gut. 1989;30:A1481.
47. Chaussade S, Denziot Y, Nicoli J et al. Presence of stool PAF-acetor in stool of patients with pouch ileoanal anastomosis and pouchitis. Gastroenterology. 1991;100:1509–14.

48. Murch SH, Braegger CP, Walker-Smith JA, MacDonald TT. Location of tumour necrosis factor α by immunohistochemistry in chronic inflammatory bowel disease. Gut. 1993;34:1705–9.
49. Kontakou M, Goldberg PA, Przemioslo RT, Nicholls RJ, Ciclitira PJ. Expression of interferon-γ, tumour necrosis factor α, and interleukins 6 and 2 in pouchitis. Gut. 1994;35:S40.
50. Sakaguchi M, Hosie K, Tudor R, Kmiot W, Keighley MRB. Mucosal blood flow following restorative proctocolectomy: pouchitis is associated with mucosal ischaemia. Br J Surg. 1989;76:1331 (abstract).
51. Warren BF, Shepherd NA. Pouch pathology. In: Nicholls RJ, Bartolo DCC, Mortensen NJMcC, editors. Restorative proctocolectomy. Oxford: Blackwell Scientific Publications; 1993:147–62.
52. Levin KE, Pemberton JH, Phillips SF, Zinsmeister AR, Pezim ME. Role of oxygen free radicals in the aetiology of pouchitis. Dis Colon Rectum. 1992;35:452–6.

32
Laparoscopic techniques: what is the role in IBD?

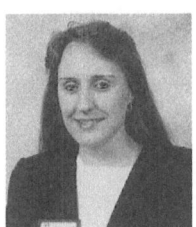

T. L. HULL

INTRODUCTION

When laparoscopic cholecystectomy was introduced in the United States many surgeons were reluctant to embrace the technique. It went against many ingrained surgical principles such as making large incisions to palpate all organs. However, fueled by public and peer pressure, surgeons were forced to consider laparoscopic surgery. In the United States, training courses quickly appeared, and any surgeon who performed cholecystectomies felt he/she had to offer this new approach to remain competitive. Subsequently, laparoscopic cholecystectomy was found to have real advantages over the traditional open technique, which include same-day surgery, 90% full activity in 1 week, minimal time off work, and minimal pain. Thus, the laparoscopic technique has quickly become the method of choice for removing most gallbladders in the United States[1-4]. Only 50 cases of laparoscopic chole-cystectomy were reported in 1989, but it has been estimated that over 500 000 cases were performed in 1993[5].

Enthusiasm for laparoscopic surgery has turned toward other organs, including the bowel. Proponents hypothesize that the advantages realized with laparoscopic cholecystectomy will be transferred to laparoscopic bowel surgery (i.e. patients will recover quicker when compared with conventional surgery)[6-8]. This remains a hypothesis, and is yet to be proven.

With laparoscopic abdominal surgery, multiple small puncture sites (10 mm or less in diameter) are strategically placed around the abdomen. Cannulas are inserted through these puncture sites. Carbon dioxide gas is insufflated through a port in the cannula and lifts the abdominal wall forward to allow better visualization of the abdominal structures. A videoscopic camera and novel laparoscopic instruments are inserted through the cannulas to perform the surgery.

It is important to realize that there are major differences that make laparoscopic bowel surgery more challenging than laparoscopic cholecystectomy. The bowel is a continuous organ so any resection must contend with either an anastomosis or stoma; the gallbladder, on the other hand, is a fixed end organ. The bowel is laden with bacteria and has an extensive (mesenteric) blood supply; the gallbladder has one artery. Laparoscopic instruments had to be redesigned to address the anatomic differences between the bowel and gallbladder, and they are still being refined to improve function and efficiency.

When considering inflammatory bowel disease, laparoscopic surgery can be divided into two areas: current and future indications for laparoscopic bowel surgery. The current indications will be discussed first.

CURRENT INDICATIONS

Diagnostic laparoscopy is probably underused by general and colorectal surgeons. In most patients it is relatively easy to insert a camera through a small puncture site to examine the abdomen. This modality is useful in patients with lower quadrant pain, especially to differentiate Crohn's disease from appendicitis or a gynecologic problem. It also can be used to investigate an intra-abdominal mass or chronic pain.

Laparoscopic bowel surgery has an important role in fecal diversion. Patients who suffer from perianal sepsis or incontinence can usually have a stoma constructed quickly with only one other small puncture site besides the stoma. This eliminates a midline incision. During the procedure the entire small bowel can also be examined. This is particularly applicable in Crohn's disease.

Limited bowel resections are being done, but the benefits have yet to be proved. Currently there are randomized prospective trials under way to evaluate the benefits of laparoscopic surgery.

Most surgeons perform extracorporeal anastomosis. The bowel is mobilized by laparoscopic techniques, then one of the small puncture sites is enlarged (to about 5 cm) to allow the bowel to be brought out onto the abdominal surface for resection and anastomosis. Intracorporeal anastomosis (resection and anastomosis totally inside the closed abdominal cavity) is feasible with new instruments and increasing skill with the technique. The resected bowel must still be removed from the abdominal cavity, so a small puncture site must be enlarged (to about 5 cm) for removal. Along with resections done extracorporeally, small bowel stricturoplasty can also be performed through the enlarged incision.

Stoma closures are also being done using laparoscopic techniques, but the overall benefit is, again, unclear when compared with conventional techniques.

FUTURE INDICATIONS

Laparoscopic subtotal colectomy is feasible, but because of its complexity requires a high level of skill. Ideally it can be attempted in selected thin patients. The bowel is mobilized with laparoscopic techniques and then one of the puncture sites is enlarged to remove the bowel. Most laparoscopic pelvic pouch procedures follow this pattern of laparoscopic mobilization followed by a small incision in the lower part of the abdomen to remove the bowel, form the ileal pelvic pouch, and perform the pouch–anal anastomosis.

Nobody really knows if the ability to use small incisions with intracorporeal mobilization followed by an extended incision to complete the procedure is beneficial to a patient's recovery. Published series in the literature reflect a mixture of highly selected patients, and are merely descriptive[6-11]. None has proven that there are any advantages in doing abdominal bowel procedures laparoscopically. Initially there was considerable enthusiasm toward laparoscopic bowel surgery, but this seems to have waned recently. Prospective randomized trials are needed to answer these questions and prove if the hypothesis of faster recovery is true.

Other concepts are also being explored for laparoscopic bowel surgery. With the redesigning of laparoscopic instruments for intracorporeal anastomosis, attention is turning toward how to get the resected bowel out of the closed abdomen. We are working on minimizing incisions through morcellation, which involves inserting the specimen in a bag then grinding the tissue until it can be pulled through the trochar. Motility studies are also under way to determine if bowel activity recovers faster after laparoscopic surgery when compared with open conventional surgery.

In conclusion, laparoscopic intestinal surgery is feasible and can be performed safely after considerable training. Results regarding its benefits are preliminary at this stage. Currently, diagnostic laparoscopy, stoma construction, terminal ileal resection with extracorporeal anastomosis, and subtotal colectomy (in selected patients) are laparascopic procedures to consider in patients with inflammatory bowel disease.

One positive aspect that has already been achieved by laparoscopic bowel surgery is to make surgeons rethink the surgical paradigms taught for generations in surgical training institutions. We now know that, with conventional surgical cases, nasogastric tubes can be removed sooner, patients can be fed sooner and sent home earlier without compromising outcome[12,13]. Even if laparoscopic bowel surgery does not become as popular as laparoscopic cholecystectomy, the positive impact it has made on conventional bowel surgery will still be substantial.

References

1. Kum CK, Wong CW, Goh PMY, Ti TK. Comparative study of pain level and analgesic requirement after laparoscopic and open cholecystectomy. Surg Laparosc Endosc. 1994;4:139–41.
2. Myers WC, Branum GD, Farouk M *et al.* A prospective analysis of 1518 laparoscopic cholecystectomies. N Engl J Med. 1991;324:1073–8.

3. Schlumpf R, Klotz HP, Wehrli H, Herzog U. A nation's experience in laparoscopic cholecystectomy. Surg Endosc. 1994;8:35–41.
4. Airan I, Appel M, Berci G, Coburg AJ *et al.* Retrospective and prospective multi-institutional laparoscopic cholecystectomy study organized by the Society of American Gastrointestinal Endoscopic Surgeons. Surg Endosc. 1992;6:169–76.
5. Health Care Investment Analyst, Inc., Baltimore, Maryland. *Statistics 1993.*
6. Zucker KA, Pitcher DE, Martin DT, Ford RS. Laparoscopic-assisted colon resection. Surg Endosc. 1994;8:12–18.
7. Scoggin SD, Frazee RC, Snyder SK, Hendricks JC *et al.* Laparoscopic-assisted bowel surgery. Dis Colon Rectum. 1993;36:747–50.
8. Proceedings of the Third International Workshop on Colorectal Cancer. Rome, Italy, 3–4 March 1994: Laparoscopic Surgery Panel (in Dis Colon Rectum. 1994;37:S144–50).
9. Wexner SD, Johansen OB, Nogueras JJ, Jagelman DG. Laparoscopic total abdominal colectomy: a prospective trial. Dis Colon Rectum. 1992;35:651–5.
10. Franklin ME, Ramos R, Rosenthal D, Schuessler W. Laparoscopic colonic procedures. World J Surg. 1993;17:51–6.
11. Milsom JW, Lavery IC, Church JM, Stolfi VM, Fazio VW. Use of laparoscopic techniques in colorectal surgery: preliminary study. Dis Colon Rectum. 1994;37:215–18.
12. Binderow SR, Cohen SM, Wexner SD, Schmitt SL, Nogueras JJ, Jagelman DG. Must early postoperative oral intake be limited to laparoscopy? Poster presentation at the American Society of Colon and Rectal Surgeons. Chicago, Illinois. 2–7 May, 1993.
13. Schmitt SL, Wexner SD, Nogueras JJ, Jagelman DG. Does laparoscopy confer an advantage over standard colectomy? Poster presentation at the American Society of Colon and Rectal Surgeons. Chicago, Illinois, 2–7 May, 1993.

Section X
Lifestyle in IBD

33
Smoking

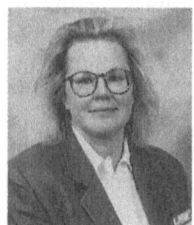

C. BENONI

INTRODUCTION

Due to the increasing incidence of inflammatory bowel disease (IBD), particularly the steep increase in Crohn's disease, a number of exogenous factors have been considered in the development of the diseases. These factors could be of importance both in the first attack and in recurrence and relapse.

During the past decade the smoking habit has been identified as a strong, perhaps the strongest, exogenous factor in IBD. Paradoxically, the diseases in this context are absolute opposites. A number of studies consistently show that smoking is associated with Crohn's disease, and nonsmoking, or former smoking, with ulcerative colitis. The smoking habit is not only associated with the first outbreak, but also seems to be of substantial importance during the clinical course of the diseases.

EPIDEMIOLOGICAL FINDINGS

In the early 1980s independent observations were made on the possible protective effects of smoking in ulcerative colitis[1-4]. It was earlier known that patients with ulcerative colitis smoked less than matched controls[5]. The author interpreted this as a consequence of the chronic disease.

Findings in a study of effects of smoking on nutritional status in IBD[6] initiated Harries and co-workers to study the smoking habit in patients with ulcerative colitis and Crohn's disease[1]. A low prevalence (8%) of smoking was found in ulcerative colitis. There were equal proportions of nonsmokers and ex-smokers. It was noted that the ex-smokers had usually given up smoking before the onset of symptoms. A Czech study by Bures and co-workers described the same association when compared to figures from the national population[2].

A male patient with ulcerative colitis who could not stop smoking due to relapses after stopping initiated our own study. We compared smoking habits in ulcerative colitis and Crohn's disease with national figures on smoking[3]. This design was chosen in order to evaluate the possible effects of the disease itself on the smoking habit. We found similar data with a low number of smokers in ulcerative colitis, but could also describe a distinct time-relationship between stopping smoking and disease onset. Gyde and co-workers reported a low number of cardiovascular and pulmonary deaths in male patients with ulcerative colitis[7]. This was followed up by the same authors in a risk factor study[4] and could, most probably, be attributed to the absence of smoking in ulcerative colitis.

The early reports of Harries stimulated others to study the relationship of smoking and ulcerative colitis in the Boston Collaborative Drug Surveillance Programme[8]. They confirmed that smoking was underrepresented in ulcerative colitis. A link between heavy smoking and lower risk was also found. Using community controls, Logan and co-workers showed an increased relative risk of 6.2 in nonsmokers of both sexes when smoking habits were examined at the onset of the disease[9]. They subsequently showed that the relative risk of ulcerative colitis in smokers was reduced to one-third of that of nonsmokers, and in ex-smokers was three-fold increased[10].

The primary interest of smoking in IBD concerned ulcerative colitis only. At the same time the first studies also pointed to a high number of smokers in Crohn's disease. In the study by Harries the positive association between smoking and Crohn's disease was not observed, probably due to the fact that the controls were chosen from patients with fractures and probably with a higher number of smokers than in the normal population[1]. We found that, compared with ulcerative colitis, smoking was significantly more common in Crohn's disease[3]. This was also the finding in a study by Holdstock *et al.*[11]. Somerville and co-workers, using the same design as in their former study on ulcerative colitis[9], described a significant positive association between smoking and Crohn's disease[12]. The association was stronger for the smoking habit before the onset of the disease than for current habits. The relative risk for smokers of both sexes at onset was nearly five times that of nonsmokers. It is worth noting that the risk for women smokers was eight times that of nonsmokers.

A number of epidemiological studies from different countries have followed. Despite different study designs the findings in all these studies are consistent. Selected studies are included in a meta-analysis by Calkins[13]. This analysis confirms that smokers have a reduced risk of ulcerative colitis and an increased risk of Crohn's disease. The study also shows an increased risk of ulcerative colitis in ex-smokers. A dose–response pattern is demonstrated in ulcerative colitis with a decreasing risk with increasing current smoking. In ex-smokers the risk increases with increasing former usage. No dose–response pattern can be demonstrated in Crohn's disease. The study also critically evaluates the findings against defined criteria for causality.

EFFECTS OF SMOKING HABIT ON THE CLINICAL COURSE

Evidence of a causal relationship between smoking habit and IBD would be further strengthened if the habit – or the changing of it – interfered with the clinical course of the diseases. Do we have further evidence of a truly beneficial effect of smoking in ulcerative colitis and a harmful effect in Crohn's disease? What is the impact of stopping smoking – and of taking it up again – in newly diagnosed or established ulcerative colitis? Does smoking influence the time of onset, the severity and the extension of the disease? In Crohn's disease, does smoking make the clinical course worse? Does it influence the distribution and localization of the inflammation? Could such an association give us any ideas on the biological explanation behind the findings?

Shortly after Harries' publication[1], case reports appeared by de Castella[14], and by Roberts and Diggle[15]. Two women with ulcerative colitis relapsed shortly after stopping smoking, and these relapses were reproducible. One patient came into remission by resuming smoking, the other by starting chewing nicotine gum. These reports arouse suspicions about the possible clinical role of stopping smoking in established ulcerative colitis, and the role of nicotine as the responsible protective agent.

Our own studies focused on the possible time-relationship between stopping smoking and disease onset in ulcerative colitis[3,16]. Such a relation in time would speak in favor of a beneficial effect of smoking. Among the ex-smokers a majority had their first attack 0–4 years after stopping. Ex-smoking was more common in men, and onsets after stopping smoking occurred at all ages. There was a male dominance among those who fell ill in the upper age groups. No time-relationship between stopping and onsets in Crohn's disease could be found.

A similar time-relationship was later demonstrated by Motley and co-workers[17]. Rudra et al. interviewed ex-smokers who had taken up smoking again, and half of them felt improvement after doing this[18].

Motley also described how the presence of a smoking history in men delayed the onset of ulcerative colitis with a mean of 15 years compared to never smoking. There was no such pattern in women[17].

Colectomy rate and hospitalization rate due to disease relapse are parameters of disease severity. Boyko and co-workers studied effects of smoking habit on the clinical course by comparing disease activity in smokers and nonsmokers measured by yearly number of hospitalizations and the need for a colectomy[19]. They found that both hospitalization and colectomy occurred more frequently in those patients who had stopped smoking before disease onset compared with smokers and never-smokers. They also found that smokers were hospitalized less often than nonsmokers, but that the colectomy rate was the same.

Irrespective of indication, we did not find any relationship between colectomy rate and smoking habit in our study, but we noted that the ex-smokers were older at the time of operation[3].

If smoking is protective in ulcerative colitis it would seem likely that it also protected against more extensive disease. When smoking habit and extension at the time of the diagnosis is considered, no correlation is found[9,16,17,20,21]. If, instead, disease extension at the time of the interview is considered, this would more adequately reflect a protective effect of smoking. This has been done in a study by Samuelsson and co-workers[22]. They showed that patients with extensive inflammation more seldom had a smoking history than those who had nonprogressive proctitis. This suggests a protective effect of cigarettes against disease extension.

If smoking is beneficial in ulcerative colitis, what evidence do we have of a harmful effect in Crohn's disease? It should be taken into consideration that the negative association between smoking and ulcerative colitis is likely to be a stronger finding than the positive association between smoking and Crohn's disease. Smoking in Crohn's disease may be associated with other lifestyle factors and those may, either by themselves or in combination with smoking, aggravate the inflammation. The use of oral contraceptives is an example of such possible interactive risk factors in Crohn's disease[23].

The effects of smoking on the clinical course in Crohn's disease have been addressed in some studies. Expressed as the frequency of relapses and the intensity of symptoms, it was demonstrated in the study by Holdstock and co-workers that smokers tended to have a more severe course compared to nonsmokers[11]. Sutherland and co-workers found that the recurrence rate, defined as the need for further surgery, was higher in smokers compared to nonsmokers[24]. This increased risk was found to be more apparent in women than in men, once again indicating sex differences. The authors also found evidence of a dose–response relationship in women which was not found in men. Lindberg and co-workers also confirm the association between heavy smoking and an increased risk of a second resection[25].

The findings of opposite smoking habits in Crohn's disease and ulcerative colitis raise the question if the presence of smoking in IBD may be associated with the localization of the inflammation. Is nonsmoking associated with isolated colonic disease and smoking with small bowel disease? There are data indicating this. In the study by Holdstock and colleagues it was found that patients with Crohn's colitis smoked less than those with small bowel disease[11]. Others also reported that small bowel disease was more frequent than isolated colonic or combined small and large bowel disease in those patients who were heavy smokers[25]. Thus, an association is reported in Crohn's disease, not only between heavy smoking and disease severity, but also between heavy smoking and small bowel disease. Whether smoking is protective to colonic disease in Crohn's disease as it is in ulcerative colitis should be evaluated further.

SMOKING AND TRENDS IN EPIDEMIOLOGY

Effects of smoking in IBD may also be seen in a wider perspective. Smoking habits have changed in society during recent decades. Men have stopped smoking and women have started smoking. These changes in smoking habits may have influenced the epidemiology in IBD during the same time. There seems to be some evidence that this might be the case. Ulcerative colitis seems to affect both sexes almost equally. Some studies, however, describe an increase in ulcerative colitis incidence in middle-aged and older men from the 1970s and onward[26,27]. The changed smoking habits in men should be considered when searching for an explanation to these findings.

Further evidence of such effects can be found in a review by Tysk and Järnerot[28]. These authors studied 60 years of epidemiologic studies in ulcerative colitis and plotted the male/female ratios. They find a change in sex distribution during these years so that ulcerative colitis, which once was a disease with a female dominance now seems to have turned to a disease with male dominance.

The increased risk of Crohn's disease in smokers is associated with female sex[13]. Studies covering IBD incidence during the last and present decades will answer the question whether the influence of smoking habit in IBD is strong enough to induce changes in epidemiology.

BIOLOGICAL ROLE OF SMOKING IN IBD

What is the biological role of smoking in IBD, and by what mechanisms does smoking exert its effects? As we do not know the pathogenesis in IBD, discussions on the biological effects of smoking remain hypothetical.

It has been proposed that Crohn's disease is a multifocal gastrointestinal infarction on the basis of a chronic mesenteric vasculitis[29]. As smoking has potent vascular injurious effects inducing a tendency for focal thrombosis, negative effects of smoking in Crohn's disease might well be explained by this[23]. Smoking in this context may also interact with other potentially disease-provoking factors in Crohn's disease; for example oral contraceptive use[23].

Smoking has a number of known effects on immune and inflammatory functions, some of which might explain a protective effect in ulcerative colitis. These studies have been done on alveolar cells or on blood cells, and the changes may not be relevant for local immune events in the gut. Effects on salivary immunoglobulins may, however, reflect general effects of smoking on mucosal immune functions.

Smoking influences both cell-mediated and humoral immunity. Light to moderate smoking increases the T-helper-inducer population while heavy smoking increases the T-suppressor cell population[30].

Smoking also lowers the circulating levels of serum immunoglobulins G, A and M[31], and also the level of salivary immunoglobulin A, which represents a mucosal immune response[32]. These effects are reversible. In addition, smoking interferes with macrophage functions as studied on alveolar macrophages obtained from bronchoalveolar lavage fluid. Smoking inhibits the release of leukotriene B4 (LTB4), thus reducing the cells' chemotactic abilities[33]; it also decreases the production of interleukin-1 from these cells[34]. In addition, smoking influences the function of circulating neutrophil leukocytes[35]. Extrinsic alveolitis and sarcoidosis are diseases which are underrepresented in smokers, possibly due to the effects of smoking on antigen presentation[34]. These effects of smoking may be representative also for immune and inflammatory response in the gut mucosa in ulcerative colitis.

Srivastava and co-workers have examined levels of immunoglobulin titres in gut lavage in smoking and nonsmoking patients with ulcerative colitis and in controls[36]. They found significantly reduced levels of IgA in lavage from smoking patients compared to controls, but no other differences. The smoking patients, however, had a low cigarette consumption, and it is possible that more substantial effects would have been seen with higher consumptions. Motley and co-workers have examined the immediate effects of smoking on the production of arachidonic acid metabolites in colonic mucosa[37]. There was a tendency, though not significant, for smokers to have a lower production. In smoking patients with ulcerative colitis Srivastava and co-workers have proposed that smoking may protect by lowering the rectal blood flow[38]. In addition, we have compared smoking habits in ulcerative colitis with 'model diseases'[39,40]. Systemic lupus erythematosus is a disorder with an accepted autoimmune pathogenesis. In rheumatoid arthritis a main event is a local infiltration of leukocytes in the synovia. Effects of smoking on immune and inflammatory function might be noticeable in the clinical course of these diseases. However, no such relationship has been reported.

Another rationale for a protective effect of smoking in ulcerative colitis may be that smoking influences intestinal permeability, and thus the uptake of potentially disease-provoking substances. This could be induced in different modes. The compositions of colonic mucus in smoking and nonsmoking patients with ulcerative colitis differed significantly in a study by Cope and co-workers[41]. Smokers were found to have a mucus production similar to control.

Principally, water-soluble substances in the gut can take two routes through the intestinal mucosa. It is proposed that PEG 400 passes transcellularly, and that $[^{51}Cr]EDTA$ passes paracellularly through the tight junctions[42]. When given orally, both substances are taken up along the small bowel. There is also, however, a significant uptake of $[^{51}Cr]EDTA$, but not of PEG 400, in the colon[42]. We have studied the effects of smoking on the urine excretion of $[^{51}Cr]EDTA$ and PEG 400[43] after an oral load. We found no differences in the 6-h urine excretions of PEG 400 between healthy smokers and never-smokers. The 24-h urine excretion of $[^{51}Cr]EDTA$, however, was significantly lower in smokers compared to never-smokers. These findings support an effect of smoking on the paracellular pathway – or an effect on colonic uptake. In an ongoing study on patients with well-defined ulcerative colitis in remission, we found a similar difference[40].

NICOTINE – THE PHARMACOLOGICALLY RESPONSIBLE AGENT?

There are thousands of substances in tobacco smoke. Which of these is responsible for the beneficial effect of smoking in ulcerative colitis? The role of nicotine was suggested early[15], and was introduced early in clinical trials.

Studies on limited unselected patient groups using chewing gum have not, however, shown any convincing effects[44]. In a recent study by Pullan and co-workers, transdermal nicotine was added to the treatment in active ulcerative colitis[45]. This study reported favorable effects both on symptoms and on endoscopic and histologic findings but requires confirmation in further trials.

So far there are indications that nicotine might be pharmacologically responsible for the biologic effects in ulcerative colitis. Even if this is so, we are still left with crucial questions. Who will benefit from nicotine treatment and when should it be started? Does it really have any advantages over traditional medical treatment in ulcerative colitis?

CONCLUSIONS AND CONSEQUENCES

A number of studies thus consistently show that smoking has profound effects in IBD both before disease onset and during its course. It is easier to understand biologically why smoking is harmful in Crohn's disease than beneficial in ulcerative colitis. Possibly this beneficial effect of smoking is exerted by nicotine, but further studies evaluating the role of nicotine in established disease are awaited.

Recent studies have described how passive smoking in childhood may be associated with IBD[46,47]. It is of the utmost importance to evaluate, clarify and confirm these findings, as they concern the information and advice that we give to our patients, as well as to their healthy relatives.

The most important consequence of the findings of an association between smoking and IBD concerns the advice given. Patients with IBD are very well informed and aware of lifestyle factors. Due to overall negative effects of smoking, the general rule must be that patients with IBD should be nonsmokers. Smokers with Crohn's disease should be offered help to stop. It would, however, seem reasonable to give individual advice to smoking patients with ulcerative colitis as to when and how they should stop smoking, taking into consideration both existing health status and existing life situation. In addition, selected ex-smokers with ulcerative colitis should be offered the possibility to try nicotine treatment instead of resuming smoking, if there is a positive history of smoking on their own clinical course.

References

1. Harries AD, Baird A, Rhodes J. Non-smoking: a feature of ulcerative colitis. Br Med J. 1982;284:706.
2. Bures J, Fixa B, Komarkova O, Fingerland A. Letter. Br Med J. 1982;285:440.
3. Benoni C, Nilsson Å. Smoking habits in patients with inflammatory bowel disease. Scand J Gastroenterol. 1984;19:824–30.
4. Gyde SN, Prior P, Alexander F et al. Ulcerative colitis: why is the mortality from cardiovascular disease reduced? Q J Med. 1984;211:351–7.
5. Samuelsson SM. Ulcerös colit och proctit. Uppsala: Department of Social Medicine, University of Uppsala, 1976 (thesis).
6. Harries AD, Jones L, Heatley RV, Rhodes J. Smoking habits and inflammatory bowel

disease: effect on nutrition. Br Med J. 1982;284:1161.
7. Gyde S, Prior P, Dew J, Saunders V, Waterhouse JAH, Allan RN. Mortality in ulcerative colitis. Gastroenterology. 1982;83:36–43.
8. Jick H, Walker AM. Cigarette smoking and ulcerative colitis. N Engl J Med. 1983;308:261–3.
9. Logan RFA, Edmond M, Somerville KW, Langman MJS. Smoking and ulcerative colitis. Br Med J. 1984;288:751–3.
10. Logan R, Langman MJS. Smoking and ulcerative colitis (Letter). Br Med J. 1984;288:1307.
11. Holdstock G, Savage D, Harman M, Wright R. Should patients with inflammatory bowel disease smoke? Br Med J. 1984;288:362.
12. Somerville KW, Logan RFA, Edmond M, Langman MJS. Smoking and Crohn's disease. Br Med J. 1984;289:954–6.
13. Calkins BM. A meta-analysis of the role of smoking in inflammatory bowel disease. Dig Dis Sci. 1989;34:1841–54.
14. De Castella H. Non smoking: a feature of ulcerative colitis (Letter). Br Med J. 1982;284:1706.
15. Roberts CJ, Diggle R. Non smoking: a feature of ulcerative colitis (Letter). Br Med J. 1982;285:440.
16. Benoni C, Nilsson Å. Smoking habits in patients with inflammatory bowel disease. A case–control study. Scand J Gastroenterol. 1987;22:1130–6.
17. Motley RJ, Rhodes J, Kay S, Morris TJ. Late presentation of ulcerative colitis in ex-smokers. Int J Colorect Dis. 1988;3:171–5.
18. Rudra T, Motley R, Rhodes J. Does smoking improve colitis? Scand J Gastroenterol. 1989;170(Suppl.):61–3.
19. Boyko EJ, Perera DR, Koepsell TD, Keane EM, Inui TS. Effects of cigarette smoking on the clinical course of ulcerative colitis. Scand J Gastroenterol. 1988;23:1147–52.
20. Tobin MV, Logan RFA, Langman MJS, McConnell RB, Gilmore IT. Cigarette smoking and inflammatory bowel disease. Gastroenterology. 1987;93:316–21.
21. Srivastava ED, Newcomb RG, Rhodes J, Avramidis P, Mayberry JF. Smoking and ulcerative colitis: a community study. Int J Colorect Dis. 1993;8:71–4.
22. Samuelsson SM, Ekbom A, Zack M, Helmick CG, Adami HO. Risk factors for extensive ulcerative colitis and ulcerative proctitis: a population based case–control study. Gut. 1991;32:1526–30.
23. Wakefield AJ, Sawyerr AM, Hudson M, Dhillon AP, Pounder RE. Smoking, the oral contraceptive pill, and Crohn's disease. Dig Dis Sci. 1991;36:1147–50.
24. Sutherland LR, Ramcharan S, Bryant H, Fick G. Effect of cigarette smoking on recurrence of Crohn's disease. Gastroenterology. 1990;98:1123–8.
25. Lindberg E, Järnerot G, Huitfeldt B. Smoking in Crohn's disease: effect on localisation and clinical course. Gut. 1992;33:779–82.
26. Nordenvall B, Broström O, Berglund M et al. Incidence of ulcerative colitis in Stockholm County 1955–1979. Scand J Gastroenterol. 1985;20:783–90.
27. Binder V, Both H, Hansen PK, Hendriksen C, Kreiner S, Torp-Pedersen K. Incidence and prevalence of ulcerative colitis and Crohn's disease in the County of Copenhagen, 1962–1978. Gastroenterology. 1982;83:563–8.
28. Tysk C, Järnerot G. Has smoking changed the epidemiology of ulcerative colitis? Scand J Gastroenterol. 1992;27:508–12.
29. Wakefield AJ, Sawyerr AM, Dhillon AP et al. Pathogenesis of Crohn's disease: multifocal gastrointestinal infarction. Lancet. 1989;2:1057–62.
30. Miller LG, Goldstein G, Murphy M, Ginns LC. Reversible alterations in immunoregulatory T cells in smoking. Analysis by monoclonal antibodies and flow cytometry. Chest. 1982;82:526–9.
31. Gerrard JW, Heiner DC, Ko CG, Mink J, Meyers A, Dosman JA. Immunoglobulin levels in smokers and non-smokers. Ann Allergy. 1980;44:261–2.
32. Barton JR, Riad MA, Gaze MN, Maran AGD, Ferguson A. Mucosal immunodeficiency in smokers, and in patients with epithelial head and neck tumours. Gut. 1990;31:378–82.
33. Tardif J, Borgeat P, Laviolette M. Inhibition of human alveolar macrophage production of leukotriene B4 by acute in vitro and in vivo exposure to tobacco smoke. Am J Respir Cell Mol Biol. 1990;2:155–61.
34. Yamaguchi E, Okazaki N, Itoh A, Abe S, Kawakami Y, Okuyama H. Interleukin-1

production by alveolar macrophages is decreased in smokers. Am Rev Respir Dis. 1989;140:397–402.

35. Noble RC, Penny BB. Comparison of leukocyte count and function in smoking and non-smoking young men. Infect Immun. 1975;12:550–5.
36. Srivastava ED, Barton JR, O'Mahony S et al. Smoking, humoral immunity and ulcerative colitis. Gut. 1991;32:1016–19.
37. Motley RJ, Rhodes J, Williams G, Tavares IA, Bennet A. Smoking, eicosanoids and ulcerative colitis. J Pharm Pharmacol. 1990;42:288–9.
38. Srivastavaa ED, Russell MAH, Feyerabend C, Rhodes J. Effect of ulcerative colitis and smoking on rectal blood flow. Gut. 1990;31:1021–4.
39. Benoni C, Nilsson Å. Smoking and inflammatory bowel disease: comparison with systemic lupus erythematosus. A case–control study. Scand J Gastroenterol. 1990;25:751–5.
40. Benoni C. Inflammatory bowel disease. Studies on the role of smoking. Doctoral dissertation, Lund University. 1991.
41. Cope GF, Heatley RV, Kelleher J. Smoking and colonic mucus in ulcerative colitis. Br Med J. 1986;293:481.
42. Travis S, Menzies I. Intestinal permeability: functional assessment and significance. Clin Sci. 1992;82:471–88.
43. Prytz H, Benoni C, Tagesson C. Does smoking tighten the gut? Scand J Gastroenterol. 1989;24:1084–8.
44. Lashner BA, Hanauer SB, Silverstein MD. Testing nicotine gum for ulcerative colitis patients. Experience with single-patient trials. Dig Dis Sci. 1990;35:827–32.
45. Pullan RD, Rhodes J, Ganesh S et al. Transdermal nicotine for active ulcerative colitis. N Engl J Med. 1994;330:811–15.
46. Persson P-G, Ahlbom A, Hellers G. Inflammatory bowel disease and tobacco smoke – a case–control study. Gut. 1990;31:1377–81.
47. Sandler RS, Sandler DP, McDonnell CW, Wurzelmann JI. Childhood exposure to environmental tobacco smoke and the risk of ulcerative colitis. Am J Epidemiol. 1992;135:603–8.

34
Nutritional advice

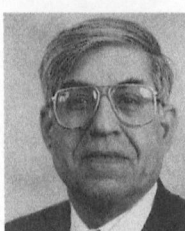

K. N. JEEJEEBHOY

INTRODUCTION

Inflammatory bowel diseases (IBD) have profound effects on nutritional status due to:

1. anorexia,
2. mechanical obstruction and motility disorders,
3. increased requirements,
4. decreased absorption,
5. gastrointestinal losses.

In a recent prospective study of 154 consecutive patients referred to the gastrointestinal clinic of a teaching hospital 11 out of 47 (23%) with Crohn's disease had significant protein–energy malnutrition. In contrast only 11 out of the remaining 107 (10%) patients with other significant gastrointestinal diseases had protein–energy malnutrition[1]. The resulting malnutrition has significant adverse effects on the clinical status and quality of life of the individual. Deficiency of micronutrients such as iron[2], folate[3], zinc[4] and vitamin B_{12} have been recognized for several years. Nutritional support has greatly improved our ability to manage acute episodes of this disease, to prevent long-term deficiency states and to treat patients with a short bowel.

EFFECT OF NUTRITION ON DISEASE ACTIVITY

In addition nutritional support may not only benefit the nutritional status of the patient but may influence the activity of Crohn's disease. It was postulated that keeping patients NPO (nil per os) should induce a remission by 'resting the bowel'. Bowel rest (no food intake) inevitably causes malnutrition, and total parenteral nutrition (TPN) was given to both rest the bowel and maintain nutrition.

EFFECTS OF TPN AND BOWEL REST ON THE ACTIVITY OF CROHN'S DISEASE

In a series of 100 patients[5] selected on the basis of not having responded to maximum medical therapy, which included several weeks of high-dose prednisone, the addition of TPN and bowel rest was effective in inducing a remission in 75% of patients. In these 100 patients taken as a whole the Crohn's disease activity index (CDAI) fell from a mean of 300–375 to below 100. Nutritionally the mean rise in serum albumin was 0.4 g/dl and weight gain was 1.6 kg.

DOES BOWEL REST WORK?

Bowel rest *per se* has no effect on the disease, but even patients resistant to prednisone improved when given nutritional support. The possibility that nutritional support may aid remission is supported by studies showing that diet counselling and better oral nutrition improve outcome[6,7].

ROLE OF ENTERAL NUTRITION IN INDUCING DISEASE REMISSION

Controlled trials[8-10] showed that enteral feeding is as effective as prednisone in inducing a remission. However, two others studies[11,12], both multicenter and based on 95 and 107 patients respectively, concluded that drug therapy was superior to enteral feeding. It is unclear how enteral diets induce a remission. The main theories include: (1) provision of nutritional support; (2) acting as a medical bypass; (3) hypoallergenicity; and (4) alteration of bowel flora.

ROLE OF ENTERAL DIETS IN AIDING DISEASE REMISSION AND GROWTH RETARDATION

Belli *et al.*[13] found that intermittent elemental diet feeding not only encouraged growth but reduced disease activity.

ROLE OF FOOD INTOLERANCE AND ELIMINATION DIETS IN THE THERAPY OF CROHN'S DISEASE

In 77 patients it was shown that by a personalized food exclusion program the annual relapse rate was only 11%[14].

ROLE OF SPECIFIC NUTRIENTS IN THE CONTROL OF INTESTINAL INFLAMMATION

Short-chain fatty acids nourish the mucosa and ω-3 fatty acids inhibit the production of proinflammatory leukotriene B_4 from arachidonic acid[15]. These substances may help control IBD.

ROLE OF NUTRITIONAL THERAPY IN IBD

It is abundantly clear that IBD, especially Crohn's disease, causes nutritional deficiency which, if associated with a short bowel or chronic obstruction, can be severe. It is also clear that nutritional support can successfully treat nutritional deficiency and improve function, promote restitution of body mass and prevent septic complications. Therefore in this context nutrition has an important therapeutic role in the management of IBD. The more contentious issue is whether nutrition can control active IBD in the same way as medications. The data are far from clear, but it is possible to arrive at a few practical (not necessarily proven) conclusions:

1. Nutritional treatment is not likely to induce a remission in patients with colitis.
2. Enteral feeding can induce disease remission in adults and children and promote growth in children.
3. The efficacy of enteral diets seems to depend upon patient acceptance and the ability to consume them for prolonged periods.
4. The data showing that TPN can induce disease remission are indirect, and their use should be reserved for patients in whom enteral feeding is impossible.
5. It remains to be determined whether the elemental nature, nutrient content, or the pharmacologic effect of nutrients are important for the success of this form of therapy.
6. The use of elimination diets, short-chain fatty acids and fish oils remains experimental.

References

1. Gee Mi, Grace MGA, Wensel RH, Sherbaniuk R, Thomson ABR. Protein–energy malnutrition in gastroenterology outpatients: Increased risk in Crohn's disease. J Am Diet Assoc. 1985;85:1466–74.
2. Child JA, Brozovic B, Dyer NH, Moller DL, Dawson AM. The diagnosis of iron deficiency in patients with Crohn's disease. Gut. 1973;14:642–8.
3. Franklin JM, Rosenberg IH. Impaired folic acid absorption in inflammatory bowel disease: Effects of salicylazosulfapyridine (Asulfadine). Gastroenterology. 1973;64:517–25.
4. Solomons NW, Rosenberg IH, Sandstead HH, Vokhactu DP. Zinc deficiency in Crohn's disease. Digestion. 1977;16:87–95.
5. Ostro MJ, Greenberg GR, Jeejeebhoy KN. Total parenteral nutrition and complete bowel rest in the management of Crohn's disease. J Parenter Enter Nutr. 1985;9:280–7.
6. Imes S, Pinchbeck B, Thomson AB. Diet counselling improves the clinical course of patients with Crohn's disease. Digestion. 1988;39:7–19.
7. Afdhal NH, Kelly J, McCormick PA, O'Donoghue DP. Remission induction in refractory

Crohn's disease using a high calorie whole diet. J Parenter Enteral Nutr. 1989;13:362–5.

8. O'Morain C, Segal AW, Levi AJ. Elemental diets as primary therapy of acute Crohn's disease: a controlled trial. Br Med J. 1984;288:1859–62.

9. Saverymuttu S, Hodgson HJF, Chadwick VS. Controlled trial comparing prednisolone with an elemental diet plus non-absorbable antibiotics in active Crohn's disease. Gut. 1985;26:994–8.

10. Gonzales-Huix F, de Leon R, Fernandez-Banares F et al. Polymeric enteral diets as primary treatment of active Crohn's disease: a prospective steroid controlled trial. Gut. 1993;34:778–82.

11. Malchow H, Steinhardt HJ, Lorenz-Meyer H et al. Feasibility and effectiveness of a defined-formula diet regimen in treating active Crohn's disease. European Cooperative Crohn's Disease Study III. Scand J Gastroenterol. 1990;25:235–44.

12. Lochs H, Steinhardt HJ, Klaus-Wentz B et al. Comparison of enteral nutrition and drug treatment in active Crohn's disease. Gastroenterology. 1991;101:881–8.

13. Belli DC, Seidman E, Bouthillier L et al. Chronic intermittent elemental diet improves growth failure in children with Crohn's disease. Gastroenterology. 1988;94:603–10.

14. Alun Jones V. Comparison of total parenteral nutrition and elemental diet in induction of remission of Crohn's disease. Long-term maintenance of remission by personalized food exclusion diets. Dig Dis Sci. 1987;32(Suppl.):100–7S.

15. Lee TH, Hoover RI, Williams JD et al. Effect of dietary enrichment with eicosapentaenoic and docosahexaenoic acids on in vitro neutrophil and monocyte leukotriene generation and neutrophil function. N Engl J Med. 1985;312:1217–24.

35
IBD, the oral contraceptive pill and pregnancy

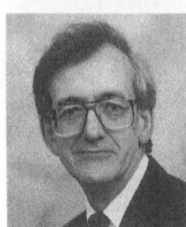

R. N. ALLAN

This chapter summarizes our current knowledge of the role of the oral contraceptive pill in the pathogenesis of inflammatory bowel disease (IBD), followed by a review of fertility in women and men. The next section considers IBD and pregnancy, including the impact on the fetus and the mother with ulcerative colitis or Crohn's disease. The chapter then considers the safety of drug treatment and the outcome of surgical treatment during pregnancy and the problems that may be encountered during pregnancy in patients with an ileostomy or ileoanal pouch. The chapter closes with a review of the short- and long-term prognosis of ulcerative colitis and Crohn's disease after parturition.

ORAL CONTRACEPTIVE PILL AND PATHOGENESIS

Several large studies have shown a small increase in the prevalence of ulcerative colitis and Crohn's disease among users of the oral contraceptive pill compared with nonusers. The differences were not large enough to reach statistical significance. For example in the study of Logan and Kay in 1989[1] the relative risk of developing Crohn's disease when users were compared with nonusers was 1.7, and for patients with ulcerative colitis was 1.3. Neither reached statistical significance.

In a study by Lesko *et al.*[2] the overall excess among patients with Crohn's disease who used the oral contraceptive pill compared with nonusers showed an overall relative risk of 1.9, but the risk was greatly increased in recent users (relative risk 4.3) compared with ex-users (relative risk 1.2). Most studies have shown that this small excess relative risk returns to normal when the oral contraceptive is discontinued.

What are we to make of these data? The overwhelming message is that the oral contraceptive pill is safe, and is only rarely associated with the development of ulcerative colitis or Crohn's disease. The data could probably be best interpreted as suggesting that a small subset of individuals develop a pill-related colitis indistinguishable from ulcerative colitis and Crohn's colitis, which resolves on withdrawing the oral contraceptive pill. The clinical message is that, for any oral contraceptive user with ulcerative colitis or Crohn's disease who has not responded to standard therapy, withdrawal of the oral contraceptive pill should be considered, provided of course that alternative contraceptive measures are offered at the same time.

FERTILITY IN WOMEN

Ulcerative colitis

Several excellent studies have shown that fertility in women with ulcerative colitis is normal and identical to that in the general population. Thus in a large series of married women with ulcerative colitis, 81% conceived normally, 12% voluntarily avoided pregnancy, 2% of husbands had oligospermia and 5% were unable to have children. These figures are equivalent to the general population, for example 10% of UK marriages are childless[3].

Crohn's disease

There is good evidence that fertility of women with Crohn's disease is impaired. Mayberry and Weterman (1986)[4] undertook an extensive European study and showed that patients with Crohn's disease had only half the number of children produced by healthy control couples.

There are several good reasons to explain this finding, but the exact explanation has not yet been defined. The possibilities include the severity of disease; avoiding pregnancy on medical advice; dyspareunia, particularly in the presence of severe perianal disease; and impaired ovulation or Fallopian tube blockage following pelvic sepsis complicating Crohn's disease.

FERTILITY IN MEN

It is well recognized that fertility may be affected in men taking sulfasalazine by both reducing the total sperm count and motility, but that this effect is reversible after withdrawing the drug[5]. The sulfapyridine moiety is probably responsible, since this problem was not found with other 5-ASA preparations. There is evidence that active Crohn's disease may cause oligospermia in some men, and thus directly account for infertility.

IMPACT OF IBD ON PREGNANCY

Ulcerative colitis – impact on the fetus

Several studies have shown that pregnancy in ulcerative colitis usually results in a normal full-term baby. Low birth weight or fetal abnormality are no greater than that expected in the general population.

Willoughby[6] summarized the 14 major studies on the outcome of pregnancy in women with ulcerative colitis and showed that among 1466 pregnancies a normal livebirth resulted in 1238 (84%). The incidence of spontaneous abortion (8%), therapeutic abortion (5%), congenital abnormalities (1%) and stillbirth (1%) was similar to that observed in the healthy population.

Ulcerative colitis – impact on the mother

In patients with established ulcerative colitis in remission at the time of conception, the disease is likely to remain quiescent throughout pregnancy and the puerperium. Active disease at the time of conception is more likely to be associated with recurrence of symptoms during pregnancy which are commonest during the first trimester of pregnancy. In the past, relapse of disease in the puerperium was accepted as a commonplace finding, but this has not been substantiated in practice. Occasionally ulcerative colitis has arisen for the first time during pregnancy.

Crohn's disease – impact on the fetus

Excellent data on Crohn's disease and pregnancy are available from a recent study from Woolfson and his colleagues (1990)[7]. They studied 78 pregnancies among 50 patients with Crohn's disease. The incidence of spontaneous abortion, babies small for dates, premature birth, respiratory distress and fetal abnormality were similar to those expected in the general population.

At the time of conception 79% had inactive Crohn's disease, and in general a poorer fetal outcome was found among patients with active disease at the time of conception. There was no evidence that appropriate medical or surgical treatment affected the outcome for the fetus.

Crohn's disease – impact on the mother

The outlook for the mother is particularly favorable if the Crohn's disease is quiescent at the time of conception, when 70% of them remain symptom-free during pregnancy and the puerperium. Individual case reports have been described of Crohn's disease presenting either during pregnancy or shortly after delivery, but both these events are distinctly unusual.

From these data, clear guidelines emerge: the overall prospects for pregnancy and Crohn's disease are good, but patients should avoid becoming pregnant when their disease is active, since it impairs the outcome of both the pregnancy and the underlying Crohn's disease.

SURGICAL TREATMENT DURING PREGNANCY

There are a number of individual case reports and small series reporting a satisfactory outcome in pregnant patients undergoing surgery for their IBD, but the reported numbers are too small to draw reliable conclusions.

PREGNANCY IN ILEOSTOMY PATIENTS

Willoughby[8] has summarized nine studies of patients who became pregnant after surgical treatment with an ileostomy for ulcerative colitis. Among 119 pregnancies the outcome for the fetus was similar to that expected in the general population. Among the 119 pregnancies there were 18 stoma problems including intestinal obstruction (nine), stoma prolapse (five), leakage from round the stoma (two), intususception (one) and one further undefined problem.

Individual case reports and small series of pouch patients who have undergone successful and uneventful pregnancy have been reported[9].

DRUG TREATMENT DURING PREGNANCY

Sulfasalazine

While high-dose sulfonamides can cause congenital abnormalities in the offspring of pregnant rats, there are no published reports of sulfasalazine-associated congenital abnormalities in humans. Indeed, extensive studies of sulfasalazine in pregnancy have shown no adverse effect on the chances of producing a normal child[10]. Recent studies of oral 5-aminosalicylic acid for IBD in pregnancy have shown that its use is safe both for the fetus and mother[11].

Metronidazole

There are no large reports of the use of metronidazole during pregnancy in patients with IBD. However, there are several large studies of pregnant patients taking metronidazole during pregnancy for trichomonas vaginalis. No adverse effect on the fetus was found. In particular, birth weight, the incidence of stillbirths and congenital abnormalities was exactly that expected in the general population[12].

Immunosuppressive therapy

There are no large studies of the use of azathioprine during pregnancy in patients with IBD. The nearest equivalent is the data analyzed from those women receiving azathioprine during pregnancy following renal transplantation. The data collected from 49 papers describe the outcome of

434 pregnancies and 375 women, of whom 356 (82%) resulted in overtly normal infants, a figure close to that expected in the general population[13].

BREAST FEEDING IN IBD PATIENTS TAKING SULFASALAZINE

Sulfasalazine and sulfapyridine are secreted into breast milk, and theoretically sulfasalazine could bind to circulating albumen and displace unconjugated bilirubin. However, it is now clear that sulfasalazine binds to albumen at sites other than high-affinity sites for bilirubin, and is not therefore a risk factor for the development of kernicterus in the breast-fed infant[14].

LONG-TERM OUTCOME AFTER PREGNANCY

Ulcerative colitis

The symptomatic pattern of ulcerative colitis in the first pregnancy cannot be used to predict the symptomatic pattern in subsequent pregnancies.

Crohn's disease

Interesting evidence is emerging that parity in women with Crohn's disease improves the long-term outcome, in that women in the postpartum period have fewer exacerbations and undergo fewer resections than nonparous controls with Crohn's disease. This beneficial effect was evident in patients with both distal ileal and colonic Crohn's disease. In nonparous patients with ileal disease, after a mean follow-up of 15 years, the mean number of resections per patient was 1.52 compared with a mean resection rate of 1.17 in those who had been pregnant prior to diagnosis. The interval from first to second resection was 10 years in nonparous patients and 13 years in parous patients. Similar data were evident in patients with colonic Crohn's disease, where the number of resections per patient was less in those who had been pregnant before diagnosis and the interval from first to subsequent resection was much longer[15]. The mechanism for this protective effect of pregnancy on the outcome of Crohn's disease is uncertain, but pregnancy could influence the natural history of Crohn's disease either by decreasing immune responsiveness or by retarding fibrous stricture formation, which is the commonest indication for surgical intervention, particularly in patients with distal ileal disease.

References

1. Logan RFA, Kay CR, Scott L. The pill, smoking and inflammatory bowel disease: results from the RCGP oral contraceptive study. Int Epidemiol. 1989;18:105–7.
2. Lesko SM, Kaufman DW, Rosenberg L et al. Evidence for an increased risk of Crohn's disease in oral contraceptive users. Gastroenterology. 1985;89:1046–9.
3. Willoughby CP, Truelove SC. Ulcerative colitis and pregnancy. Gut. 1980;21:469–74.

4. Mayberry JF, Weterman IT. European survey of fertility and pregnancy in women with Crohn's disease: a case-control study by European collaborative group. Gut. 1986;27:821–5.

5. Cann PA, Holdsworth CD. Reversal of male infertility on changing treatment from sulphasalazine to 5 amino salicylate. Lancet. 1984;1:1119.

6. Willoughby CP. Fertility, pregnancy and inflammatory bowel disease. In: Allan RN, Keighley MRB, Hawkins CF, Alexander-Williams J, editors. Inflammatory bowel diseases, 2nd edn. Edinburgh: Churchill Livingstone; 1990:547–58.

7. Woolfson K, Cohen Z, McLeod RS. Crohn's disease and pregnancy. Dis Col Rectum. 1990;33:869–73.

8. Willoughby CP. Fertility, pregnancy and inflammatory bowel disease. In: Allan RN, Keighley MRB, Hawkins CF, Alexander-Williams J, editors. Inflammatory bowel diseases, 2nd edn. Edinburgh: Churchill-Livingstone; 1990:555.

9. Metcalf A, Dozois RR, Beart RW, Wolff BG. Pregnancy following ileal pouch–anal anastomosis. Dis Colon Rectum. 1985;28:859–61.

10. Nielson OH, Andreasson B, Bondesen S, Jacobson O, Jarnum S. Pregnancy in Crohn's disease. Scand J Gastroenterol. 1984;19:724–32.

11. Habal FM, Hui G, Greenberg GR. Oral 5-aminosalicylic acid for inflammatory bowel disease in pregnancy: safety and clinical course. Gastroenterology. 1993;105:1057–60.

12. Piper JM, Mitchell EF, Ray WA. Prenatal use of metronidazole and birth defects: no association. Obstet Gynaecol. 1993;82:348–52.

13. Davies PM. Azathioprine in pregnancy. Wellcome Foundation, personal communication.

14. Jarnerot G, Anderson S, Esbjorner E, Sandstrom B, Brodersen R. Albumin reserve for binding of bilirubin in maternal and cord serum under treatment with sulphasalazine. Scand J Gastroenterol. 1981;16:1049–55.

15. Nwokolo CU, Tan WC, Andrews HA, Allan RN. Surgical resections in parous patients with distal ileal and colonic Crohn's disease. Gut. 1994;35:220–3.

36
The social toll of IBD

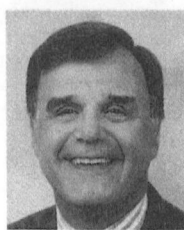

R. G. FARMER

The 'human cost' of inflammatory bowel disease (IBD) is not easily assessed or quantified. The most obvious measure would be death, but this occurs in fewer than 5% of IBD patients[1]. The second most obvious measure would be the number of operations, or some assessment of disease severity. However, as is well known[2,3], IBD – both ulcerative colitis (UC) and Crohn's disease (CD) – is characterized by unpredictability of exacerbation and remission. Since the majority of patients afflicted are diagnosed between the ages of 15 and 35[4], and with the low mortality rate, efforts have been made to quantify various elements which are associated with morbidity. Since patients with IBD are often found in a higher socioeconomic level than the general public[5], the loss of work and income can also be used; however, as can be easily seen, these measures are exceedingly difficult to assess.

In recent years attempts have been made to quantify the disease activity as well as the quality of life assessment for patients with IBD[6-8]. These measures have proved elusive, as they are usually from the medical (or the physician's) perspective, and emphasis is often placed on symptoms and clinical findings[9,10]. A major complicating factor in such assessments has been the unpredictable nature of the disease on the one hand, and presumed psychological aspects on the other[11].

Currently, there have been attempts to define more accurately and scientifically the various aspects of quality of life for patients with IBD. Garrett and Drossman[12] defined the 'biological and behavioral considerations' of the health status of patients with IBD to include the following: disease activity, psychological state, cultural influences, social support, effects of complications, previous surgery, and medications. Drossman *et al.* also described the 'functional states and patient worries' in IBD using a specific

Table 1 IBD: costs of illness

Crohn's disease – average annual medical cost per patient, 1990, US = $6561.00
Total annual medical cost, US = $1.0–1.2 billion
Ulcerative colitis – annual medical cost per patient, 1990, US = $1488
Total annual medical cost, US = $0.4–0.6 billion
Adjusting for productivity losses – annual economic cost for IBD, US = $1.8–2.6 billion
Top 2% of Crohn's patients accounted for 34.3% of total amount

Data from ref. 14

instrument for detection[13]. They observed that IBD patients experienced moderate functional impairment, but more in the social and psychological sphere than in the physical dimensions, CD patients have more psychological dysfunction than UC patients, and IBD patients generally have their greatest concerns regarding the need for surgery, their degree of energy, and their body image. Drossman et al.[13] concluded that the functional status and patient concerns correlate better than physician rating of symptoms.

Likewise, there has beeen an attempt to quantify the economic cost for patients with IBD. This was estimated by Hay and Hay[14] as having an economic impact in the USA of more than two billion dollars per year. An important observation was that the top 2% of CD patients accounted for more than one-third of the total health-care expenditures for patients with IBD (Table 1). However, as one assesses this ability for patients with IBD, European studies have demonstrated that only 3% of patients with IBD are permanently disabled[11,15]. In a German study it was noted that this ability was twice that among young females as it was for either male patients or older persons with IBD; however, the vast majority of patients remained employed, although functioning suboptimally.

In attempts to define and quantify the quality of life for patients with IBD, attention has focused primarily on the results of surgery, particularly with patients with UC. McLeod et al.[16] showed that there was no significant difference for quality of life for the type of operation for patients with UC (pouch or standard ileostomy) but that generally quality of life improved after surgery. Likewise Sagar et al.[17] noted that, in comparison with medically treated patients with UC, those who had undergone (presumably curative) surgery had a better quality of life, and there was more depression and limitation of social activity by patients who were treated medically.

The pelvic pouch operation had understandably received specific attention in terms of quality of life assessment, and Tjandra et al. from the Cleveland Clinic described similar functional results among patients who had undergone this procedure for UC and those for familial polyposis[18]. In a large study from the Mayo Clinic[19], encompassing 240 patients over an 8-year period, it was noted that overall quality of life was satisfactory, and patients were able to function reasonably well by comparison with their peers 90% of the time[19].

Assessment of the quality of life for patients following medical therapy has been more difficult to accomplish, and Irvine and her colleagues at McMaster University in Hamilton, Ontario have had a particular interest in assessing the results of clinical trials[8,9]. In a recent study of 305 patients with IBD, a multicenter study of cyclosporine vs. placebo was carried out using a quality-of-life instrument as a measure of therapeutic efficacy. This study[20] showed that quality-of-life assessment compared well with the CDAI[6], and also correlated with the clinical assessment quite satisfactorily. Thus, a number of recent studies have indicated the value of quality-of-life assessment, but the optimal instrument to assess and quantify the quality of life continues to be a challenge.

Because of a long-term interest in IBD[21], and a registry of patients developed over 15–20 years, we were able to develop cohorts of patients followed at the Cleveland Clinic Foundation whose quality of life could be measured[22]. The study group consisted of 164 patients with IBD, both UC and CD, with or without operation. Patients selected had IBD for approximately 10 years, with disease onset at about age 20.

To ensure applicability to outpatient care the survey questionnaire was designed for use with ambulatory patients who are functioning in society; this characterizes most patients with IBD[3,4]. Therefore, questions assess activities of daily living rather than focusing on either medical or psychological issues.

Four broad categories of questions were developed for the IBD questionnaire (Table 2).

1. Functional/economic – the ability to function in work, school, and home, to support self and others, and to advance professionally.
2. Social/recreational – interpersonal relationships including those with spouse or significant other and family, sexual relationships, relationships in social settings, and ability to perform recreational, leisure and social activities.
3. Affect/life in general – attitude toward life and health, presence of optimism or pessimism (e.g. depression) and ability to plan for the future.
4. Medical – gastrointestinal and other symptoms, use of medication, history of surgery, interaction with health-care professionals and relationship with physician.

Answers were scored using the Likert scale of 1–5 (strongly agree to strongly disagree). Questions were phrased both positively and negatively, to avoid repetition of answers.

The survey was administered during a 2-month period in 1988 and was repeated as a 1-year follow up in 1989. Our experience with long-term follow-up studies discouraged us from using physicians to administer the survey, because of their orientation toward clinical manifestations of disease and treatment. The 47 questions were administered by nonphysician interviewers in person or by telephone. Questions were short, grammatically simple and free from clinical terminology. Completion took 15–20 min. The instrument could also be used as a self-administered questionnaire.

Univariate analysis of 45 instrument questions to determine whether scores differed by group (UC, surgery; UC, no prior surgery; CD, surgery; CD, no prior surgery) resulted in 18 questions yielding statistically significant or marginally significant results[22]. The other two questions listed multiple physical activities and medications, and were reported descriptively. The

Table 2 IBD: quality-of-life questionnaire

Category	First year	Follow-up year
I. Functional/economic		
1. I have been able to fulfil my educational goals		
2. I am able to support myself and my family		
3. I am receiving financial support from a source other than from my employment		
4. I am having difficulty getting insurance		
5. I feel that I am able to get through each day as well as others	+ +	+ +
6. My earnings are as good as others in similar jobs or activities		
7. My disease has made it difficult for me to obtain a job	+ +	
8. My symptoms interfere with my job or activities		+
9. In comparing myself to others, I feel I have less energy	+ +	+ +
10. I am able to carry out my regular activities in a way satisfying to me	+	
11. I feel I have been able to move ahead in my job, family responsibilities or school		
12. My growth and physical development were affected by my illness		
II. Social/recreational		
1. I am able to enjoy activities with my family	+ +	+ +
2. I have someone to talk to about the way I feel		+
3. I feel isolated because of my disease	+	+
4. I cancelled an activity/activities this past month because of symptoms	+	+ +
5. I feel frightened by the future	+	+
6. I can participate in social activities with friends		
7. I can depend on my family or friends for support		
8. I am able to participate in a recreational/sport activity regularly	+ +	
9. The physical activity I participate in at least once a week is [fill in]:		
10. I belong to and participate regularly in a club/church/professional organization		
11. I feel satisfied with my relationship with my spouse or significant other		
12. I feel satisfied about the way I participate in family activities	+	
13. My disease has made it difficult for me to have a family	+ +	+ +
14. My condition has made it difficult for me to share intimate relationships		+
15. I participate in a hobby or special interest in addition to my other tasks		
III. Affect/life in general		
1. I have made plans for things to do next month		
2. Most of the time I sleep through the night	+ +	+ +
3. I have made plans for things I will be doing a year from now	+ +	
4. My life is going along pretty much as I had planned		
5. When compared with other persons of my age, I feel pleased with my accomplishments		

continued

Table 2 *continued*

Category	First year	Follow-up year
6. I feel frustrated with my health problems	+	+
7. I look forward to each day		
8. I frequently worry about my health		
9. In comparison to other people, I feel I become more easily discouraged		
10. I find that I need mood-elevating medications to help get me through the day		
11. Others see me as chronically ill		
IV. Medical/symptoms		
1. I would describe my general physical condition in comparison to others as [fill in]:		
2. I find myself preoccupied with what I eat		
3. My symptoms significantly affect the way I function each day	+	+
4. I have abdominal pain frequently	+	
5. My diarrhea is disruptive [i.e. does it interfere with your daily life?]	+	+
6. I have difficulty maintaining my weight	+	
7. I take medications		
8. I take the following medications once a day [fill in]:		
9. Do you feel your doctor has been supportive and understanding of your feelings?		

This table is copyright 1989, Richard G. Farmer, MD, Cleveland Clinic Foundation. +, Response marginally significant ($0.05 \leq p \leq 0.01$); + +, Response statistically significant ($p \leq 0.01$)

scores indicate that:

1. Patients with UC have a better quality of life than patients with CD ($p < 0.009$). (Additionally, surgery impacted the score ($p < 0.003$); there was no interactive effect between disease and surgery.)
2. Nonsurgical UC patients have a better quality of life than surgical UC patients and CD patients regardless of whether the latter group has undergone surgery.
3. Nonsurgical CD patients have a better quality of life than surgical CD patients.
4. CD patients who have unergone surgery have the worst quality of life compared with the other three categories.
5. The score by disease group suggests a possible need for closer surveillance for surgical CD patients (compared to the other groups).

Subsequent to the completion of the assessment of the quality of life of ambulatory patients with IBD, further comparisons were made with patients similar in age and other chronic diseases, using the same survey instrument. Comparison using the quantifiable quality of life for patients with rheumatoid arthritis and multiple sclerosis (MS) was completed[23]; comparison was made among patients whose chronic illness had begun at approximately age 20 and had been present for approximately 10 years, thus enabling general comparison among the three groups. It was observed that the quality of life for patients with MS was the poorest, patients with rheumatoid arthritis was next, and the quality of life of patients with IBD was the best among the three groups studied. It was further noted that there was a discrepancy between the functional assessment by the physician and the quality of life by the patient, particularly in MS, observed previously in IBD[12,22].

Thus, while the survey instrument was designed specifically for patients with IBD, the impact on the quality of life of patients with other chronic illnesses can also be assessed, and can provide the physician and other members of the health-care team (particularly nurses, physical and occupational therapists, and social workers), with helpful information regarding the response to therapy, the overall functioning of the patient, and an assessment of the 'natural history' of these important chronic diseases.

In summary, attempts to quantify the quality of life for patients with IBD (and other chronic illnesses) can provide valuable information not generally recognized by health-care professionals or assessed by physicians both in terms of assessing the results of medical and surgical therapy as well as attempting to define the 'natural history' of the diseases. Quality-of-life measurement can be useful, and can provide additional information not usually obtained in the course of medical follow-up studies.

References

1. Farmer RG, Hawk WA, Turnbull RB. Clinical patterns in Crohn's disease. A statistical study of 615 patients. Gastroenterology. 1975;68:627–35.
2. Farmer RG, Whelan G, Fazio VW. Long-term follow-up of patients with Crohn's disease. Gastroenterology. 1985;88:825–33.
3. Farmer RG. Ulcerative colitis: history and epidemiology; clinical features; endoscopy; clinical types and differential diagnosis; complications; medical management. In: Haubrick WS, Kalser MH, Roth JLA, Schaffner F, editors. Bockus gastroenterology, 4th edn. Philadelphia: WB Saunders; 1985:2137–9, 2153–7, 2179–207.
4. Hellers G. Crohn's disease in Stockholm County, 1955–1974. A study of epidemiology, results of surgical treatment and long term prognosis. Acta Chir Scand. 1979;490(Suppl.):1–84.
5. Gazzard BG. The quality of life in Crohn's disease. Gut. 1987;28:378–81.
6. Best WR, Becktel JM, Singleton JW. Development of a Crohn's disease activity index: national Cooperative Crohn's Disease Study. Gastroenterology. 1976;70:439–44.
7. Drossman DA, Patrick DL, Mitchell CM, Zagami EA, Applebaum I. Health related quality of life in inflammatory bowel disease: Functional status and patient worries and concerns. Dig Dis Sci. 1989;34:1379–86.
8. Mitchell A, Guyatt G, Singer J et al. Quality of life in patients with inflammatory bowel disease. J Clin Gastroenterol. 1988;10:306–10.
9. Guyatt G, Mitchell A, Irvine EJ et al. A new measure of health status for clinical trials in inflammatory bowel disease. Gastroenterology. 1989;96:804–10.
10. Scholmerich J, Sedlak P, Hoppe-Seyler P. The information needs and fears of patients with inflammatory bowel disease. Hepatol Gastroenterol. 1987;34:182–5.
11. Sorensen VZ, Olsen BG, Binder V. Life prospects and quality of life in patients with Crohn's disease. Gut. 1987;28:382–5.
12. Garrett JW, Drossman DA. Health status in inflammatory bowel disease: biological and behavioral considerations. Gastroenterology. 1990;99:90–6.
13. Drossman DA, Patrick DL, Mitchell CM et al. Health-related quality of life in inflammatory bowel disease. Functional status and patient worries and concerns. Dig Dis Sci. 1989;34:1379–86.
14. Hay JW, Hay AR. Inflammatory bowel disease: costs of illness. J Clin Gastroenterol. 1992;14:309–17.

15. Sonnenberg A. Disability and need for rehabilitation among patients with inflammatory bowel disease. Digestion. 1992;51:168.
16. McLeod RS, Churchill DN, Lock AM *et al*. Quality of life of patients with ulcerative colitis, pre-operatively and post-operatively. Gastroenterology. 1991;101:1307–13.
17. Sagar PM, Lewis W, Holdsworth PJ. Quality of life after restorative proctocolectomy with a pelvic ileal reservoir compares favorably with that of patients with medically treated colitis. Dis Colon Rectum. 1993;36:584.
18. Tjandra JJ, Fazio VW, Church JM *et al*. Similar functional results after restorative proctocolectomy in patients with familial adenomatous polyposis and mucosal ulcerative colitis. Am J Surg. 1993;165:322.
19. Kohler LW, Pemberton JH, Hodge DO *et al*. Long term functional results and quality of life after ileal pouch–anal anastomosis and colectomy. World J Surg. 1992;16:1126–31.
20. Irvein EJ, Feagan B, Rochon J *et al*. Quality of life: a valid and reliable measure of therapeutic efficacy in the treatment of inflammatory bowel disease. Gastroenterology. 1994;106:287–96.
21. Farmer RG. Inflammatory bowel disease in tertiary referral center: the Cleveland Clinic experience. Can J Gastroenterol. 1988;2S:89–94.
22. Farmer RG, Easley KA, Farmer JM. Quality of life assessment of patients with inflammatory disease. Cleve Clin J Med. 1992;59:35–42.
23. Rudick RA, Miller D, Clough JD *et al*. Quality of life in multiple sclerosis, comparison with inflammatory bowel disease and rheumatoid arthritis. Arch Neurol. 1992;49:1237.

37
Insurance rating of patients with IBD: a report of a conference on morbidity and mortality

I. T. BECK, D. J. LEDDIN, S. E. LEMIRE,
E. A. SHAFFER, L. R. SUTHERLAND,
A. B. R. THOMSON and G. TREMBLAY

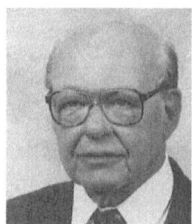

I. T. BECK

INTRODUCTION

The Crohn's and Colitis Foundation of Canada (CCFC) (previously the Canadian Foundation for Ileitis and Colitis – CFIC) supports medical research in inflammatory bowel disease (IBD), undertakes education of physicians and patients, and advocates support for some specific needs of patients with IBD. The Foundation has a Lay Board and a Medical Advisory Board (MAB). The Lay Board is involved in the administration of the Foundation and in organizing drives to obtain charitable donations. The MAB has three major committees: the Research Committee, the Education Committee and the Patient Advocacy Committee. The Research Committee reviews research applications and advises the Lay Board on the distribution of funds to support research. The Education Committee provides educational material for patients and physicians.

Issues of concern to patients with IBD range from provincial funding of costly drugs and nutrients, the availability of insurance benefits for persons with IBD, to the human rights of persons suffering from IBD. Because of this a Patient Advocacy Committee was established in 1986. This Committee was charged to establish representations to Provincial Governments, to approach the insurance industry and to deal with other relevant issues. The first chairman of this new committee was Dr Edward Prokipchuk. During his chairmanship the committee was able to get approval for total parenteral nutrition, and the inclusion of some liquid nutrients into the drug lists of several provinces. At the 20 September, 1991, meeting of the Medical Advisory Board, the second chair of this committee, Dr Suzanne Lemire, presented a report addressing the problems being faced by those with IBD seeking life insurance coverage. Examples of the current rating methods based on the 1985 edition of Brackenridge's[1] text on life risks suggested that there may be a great deficiency in the data upon which such rating is based, and thus it appeared that most of the data used were outdated.

A book written in 1985 could not have included morbidity and mortality data published after 1982. Any report published in 1982 would deal with cases that were collected during the 1970s. Because of the improved diagnostic techniques, improved medical and nutritional support, and safer and less complex surgery in the 1980s, the MAB of the CCFC assumed that the mortality and morbidity figures must have improved since the publication of Brackenridge's text.

Therefore, the MAB of the CCFC decided to organize a conference to review recent data on the morbidity and mortality of IBD. An Organizing Committee consisted of Drs Ivan T. Beck, Kingston (Chair); Desmond J. Leddin, Halifax; Suzanne E. Lemire, Quebec; Eldon A. Shaffer, Calgary; Lloyd R. Sutherland, Calgary and Alan B. R. Thomson, Edmonton. The meeting was fully supported by the Lay Board, and Mr Raymond J. van Berkel, Executive Director of the CFIC from Toronto, was made an ex-officio member of the Organizing Committee. The Lay Board was also represented at the Conference by Dr Ted Hannah, Liaison Chairman of the Lay Board to the Medical Advisory Board. The advice of Dr Guy Tremblay, Past-President, Canadian Life Insurance Medical Officers Association, was obtained at the first meeting of this committee.

Because the CFIC is a charitable organization there were only limited funds available to arrange this meeting; therefore the Organizing Committee decided to hold the conference in combination with a major symposium on IBD. This allowed us to draw on the expertise of some of the well-known international investigators who attended the other meeting. Starting with a reception on the evening of 20 May 1992, the Falk Symposium on 'Trends in Inflammatory Bowel Disease Therapy' was held in Quebec-City between 21 and 23 May. The CCFC was fortunate to be able to organize its conference on morbidity and mortality during the day of 20 May 1992. This is how we could attract Dr Richard Farmer (previously from the Cleveland Clinic, presently the Medical Advisor to the Agency of International Development, Washington, DC, USA); Dr Goran Hellers (from the Department of Surgery, Karolinska Institute, Huddinge University Hospital, Huddinge, Sweden); and Vibeke Binder (from the Medical Gastroenterology Department of Herlev Hospital, University of Copenhagen, Herlev, Denmark). In addition to these speakers we were fortunate to have Rod Riley from the Canadian Centre for Health Information, Statistics Canada, to talk on the Canadian experience on morbidity and mortality of Crohn's disease and ulcerative colitis. Most importantly we had to find an outstanding clinician, who has in-depth knowledge of insurance matters, and who could interact with the speakers and the audience. Dr Guy Tremblay, an academic cardiologist and

Table 1 Program of the meeting

Part One	
Welcome	S. Lemire
Objective of conference	I. T. Beck
Results of patients' survey questionnaire on insurance	L. R. Sutherland
Process by which life insurance applications are rated	G. Tremblay
The human cost of IBD	R. G. Farmer
Crohn's disease and ulcerative colitis – morbidity and mortality, the Canadian experience	R. Riley
Morbidity and mortality in Crohn's disease	G. Hellers
Overview of morbidity and mortality in ulcerative colitis	V. Binder
Panel discussion	
Part Two – Report on group discussions	
Ulcerative colitis	Summarizer
	D. J. Leddin
Crohn's disease before surgery	Summarizer
	L. R. Sutherland
Crohn's disease after surgery	Summarizer
	A. B. R. Thomson
Summary, conclusions and recommendations	I. T. Beck

a Past President of the Canadian Life Insurance Medical Officers Association, joined us at our first organizational meeting. He was extremely helpful, not only as a speaker during the conference, but also by giving us advice as to what questions we should address and discuss in detail.

In addition to the speakers, 19 Canadian gastroenterologists and surgeons were invited to participate in the conference. The total number of participants was 30. The invited guests represented a broad spectrum of individuals with specific interests. There was a good scattering of age and of geographic location. There was a mix of academic and non-academic physicians and surgeons. Two of the invited practising gastroenterologists were also insurance medical officers.

The possibility of bias in the assessment of the Lay Board was considered by the Organizing Committee. It was possible that patients who encounter difficulties would call the CCFC and talk about the rejection of their application, but those who had no problems may never discuss the issue. Therefore, the organizing committee decided that, before embarking on the conference, it was necessary to ascertain whether the impression of the Lay Board of the CCFC was correct in assuming that patients with IBD have difficulties in obtaining insurance. Dr Sutherland was charged to obtain data on this, and to report to the conference on his findings.

The conference lasted one day (Table 1). In the morning lectures were given, and in the afternoons small group sessions were held. The invited audience was divided into three small groups for discussion (Table 2). The groups reviewed designated specific subjects of IBD. Dr Leddin chaired and summarized the session on morbidity and mortality of ulcerative colitis, Dr Sutherland on Crohn's disease before surgery, and Dr Thomson on Crohn's disease after surgery. After the 2-h small-group sessions the summarizer reported to the plenary session for final discussion and conclusion. The recommendations of this meeting are based on the results of these discussions.

Table 2 Discussion groups

Group I – Ulcerative colitis. *Chair:* Dr D. Leddin
Participants
Dr V. Binder
Dr H. Freeman
Dr J. Irvine
Dr J. W. D. McDonald
Dr C. A. Ottaway
Dr R. Preshaw
Dr N. Williams

Group II – Crohn's before surgery. *Chair:* Dr L. Sutherland
Participants
Dr L. DaCosta
Dr D. Daly
Dr R. Farmer
Dr B. Feagan
Dr F. Martin
Dr R. Riley
Dr M. Ste. Marie
Dr G. Thompson

Group III – Crohn's after surgery. *Chair:* Dr A. B. R. Thomson
Participants
Dr J. R. Bourdages
Dr W. Depew
Dr O. Gagnon
Dr H. Haddad
Dr G. Hellers
Dr R. C. Lapointe
Dr E. Prokipchuk
Dr J. Sidorov

SYNOPSIS OF THE LECTURES

Dr Lloyd Sutherland: Results of patient's survey questionnaire on insurance[2]

The database consisted of questionnaires filled out by patients of the Organizing Committee. As Toronto was not represented amongst the organizers, Dr Prokipchuk of Toronto was also asked to send out the questionnaires. Drs Beck, Leddin, Prokipchuk, Thomson and Sutherland sent questionnaires to 50 randomly selected patients under their care, while Dr Lemire, whose cases represented the experience of the French–Canadian population, sent questionnaires to 70 patients with IBD. Of the 320 questionnaires 206 responded, providing a 66% response rate. The results for straight life insurance indicate a high rejection rate for both diseases. For ulcerative colitis the percentage acceptance without premium was only 31%. Thirty-seven percent were rated and 32% were rejected. For Crohn's disease the acceptance, rating and rejection, in percentages, were as follows: 18% (accepted), 44% (rated) and 38% (rejected), respectively. Rejection and special rating for disability insurance showed similar results. Interestingly, group life was refused in 35% of patients with ulcerative colitis and 17% of patients with Crohn's disease. At the discussion of his data Dr Sutherland indicated that there was a possibility of selection bias. Patients who were rejected may have responded more readily than those who had obtained insurance without difficulty. On the other hand patients who were well, and would have obtained insurance without rating, may not have applied because they believed that they would be rejected. Another problem was that there were no controls. However, even without controls, the rejection rate of patients with IBD was higher than that of the normal population in whom straight life insurance is refused to only about 5% of applicants[1].

Considering all the shortcomings of a one-time mail questionnaire, this study provides reasonable evidence that patients with IBD have considerable difficulties in obtaining insurance.

Dr Guy Tremblay: Process by which life insurance applications are evaluated/rated[3]

In this lecture Dr Tremblay explained how insurance companies work. He pointed out that because individuals who have recognizable diseases have already been excluded when they applied for their insurance, the life expectancy of the insured population is one-half to one-third better than that of the general population. This difference is obvious up to the first 7–8 years, but persists for 15 years after obtaining insurance.

Dr Tremblay pointed out that the insurance business is competitive and companies want to sell insurance. For this reason, the medical director is responsible for the updating of his company's selection procedure. Similarly to that of other specialists, he attends many continuing medical education meetings to ensure that his knowledge is updated. Many medical directors are in clinical academic practice and apply their knowledge to the insurance screening and rating of applications. Therefore patients with IBD may have a better chance of obtaining insurance at a lower additional rate if they shop around among several insurance companies. Furthermore, the insurability of patients improves after periods of good health; therefore patients should be encouraged to reapply after periods of remission.

Most importantly, patients will do better if their physician helps the medical director to evaluate the risk. Dr Tremblay advised that clinicians should write a letter, rather than just fill out a form and, if applicable, the treating physician should mention the period of remission, the fact that the patient is reliable, is not disabled from working and is under ongoing follow-up. Medications used should be mentioned, especially if the patient is not on steroids or immunosuppressive agents. He suggested that patients who have group insurance coverage at their work should be advised not to change their jobs, as they may lose their group insurance by moving to another company. Furthermore, to obtain individual insurance, an important factor is the patient's ability to function, and his/her ability to maintain the same job for a certain length of time.

Dr Richard Farmer: Human cost of IBD[4]

One hundred and sixty-four patients with IBD, followed at the Cleveland Clinic, were studied. Only those patients whose diseases started around the age of 20, and whose follow-up was over 10 years, were included in the study. The questionnaire was designed to assess their (a) ability to function, (b) social and recreational activities, (c) attitude toward life and health and (d) medical status. The questions on the ability to support themselves dealt with work and family support; those on social and recreational activities with relationship to family, sexual, social and recreational habits. Questions on attitude toward life and health assessed depression, optimism, etc.; while medical questions dealt directly with symptoms, medication, surgery, etc.

Dr Farmer concluded that patients with ulcerative colitis have a better quality of life than those with Crohn's disease. The quality of life of patients with both diseases was better before than after surgery. Most patients with IBD have a close to normal lifestyle, with 44% functioning well and being able to maintain a working capacity close to normal, 50% function suboptimally, but most of them are still able to work. Only 6% had severe disabling disease.

Rod Riley: Crohn's disease and ulcerative colitis – morbidity and mortality data, the Canadian experience[5]

The data were obtained from hospital discharges between 1971 and 1989. In Canada, discharge diagnoses are filled out in every hospital. These forms are submitted to the Provincial Ministries of Health, which then forwards these annually to the Canadian Centre for Health Information. As patients may be admitted several times a year, the discharge statistics collected at the Centre of Health, Information, Statistics Canada do not provide data on incidence or prevalence. They are, however, useful to assess the general trends and provide accurate mortality statistics. In Canada, similar to that in other Western countries, Crohn's disease was on the rise. The discharge rose from 11.2/100 000 between 1971 and 1974 to 30.2/100 000 between 1987 and 1989. The rate of discharge for ulcerative colitis remained unchanged in Canada (12.3/100 000 between 1971 and 1974 and 14.1/100 000 between 1987 and 1989).

For IBD as a whole, there is a greater increase in the prevalence in the elderly. It is possible, however, that this increase in the elderly may be due to the inclusion of patients with ischemic bowel disease.

The mortality rate for IBD was steadily decreasing between 1971 and 1989. Mortality due to ulcerative colitis was 1.5/million and for Crohn's disease 2/million (Fig. 1). The mortality in the young was extremely low. The somewhat higher mortality in the elderly (Table 3) may be due to the fact that many of them have had multisystem diseases or may have suffered from ischemic bowel disease rather than from IBD.

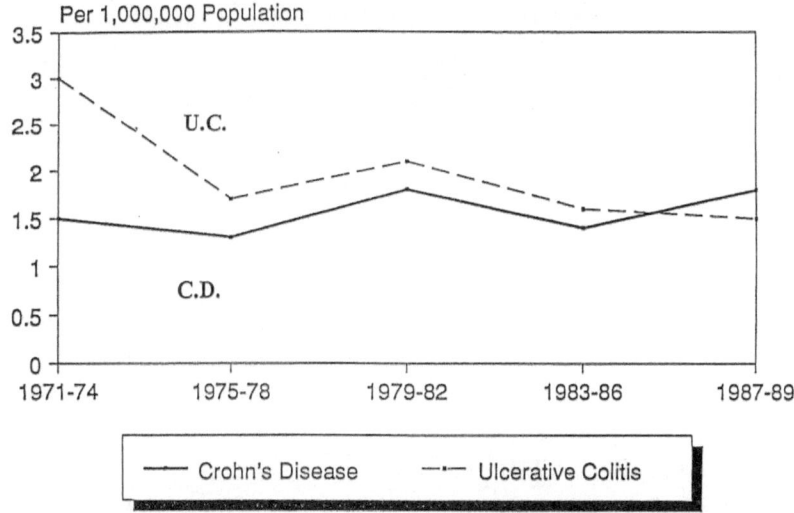

Fig. 1 Changes in Canadian mortality rates of IBD patients between 1971 and 1989 (reproduced from ref. 5)

Table 3 Inflammatory bowel disease, ratio of discharges to deaths in Canadian hospitals

	< 24	25–44	45–64	65 +	Total
Crohn's disease					
1971–74	166	152	34	18	76
1975–78	287	337	69	18	123
1979–82	1800	291	73	16	127
1983–86	1068	953	92	23	191
1986–89	—	623	105	19	172
Ulcerative colitis					
1971–74	136	100	33	7	42
1975–78	367	282	50	16	70
1979–82	484	234	65	13	61
1983–86	1042	384	92	17	83
1986–89	2388	440	101	20	96

— No deaths
Reproduced from ref. 5

Dr Goran Heller: Morbidity and mortality in Crohn's disease[6]

Early studies on Crohn's disease indicate a higher mortality rate than that expected for the general population (Fig. 2)[7]. Later studies, for instance by Dr Vibeke Binder[8], which included patients up to the year of 1985, indicated that mortality for Crohn's disease was equal to that expected in non-IBD patients (Fig. 3). Dr Heller also reported on the standard incidence ratio of cancer in Crohn's disease. In younger patients there is an increased excess mortality due to cancer. This is not the case in the older population, where the cancer rate in the general population increases. After the age of 30, the

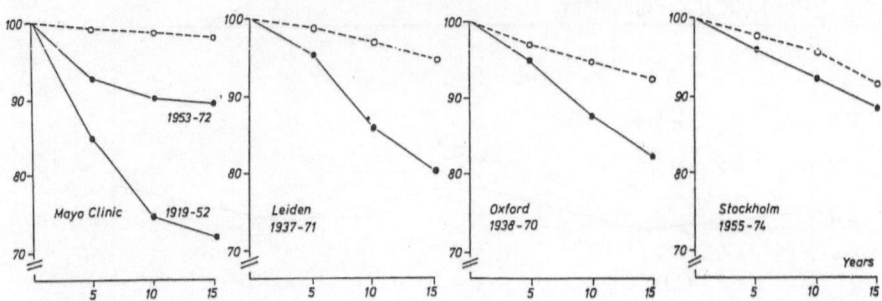

Fig. 2 Early studies on mortality in Crohn's disease (reproduced from refs 6 and 7). The expected (dashed line) and observed (solid line) mortality in studies from different time periods

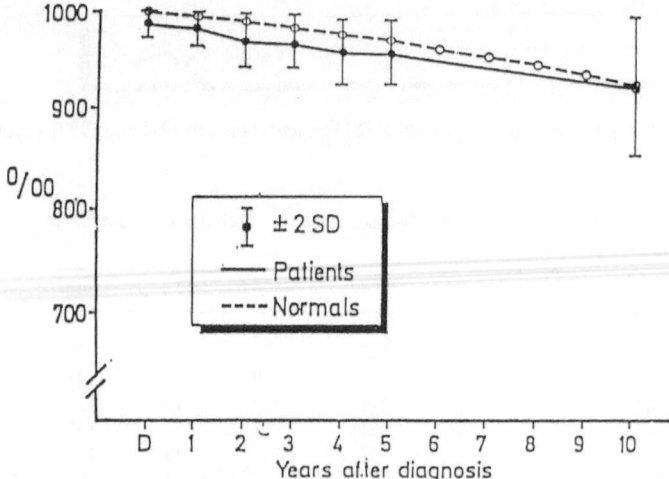

Fig. 3 A later study on mortality in Crohn's disease (reproduced from ref. 8). Survival of patients with Crohn's disease compared with the age- and sex-matched background population

ratio of cancer in Crohn's disease is 1.5, which is similar to that of the general population.

Dr Vibeke Binder: Morbidity and mortality of ulcerative colitis[9]

This study included ulcerative colitis patients seen in Copenhagen County between 1962 and 1987[9]. The total number of patients was 1161. The median observation time was 11.7 years (1–25 years). There was a slight increase in mortality in the first year after diagnosis. However, once the patient survived the first year of illness, the mortality rate fell to that of the background population. The quality of life of patients with ulcerative colitis regarding their working capacity, professional life, private, family and sexual adjustment was similar to that of the general population. Cancer incidence was investigated on 600 patients who were followed for over 7 years. The calculated lifetime cancer risk for ulcerative colitis (3.6%) was not different from that of the Danish population (3.7%).

REPORTS OF THE DISCUSSION GROUPS

After these presentations, the Conference broke up into three groups (Table 2). In order to update our statistical data, prior to the meeting, participants of each group were requested to review the literature on morbidity and mortality of the area designated to them. Furthermore, the chairman of each group was instructed to come forward with recommendations regarding the education of patients and physicians on the working of insurance companies. At the end of the group meetings the chair of each session summarized the discussion and reported to the general session.

Ulcerative colitis (Chaired by Dr D. Leddin)

The group reviewed the appropriate section of the volume *Medical selection of life risks* by R. D. C. Brackenridge, 1985[1]. They agreed with the classification and the approach used in this volume to divide ulcerative colitis into mild, moderate and severe forms, but found that the data were out of date on mortality. Several suggestions regarding the patient's and physician's approach to insurance companies were brought forward by this section, and these are incorporated below with the recommendations of the two other groups.

Crohn's disease before surgery (Chaired by Dr L. Sutherland)

Dr Sutherland reported that, since most patients eventually go to surgery, there is very little known about the morbidity and mortality of unoperated Crohn's disease. There are no predictors as to whether a patient will or will not have surgery in the future. One of the members of the group, Dr Don Daly, a gastroenterologist and a medical officer of Prudential of England, provided for review the text 'M & G Underwriting', which is used by the above company for insurance rating. Patients whose Crohn's disease was localized solely to the small or to the large bowel paid lower premiums than those with ileocecal involvement. Patients with jejunitis were rejected irrespective of the severity of the disease. This was astonishing, and the group wondered whether jejunal Crohn's was confused with 'ulcerative jejunitis', which has more severe consequences than Crohn's disease involving the jejunum. The recommendations of this group will be discussed below.

Crohn's disease after surgery (Chaired by Dr A. B. R. Thomson)

Surgical expertise to this group was provided by Dr Gorman Hellers. Due to the modern surgical and postsurgical techniques, morbidity and mortality

Table 4 Recommendations of the Conference to the CCFC

---

1. The CCFC should develop an educational booklet for patients to:
   Explain how insurance companies rate applicants
   Encourage patients to reapply after having been in remission
   Suggest that patients try to stay in the same job to maintain group insurance
   Have regular follow-up because individuals under regular medical supervision are better rated
   Develop a form with the information that is important to provide to insurance companies to obtain a more favourable rating. Patients could take this form to their physician when they request that they write a letter to an insurance company

2. The CCFC should identify insurance brokers who have an understanding of IBD

---

of surgery in Crohn's disease has improved; patients are therefore sent earlier, and in better condition, to the operating room. Dr Heller stated that, taking the general risk of surgery as a basis, there is no additional surgical mortality related to Crohn's disease. Previous surgery does not increase the risk of a second or third operation. The re-operation rate is only 4% per year; therefore previous surgery should not be considered for extra rating for life insurance. However, previous surgery may be a factor in disability insurance. The recommendations of this session are discussed below in conjunction with those of the other two groups.

RECOMMENDATIONS

The composite recommendation of the three groups to the CCFC was that the Patient Advocacy Committee should develop educational material, which should explain to patients how insurance companies rate applicants. The pamphlet should emphasize that patients should reapply after a period of remission. To maintain group insurance, patients should try to stay in the same job, as they may have difficulties in being accepted in a new group insurance plan. Patients should be told that they may get a better insurance rating if they are regularly followed up. The CCFC should develop a form which provides information as to what physicians should convey to insurance companies in order to obtain a better rating. Patients could take this to their physician as a guideline. Simultaneously, in the different communities, the CCFC should identify insurance brokers who have a better understanding of this disease (Table 4).

It was suggested that the Canadian Association of Gastroenterology should start an educational program to enlighten physicians about the methods of rating by insurance companies. Clinicians should learn to interact directly with the medical officers of insurance companies and, rather than filling out a form, they should write a detailed letter about their patients. If applicable, the patient's physician should indicate that he/she has constant careful follow-up, is compliant and is on maintenance therapy, and does not require total parenteral nutrition or long term steroid or immunosuppressive therapy. They should indicate that he/she has lost little time from work. As at least one undewriting text considered jejunitis a cause for complete

Table 5 Recommendations of the Conference to the Canadian Association of Gastroenterology

This organization should embark on an educational campaign to enlighten physicians about insurance companies and their ratings

Specifically:
1. Clinicians should be encouraged to interact with insurance company physicians
2. They should be requested to write a letter about the patient's condition, rather than just filling out a form
3. If applicable, to point out that the patient:
   Has lost little time from work
   Has constant careful follow-up
   Is on maintenance therapy
   Has no jejunal disease, is not on TPN or long-term steroid therapy
4. Propose methods to investigate why jejunal disease is considered so deleterious that it excludes patients from insurance

Table 6 Rating of patients with ulcerative colitis

Time since diagnosis	Rating
Less than 1 year	+100 to +250[a] and 5 per mil for 2 years
Second year	+75 to +200[a] and 2.5 per mil for 1 year
Thereafter	+50 to +150[a]

[a]Depending on the extent and severity of disease, frequency of relapses and quality of cancer surveillance. Additional rating of +50 for corticosteroid therapy (continuous or repeated)
Normal expected mortality rate = 100. +100 means insured pays twice the normal rate. +150 means insured pays normal +1.5 × normal rate. x/mil = insured pays x units of currency per 1000 units of amount insured
Reproduced from ref. 10

rejection, the clinician should mention that the patient does not have jejunal disease. Furthermore, it would be of interest to find out from underwriting companies why jejunal disease should exclude Crohn's disease patients from insurance (Table 5).

RECENT DEVELOPMENTS

Several events have occurred since the conclusion of this conference. The third edition of Brackenridge was published in 1992[10]. This volume updated the literature on mortality of IBD and provided references up to 1991[11-13]. As all these papers indicated that during the last year there was a decrease in mortality, the new edition of Brackenridge states (p. 611), that 'long-term prognosis in both ulcerative colitis and Crohn's disease had significantly improved within the last decade and has become nearly similar in the two diseases'. In spite of this, there was no considerable improvement in the ratings for ulcerative colitis (Table 6) and the ratings for Crohn's disease (Table 7) have not been improved.

A recent study on 140 patients with IBD and 100 controls, carried out by Drs Leddin, Christie and VanZanten (personal communication) indicates that, in the Halifax area, Nova Scotia, a significantly greater number of patients with IBD were refused life insurance (17%) as compared to the

Table 7 Rating of patients with Crohn's disease

Time since diagnosis	Rating
Less than 1 year	+100 to +250[a] and 5 per mil for 3 years
Second year	+75 to +200[a] and 2.5 per mil for 2 years
Thereafter	+50 to +150[a]

[a]Depending on age at onset (worse for onset before age 20), severity of disease, frequency of relapses and evidence of complications. Additional rating of +50 for corticosteroid therapy (continuous or repeated)
With surgery – no additional rating, but refer to medical director if complex
Reproduced from ref. 10

controls (7%; $p = 0.04$). However, the majority (62%) of patients with IBD were able to obtain life insurance, and this was not significantly different (73%) from that of the control population.

At the North American scene, excellent contacts were established with physicians specializing in insurance medicine. For instance Dr Beck was asked to discuss ulcerative colitis and Crohn's disease in general, and the results of the Conference on IBD at the combined annual meeting of the American Academy of Life Insurance Medicine and the Canadian Life Insurance Medical Officers Association. Our colleagues were impressed by the approach that our specialty has taken toward the specialty of insurance medicine. A letter received from a member of the audience, Dr Daniel M. Fleming, Vice-President and Chief Medical Director of North-American Life Insurance Company, states, 'Once again, thank you for updating our understanding of this complex disorder. Your educational campaign to include the insurance physicians will undoubtedly be successful in the long run. Knowledge based on risk selection results in competitive insurance offers to your patients and our policyholders'. This response from our colleagues in insurance medicine suggests that similar cooperation has to be maintained in the future. Hopefully the Patient Advocacy Committee of the CCFC will prepare its brochure based on the recommendations of the Conference, and it may be advisable to prepare these brochures in co-operation with members of the executive of the Canadian Life Insurance Medical Officers Association.

CONCLUSION

Patients with IBD have considerable difficulty in obtaining straight life and disability insurance. This is in spite of the fact that the quality of life of most patients with IBD is not very different from that of the general population, and the mortality rate of patients with IBD is decreasing and presently not different from that of the general population. However, members of the Conference learned from representatives of the insurance industry that the mortality rate of the general population is higher during the first 15 years than that of an insured population. Members of the Conference learned that patients with IBD had a better chance to obtain insurance if there is close co-operation between the treating physician and the medical officer of the insurance company. Some changes have occurred since the conference was held in May 1992. In comparison to the 1985 edition the recent third edition of Brackenridge (1992) provides a better prognosis, but as yet basically unchanged ratings for patients with IBD. Excellent contacts have been established with the Canadian Insurance Medical Officers, and further close co-operation of the Patient Advocacy Committee with the executive of the Canadian Life Insurance Medical Officers Association may further improve the insurance rating of patients with IBD.

References

1. Brackenridge RDC. Medical selection of life risks, a comprehensive guide to life expectancy for underwriters and clinicians. 1985. New York: H.L. Press.
2. Sutherland LR. Results of patient's survey on insurability. Can J Gastroenterol. (In press).
3. Tremblay G. Process by which life insurance applications are evaluated/rated. Can J Gastroenterol. (In press).
4. Farmer RG. Human cost of inflammatory bowel disease. Can J Gastroenterol. (In press).
5. Riley R. Crohn's disease and ulcerative colitis – morbidity and mortality, the Canadian experience. Can J Gastroenterol. (In press).
6. Hellers G. Morbidity and mortality of Crohn's disease. Can J Gastroenterol. (In press).
7. Hellers G. Crohn's disease in Stockholm county 1955–74. A study of epidemiology, results of surgical treatment and long term prognosis. Acta Chir Scand. 1979;490(S):1–84.
8. Binder V, Hendriksen C, Kreiner S. Prognosis in Crohn's disease – based on the results from a regional patient group from the county of Copenhagen. Gut. 1985;26:146–50.
9. Binder V. Overview of morbidity and mortality in ulcerative colitis. Can J Gastroenterol. (In press).
10. Brackenridge RDC, Elder JW. Medical selection of life risks, 3rd edn. New York: Stockton Press; 1992.
11. Andrews HA, Lewis P, Allan RN. Mortality in Crohn's disease – a clinical analysis. Q J Med. 1989;71:399–05.
12. Weterman IT, Biemond I, Pena AS. Mortality and causes of death in Crohn's disease: review of 50 years' experience in Leiden University Hospital. Gut. 1990;31:1387–90.
13. Hiwatashi N, Yamazaki H, Kimura M et al. Clinical course and long-term prognosis of Japanese patients with ulcerative colitis. Gastroenterol Jpn. 1991;26:312–18.

Section XI
Therapeutics

38
Overview of 5-ASA in the therapy of IBD

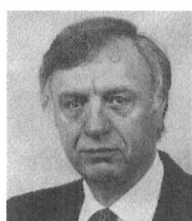

C. N. WILLIAMS

Sulfasalazine (SAS) was developed in the early 1940s[1] as an anti-inflammatory antibiotic for use in rheumatoid arthritis, then thought to have an infectious etiology. 5-Aminosalicylic acid (5-ASA) is the active principle of the drug sulfasalazine. 5-ASA is available in carrier-mediated form. Here, the prodrug is delivered to the large intestine, where bacterial action breaks an azo-bond[2] and releases the active principle. For sulfasalazine the release is of the active principle, 5-ASA, and inactive sulfapyridine[3,4]. For olsalazine (Dipentum), splitting the azo-bond releases two molecules of 5-ASA. Other prodrugs, balsalazide and ipsalazide, are not available in Canada[5]. Enteric-coated, slow-release, pH-dependent forms of 5-ASA are available in North America; Asacol, Salofalk, Rowasa (Table 1). These preparations avoid excessive upper intestinal absorption, and theoretical renal damage[6]. Salofalk and Rowasa are released in the distal ileum, Asacol in the right colon[7]. Another preparation, Pentasa, is a formulation of 5-ASA granules covered with ethyl cellulose. This allows slow release starting in the proximal small bowel[8].

While SAS inhibits both the lipoxygenase and cyclooxygenase arachidonic acid pathways, 5-ASA inhibits leukotriene production by inhibiting 5-lipoxygenase in the cyclooxygenase pathway[9]. 5-ASA acts on soluble mediator production. It modulates leukocyte function. It is an inhibitor of prostaglandins, thromboxanes, platelet-activating factor, tumor necrosis factor, interleukin-1, intestinal mast cell and basophil-stimulated histamine release. It is an effective scavenger of free oxygen radicals[10]. The relative importance of these actions is not known.

5-ASA is metabolized to one end-product only in humans, *N*-acetyl-5-

Table 1 5-ASA drugs available in North America

Drug	Company	Coating	Delivery mechanisms
Salofalk 250, 500, 750 mg	Axcan	Eudragit L	pH > 6.0
Mesasal 250, 500 mg	Smith Kline Beecham	Eudragit L	pH > 6.0
Asacol 400 mg	Norwich Eaton	Eudragit S	pH > 7.0
Rowasa 250, 500 mg	Reid-Rowell	Eudragit LH	pH > 6.0
Pentasa 250 mg	Nordic	Ethyl cellulose	Slow release
Dipentum, olsalazine 250 mg capsule, 500 mg tablet	Pharmacia	Gelatin capsule, Ec tablet	Bacterial cleavage
Sulfasalazine 500 mg	Pharmacia	Regular and Ec tablet	Bacterial cleavage

ASA[11], and is independent of acetylation phenotype[12]. This probably occurs by bacterial action in the colonic lumen as well as in the mucosal cell[13] and the hepatocyte[14]. N-acetyl-5-S is believed to have no biologic action[15] and is excreted by the kidneys. Factors affecting oral 5-ASA disposition include food intake, omeprazole, luminal pH, intestinal transit time, colon flora and antibiotics. The disease itself alters 5-ASA absorption and is reversed toward normal after effective treatment[16]. There are few available studies of intestinal pH in patients with IBD. However, using serum, urine and stool measurements, increasing proportions of non-metabolized 5-ASA reaches the colon from the slow-release (Pentasa) through the enteric-coated (Salofalk, Asacol) to the prodrugs (olsalazine, sulfasalazine). Topical formulations of 5-ASA are available as enemas, suppositories and foams.

The prodrug SAS is associated with an approximate 30% incidence of side-effects, predominantly related to the sulfapyridine component[17]. Desensitization is helpful for some, but not for hypersensitivity reactions such as agranulocytosis, hemolysis or aplastic anemia. Other rare side-effects include male infertility and folate deficiency. Side-effects associated with 5-ASA tend to be dose-related and infrequent in number; headache, nausea, epigastric distress and diarrhea are common[18]. Rare complications of 5-ASA include acute pancreatitis[19], pericarditis[20], myocarditis[21], thrombocytopenia[22] and renal tubular damage[23]. Rarely, both drugs may exacerbate the IBD itself[24,25].

5-ASA is recommended for the treatment of patients with mild to moderate IBD. The type of 5-ASA used depends on the type of disease (Crohn's disease or ulcerative colitis), and the site and extent of disease. The oral 5-ASA drugs, including the prodrugs, are probably equally effective when universal ulcerative colitis is present. Suppositories are the treatment of choice for distal disease of 20 cm or less; enemas are used when there is 20–40 cm of disease. Enemas are particularly effective in universal colitis, together with an oral 5-ASA, when rectal symptoms predominate. 5-ASA is particularly useful in Crohn' disease with colonic involvement with or without limited ileal disease. Pentasa is probably the theoretical drug of choice in more proximal small-bowel disease because of its mechanism, but this remains to be shown by clinical trial. 5-ASA appears to induce remission more slowly than corticosteroids and is more expensive. However, patient tolerability, especially for the topical formulations, is high and there is less toxicity.

5-ASA is effective in treating inflammatory bowel disease[26]. Its exact efficacy is difficult to ascertain from careful literature review due to lack of accurate definitions of remission versus improvement; failure to define the exact type or extent of IBD; whether placebo or active drugs are used for controls; different end-points, clinical, endoscopic or histologic; use of different scoring systems; varying doses; different treatment periods; and the absence of power calculations for accurate estimates of number of patients required. Placebo responses in acute ulcerative colitis range from 5% to 38%, and active drug dose responses from 24% to 63%, using doses up to 4.8 g over 3–8-week periods[27-30]. Using the same dose for different time periods shows a tendency for increased efficacy in clinical response, but not to endoscopic response[31]. In maintenance therapy for ulcerative colitis, comparisons of SAS versus placebo over a 6–12-month period reveals a therapeutic gain of 43–50%[32,33], with a therapeutic gain of 24% using increasing doses of SAS[34]. There are many studies showing equal efficacy in maintaining remission between SAS and another prodrug, Dipentum[35], as well as between SAS and enteric-coated 5-ASA[36]. Meta-analyses have shown that 5-ASA is equivalent to SAS in mild to moderate acute ulcerative colitis and in maintenance therapy[37,38]. Similarly, the use of topical 5-ASA in ulcerative colitis is very effective for enemas, 85–90% using 4 g at nighttime for 4–12 weeks[39,40], and for suppositories similar efficacy using either 500 mg twice or three times a day for 6 weeks[41,42]. For maintenance therapy, 1 g at nighttime for enemas, and 0.5 g every second night for suppositories, are effective treatments. Recent meta-analysis of topical 5-ASA in ulcerative colitis confirms significant benefits over placebo for both active disease and maintenance therapy[43].

5-ASA is effective in active Crohn's disease. There is a 32% therapeutic gain when SAS, 3 g/day, is compared to placebo over a 4-month period[44]. This was later confirmed in the National Cooperative Crohn's Disease Study where a subgroup with colitis responded better[45]. In a recent study, a 25% therapeutic gain of Pentasa over placebo was seen in 310 patients randomized to various doses over a 16-week period[46]. There was no difference between placebo, 1 g or 2 g doses in this study. In maintenance therapy, Pentasa is beneficial, when compared to placebo, in a subgroup of patients who had relapsed within 3 months prior to enrollment[47]. Other studies have shown no effect when either Pentasa[48] or SAS[49] was compared to placebo. However, in a large group of patients treated with SAS followed up to 2 years, there was a therapeutic gain of 25%[50], and in another study of 12 months duration, patients randomized to Claversal experienced a 24% therapeutic gain over those randomized to placebo[51]. Patients with Crohn's disease had remission rates on placebo varying from 35% to 54%, compared to 60% on SAS and 78% on Claversal over 12 months. These findings are confirmed in a recent meta-analysis where maintenance therapy with 5-ASA or SAS reduces the likelihood of clinical relapse at 1 year[52].

5-ASA is a well-tolerated medication with few side-effects, allowing increase in effective dosage. It is recommended that 4 g 5-ASA be given orally for active IBD, with increases as necessary. It is uncertain whether continuous active treatment should be advised for maintenance therapy; i.e. 4 g/day or the standard 2 g/day. Different preparations can be used to target the site of disease and, when given orally, appear to be equally as effective in maintaining remission as SAS. However, SAS is much cheaper and, when tolerated, is effective therapy. 5-ASA given to SAS-intolerant patients is of therapeutic benefit in most, with the caveat of occasional allergic reactions to 5-ASA itself.

References

1. Svartz N. Salazopyrin, a new sulfanilamide preparation: A. Therapeutic results in rheumatic polyarthritis. B. Therapeutic results in ulcerative colitis. C. Toxic manifestations in treatment with sulfanilamide preparations. Acta Med Scand. 1942;110:577–98.
2. Peppercorn MA, Goldman P. Distribution studies of salicylazosulfapyridine and its metabolites. Gastroenterology. 1973;64:240–5.
3. Azad Khan AK, Piris J, Truelove SC. An experiment to determine the active therapeutic moiety of sulphasalazine. Lancet. 1977;2:891–5.
4. van Hees PAM, Bakker JH, van Tongeren JHM. Effect of sulphapyridine, 5-aminosalicylic acid and placebo in patients with idiopathic proctitis: a study to determine the active therapeutic moiety of sulphasalazine. Gut. 1980;21:632–5.
5. Chan RP, Pope DJ, Gilbert AP et al. Studies of two novel sulfasalazine analogs, ipsalazide and balsalazide. Dig Dis Sci. 1983;28:609–15.
6. Lauritzen K, Laursen LS, Rask-Madsen J. Review of oral salicylates in the treatment of inflammatory bowel disease. In: Shaffer EA, editor. Proceedings, Medical Management of IBD. Montreal: Medicopea International; 1992:68–90.
7. Dew MJ, Hughes PJ, Lee MG, Evans BK, Rhodes J. An oral preparation to release drugs in the human colon. Br J Clin Pharmacol. 1982;14:405–8.
8. Keller J, Layer P, Klotz U, Goebell H. Small intestinal transit of oral mesalazine (5-ASA) from a microsphere preparation in humans. Proceedings, Falk Symposium (67). In: Scholmerich J, Goebell H, Kruis W, Hohenberger W, editors. Inflammatory bowel diseases. Dordrecht: Kluwer; 1992:540–1.
9. Lauritsen K, Staerk Laursen L, Buhave K, Rask-Madsen J. Longterm olsalazine treatment: pharmacokinetics, tolerance and effects on local eicosanoid formation in ulcerative colitis and Crohn's disease. Gut. 1988;29:974–82.
10. Ahnfelt-Ronnel, Hielsen OH, Christensen A, Langholz E, Binder V, Ris P. Clinical evidence supporting the radical scavenger mechanism of 5-ASA. Gastroenterology. 1990;98:1162–9.
11. Nielsen OH, Bondesen S. Kinetics of 5-aminosalicylic acid after jejunal installation in man. Br J Clin Pharmacol. 1983;16:738–40.
12. Allgayer H, Ahnfeldt NO, Frank K, Soderberg HNA, Kruis W, Paumgartner G. Acetylation phenotype independent colonic N-acetylation of 5-aminosalicylic acid: an example for intestinal drug metabolism. Gastroenterology. 1985;88:133(abstr.).
13. Ireland A, Priddle JD, Jewell DP. Acetylation of 5-aminosalicylic acid by human colonic epithelial cells. Gastroenterology. 1986;90:1471(abstr.).
14. Myers B, Evans DNW, Rhodes J et al. Metabolism and urinary excretion of 5-aminosalicylic acid in healthy volunteers when given intravenously or released for absorption at different sites in the gastrointestinal tract. Gut. 1987;28:196–200.
15. van Hogezand RA, van Hees PAM, Van Gorp JPWM et al. Double-blind comparison of 5-aminosalicylic acid and acetyl-5-aminosalicylic acid suppositories in patients with idiopathic proctitis. Aliment Pharmacol Ther. 1988;2:33–40.
16. Williams CN. Pharmacokinetics of 5-aminosalicylic acid enteral suspension in Crohn's disease and in healthy volunteers. Can J Gastroenterol. 1990;4:458–62.
17. Watkinson G. Sulphasalazine: a review of 40 years experience. Drugs. 1986;32:1–11.
18. Allgayer H. Sulphasalazine and 5-ASA compounds. Gastroenterol Clin N Am. 1993;21:643–

58.

19. Deprez P, Descamps C, Fiasse R. Pancreatitis induced by 5-aminosalicylic acid. Lancet. 1989;2:445–6.
20. Agnholt J, Sorensen HT, Rasmussen SN, Gotzsche CO, Halkier P. Cardiac hypersensitivity to 5-aminosalicylic acid. Lancet. 1989;2:1135.
21. Kristensen KS, Hoegholm A, Bohr L, Friis S. Fatal myocarditis associated with mesalazine. Lancet. 1991;335:605.
22. Daneshmend TK. Mesalazine-associated thrombocytopenia. Lancet. 1991;337:1297–8.
23. Zehnter E, Dorhofer H, Ziegenhagen DJ, Scheurlen C, Baldamus CA, Kruis W. Renal damage in patients with IBD treated with 5-aminosalicylic acid and sulphasalazine. Gastroenterology. 1991;100:A264(abstr.).
24. Schwartz AG, Targan SR, Saxon A, Weinstein WM. Sulfasalazine-induced exacerbation of ulcerative colitis. N Engl J Med. 1982;306:409–12.
25. Austin CA, Cann PA, Jones TH, Holdsworth CD. Exacerbation of diarrhea and pain in patients treated with 5-aminosalicylic acid for ulcerative colitis (letter). Lancet. 1984;1:917–18.
26. Williams CN. Efficacy of corticosteroid and mesalazine (5-aminosalicylate) in inflammatory bowel disease. In: Hadziselimovic F, Herzog B, editors. Pediatric gastroenterology; inflammatory bowel diseases and morbus Hirschsprung. Dordrecht: Kluwer; 1992:137–46.
27. Schroeder KW, Tremaine WJ, Istrup DM. Coated oral 5-aminosalicylic acid therapy for mildly to moderately active ulcerative colitis; randomized study. N Engl J Med. 1987;317:1625–9.
28. Sutherland LR, Martin F, Greer S et al. 5-Aminosalicylic acid enema in the treatment of distal ulcerative colitis, proctosigmoiditis and proctitis. Gastroenterology. 1987;92:1894–8.
29. Meyers S, Lever PK, Feuer EJ, Johnson JW, Janowitz HD. Predicting the outcome of corticosteroid therapy for acute ulcerative colitis; results of a prospective, randomized, double-blind trial. J Clin Gastroenterol. 1987;9:50–4.
30. Hanauer S, Beshears L, Wilkinson C et al. Induction of remission in a dose-raning study of oral mesalamine capsules (Pentasa) Gastroenterology. 1990;98:A174(abstr.).
31. Rachmilewicz D (On behalf of an international study group). Coated mesalazine 5-aminosalicylic acid versus sulphasalazine in the treatment of active ulcerative colitis; a randomized trial. Br Med J. 1989;298:82–6.
32. Misiewicz JJ, Lennard-Jones JE, Connell AM, Baron GH, Avery-Jones F. Controlled trial of sulphasalazine in maintenance therapy of ulcerative colitis. Lancet. 1965;1:185–8.
33. Dissanayake AS, Truelove SC. A controlled, therapeutic trial of long-term maintenance treatment of ulcerative colitis with sulphasalazine (Salazopyrine). Gut. 1973;14:923–6.
34. Azad-Khan AK, Hows DT, Piris J, Truelove SC. Optimal dose of sulphasalazine for maintenance treatment in ulcerative colitis. Gut. 1980;21:232–40.
35. Ireland A, Mason CH, Jewell DP. Controlled trial comparing olsalazine and sulphasalazine for the maintenance treatment of ulcerative colitis. Gut. 1988;29:835–7.
36. Rutgeerts P. Comparative efficacy of coated oral 5-aminosalicylic acid (Claversal) and sulphasalazine for maintaining remission of ulcerative colitis. Alim Pharmacol Ther. 1989;3:183–92.
37. Rosellini SR, Valipani D, Spada M, Miglio F, Tragnone A, Lanfranchi GA. 5-aminosalicylic acid and sullphasalazine in acute and maintenance treatment of ulcerative colitis; a meta analysis of comparative, randomized trials. Gastroenterology. 1991;100:A243(abstr.).
38. Sutherland LR, May GR, Shaffer EA. Sulphasalazine revisited: a meta-analysis of 5-aminosalicylic acid in the treatment of ulcerative colitis. Ann Intern Med. 1993;118:540–9.
39. Robinson SG, Decktor DL. Efficacy of 5-aminosalicylic acid enemas in the treatment of distal ulcerative colitis. Can J Gastroenterol. 1990;4:468–71.
40. Biddle WL, Miner PB. Long-term use of mesalamine enemas to induce remission in ulcerative colitis. Gastroenterology. 1990;99:113–18.
41. Williams CN, Haber G, Aquino J. Double-blind, placebo-controlled evaluation of 5-ASA suppositories in active distal proctitis and measurement of extent of spread using ^{99m}Tc-labelled 5-ASA suppositories. Dig Dis Sci. 1987;32:31–5S.
42. Williams CN. Efficacy and tolerance of 5-aminosalicylic acid suppositories in the treatment of ulcerative colitis; two double-blind, multicentre, placebo-controlled trials. Can J Gastroenterol. 1990;472:5.

43. Irvine EJ, Marshall JK. A meta-analysis of topical 5-ASA's for distal ulcerative colitis. In: Sutherland LR, Collins SM, Martin F et al, editors. Inflammatory bowel disease: basic research, clinical implications and trends in therapy. Lancaster: Kluwer Academic Publishers; 1994.
44. Anthonisen T, Barany F, Folkenborg O et al. The clinical effect of salazosulphapyridine (Salazopyrine) in Crohn's disease; a controlled, double-blind study. Scand J Gastroenterol. 1974;9:549–54.
45. Summers RW, Switz DM, Sessions JR et al. National Cooperative Crohn's Disease Study; results of treatment. Gastroenterology. 1979;77:847–69.
46. Singleton JW, Hanauer SB, Gitnick GL et al. Mesalamine capsules for the treatment of active Crohn's disease: results of a 16 week trial. Gastroenterology. 1993;104:1293–301.
47. Gendre JP, Marrie JY, Florent C et al. Does Pentasa prevent relapses in quiescent Crohn's disease? A multicentre, placebo-controlled trial (161 patients). Gastroenterology. 1990;98:A171(abstr.).
48. Bondesen S and the Danish 5-ASA group. Mesalazine (Pentasa) as prophylaxis in Crohn's disease; a multicentre, controlled trial. Scand J Gastroenterol. (Suppl.). 1991;26:68(abstr.).
49. Lennard-Jones JE. Sulphasalazine in asymptomatic Crohn's disease; a multicentre trial. Gut. 1977;18:69–72.
50. Malchow H, Hewe K, Brandes JW et al. European Cooperative Crohn's Disease Study (E.C.C.D.S.); results of drug treatment. Gastroenterology. 1984;86:249–66.
51. Thomson ABR, with International Mesalazine Study Group. Coated, oral 5-aminosalicylic acid versus placebo in maintaining remission of inactive Crohn's disease. Aliment Pharmacol Ther. 1990;4:55–64.
52. Steinhart AH, Hemphill DJ, Greenberg GR. Sulphasalazine and mesalamine for the maintenance therapy of Crohn's disease: a meta-analysis. In: Sutherland LR, Collins SM, Martin F et al, editors. Inflammatory bowel disease: basic research, clinical implications and trends in therapy. Lancaster: Kluwer Academic Publishers; 1994.

39
Immunosuppressive agents in IBD: current status and future prospects

F. SHANAHAN, G. C. O'SULLIVAN and J. K. COLLINS

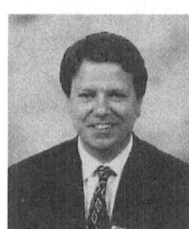

F. SHANAHAN

INTRODUCTION

Inflammatory bowel disease (IBD) has become an exciting area for both the clinician investigator and the basic researcher. Because of improvements in our understanding of the mechanisms and mediators involved in the immune-mediated tissue injury, new and exciting forms of immunotherapy are emerging[1-3]. The interacting elements that contribute to the pathogenesis of Crohn's disease and ulcerative colitis are summarized in Fig. 1. Central to this schema is the concept that the tissue damage is mediated by the mucosal immunoinflammatory response[4,5], and therein lies the rationale for the therapeutic use of immunomodulatory agents in these conditions. The various immunomodulatory strategies that have been reported in patients with IBD have been comprehensively reviewed elsewhere[2]. What follows here is a brief

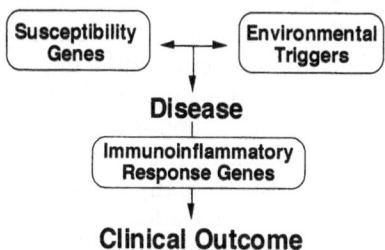

Fig. 1 Factors that contribute to the pathogenesis of IBD

overview of the current status of immunosuppressive therapy in these disorders and a commentary on future prospects.

PURINE ANALOGS

The efficacy of the immunosuppressive purine analogs, azathioprine and its active metabolite, 6-mercaptopurine, is now generally accepted in both Crohn's disease and ulcerative colitis. Although a statistically significant benefit was not obtained in early studies, including the National Cooperative Crohn's Disease Study, this can be attributed in large part to the relatively short duration of the trials[6]. The latency or delayed onset of clinical efficacy of the purine analogs is now recognized. For both Crohn's disease and ulcerative colitis, their role in the treatment of active disease[7,8] and maintenance of remission[9,10] has been convincingly demonstrated in well-designed controlled trials.

In practice these drugs are particularly useful in chronically active Crohn's disease that is uncontrolled by corticosteroids, and in patients requiring persistently high doses of steroids for control of disease activity[8]. The chief limitation to the clinical use of these drugs is that they are slow-acting, having a mean response time of approximately 3 months. Because of this they have no role in the management of acutely ill patients; also, when these drugs are prescribed it is necessary to continue steroid therapy until sufficient time has elapsed for the immunosuppressant effect to become established.

Although doses of up to 2 mg/kg per day were initially used, most clinicians now use a single dose of 50–100 mg/day of 6-mercaptopurine or 100 mg/day of azathioprine. At these low doses the purine analogs are remarkably well tolerated by patients with IBD and bone marrow suppression is uncommon[11,12]. Indeed, a very low frequency of adverse effects was found in a study of 396 patients with IBD followed for up to 18 years with a mean duration of follow-up of 5 years[13]. Pancreatitis occurs in approximately 3% of patients. This is probably a hypersensitivity event and precludes further use of either form of purine analog. Occasionally these drugs produce a debilitating flu-like illness that also appears to be a hypersensitivity phenomenon. The most important potential drug interaction is that which may occur if purine analogs are given to patients taking the xanthine oxidase inhibitor, allopurinol. Purine analogs are metabolized by this enzyme and the concomitant use of allopurinol leads to dangerously high drug levels.

While opportunistic infections are uncommon in patients taking low dose 6-mercaptopurine, the most worrisome potential hazard of long-term usage of purine analogs is the possibility of opportunistic neoplasia. Whether this is a real or theoretical risk is unclear. It may not be a significant problem with the low doses currently used[13]. Many clinicians feel that it is wise to provide patients with a pamphlet that attempts to place in perspective the theoretical risks associated with these drugs in addition to their well-established benefits.

METHOTREXATE

The folic acid antagonist, methotrexate, has been found to have clinical efficacy in a variety of immunologically mediated disorders. The molecular mechanism by which methotrexate suppresses inflammation has recently been clarified[14]. Its action involves a series of biochemical steps that promote the local release of adenosine. Adenosine has a variety of receptor-mediated immunomodulatory properties and inhibits the generation of toxic oxygen metabolites from neutrophils[14].

In an open study of patients with IBD, methotrexate was found to have a marked beneficial effect in some patients, particularly those with Crohn's colitis[15]. Some of these patients were refractory to other treatments including steroids and 6-mercaptopurine, and responded to high-dose methotrexate (25 mg/i.m.) over a 12-week period. Lower doses of methotrexate may also have a steroid-sparing effect[16]. However, the clinical usefulness of methotrexate is limited by adverse effects which include leukopenia, gastro-intestinal toxicity, hypersensitivity pneumonitis and hepatic dysfunction. For this reason methotrexate is probably best reserved for patients who are refractory to, or are intolerant of, purine analogs.

CYCLOSPORINE

The delayed induction of clinical response associated with the purine analogs and methotrexate prompted an investigation of other immunomodulatory agents that might have a more rapid onset of clinical efficacy in acutely ill patients with IBD[17-19]. Cyclosporine has a rapid onset of action, and is thought to suppress the induction and amplification of the immune response by inhibiting cytokine gene activation, particularly interleukin-2[2,19,20]. More recently, evidence for an additional mode of action has emerged that may have particular relevance in IBD. The cyclosporine-binding protein, cyclophilin, which had hitherto been considered to be an intracellular protein, has recently been shown to be a secretory product of activated macrophages. Furthermore, it has cytokine-like, proinflammatory activity with chemotactic effects on neutrophils and eosinophils[20-22]. It has been proposed that this, rather than inhibition of cytokine production, may be the primary immunomodulatory mechanism of action of cyclosporine[23].

One placebo-controlled study of oral cyclosporine in patients with Crohn's disease who were intolerant of or resistant to corticosteroids has been published[24]. Of 37 patients, 22 (59%) improved on cyclosporine (5–7.5 mg/kg per day for 3 months), compared with 11 of 34 (32%) receiving placebo. The improvement was evident after only 2 weeks. However, the preliminary results of a second placebo-controlled trial that have been reported in abstract form suggest a cautious approach to the use of cyclosporine in Crohn's disease[25]. This large ongoing Canadian study found that cyclosporine at a dosage of 4.8 mg/kg is ineffective as therapy of Crohn's disease, and may even have an adverse effect on disease activity in patients in remission.

Several factors limit the long-term use of cyclosporine. These include its wide range of serious toxic side-effects, the need for close monitoring of blood levels, the variable bioavailability when given by the oral route, and the frequency of drug interactions[2]. Many clinicians regard the role of cyclosporine in acute Crohn's disease as a short-term measure at best. Whether it has an interim role, before more slow-acting drugs such as 6-mercaptopurine take full effect, needs to be assessed.

In contrast to Crohn's disease, cyclosporine appears to have a rapid and dramatic beneficial effect in patients with acute severe ulcerative colitis[26,27]. In a preliminary open study of patients with severe ulcerative colitis who had failed to respond to 10 days of intravenous steroids, treatment was supplemented with intravenous cyclosporine (4 mg/kg per day). Remission was achieved in about 80% of the patients such that surgery was avoided[26]. Similar results were found in a subsequent double-blind trial; the trial was halted after 82% of the patients on cyclosporine responded, whereas none of those on placebo improved[27]. For patients with severe colitis who have not responded to traditional treatment with steroids, and who are either not suited or not psychologically ready for colectomy, cyclosporine offers a welcome new option.

Topical enema preparations of cyclosporine have also been used in patients with resistant proctitis[17,28]. However, although several open studies have been encouraging, a recent controlled trial of cyclosporine enemas in patients with mild to moderate ulcerative colitis failed to show a significant therapeutic benefit[29].

OTHER IMMUNOMODULATORY STRATEGIES

The introduction of newer immunosuppressive drugs such as the macrolides, rapamycin and FK506, may eclipse cyclosporine in clinical use during the next decade[2,30]. Studies of FK506 in IBD are already under way[31]. Its mode of action is similar to that of cyclosporine but it is approximately 100-fold more potent. Toxicity is likely to be similar also, although early data have suggested that it occurs with a lower frequency than with cyclosporine. Its efficacy in intestinal transplantation has been particularly impressive, but whether this implies a greater specificity for the intestinal mucosal immune system than occurs with cyclosporine is not yet clear[32].

Intravenous immunoglobulin therapy appears to have a beneficial effect in a variety of immunologically mediated disorders, although its mechanism of action is uncertain. In a recent open study of patients with IBD, some patients appeared to benefit[33]. This is a cumbersome and expensive form of therapy and is unlikely to eclipse other therapeutic strategies. The same limitations apply to the use of T-cell apheresis, even though its efficacy in Crohn's disease appears impressive from the results of a recent open study[34]. A similar outcome can now be achieved with monoclonal antibodies to specific T cell subsets[35].

Cytokine modulation and antagonism is perhaps one of the more exciting recent approaches to therapeutic immunomodulation. Cytokines are the regulatory and effector intercellular messenger molecules of the immune response. They are thus ideal targets for selective immunotherapy[36]. Encouraging preliminary results of cytokine antagonism directed against interleukin-1 in animal models of intestinal inflammation[37,38], and against tumor necrosis factor in humans with IBD[39], have already been reported.

PROSPECTS AND PREDICTIONS

It is likely that the pharmaceutical industry will continue to introduce modifications that improve either the biologic activity or the delivery systems for most of the traditional immunosuppressive drugs. For example, newer purine analogs are already in use for certain leukemias[40]. Whether these agents will have a role in the management of chronic inflammatory disease is unknown. There is also the potential and rationale for developing another generation of cyclosporine-like drugs. As discussed earlier, cyclosporine and related drugs may act primarily by inhibiting the chemotactic activity of secreted cyclophilin. It has been proposed that this mechanism, rather than inhibition of interleukin-2 synthesis, is responsible for the therapeutic effect in both organ graft survival and chronic inflammatory disorders[23]. If this is true, it would be desirable to develop novel agents including cyclosporine derivatives that are potent inhibitors of chemotaxis with less effect on cytokine synthesis by T cells. The potential for selectively removing subsets of T cells by monoclonal antibodies has been facilitated by the ability to engineer 'humanized' antibodies[41], and by the identification of several new receptor/ligand interactions on the T-cell surface that influence activation and physiological cell death[35,42]. For example, rather than targeting an entire CD4 subpopulation, it may be more appropriate to use monoclonal antibodies directed to molecules on the T cell surface that are responsible for physiological cell death and termination of autoreactive lymphocytes during development. Thus, an antibody directed toward the Apo-1/Fas antigen may selectively eliminate a subset of activated T cells by apoptosis[43,44]. Thus, it may be possible to exploit endogenous mechanisms for lymphocyte cell death for beneficial effect in chronic inflammatory disorders with minimal collateral damage or toxicity.

From a clinical perspective, immunosuppressive strategies are likely to be used more widely. The traditional use of drugs on an empiric basis has been replaced by approaches that have a sound rationale and are based on improved understanding of the pathogenesis of IBD. Because of the remarkable reserve of mediators within the inflammatory cascade, it is likely that combination therapy should be used rather than a stepwise approach. Unlike rheumatologists, gastroenterologists have been slow to adopt this concept, and may have much to benefit by earlier use of disease-modifying drugs such as immunosuppressives for chronic inflammatory disease. Finally, future immunomodulatory strategies should target the mucosal immune system rather than the systemic immune response, and should focus on maintenance of disease remission rather than treatment of relapse.

References

1. Bernstein CN, Shanahan F. Immunosuppressive and immunomodulatory therapy for inflammatory bowel disease. Can J Gastroenterol. 1993;7:115–20.
2. Bernstein CN, Shanahan F. Immunomodulatory therapy in inflammatory bowel disease. In: Targan S, Shanahan F, editors. Inflammatory bowel disease: from bench to bedside. Baltimore: Williams & Wilkins; 1994:503–23.
3. Shanahan F, Targan S. Medical treatment of inflammatory bowel disease. Annu Rev Med. 1992;43:125–33.
4. Shanahan F, Targan S. Mechanisms of tissue injury in inflammatory bowel disease. In: Targan S, Shanahan F, editors. Inflammatory bowel disease: from bench to bedside. Baltimore: Williams & Wilkins; 1994:78–88.
5. Shanahan F. Pathogenesis of ulcerative colitis. Lancet. 1993;342:407–11.
6. Summers RW, Switz DM, Sessions JT Jr et al. National Cooperative Crohn's Disease Study: results of drug treatment. Gastroenterology. 1979;77:847–69.
7. Present DH, Korelitz BI, Wisch N, Glass JL, Sacher DB, Pasternack BS. Treatment of Crohn's disease with 6-mercaptopurine. A long term randomized double blind study. N Engl J Med. 1989;302:981–7.
8. Ewe K, Press AG, Singe CC et al. Azathioprine combined with prednisolone or monotherapy with prednisolone in active Crohn's disease. Gastroenterology. 1993;105:367–72.
9. O'Donoghue DP, Dawson AM, Powell-Tuck J, Brown RL, Lennard-Jones JE. Double-blind withdrawal trial of azathioprine as maintenance treatment of Crohn's disease. Lancet. 1978;2:955–7.
10. Hawthorne AB, Logan RFA, Hawkey CJ et al. Randomized controlled trial of azathioprine withdrawal in ulcerative colitis. Br Med J. 1992;305:20–2.
11. Bernstein CN, Artinian L, Anton PA, Shanahan F. Low dose 6-mercaptopurine in inflammatory bowel disease is associated with minimal hematologic toxicity. Dig Dis Sci. 1994 (In press).
12. Connell WR, Kamm MA, Ritchie JK, Lennard-Jones JE. Bone marrow toxicity caused by azathioprine in inflammatory bowel disease: 27 years of experience. Gut. 1993;34:1081–5.
13. Present DH, Meltzer SJ, Krumholz MP, Wolke A, Korelitz BI. 6-Mercaptopurine in the management of inflammatory bowel disease: short- and long-term toxicity. Ann Intern Med. 1989;111:641–9.
14. Cronstein BN, Naime D, Ostad E. The antiinflammatory mechanism of methotrexate. Increased adenosine release at inflamed sites diminishes leukocyte accumulation in an in vivo model of inflammation. J Clin Invest. 1993;92:2675–82.
15. Kozarek RA, Patterson DJ, Gelfand MD, Botoman VA, Ball TJ, Wilske KR. Methotrexate induces clinical and histologic remission in patients with refractory inflammatory bowel disease. Ann Intern Med. 1989;110:353–6.
16. Baron TH, Truss CD, Elson CO. Low-dose oral methotrexate in refractory inflammatory bowel disease. Dig Dis Sci. 1993;38:1851–6.
17. Brynskov J. Cyclosporin for inflammatory bowel disease: mechanisms and possible actions. Scand J Gastroenterol. 1993;28:849–57.
18. Sandborn WJ, Tremaine WJ. Cyclosporine treatment of inflammatory bowel disease. Mayo Clin Proc. 1992;67:981–90.
19. Sigal NH, Dumont FJ. Cyclosporin A, FK-506 and rapamycin: pharmacologic probes of lymphocyte signal transduction. Annu Rev Immunol. 1992;10:519–60.
20. Schrieber SL, Crabtree GR. The mechanism of action of cyclosporin a and FK506. Immunol Today. 1992;13:136–42.
21. Sherry B, Yarlett N, Strupp A, Cerami A. Identification of cyclophilin as a proinflammatory secretory product of lipopolysaccharide-activated macrophages. Proc Natl Acad Sci USA. 1992;89:3511–15.
22. Xu Q, Leiva MC, Fischkoff SA, Handschumacher RE, Lyttle CR. Leukocyte chemotactic activity of cyclophilin. J Biol Chem. 1992;267:11968–71.
23. Erlanger BF. Why cyclosporin is an effective drug. Immunol Today. 1993;14:369(Letter).
24. Brynskov J, Freund L, Rasmussen SN et al. A placebo-controlled double-blind randomized trial of cyclosporine therapy in active chronic Crohn's disease. N Engl J Med. 1989;321:845–50.

25. Archambault A, Feagan B, Fedorak R et al. The Canadian Crohn's relapse prevention trial (CCRPT). Gastroenterology. 1992;102:A591.
26. Lichtiger S, Present DH. Preliminary report: cyclosporin in the treatment of severe active ulcerative colitis. Lancet. 1990;336:16–19.
27. Lichtiger S, Present DH, Kornbluth A, Hanauser SB. Cyclosporine A in the treatment of severe refractory ulcerative colitis: a double blinded placebo controlled trial. Gastroenterology. 1993;104:A732.
28. Brynskov J, Freund L, Thomsen OO et al. Treatment of refractory ulcerative colitis with cyclosporin enemas. Lancet. 1989;1:721–2.
29. Sandborn WJ, Tremaine WJ, Schroeder KW et al. A randomized, double-blind, placebo-controlled trial of cyclosporine enemas for mildly to moderately active left-sided ulcerative colitis. Gastroenterology. 1993;104:A775(bstr.).
30. Macleod AM, Thomson AW. FK506: an immunosuppresant for the 1990s? Lancet. 1991;337:25–7.
31. Reynolds JC, Trellis DR, Abu-Elmgd K, Fung J. The rationale for FK506 in inflammatory bowel disease. Can J Gastroenterol. 1993;7:208–10.
32. Todo S, Tzakis A, Teyes J et al. Intestinal transplantation in humans under FK506. Transplant Proc. 1993;25:1198–9.
33. Levine DS, Fischer SH, Haggitt RC, Christie DL, Ochs HD. Intravenous immunoglobulin therapy for active, extensive, and medically refractory idiopathic ulcerative colitis or Crohn's colitis. Am J Gastroenterol. 1992;87:91–100.
34. Bicks RO, Groshart KD. The current status of T-lymphocyte apheresis (TLA) treatment of Crohn's disease. J Clin Gastroenterol. 19898;11:136–8.
35. Waldmann TA. Immune receptors: targets for therapy of leukemia/lymphoma, autoimmune diseases and for the prevention of allograft rejection. Annu Rev Immunol. 1992;10;675–704.
36. Waldmann TA, Grant A, Tendler C et al. Lymphokine receptor-directed therapy: a model of immune intervention. J Clin Immunol. 1990;10:19–28S.
37. Cominelli F, Nast CC, Clark BD et al. Interleukin-1 gene expression, synthesis and effect of special IL-1 receptor blockade in rabbit immune complex colitis. J Clin Invest. 1990;86:972–80.
38. Sartor RB, Holt LC, Bender DE, Murphy ME, McCall RD, Thompson RC. Prevention and treatment of experimental enterocolitis with a recombinant interleukin-1 receptor antagonist. Gastroenterology. 1991;100:A613.
39. Derkx B, Taminiau J, Radema S et al. Tumor necrosis factor antibody treatment in Crohn's disease. Lancet. 1993;342:173–4.
40. Saven A, Piro L. Newer purine analogues for the treatment of hairy-cell leukemia. N Engl J Med. 1994;330:691–7.
41. Winter G, Harris WJ. Humanized antibodies. Immunol Today. 1993;14:243–6.
42. Adorini L, Guery J-C, Rodriguiz-Targduchy G, Trembleau S. Selective immunosuppression. Immunol Today. 1993;14:285–9.
43. Trauth BC, Klas C, Peters AMJ et al. Monoclonal antibody-mediated tumor regression by induction of apoptosis. Science. 1989;245:301–5.
44. Suda T, Takahashi T, Goldstein P, Nagata S. Molecular cloning and expression of the Fas ligand, a novel member of the tumor necrosis factor family. Cell. 199375:1169–78.

40
Novel targets for anti-inflammatory therapy in IBD

J. L. WALLACE

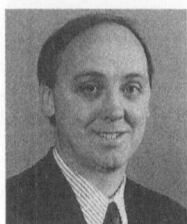

INTRODUCTION

At least in the short term, advances in the treatment of inflammatory bowel disease (IBD) will likely come from improvements in the delivery of existing drugs to the affected region of the intestinal tract, or from improvements in the effectiveness of anti-inflammatory therapy. Over the past decade much attention has been focused on the prospect of targeting specific inflammatory mediators for the therapy of IBD. For example, it has been suggested that inhibiting the synthesis or actions of leukotrienes[1,2], platelet-activating factor (PAF)[3,4] or interleukin-1[5] may be rational approaches to the treatment of IBD. It remains to be seen if any of these approaches will lead to significant improvement in therapy of IBD. An important question that will be answered by clinical studies is whether it is better to have a highly selective anti-inflammatory drug (i.e. one targeted at a single inflammatory mediator) or, because of the redundancy of inflammatory mediators, if a less specific anti-inflammatory drug is more appropriate. For example, is the success of a glucocorticoid in the treatment of IBD attributable to its lack of specificity (it inhibits production of many inflammatory mediators and cytokines, blocks expression of adhesion molecules, etc.)?

This chapter will review the evidence pertinent to three of the possible targets for anti-inflammatory therapy in IBD which have been explored either in animal models or in small clinical trials; these are: (a) nerves and neuropeptides, (b) coagulation and thrombosis, and (c) adhesion molecules on leukocytes and endothelial cells.

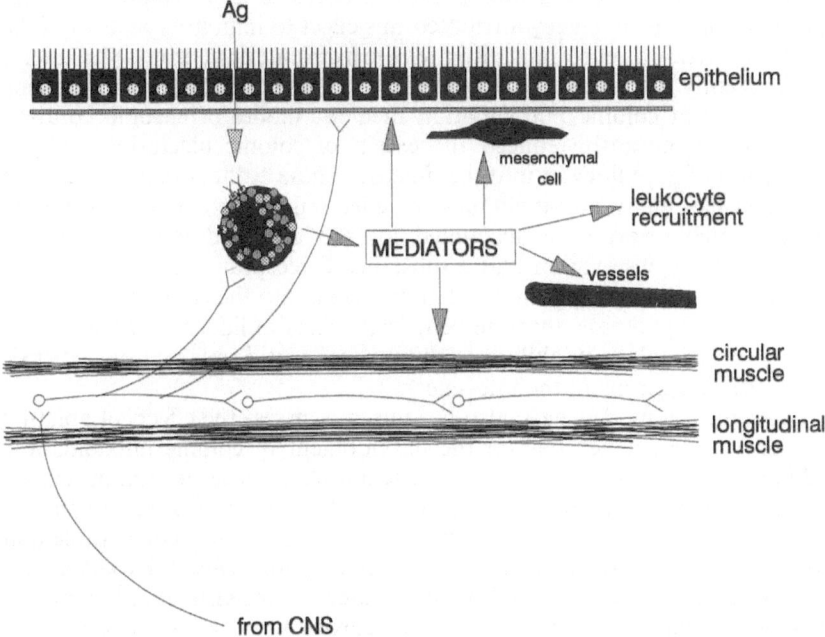

Fig. 1 Possible role of enteric and extrinsic neurons in modulating intestinal inflammation. Immunocytes, including mast cells, are in close contact with mucosal neurons and it is possible that neural activation can lead to activation of the immunocytes to release soluble mediators. These mediators exert effects on the epithelium, mesenchymal cells, vasculature and muscle, as well as recruiting granulocytes into the tissue. The nerves themselves can also release chemotactic mediators (e.g. substance P)

NERVES AND NEUROPEPTIDES

Among the mediators implicated in the pathogenesis of IBD are the neuropeptides released from enteric and sensory afferent neurons[6] (Fig. 1). These peptides, which include substance P, vasoactive intestinal polypeptide and calcitonin gene-related peptide, have been shown to modulate many aspects of mucosal function, including blood flow and secretion, and may also play a role in the recruitment of granulocytes and lymphocytes[7] and in the modulation of immune function[8,9]. Lymphocyte function may also be modulated by neurons within the colonic mucosa, since these cells have receptors for a number of neuropeptides and noradrenaline[10]. Changes in the density and neurotransmitter content of enteric neurons in patients with IBD are well documented[10-12]. A role for the enteric nervous system in the pathogenesis of IBD is further supported by the demonstration that colitis in experimental animals can be initiated or exacerbated by stress[13,14]. Further evidence for a contribution of neuropeptides to the pathogenesis of IBD comes from the study of Björck et al.[15]. They tested the effects of twice-daily lidocaine enemas on 100 patients with ulcerative proctitis, two-thirds of whom were resistant to previous therapy with sulfasalazine or steroids.

Over the course of 3–32 weeks, 90% of the patients responded, with symptomatic improvement and a marked decrease in T lymphocyte infiltration of the mucosa. They attributed this effect to inhibitory actions of the local anesthetic on neurotransmitter release from enteric neurons. McCafferty et al. recently confirmed the effectiveness of lidocaine enemas in reducing the severity of colonic inflammation in a rat model of chronic colitis[16]. Lidocaine significantly reduced the extent of colonic ulceration and the infiltration of granulocytes into the mucosa. These authors pointed out that lidocaine has many anti-inflammatory effects unrelated to its actions on nerves which could have accounted for the observed beneficial effects. However, their observation that a substance P receptor antagonists (NK-1) was capable of reducing granulocyte infiltration into the colon in this model supports the hypothesis that the beneficial effects of lidocaine were at least in part attributable to its ability to inhibit neuropeptide release from extrinsic and intrinsic neurons in the intestine[16].

Experimental models have also been used to assess the effects of ablation of sensory afferent neurons on the development of colonic inflammation. Administration of the neurotoxin capsaicin leads to degeneration of sensory afferent neurons. If these neurons, through the release of proinflammatory neuropeptides, contribute to the inflammatory process, it is conceivable that ablation of the neurons will have anti-inflammatory effects. However, this question has not been thoroughly investigated. Evangelista et al.[17] reported that prior ablation of sensory afferent neurons with capsaicin resulted in exacerbation of colitis in a rat model. However, one must interpret these data carefully. Capsaicin-sensitive neurons play an important role in modulating mucosal blood flow through the gastrointestinal tract. By ablating these neurons an important component of mucosal defense is removed. As the model used by Evangelista et al. involves intraluminal application of a cytotoxic solution, it is likely that capsaicin-induced ablation of sensory afferent neurons greatly increased the extent of mucosal injury. Another recent publication from the same group suggested that capsaicin could protect the colonic mucosa from injury induced by a cytotoxic solution[18]. Co-administration of capsaicin with the agent used to induce colitis (trinitrobenzene sulfonic acid in a vehicle of 50% ethanol) resulted in a diminution of the extent of mucosal injury. One possible explanation for these results is that capsaicin, by activating sensory afferent neurons, increased colonic mucosal blood flow, thereby increasing the resistance of the colonic mucosa to damage induced by the cytotoxic solution. Thus, in both of the published studies on the effects of capsaicin in experimental colitis, interpretation of the data is made difficult by the possibility that capsaicin administration has an impact on the induction of colitis in the model used. The question of whether or not capsaicin can modulate colonic inflammation has not yet been adequately addressed. Of greatest interest would be a study of the effects of intracolonic capsaicin administration after colitis is established.

COAGULATION AND THROMBOSIS

The recent work of Wakefield and his colleagues has stimulated many investigators to re-examine the relationship between coagulation and inflammation as it pertains to the pathogenesis of IBD. Wakefield *et al.*[19,20] suggested that activation of the mesenteric microvascular endothelium is a central step in the development of vasculitis, and that this is an early step in the pathogenesis of Crohn's disease (CD) since it is detectable before mucosal inflammation and microscopic ulceration can be seen. This group reported the presence of platelet thrombi in a significant proportion of CD patients prior to the development of ulceration[21]. They have also demonstrated that mimicking the development of thrombi within the mesenteric circulation, through local injection of microspheres into the submucosal collateral plexus of the ferret, led to the development of intestinal injury which was histologically similar to that seen in CD[22].

For decades there have been reports of a hypercoagulable state in IBD, and a relatively high incidence of thromboembolism. For example, clinical thromboembolic complications have been reported in 2–4% of patients with IBD[23], and in one post-mortem study, evidence of thromboembolism was found in 39% of IBD cases[24]. Active CD has been associated with elevated levels of plasma fibrinogen, factors V and VIII and platelet count, suggesting a hypercoagulable state[25–27]. Hudson *et al.*[28] reported elevated levels of many prothrombotic factors (fibrinopeptide A, prothrombin fragments) in the blood of CD patients. There is also evidence of impaired fibrinolysis in IBD[29–31]. Lam *et al.*[26] reported low antithrombin III levels in IBD patients, and noted that even a modest decrease in blood levels of this factor is considered a risk for thromboembolism. Taken together, the data from these studies and numerous others suggest that a disorder of coagulation may contribute to the pathogenesis of IBD.

In addition to its central role in thrombosis, the platelet is increasingly being recognized as an important inflammatory cell. There is evidence for the involvement of platelet in the thromboembolic disorders reported in IBD patients. Webberley *et al.*[32] recently reported that in a study of 104 patients with IBD (eight of whom had previously had thromboembolism), 30% had spontaneous platelet aggregation, and a further 20% exhibited a hypersensitivity to low concentrations of aggregating agents. Plasma thromboxane and β-thromboglobulin levels were also significantly elevated, suggesting activation of platelets.

The difficulty in interpreting these studies of platelet function in IBD is that it is not clear if these changes predated the development of IBD, or occurred as a consequence of IBD. It is also difficult to assess the contribution of these changes to the pathogenesis of IBD and the development of tissue injury. Moreover, the use of various anti-inflammatory drugs by the IBD patients may have contributed to the observed changes in platelet function.

A recent clinical trial suggests that the coagulative disorders associated with IBD may indeed contribute to the disease process and the development of symptoms. Gaffney *et al.*[33] reported improvement in 10 ulcerative colitis patients treated with anticoagulant doses of heparin. Nine of the 10 patients were poorly controlled on sulfasalazine and prednisolone, while the other was not taking medication. The patients self-administered heparin daily and continued to take sulfasalazine, while the prednisolone was tapered to a stop.

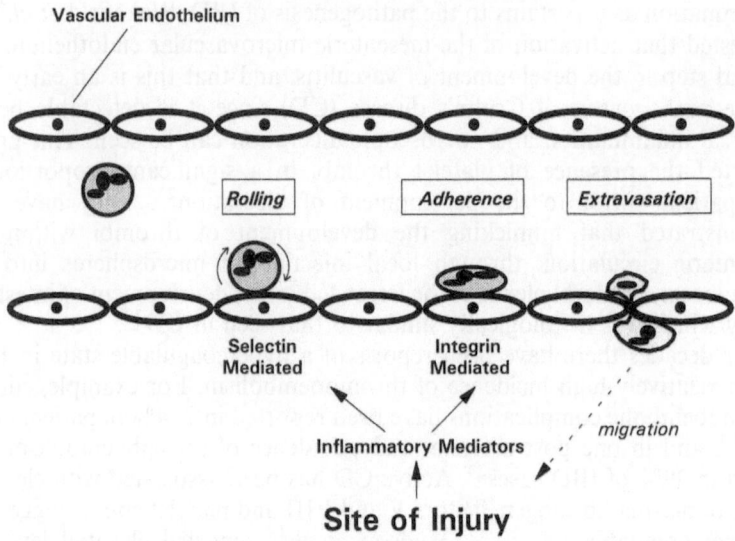

Fig. 2 Leukocyte rolling, adherence and emigration in response to an inflammatory signal. Rolling of leukocytes is mediated by 'selectins' on the endothelium and the leukocyte. Adherence and possibly emigration are mediated by adhesion molecules on the leukocyte and on the endothelium

Nine patients became asymptomatic, and the other had persistent symptoms, but with a 40% reduction in severity. Paradoxically, rectal bleeding decreased during heparin therapy.

It is important to note that heparin can exert anti-inflammatory effects and influence endothelial function through mechanisms unrelated to its anticoagulant properties[34]. Evidence that heparin can block anaphylactic reactions dates back to the 1920s[35]. Seeds et al.[36] reported anti-inflammatory effects of heparin on allergen or PAF-induced eosinophil infiltration of the guinea-pig lung. Interestingly, these effects were observed with a low molecular weight heparin-like molecule which did not exert anticoagulant effects, but not with polyglutamic acid or high molecular weight dextrans that share the property of heparin of being polyanionic.

ADHESION MOLECULES

Infiltration of the intestinal mucosa by neutrophils, macrophages, lympho-cytes and other leukocytes is a hallmark feature of IBD. Moreover, this infiltration almost certainly accounts for a significant amount of the mucosal injury associated with IBD. The movement of leukocytes from the blood stream into a tissue occurs in several steps (Fig. 2). The leukocyte first leaves the main flow of blood and begins to roll along the vascular endothelium. Next, the leukocyte becomes firmly adherent to the endothelium. The leukocyte then slowly migrates to the junction between adjacent endothelial cells and begins to crawl through this junction and into the underlying tissue.

Each of these steps in leukocyte emigration involves tightly regulated interactions between specific adhesion molecules on the leukocyte and the endothelium. By interfering with these interactions it is possible to inhibit the movement of leukocytes from the blood stream to an inflamed tissue and, in doing so, to reduce the extent of tissue injury.

Rolling of leukocytes along the endothelium is mediated by a group of adhesion molecules called 'selectins'. These molecules have carbohydrate domains which are critical to their function in mediating intercellular adhesive interactions. The selectins on leukocytes are not yet completely characterized. 'E-selectin' and 'P-selectin' are examples of selectins expressed on the surface of vascular endothelial cells. It is possible to inhibit leukocyte rolling on the endothelium by administering monoclonal antibodies directed against these molecules[37]. If leukocytes are prevented from rolling on the endothelium, firm adherence and migration out of the vessel are also prevented.

Firm adherence of leukocytes to the endothelium is mediated by another group of adhesion molecules. On the endothelium these include intercellular adhesion molecule-1 and -2 (ICAM-1 and -2, respectively), and vascular cell adhesion molecule-1 (VCAM-1). There are numerous types of adhesion molecules on the leukocytes which bind to the integrins. For example, the principal group of adhesins on neutrophils are termed CD11/CD18. Adherence and subsequent emigration of leukocytes can be blocked by monoclonal antibodies directed against these integrins or against the endothelial adhesion molecules. Such antibodies have been tested in experimental models of intestinal inflammation. For example, the increased epithelial permeability associated with a rabbit model of colitis could be reduced by ~70% by treating the animals with an antibody directed against CD18[38]. This antibody completely suppressed granulocyte infiltration into the mucosa. These data support the hypothesis that granulocyte recruitment into the mucosa and across the epithelium accounts for a significant portion of epithelial injury. Podolsky et al.[39] recently reported dramatic beneficial effects of treatment of colitis in cottontop tamarins with an antibody directed against an adhesion molecule found on monocytes and lymphocytes (VLA-4).

While adhesion molecules represent a relatively new target for anti-inflammatory drug development, many of the anti-inflammatory drugs that have been in use for decades exert at least a part of their beneficial actions through effects on adhesion molecule expression. For example, glucocorticoids inhibit the expression of a number of adhesion molecules, including ICAM-1 and E-selectin[40]. Indeed, the down-regulation of expression of these adhesion molecules by glucocorticoids likely accounts for the well-documented observation of leukopenia following administration of these drugs. When expression of ICAM-1 and E-selectin is inhibited, the pool of leukocytes that under normal conditions are rolling or adherent to the endothelium become detached and re-enter the circulation. Heparin is another drug which exerts anti-inflammatory properties that may in part be related to effects on adhesion molecules. Nelson et al.[41] recently demonstrated that various preparations of heparin could block L-selectin and P-selectin, and therefore could block binding of neutrophils to endothelium and platelets.

The development of drugs which will interfere with the function of adhesion molecules is a considerable challenge. While many monoclonal antibodies have been developed which will block the interactions mediated by these molecules, the utility of these substances for treatment of IBD is limited by the need for systemic administration. Moreover, despite attempts to 'humanize' the antibodies, immunogenicity remains a problem, especially when the antibodies have to be administered repeatedly. A further problem is that blockade of the ability of leukocytes to adhere renders the patient more susceptible to infections, although there is evidence that adequate antibiotic coverage during the period of treatment will greatly reduce the risk of infection. Since many of the adhesion molecules, particularly selectins, have carbohydrate residues that are critical to their activity, some pharmaceutical companies are attempting to develop carbohydrate-based drugs which will interfere with leukocyte adherence to these molecules. Attempts are also being made to better understand the signal transduction pathways involved in the regulation of adhesion molecule expression, in the hope that this may be a target for modulation of the activity of these molecules.

SUMMARY

There are numerous potential targets for anti-inflammatory therapy in IBD. In this review I have focused on only three of these targets. Improvements in anti-inflammatory therapy can be achieved in two major ways: first, it may be possible to develop more effective therapies; secondly, it may be possible to develop therapies that are equally effective as existing drugs, but have a better adverse effect profile. For example, if glucocorticoids produce their desired anti-inflammatory effects through inhibition of expression of adhesion molecules, it should be possible to produce novel molecules that achieve this more effectively and selectively, thereby yielding fewer side-effects. On the other hand, it is possible that the anti-inflammatory effects of glucocorticoids are not attributable to a single action, but to the ability of these drugs to interfere with the inflammatory cascade at many different steps. If this latter possibility is the case it may be difficult to improve on anti-inflammatory effectiveness and at the same time reduce the adverse effect profile.

The anti-inflammatory properties of heparin have been recognized for over 60 years. There is a growing body of evidence suggesting that the anti-inflammatory and anticoagulant properties of this substance can be separated. There are intriguing preliminary studies suggesting that heparin is very effective in reducing the severity of ulcerative colitis. The novel heparin derivatives which lack anticoagulant activity will be powerful tools to determine to what extent the beneficial effects of heparin are attributable to its anticoagulant effects.

Evidence for a neural component of the pathogenesis of IBD, while primarily anecdotal in nature, is still compelling. In particular there is a wealth of data suggesting that the central and enteric nervous systems can markedly alter mucosal immune function. The demonstration of the effectiveness of lidocaine enemas in the treatment of proctitis is fascinating, but these studies need to be repeated in a more controlled manner (recognizing that a placebo control may not be feasible). Specific receptor antagonists for many of the neuropeptides are now becoming available, and should prove to be useful for dissecting out the contribution of some of these mediators to the inflammatory response in IBD.

Acknowledgements

Dr Wallace is a Medical Research Council of Canada (MRC) Scientist and an Alberta Heritage Foundation for Medical Research Scientist, supported by grants from the MRC and the Crohn's and Colitis Foundation of Canada.

References

1. Sharon P, Stenson WF. Enhanced synthesis of leukotriene B_4 by colonic mucosa in inflammatory bowel disease. Gastroenterology. 1984;86:453–60.
2. Wallace JL. 5-Lipoxygenase: a rational target for therapy of inflammatory bowel disease. Trends Pharmacol Sci. 1990;11:51–3.
3. Wallace JL. Release of platelet-activating factor (PAF) and accelerated healing induced by a PAF antagonist in an animal model of chronic colitis. Can J Physiol Pharmacol. 1988;66:422–5.
4. Eliakim R, Karmeli F, Razin E, Rachmilewitz R. Role of platelet activating factor in ulcerative colitis. Enhanced production during active disease and inhibition by sulfasalazine and prednisolone. Gastroenterology. 1988;95:1167–72.
5. Cominelli F, Nast CC, Duchini A, Lee M. Recombinant interleukin-1 receptor antagonist blocks the proinflammatory activity of endogenous interleukin-1 in rabbit immune colitis. Gastroenterology. 1992;103:65–71.
6. Sharkey KA. Substance P and calcitonin gene-related peptide (CGRP) in gastrointestinal inflammation. Ann NY Acad Sci. 1992;664:425–42.
7. Kubota Y, Petras RE, Ottaway CA, Tubbs RR, Farmer RG, Fiocchi C. Colonic vasoactive intestinal peptide nerves in inflammatory bowel disease. Gastroenterology. 1992;102:1242–51.
8. Bienenstock J, Croitoru K, Ernst PB, Stanisz AM. Nerves and neuropeptides in the regulation of mucosal immunity. Adv Exp Med Biol. 1990;257:19–26.
9. Shanahan F, Denburg JA, Fox K, Bienenstock J, Befus D. Mast cell heterogeneity: effects of neuroenteric peptides on histamine release. J Immunol. 1985;135:1331–7.
10. Felton DL, Felton SY, Carlsson SL, Olschowka JA, Livnat S. Noradrenergic and peptidergic innervation of lymphoid tissue. J Immunol. 1985;135:755–65.
11. Kyosola K, Penttila O, Salaspuro M. Rectal mucosal adrenergic innervation and enterochromaffin cells in ulcerative colitis and irritable colon. Scand J Gastroenterol. 1977;12:363–7.
12. Mantyh CR, Gates TS, Zimmerman RP et al. Receptor binding sites for substance P, but not for substance K or neuromedin K, are expressed in high concentrations by arterioles, venules, and lymph nodules in surgical specimens obtained from patients with ulcerative colitis and Crohn's disease. Proc Natl Acad Sci. 1988;85:3235–9.
13. McHugh K, Weingarten HP, Khan I, Riddell R, Collins SM. Stress-induced exacerbation of experimental colitis. Gastroenterology. 1993;104:A803(abstr.).
14. Wood JD, Peck OC, Sharma HM et al. Stress-induced inflammatory changes in the colon of the cotton-top tamarin model for spontaneous colitis and colon cancer. Gastroenterology. 1993;104:A803(abstr.).
15. Björck S, Dahlström A, Johansson L, Ahlman H. Treatment of the mucosa with local anaesthetics in ulcerative colitis. Agents Actions. 1993;35(Suppl.):C60–72.

16. McCafferty DM, Sharkey KA, Wallace JL. Beneficial effects of local and systemic lidocaine in experimental colitis. Am J Physiol. 1994 (In press).
17. Evangelista S, Meli A. Influence of capsaicin-sensitive fibres on experimentally-induced colitis in rats. J Pharm Pharmacol. 1989;41:574–5.
18. Goso C, Evangelista S, Tramontana M, Manzini S, Blumberg PM, Szallasi A. Topical capsaicin administration protects against trinitrobenzene sulfonic acid-induced colitis in the rat. Eur J Pharmacol. 1993;249:185–90.
19. Wakefield AJ, Sankey EA, Dhillon AP et al. Granulomatous vasculitis in Crohn's disease. Gastroenterology. 1991;100:1279–87.
20. Wakefield AJ, Sawyerr AM, Dhillon AP et al. Pathogenesis of Crohn's disease: multifocal gastrointestinal infarction. Lancet. 1989;2:1057–62.
21. Dhillon AP, Anthony A, Sim R et al. Mucosal capillary thrombi in rectal biopsies. Histopathology. 1992;21:127–33.
22. Hudson M, Piasecki C, Sankey EA et al. A ferret model of acute multifocal gastrointestinal infarction. Gastroenterology. 1992;102:1591–6.
23. Talbot RW, Heppell J, Dozois RR, Beart RW. Vascular complications of inflammatory bowel disease. Mayo Clin Proc. 1986;61:140–5.
24. Graef V, Baggenstoss AH, Sauer WG, Spittell JL. Venous thrombosis occurring with nonspecific ulcerative colitis. Arch Intern Med. 1966;117:277–82.
25. Lake AM, Stauffer JQ, Stuart MJ. Haemostatic alterations in inflammatory bowel disease. Am J Dig Dis. 1978;23:897–902.
26. Lam A, Borda LT, Inwood MJ, Thompson S. Coagulation studies in ulcerative colitis and Crohn's disease. Gastroenterology. 1975;68:245–51.
27. Lee JCL, Spittell J, Sauer WG, Owen CA, Thompson JH. Hypercoagulability associated with chronic ulcerative colitis: changes in blood coagulation factors. Gastroenterology. 1968;54:76–84.
28. Hudson M, Hutton RA, Wakefield AJ, Sawyerr AM, Pounder RE. Evidence of activation of coagulation in Crohn's disease. Blood Coag Fibrin. 1992;3:773–8.
29. Conlan MG, Haire WD, Burnett DA. Prothrombotic abnormalities in inflammatory bowel disease. Dig Dis Sci. 1989;34:1089–93.
30. de Bruin PAF, Crama-Bohbouth G, Verspaget H et al. Plasmogen activators in the intestine of patients with inflammatory bowel disease. Thromb Haemost. 1988;60:262–6.
31. Gris JC, Schved JF, Raffanel C et al. Impaired fibrinolytic capacity in patients with inflammatory bowel disease. Thromb Haemost. 1990;63:472–5.
32. Webberley MJ, Hart MT, Melikian V. Thromboembolism in inflammatory bowel disease: role of platelets. Gut. 1993;34:247–51.
33. Gaffney PR, Doyle CT, Hogan J, Gaffney A. Paradoxical response to heparin in 10 patients with ulcerative colitis. Gastroenterology. 1993;A703.
34. D'Amore PA. Heparin–endothelial cell interactions. Haemostasis. 1990;20(Suppl. 1):159–65.
35. Van der Carr RF, Williams OB. Further studies on the influence of heparin on anaphylactic shock in the guinea pig. J Immunol. 1928;15:13–20.
36. Seeds EAM, Hanss J, Page CP. The effect of heparin and related proteoglycans on allergen and PAF-induced eosinophil infiltration. J Lipid Mediators. 1993;7:269–78.
37. Mulligan MS, Watson SR, Fennie C, Ward PA. Protective effects of selectin chimeras in neutrophil-mediated lung injury. J Immunol. 1993;151:6410–17.
38. Wallace JL, Higa A, McKnight GW, MacIntyre DE. Prevention and reversal of experimental colitis by a monoclonal antibody which inhibits leukocyte adherence. Inflammation. 1992;16:343–54.
39. Podolsky DK, Lobb R, King N et al. Attenuation of colitis in the cotton-top tamarin by anti-α4 integrin monoclonal antibody. J Clin Invest. 1993;92:372–80.
40. Cronstein BN, Kimmel SC, Levin RI, Martiniu F, Weissmann G. A mechanism for the antiinflammatory effects of corticosteroids: the glucocorticoid receptor regulates leukocyte adhesion to endothelial cells and expression of endothelial–leukocyte adhesion molecule 1 and intercellular adhesion molecule 1. Proc Natl Acad Sci USA. 1992;89:9991–5.
41. Nelson RM, Cecconi O, Roberts WG, Aruffo A, Linhardt RJ, Bevilacqua MP. Heparin oligosaccharides bind L- and P-selectin and inhibit acute inflammation. Blood. 1993;82:3253–8.

Section XII
Therapy in IBD in 1994

41
A gastroenterologist's perspective of the medical management of patients with Crohn's disease and ulcerative colitis

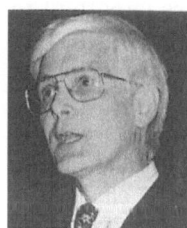

A. B. R. THOMSON

INTRODUCTION

The reasons for the chronic relapsing nature of Crohn's disease (CD) and chronic idiopathic ulcerative colitis (UC) are unknown. Certain factors have been described in association with symptomatic recurrences, such as the use of nonsteroidal anti-inflammatory drugs (NSAID), an intercurrent viral illness, emotional stress, pregnancy, development of diarrhea masquerading as active disease in a patient on antibiotics, the rare worsening of symptoms with sulfasalazine, the discontinuation of maintenance therapy, and a change in smoking habits. It is important to establish the cause of recurrences. It is, however, recognized that many more persons will have endoscopically active CD after a previous surgical resection, than those who have symptoms (Rutgeerts *et al.*, 1990). It is unclear whether the object of therapy should be to control symptoms or to control disease activity (as measured endoscopically, microscopically or biochemically). Knowing what are the pathophysiological factors responsible for causing the inflammation, or causing the inflammation to become symptomatic, would be useful considerations.

Several clinical indices have been developed to assess the activity of CD, such as the widely used Crohn's disease activity index (CDAI) (Best *et al.*, 1979). The uses and limitatons of these indices have been reviewed (Sutherland,

1991). Clinical indices have also been developed for patients with UC. Objective markers of continued disease activity need to be developed and used to predict future clinical recurrences. For example, intestinal permeability is abnormal in patients with active CD, and may return towards normal when the disease becomes clinically inactive. Should medical treatment be continued until this altered permeability is normalized? What does the increased permeability tell us about the underlying immunological or vascular abnormalities? Furthermore, it is difficult to know how best to define relapse: symptoms, laboratory values, endoscopic appearances (Sutherland, 1991). Consider, for example, that it is unknown whether abnormal laboratory measures of disease activity should be treated in asymptomatic individuals, or should be used as an endpoint for therapy rather than attempting to achieve the rather arbitrary reduction in the CDAI to less than 150 units.

It is important to consider several concepts: (1) Treating symptoms does not necessarily alter disease activity, prevent complications, or change the natural history of inflammatory bowel disease (IBD); (2) it is important to distinguish between the treatment of active disease and continuous disease activity suppression – versus true maintenance of remission; (3) predictors of recurrence versus predictors of continued disease activity need to be developed; (4) improved quality of life (QOL) is likely to be achieved with treatments which reduce the frequency and severity of symptoms, so that changes in disease activity indices should be correlated with changes in indices of QOL; and (5) the cost-effectiveness of all medical and surgical treatments for IBD need to be assessed against the background of improving QOL. Let us consider each of the major therapeutic options available for the medical management of patients with UC or CD. These include the anti-inflammatories (sulfasalazine, mesalamines, 5'-lipoxygenase inhibitors and ω-3 fatty acids), antibiotics, glucocorticosteroids, immunomodulators (aza-thioprine, 6-mercaptopurine [6-MP], cyclosporin, methotrexate, immuno-globulin and K76), nutritional therapy, lifestyle modification, and numerous as yet unproven experimental agents.

ANTI-INFLAMMATORIES

Sulfasalazine

Sulfasalazine (SASP), composed of a sulfa moiety (a sulfonamide, sulfapyridine [SP]), is covalently bonded through an azo-bond to an aspirin analogue, mesalamine (5-aminosalicylic acid, 5-ASA). SASP is cleaved by the enzyme azoreductase, found in enteric bacteria, to yield its constituent moieties, SP and 5-ASA. While the SP is often viewed as an inactive 'carrier', it may in fact partially contribute to the clinical effectiveness of SASP. Mesalamine confers its anti-inflammatory activity largely as the result of a local action on the bowel. Mesalamine inhibits interleukin production, platelet-activating factor, and chemotaxis of neutrophils and monocytes; also, it is a potent scavenger of oxygen free radicals, and affects the inflammatory process through leukotrienes and prostaglandins[4]. Although there are many actions of 5-ASA, it is unknown which ones are important for the therapeutic response in patients with IBD.

A major advance in the management of patients with UC was the introduction of SASP for maintenance therapy. A detailed meta-analysis has reviewed the efficacy of SASP in the management of patients with a mild–moderate attack of UC, and in the maintenance of clinical remission (Sutherland et al., 1993). For example, a relapse rate of 14% over 3 years was observed using 2 g/day SASP, much lower than with placebo (56%) (Dissanayake and Truelove, 1973). Adverse effects to SASP occur in at least 15% of patients using SASP, and these adverse effects may vary from a minor inconvenience to a major allergic reaction.

The use of SASP in CD is limited to the relatively modest effect in patients with colonic or ileo-colonic disease (National Cooperative Crohn's Disease Study [NCCDS]) (Summers et al., 1979) or to colonic and ileal disease (Malchow et al., 1984). In the NCCDS SASP was not found to be effective in the prevention of relapse of CD (Best et al., 1976). On the other hand, SASP 3 g/day for 2 years appears to be beneficial to prevent postoperative recurrences of CD (Ewe et al., 1989).

Mesalamine by mouth

The topic of the use of the new 5-ASA preparations in patients with CD and UC has been reviewed (Greenfield et al., 1993; Riley and Turnberg, 1991). It is generally accepted that mesalamine is therapeutically equivalent to SASP for treatment of active UC and for maintaining remission in this disease (Kulerich et al., 1992; Rijk et al., 1992; Record and Macrae, 1992; Courtney et al., 1992; Nakashabendi et al., 1992; Giaffer et al., 1992; Green et al., 1992). It must be stressed that the mesalamine products have different delivery properties, and they are not necessarily equivalent in beneficial action. Thus, efficacy proven from a clinical trial of one mesalamine compound cannot necessarily be compared directly with another 5-ASA compound with a different coating. Both SASP and mesalamine may be useful to treat active CD, and mesalamine, but not SASP, is effective maintenance therapy in CD (Hemphill et al., 1993; International Mesalamine Study Group, 1990).

Asacol® has been used in patients with mild attacks of UC: there is a clear benefit of 4.8 g/day (Schroeder et al., 1986). Miglioli et al. (1990) compared the efficacies of 1.2, 2.4 and 3.6 g/day of Asacol® in a multicenter trial including 73 UC patients with mild attacks. After 1 month treatment, 46% were in remission with 3.6 g/day, compared with 12% of those receiving 1.2 g/day. Although the 3.6 g/day dose was superior, this is still only a modest response rate. Sninsky et al. (1991) obtained approximately comparable results.

Doses of Asacol® of 3.2 g/day by mouth are equivalent to low-dose topical steroid enemas (prednisolone 20 mg/day) over a 4-week interval for the treatment of patients with distal colitis (Zaytoun et al., 1991). This allows patients to choose between an oral or a topical approach for the treatment of mild disease.

Olsalazine (Dipentum®), 3 g/day, is superior to placebo for the treatment of mild attacks of active UC (Zinberg et al., 1990). Olsalazine 1 g/day in 114 UC patients was compared with SASP 2 g/day in 112 patients for maintenance therapy (Killerich et al., 1992). Patients were admitted to the study within 1 month of remission after an attack: rates were similar in both groups, about 45% in a year. On the other hand, it has been suggested that relapse rates are lower in UC patients treated with olsalazine than with SASP or other mesalamines (Courtney et al., 1992; Record and Macrae, 1992; Rijk et al., 1992). The issue is really whether SASP is more effective than an equivalent amount of 5-ASA, whether higher doses of 5-ASA may be used to achieve even lower relapse rates, and whether one 5-ASA preparation is superior to another in the equivalent clinical setting.

The topic of the bioavailability, plasma level and excretion of the slow-release 5-ASA preparations has been reviewed (Rasmusson et al., 1982; Thomson, 1991). Absorption of delayed-release oral mesalamine is not modified by dietary fiber intake (Riley et al., 1991). The dispositions of Asacol®, Salofalk®, Pentasa® and Dipentum® have been compared when given as 2 g/day for 5 days in 14 patients with UC in remission (Laursen et al., 1990). The mesalamine concentration in the colonic lumen (estimated with the rectal dialysis technique) was doubled after olsalazine as compared with Pentasa® or Salofalk®, but was not greatly different for Asacol®. Conversely, systemic concentrations of mesalamine were lower with olsalazine than with Salofalk® or Pentasa®, with results similar to those of another comparative study (Christensen et al., 1990). De Vos et al. (1992) evaluated intramucosal (as contrasted with intraluminal) mesalamine and acetylated mesalamine concentrations in ileocolonic biopsy specimens in 61 patients with IBD who took different preparations of mesalamine for 1 week. The highest concentrations of native and acetylated mesalamine were seen after administration of Asacol®, with lower concentrations after SASP or Dipentum®. This information is useful to select a new 5-ASA for colonic delivery for patients in remission, but mesalamine release may not necessarily be as favorable with azo derivatives as it is in patients in remission (Rijk et al., 1989).

Oral mesalamines have shown favorable results in patients with active CD in an American multicenter study of 310 patients who received 1, 2 or 4 g/day of Pentasa® for 16 weeks, compared with placebo (Singleton et al., 1993): 64% of CD patients went into remission on 4 g/day. It was surprising that there was no clear-cut dose-dependent response in this study (Fig. 1). It is in dispute whether Pentasa® 1.5 g/day is (Rasmussen et al., 1982) or is not (Mihida and Jewell, 1990) useful to treat patients with active CD. Salofalk® 3 g/day is comparable over 12 weeks to prednisone (40 mg/day for 2 weeks with subsequent dose reduction) in the treatment of active CD, although the initial clinical response was faster with prednisone (Martin et al., 1990) (Fig. 2).

Patients given Mesasal® (also known as Claversal® or Salofalk®) 1.5 g/day versus placebo in patients with CD, in a 1-year study, showed lower relapse rates, especially in those persons with ileal disease, in males,

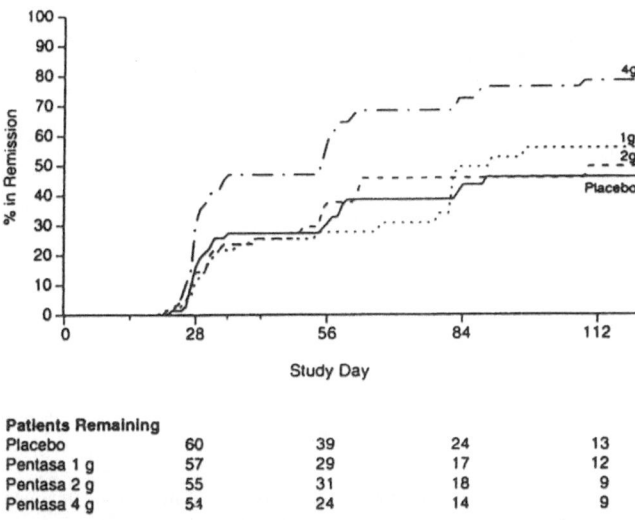

Patients Remaining				
Placebo	60	39	24	13
Pentasa 1 g	57	29	17	12
Pentasa 2 g	55	31	18	9
Pentasa 4 g	54	24	14	9

Fig. 1 Mesalamine life table plot: percentage of patients achieving remission in each treatment group at each study visit (Kaplan–Meier method) (Singleton *et al.*, 1993)

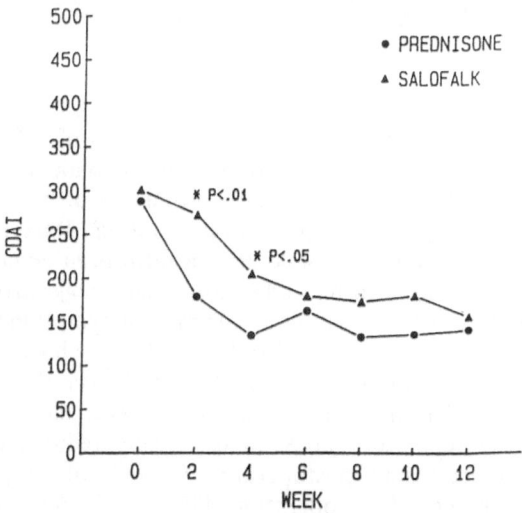

Fig. 2 Mean Crohn's disease activity index (CDAI) score changes obtained at each 2-week visit in all studied patients in a multicentre controlled trial of 5-aminosalicylic acid versus prednisone (Martin *et al.*, 1990)

or following ileal resection (International Mesalamine Study Group, 1990). A large multicentre study with Claversal® 3 g/day (unpublished observations, 1994) versus placebo has been completed; but the results are not yet available. A French multicentre study with Pentasa®, 2 g/day, showed benefit only in CD patients admitted with a flare-up of disease within the last 3 months

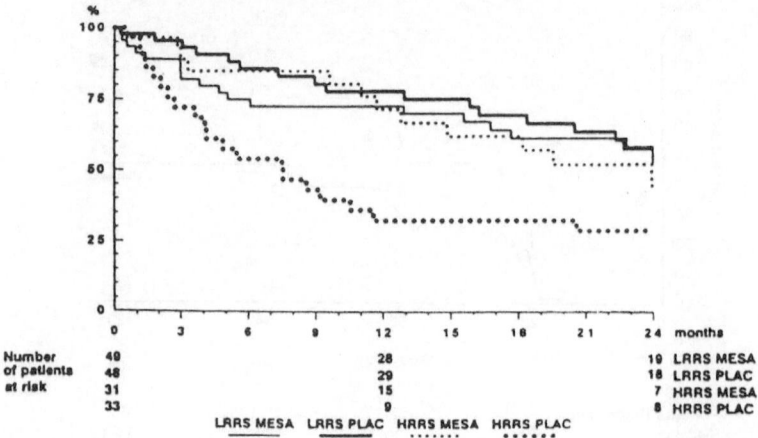

Fig. 3 Kaplan–Meier life-table curves of maintaining remission in the four treatment groups. MESA, mesalamine; PLAC, placebo (Gendre *et al.*, 1993)

(Gendre *et al.*, 1990) (Fig. 3). In contrast, a 1-year Danish multicenter study using Pentasa® 1.5 g b.i.d. or placebo in 202 patients with inactive CD showed no benefit of the 5-ASA treatment (Bandesen *et al.*, 1991). A recently completed Canadian maintenance study with Pentasa® 3 g/day proved to be superior to placebo (Sutherland *et al.*, 1994). An open study has suggested that Pentasa® may be useful to treat patients whose CD is active or in remission (Hanauer *et al.*, 1993). In an Italian multicenter placebo-controlled study of 125 CD patients with a CDAI lower than 150, patients on Asacol® 800 mg t.i.d. had a yearly relapse rate of 34% versus the 55% 1-year relapse rate observed in the patients on placebo (Prantera *et al.*, 1992) (Fig. 4). The efficacy of long-term use of oral mesalamine has also been demonstrated in asymptomatic CD patients who had laboratory signs suggestive of disease activity (Brignola *et al.*, 1992), with fewer subsequent symptomatic relapses of patients on mesalamine. Caprilli and Italian colleagues have reported the benefit of Asacol® 2.4 g/day to reduce recurrences postoperatively in patients with Crohn's disease (Caprilli *et al.*, 1994), and McLeod and her colleagues (1994) have recently reported that Salofalk 3 g/day reduces clinical and endoscopic signs of recurrent postoperative Crohn's disease, as well as complications and the need for reoperation. The use of 5-ASA preparations for maintenance therapy in CD has been thoughtfully questioned (Tremaine, 1992). However, two meta-analyses have been performed on published data, and confirm clinical efficacy of mesalamine but not SASP in the maintenance of remission of patients with CD (Hemphill *et al.*, 1993; Messori *et al.*, 1994). With a therapeutic gain of approximately 30% (i.e. about 30% fewer patients with CD will have a symptomatic recurrence when treated with mesalamine for 12 months), and with the clinical remissions often being milder, the issue remains open for discussion and review. Maintenance therapy with 5-ASA in CD certainly looks favorable, and cost-efficacy should be evaluated. Attempts should also be made to determine what characteristics of the

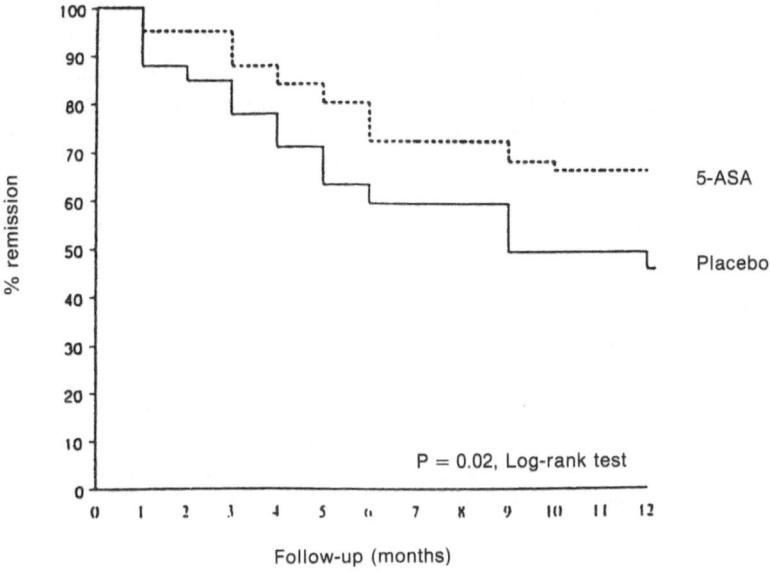

Fig. 4 Life table estimate of maintaining remission during treatment with 5-ASA or placebo (Prantera *et al.*, 1992)

patient and her/his CD best predicts response to maintenance therapy.

The only obvious clinical benefit of mesalamine versus SASP in the treatment of active UC or CD is the lower prevalence (3% versus 30%, approximately) of adverse effects, including fewer serious side-effects, and equivalent cost for some but not all mesalamine preparations (Thomson, 1991). Thus, a favorable safety profile is the primary advantageous characteristic of the mesalamines, whose use has almost completely eradicated dose-dependent side-effects, including male infertility. Allergic reactions have also been greatly reduced, but other side-effects such as pancreatitis (Fiorentini *et al.*, 1990) and interstitial nephritis (Mehta, 1990) are still described, but are very uncommon events. Thus, the mesalamine compounds have approximately comparable clinical efficacy with SASP, with generally fewer adverse effects (Mulder *et al.*, 1988; McIntyre *et al.*, 1988; Riley *et al.*, 1988). This was not observed in one study with olsalazine (Ireland *et al.*, 1988), whereas in another study olsalazine was beneficial and free of side-effects in nearly 87% of patients intolerant to SASP (Sandberg-Gertzen *et al.*, 1986). Both SASP and mesalamine appear to be safe to be used in pregnancy (Habel *et al.*, 1993).

The new 5-ASA compounds are clearly superior to placebo in the treatment of patients with active ulcerative colitis (Fig. 5), whereas only the higher dose of Pentasa® is superior to placebo in the treatment of patients with active Crohn's disease (Fig. 6). The 5-ASA are comparable to equivalent doses of SASP to maintain a remission in ulcerative colitis (Fig. 7), whereas three of six trials demonstrate superiority of 5-ASA versus placebo in the maintenance of remission in patients with Crohn's disease (Fig. 8).

Is there a role for combination therapy of SASP/5-ASA with another class of drug? A Dutch trial compared the value of SASP alone (4–6 g/day) versus a combination of the same dose of SASP plus prednisolone (30 mg/day for 2 weeks, then reduced) for a 16-week double-blind study using the Van Hees Activity Index (VHAI) and the CDAI (Rijk et al., 1991) as the primary outcome variables (Fig. 9). Of the 60 patients who completed the study, those who received the combined treatment manifested a significantly faster initial 6-week clinical improvement (according to the VHAI only), but shared results similar to SASP alone at the end of the study (using both the CDAI and the VHAI). Some critical questions have been asked regarding the use of combination therapy, such as differences in baseline conditions, the relatively small number of patients, and the lack of a placebo-controlled group (Hanauer et al., 1991). Nonetheless, once a decision has been made to use glucocorticosteroids (GS), the addition of SASP to GS appears to offer the patient some potential therapeutic advantage. Although not specifically studied, it is likely that the combination of GS plus 5-ASA will be as useful as GS plus SASP.

Mesalamine by enemas or suppositories

Topical mesalamine is established therapy for the treatment of active disease as well as maintenance of remission in left-sided UC or proctitis (Campieri et al., 1990a,b,c; 1991a,b). Mesalamine enemas are efficacious in the treatment of disease extending to the level of the splenic flexure. The response to mesalamine enemas is typically about 80%, with onset of clinical improvement observed in 3–21 days (Linn and Peppercorn, 1992). A recent meta-analysis of 17 randomized, double-blind controlled trials of ulcerative colitis distal to the splenic flexure demonstrated dramatic improvement with topical 5-ASA as compared with placebo, with odds ratios 7.36–10.59 for active disease, and 16.22 for quiescent disease (Irvine and Marshall, 1994).

To attempt to determine the optimal dosage of topical treatment, a dose-ranging study using enemas containing 1, 2 or 4 g of mesalamine and placebo was carried out in 113 patients with mild to moderate attacks of UC (Campieri et al., 1981). After 1 month all patients treated with mesalamine enemas were significantly better than were those on placebo. No difference was found in relation to the three concentrations of mesalamine, so that doses as low as 1 g/day appear to be effective. In 90 patients with left-sided UC unresponsive to conventional medical therapy with corticosteroids and SASP, 87% improved by at least one grade of endoscopic inflammation after 12 weeks of mesalamine enemas (Biddle and Miner, 1990). Mesalamine foams are at least as good as enemas (Campieri et al., 1991a).

The topic of the role of mesalamine suppositories has been reviewed (Williams, 1990). Campieri et al. (1990a) carried out a multicenter study in which the efficacies of suppositories of mesalamine 500 mg b.i.d. and t.i.d. were compared; both active treatment arms were comparable (about 70% improvement at 1 month), and both were superior to placebo. Similarly,

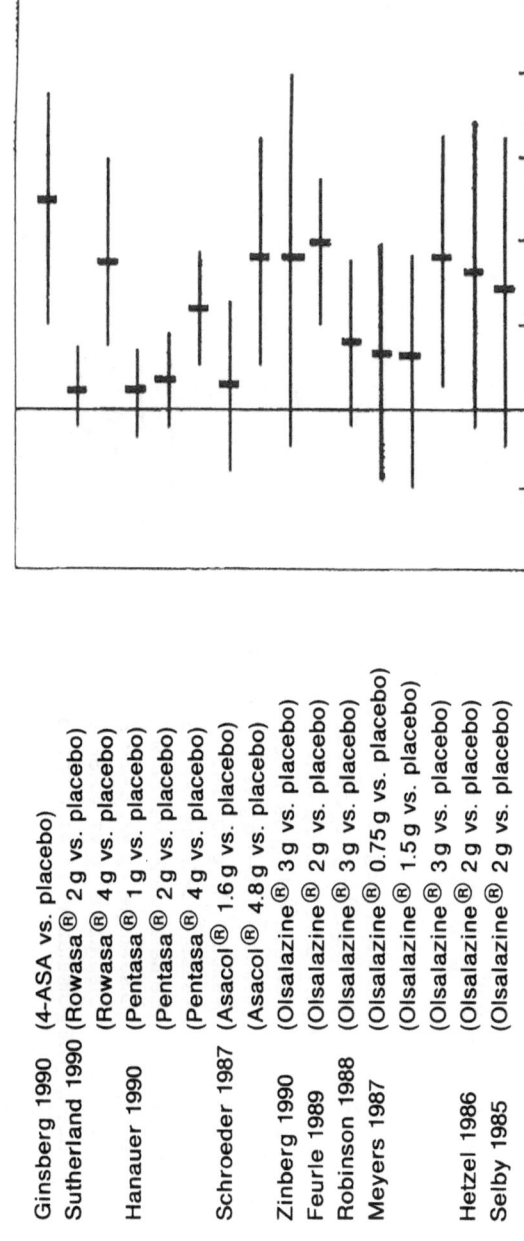

Ginsberg 1990 (4-ASA vs. placebo)
Sutherland 1990 (Rowasa® 2 g vs. placebo)
(Rowasa® 4 g vs. placebo)
Hanauer 1990 (Pentasa® 1 g vs. placebo)
(Pentasa® 2 g vs. placebo)
(Pentasa® 4 g vs. placebo)
Schroeder 1987 (Asacol® 1.6 g vs. placebo)
(Asacol® 4.8 g vs. placebo)
Zinberg 1990 (Olsalazine® 3 g vs. placebo)
Feurle 1989 (Olsalazine® 2 g vs. placebo)
Robinson 1988 (Olsalazine® 3 g vs. placebo)
Meyers 1987 (Olsalazine® 0.75 g vs. placebo)
(Olsalazine® 1.5 g vs. placebo)
(Olsalazine® 3 g vs. placebo)
Hetzel 1986 (Olsalazine® 2 g vs. placebo)
Selby 1985 (Olsalazine® 2 g vs. placebo)

ASA: aminosalicylic acid

Fig. 5 5-ASA in ulcerative colitis acute treatment

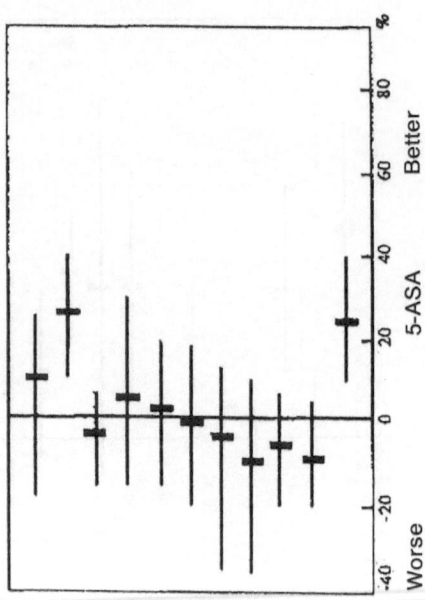

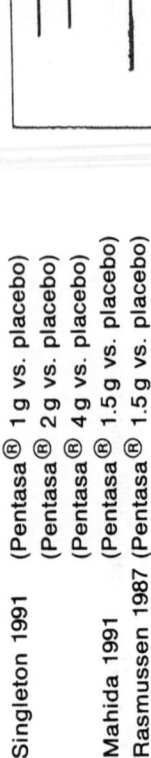

Singleton 1991   (Pentasa® 1 g vs. placebo)
                  (Pentasa® 2 g vs. placebo)
                  (Pentasa® 4 g vs. placebo)

Mahida 1991   (Pentasa® 1.5 g vs. placebo)
Rasmussen 1987 (Pentasa® 1.5 g vs. placebo)

5-ASA: 5-aminosalicylic acid

Fig. 6 5-ASA in Crohn's disease active treatment

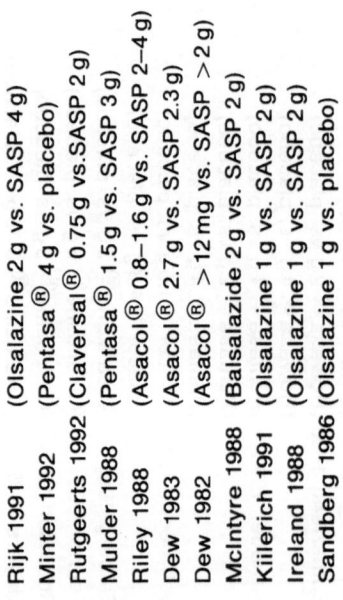

Rijk 1991   (Olsalazine 2 g vs. SASP 4 g)
Minter 1992   (Pentasa® 4 g vs. placebo)
Rutgeerts 1992 (Claversal® 0.75 g vs.SASP 2 g)
Mulder 1988   (Pentasa® 1.5 g vs. SASP 3 g)
Riley 1988   (Asacol® 0.8–1.6 g vs. SASP 2–4 g)
Dew 1983   (Asacol® 2.7 g vs. SASP 2.3 g)
Dew 1982   (Asacol® > 12 mg vs. SASP > 2 g)
McIntyre 1988   (Balsalazide 2 g vs. SASP 2 g)
Kiilerich 1991   (Olsalazine 1 g vs. SASP 2 g)
Ireland 1988   (Olsalazine 1 g vs. SASP 2 g)
Sandberg 1986 (Olsalazine 1 g vs. placebo)

5-ASA: 5-aminosalicylic acid
SASP: sulfazalazine

Fig. 7 5-ASA in ulcerative colitis remission maintenance

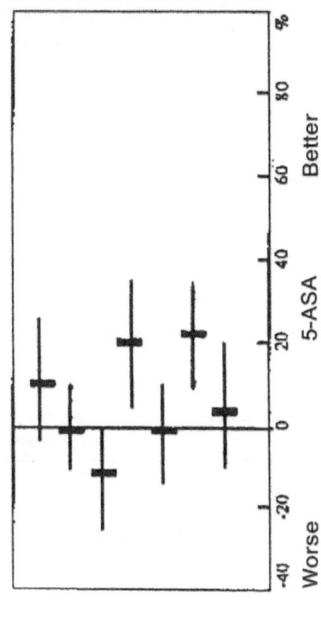

Brignola 1992 (Pentasa® 2 g vs. placebo)
Schreiber 1992 (Claversal® 1.5 g vs. 4-ASA 1.5 g)
Florent 1992 (Claversal® 3 g vs. placebo)
Prantera 1991 (Asacol® 2.4 g vs. placebo)
Bondesen 1991 (Pentasa® 3 g vs. placebo)
Thomson 1990 (Claversal® 1.5 g vs. placebo)
Gendre 1990 (Pentasa® 2 g vs. placebo)

ASA: aminosalicylic acid

Fig. 8 5-ASA in Crohn's disease remission maintenance

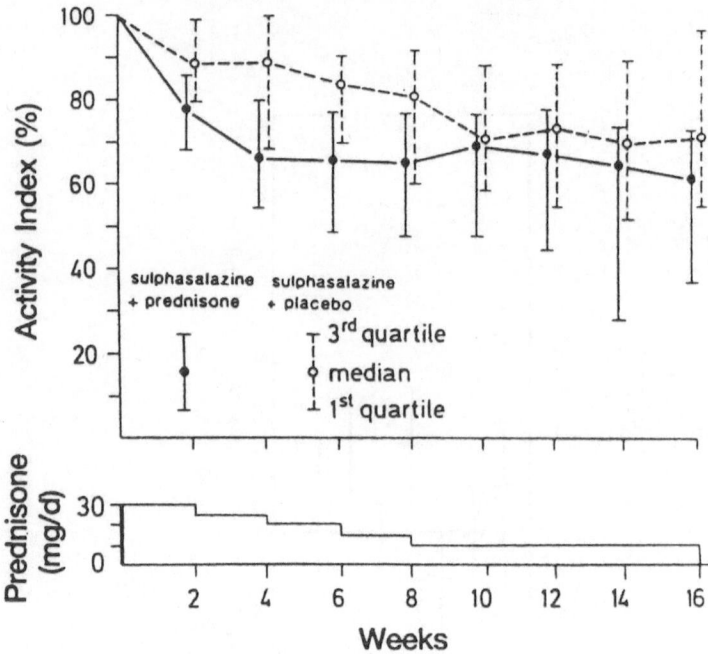

Fig. 9 The Van Hees Activity Index as a proportion of the initial value in patients treated with sulfasalazine and prednisone or sulfasalazine and placebo. The daily dose of prednisone in the patients treated with sulfasalazine and prednisone is shown in the bottom panel. Data are presented as medians and quartiles. The median and the first and third quartiles of a sample are the values which include 50%, 25% and 75% of the observations, respectively (Rijk *et al.*, 1991)

D'Arienzo *et al.* (1990) demonstrated the superiority of mesalamine suppositories 400 mg b.i.d. versus placebo. Gionchetti *et al.* (1990) also demonstrated the beneficial role of mesalamine suppositories in patients with proctitis. The optimal dose or dosage of mesalamine to be given by suppositories is not known; neither is the comparative efficacy against oral therapy or enemas.

There is the possibility of the need for long-term treatment with mesalamine enemas in patients with distal UC, and with suppositories in ulcerative proctitis (D'Arienzo *et al.*, 1990). Treatment usually needs to be continued for at least 1 month; longer periods of treatment may be necessary, and many patients need to continue indefinitely on mesalamine enemas or suppositories taken every 1, 2 or 3 days.

5'-Lipoxygenase inhibitors

Elevated levels of leukotriene B_4 (LTB_4) and prostaglandin E_2 (PGE_2) have been reported in the rectal dialysates of patients with active UC, falling or returning to normal with clinical disease remission. Selective 5'-lipoxygenase inhibitors and leukotriene receptor antagonists have been developed. Zileuton® at a dose of 800 mg/day for 28 days was studied in 11 active UC patients; this demonstrated improved symptoms, with endoscopic improvement in eight persons (Collawn et al., 1992). Zileutron® was tested in a clinical trial in 71 patients with active UC who received 800 mg/day orally or a placebo for 28 days. Significantly better results were obtained only in Zileutron®-treated UC patients free of previous SASP treatment (Stenson et al., 1991).

In vitro the 5′-lipoxygenase inhibitor BW-A4C reduces LTB_4 in rectal biopsies of patients with IBD, without affecting PGE_2 or thromboxane B_2 synthesis. The clinical use of BW-AYC is unknown.

ω-3 Fatty acids

Fish oils are rich in omega-3 fatty acids such as eicosapentaenoic acid (EPA) and docosahexanoic acid (DHA). These fatty acids are metabolized by the enzyme 5′-lipoxygenase to form leukotriene B_5 (LTB_5) and prostaglandin E_3, with subsequent reduction of LTB_4 levels. LTB_5 does not possess as many of the pro-inflammatory properties as does LTB_4. Oral supplementation with ω-3 fatty acids or EPA has been examined in patients with active UC. In a multicenter, randomized, double-blind, placebo-controlled, crossover trial with 4-month treatment periods separated by a 1-month washout in 24 patients with UC, Stenson et al. (1992) gave 18 Maxepa capsules daily (3.2 μg EPA, and 2.6 μg DHA). Rectal dialysate levels of LBT_4 fell, as did histological abnormalities of UC. Aslan and Triadafilopoulos (1992) gave 15 Maxepa tablets or placebo in an 8-month, double-blind, placebo-controlled, crossover trial in patients with UC: disease activity fell, but there was no change in histology and no change in LBT_4 levels. McCall et al. (1992), in a small open study in six patients with UC, administered 3–4 g/day of EPA for 12 weeks. The patients showed improvement of symptoms and histological appearance of the rectal mucosa, and decreased LTB_4 levels in peripheral blood neutrophils. Solomon et al. (1990) treated 10 patients with mild to moderate attacks of UC in whom conventional therapy had failed. They had dietary supplementation with 2.75 g/day of EPA for 8 weeks. There was marked improvement in seven, and four of five who continued with glucocorticosteroids could reduce the dose. The mechanism of action of this steroid-sparing effect is unknown. Thus, fish oil may be useful to manage those patients with active UC who do not respond to standard therapy.

EPA is of no benefit in maintenance therapy treatment in UC (Hawthorne et al., 1992), and the role of EPA in the treatment of patients with active or remitted CD remains unproven.

ANTIBIOTICS

In a multicenter American–Canadian study, metronidazole (Flagyl®) was given as approximately 10 or 20 mg/kg per day for 16 weeks, versus placebo, in patients with active CD (Sutherland et al., 1991). Both doses of metronidazole were superior to placebo, especially in patients with colonic disease. The basis for this beneficial effect is unknown. Some patients with CD have bacterial overgrowth secondary to strictures, fistulae and hypomotility, and this may provide the basis for a portion of the symptomatic benefit achieved with some antibiotics. Metronidazole, 400 mg b.i.d., is similar in effectiveness to SASP in active CD (Ursing *et al.*, 1982), and is useful for treating abscesses, fistulae and perianal lesions.

Pouchitis is a syndrome of unknown cause that develops specifically in patients operated on for UC, leaving them with an ileal pouch. Metronidazole has been used with satisfactory results in combination with antidiarrheal agents in the treatment of pouchitis (Tytgat and Van Deventer, 1988). Enemas containing mesalamine have also been shown to give satisfactory results in the treatment of pouchitis (Miglioli *et al.*, 1989). The mechanism of action of these medications in treating pouchitis is unclear.

Clofazimine, 100 mg/day, has been administered together with prednisone, 45 mg/day, to 25 patients with active CD (Afdhal *et al.*, 1991), and the results compared with prednisone alone. There was no added benefit for acute therapy, but when clofazimine was continued without prednisone for 8 months, patients had fewer relapses than those off prednisone and maintained on placebo. This interesting and important possibility of the use of clofazimine for maintenance therapy in CD needs to be confirmed.

Rutgeerts *et al.* (1992) tested the efficacy of rifabutin and ethambutol in combination for their ability to heal severe recurrent CD at the neoterminal ileum. No patients who received treatment demonstrated improvement, either endoscopically or clinically.

In acute UC, adding oral tobramycin to the standard acute regimen may be of benefit (Burke *et al.*, 1990), but the addition of tobramycin plus metronidazole to intravenous hydrocortisone is of no added benefit in patients with acute, severe ulcerative colitis (Mantzaris *et al.*, 1994).

GLUCOCORTICOSTEROIDS

Intravenous

The outcome of medical treatment in patients with severe attacks of UC is worse in those with more extensive disease and with the early presence of gas in the small bowel (Truelove and Jewell, 1974a,b). An old and tried regimen of intravenous (i.v.) fluids, 60 mg/day i.v. prednisolone, an antibiotic (tetracycline was initially used), as well as achievement of blood and electrolyte balance (Jewell *et al.*, 1974) is used for 5–10 days; the response rate is about two patients in three, with a mortality rate of about 1%. Thus, the use of high-dose i.v. glucocorticosteroids (GS) for at least 5 days represented a major therapeutic step for patients with severe attacks of UC. The value of this protocol, which has been partially modified by excluding antibiotics and prolonging the period of treatment up to 10 days, has been confirmed more recently (Jarnerot *et al.*, 1985, 1991). In an attempt to improve the outcome of patients with severe attacks of UC, GS were given as a pulse dosage of methylprednisolone 1 g/day for 3 days (Rosenberg *et al.*, 1990), followed by 100 mg of hydrocortisone every 6 h for 2 days, together with topical GS treatment. The success rate was about 60%, not different from that obtained in previous studies by the same group. The regimen followed for patients with severely active CD is usually the same as for UC, but controlled trials have not yet been done to prove the expected efficacy of this intensive regimen.

What is there to do immediately with the UC patients who do not respond to this intensive regimen? Correct timing for early surgery is paramount (Jewell *et al.*, 1991). The use of i.v. cyclosporin remains promising, but this is at an early stage of development for possible use as adjunct therapy for persons with severely active UC not responding to i.v. GS (see later).

There is no widely accepted definition for refractory disease, either in terms of accepted dose and duration of treatment, or in terms of an acceptable outcome measure. A pragmatic approach to refractory distal UC has been published (Jarnerot *et al.*, 1991), but there are no scientific data on which approach is optimal, or on what constitutes disease refractory to oral or intravenous therapy.

Oral

The orally administered GS act systemically and locally. The first-used GS, prednisone and prednisolone, are systemically active. Prednisone, 0.5–0.75 mg/kg per day orally, is effective in treating moderately active CD, as shown by the National Cooperative Crohn's Disease Study (NCCDS) (Summers *et al.*, 1979) and by the European Cooperative Crohn's Disease Study (ECCDS) (Malchow *et al.*, 1984). GS work best in patients with ileal or ileocolonic disease, and when used in tapering doses over at least 4 months. The response of active symptomatic disease to prednisone or sulfasalazine was significantly better than to placebo; the difference achieved with azathioprine was not statistically significant (Summers *et al.*, 1979) (Fig. 10). In the European Cooperative Crohn's Disease Study (Malchow *et al.*, 1984), 6-methylprednisolone was the most effective drug in overall comparison in all patients (in previously treated patients, and in those with small bowel or small bowel plus colonic disease). The combination of 6-methylprednisolone and SASP was the most effective regimen in previously untreated patients, and when disease was localized to the colon. In patients with colonic involvement, prednisone 1 mg/kg per day exerts only a minor benefit on colonic mucosal endoscopic biopsies, perhaps because of the transmural depth of the lesions (Modigliani *et al.*, 1990). Nonetheless, patients with moderately active colonic CD are usually not denied a trial of prednisone after the colonically active anti-inflammatory agents such as mesalamine have been tried and have failed.

The GS have mainly an effect on symptoms, without a clearly associated improvement in the inflammatory process: this statement is supported from the results of two endoscopically controlled studies. In the first, Oliason *et al.* (1992) followed eight CD patients with recurrent preanastomotic ileal

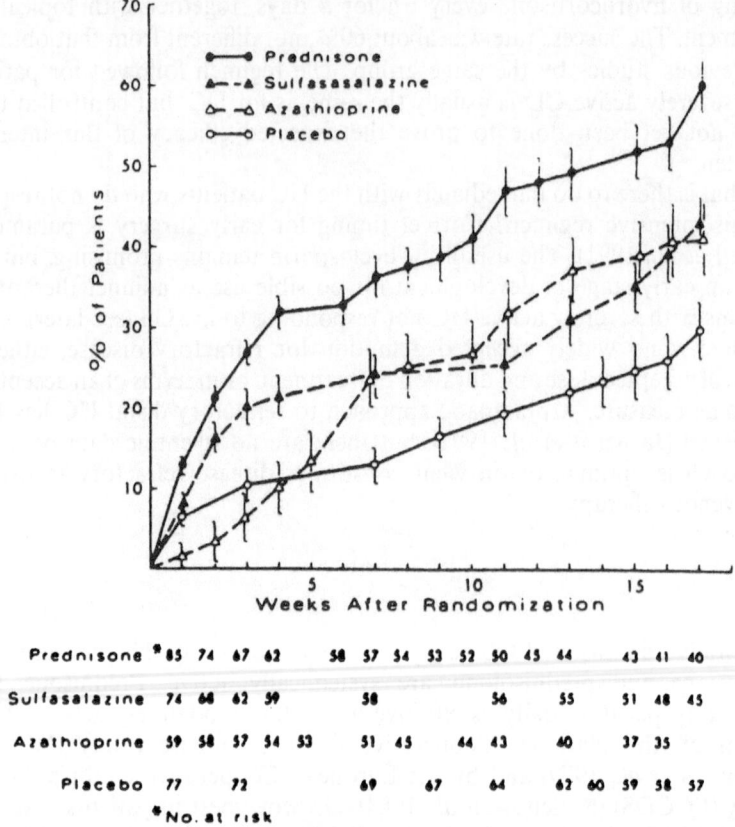

Prednisone °85 74 67 62   58 57 54 53 52 50 45 44   43 41 40

Sulfasalazine 74 68 62 59   58   56   55   51 48 45

Azathioprine 59 58 57 54 53   51 45   44 43   40   37 35

Placebo 77   72   69   67   64   62 60 59 58 57

(A)   *No. at risk

Fig. 10 A: Cumulative percentage of patients in remission week-by-week. Remission is defined as CDAI less than 150 and continuing below 150 through week 17. Brackets indicate standard errors of the mean. Life table using Kaplan–Meier method (Summers *et al.*, 1979). B:Mean CDAI week-by-week of patients in each treatment group who completed 17 weeks on-study. Brackets give standard errors of the mean (Summers *et al.*, 1979)

inflammation who had received 20–30 mg/day of prenisolone for 6–9 weeks. All patients showed clinical improvement, but endoscopic examination was unable to show objective evidence of decreased inflammation. Modigliani *et al.* (1990) studied 142 patients with symptoms of active CD, increases in their ESR, and with colonoscopic signs of inflammation. Treatment was with prednisolone 1 mg/kg per day for 7 weeks, with symptomatic improvement in 63% of patients at 4 weeks, and 92% at 7 weeks. This clinical outcome was parallelled by a decrease in laboratory parameters suggesting biological activity, but only 29% of patients in clinical remission showed colonoscopic remission as well.

It is generally accepted that GS have no use as maintenance therapy in patients with UC or CD, although the NCCDS showed that about one-third of patients with active CD started on prednisone will need to remain on prednisone to suppress continued active disease. In the ECCDS (Malchow

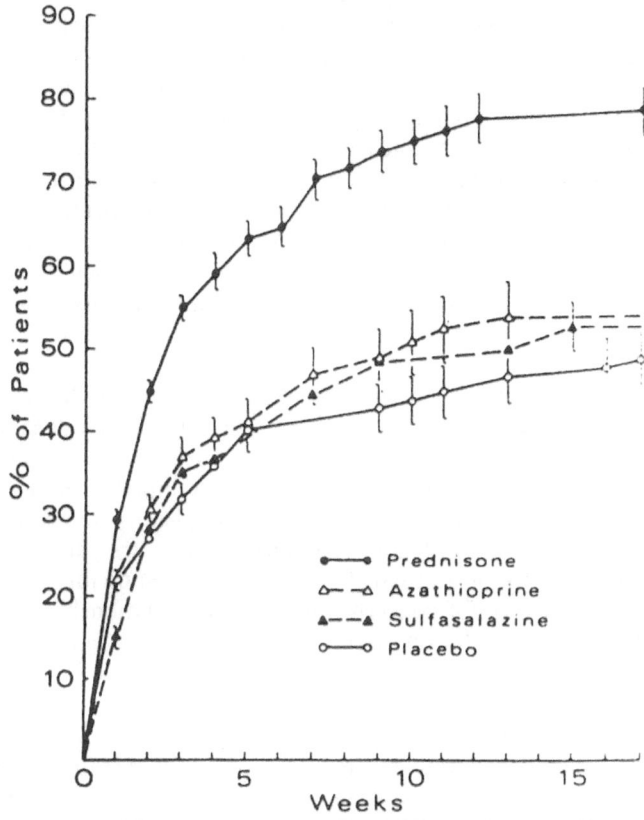

Prednisone *85 60 47 38 35 31 30 25 24 22 21 20

Azathioprine 59 46 41 37 36   35   31 30 29   28

Sulfasalazine 74 63 53 48   47   41   38   37

Placebo 77 60 56 52 49   46 44 43   42   41 40

(B)   *No. at risk

Fig. 10 *continued*

et al., 1984), drug treatment was of no significant benefit to patients with quiescent disease, whereas continuous administration of low-dose 6-methylprednisolone or the combination of 6-methylprednisolone plus sulfasalazine was beneficial in patients who responded initially to treatment of active disease. In a small group of patients with inactive CD (CDAI < 150) and yet with abnormal laboratory parameters, GS used at a low dose (0.25 mg/kg per day) for 6 months showed a reduced risk of clinical relapses as compared with placebo (Brignola *et al.*, 1986, 1988).

In a retrospective study, the use of an alternate-day prednisone treatment regimen (25 mg every other day) sustained clinical remission in 60% of 33 treated CD patients, with a mean follow-up of 6.6 years (Bello *et al.*, 1991). There is difficulty in determining if in patients with asymptomatic CD there is an active inflammatory process, and whether maintenance therapy is really just lower-dose suppressive therapy for lesser degrees of inflammation. These issues of defining continued active inflammation, and whether suppression of this activity leads to a better prognosis, need to be resolved before embarking on maintenance studies with newer therapeutic agents. It is necessary to determine whether the endpoint of therapy should be improved clinical symptoms, or improved laboratory measures such as markers of increased intestinal permeability, LTB_4 levels, immune markers, or serum concentrations of acute-phase reactants such as orosomucoid or C-reactive proteins.

There are two main categories of adverse effects seen with the use of GS: those related to withdrawal and those related to high-dose treatment (Kusunoki *et al.*, 1992). There are numerous adverse effects from GS, and while these may be uncommon, when they develop they may be serious and/or unpleasant for the patient. For example, an increase in mean intraocular pressure (IOP) has been reported when 109 young people (age 7–21 years) with IBD were treated with oral prednisone for 1–104 months (Tripathi *et al.*, 1992). Of concern, there was no relationship between the IOP and the total prednisone dose, duration of treatment, or number of days on high-dose prednisone. The increased IOP fell in some patients when the dose of prednisone was decreased, but three persons had increased IOP while on only 5 mg/day of prednisone.

There has been major research to develop rapidly metabolized GS in an effort to limit availability of active GS components to the inflamed intestinal tissue, in an effort to minimize the prevalence of GS side-effects (Tripathi *et al.*, 1992). Tixocortol pivalate, beclomethasone, and budesonide are examples of rapidly metabolized GS. These have been used as enemas or as tablets. Oral fluticasone propionate, in a dose of 5 mg q.i.d., is no better than placebo in the treatment of distal UC (Angus *et al.*, 1992). A European (Rutgeerts *et al.*, 1993) and a Canadian (Greenberg *et al.*, 1993) study of over 475 patients with active CD has proven the clinical efficacy of budesonide in an oral controlled release formulation when compared versus prednisolone or versus placebo, respectively. Adverse effects were much less prevalent with budesonide than with prednisone, and the suppression of the adrenal axis was also much less. Interestingly, some CD patients treated with placebo reported prednisone-associated adverse effects, such as moon-face! In addition, oral budesonide 6 mg/day for up to 1 year is significantly more efficacious than placebo in delaying relapse in ileocecal CD, with only minor systemic effects (Löfberg *et al.*, 1994). This represents a potential breakthrough in the therapy of patients with IBD.

Topical: enemas and suppositories

Beclomethasone enemas (0.5 mg/day) were compared with 5 mg betamethasone enemas (5 mg/day) for 28 days in 32 patients with acute UC

(Halpern *et al.*, 1991): both enema preparations were similarly effective, but beclomethasone dipropionate did not depress plasma cortisol levels (Danielsson *et al.*, 1987). These results were confirmed in an Italian multicenter study of 44 patients using either budesonide (2 mg/100 ml) or prednisolone (20 mg/100 ml) enemas for 1 month (Bianchi *et al.*, 1991). Budesonide enemas are superior to placebo for the treatment of distal colitis or proctitis when given over a 4-week period (Danielsson *et al.*, 1992). In a multicenter Danish trial, 146 UC patients were given (for 2 weeks) 100 ml enemas containing 1, 2 or 4 mg budesonide or 25 mg prednisolone (Danish Budesonide Study Group, 1991); the 2 mg dose was the most uniformly effective enema. Plasma cortisol levels do not change in the budesonide-treated patients. A Swedish group compared intrarectal budesonide 2 mg/day versus prednisolone 25 mg/day in 100 patients with distal UC (Löfberg *et al.*, 1993); the two treatments were similarly efficacious. Importantly, budesonide did not suppress plasma cortisol, as did prednisolone, and after 8 weeks of treatment the decrease in S-osteocalcin was lower with budesonide than with predniso-lone. Budesonide enemas have recently been released for use in Canada.

Mesalamine enemas of 1–4 g/day are at least as effective as GS (Azad Khan *et al.*, 1977; Campieri *et al.*, 1981; Danish 5-ASA Group, 1987). Mesalamine and 'new' steroid enemas have been compared in a Dutch multicenter trial (Lamers *et al.*, 1991), in which patients received 2 mg/100 ml of buclosamide or 4 g/60 ml mesalamine for 1 month; there were similar treatment outcomes.

Oral versus topical treatment appear to be comparable in the treatment of distal UC, and the choice of one route versus another will depend upon patient preference, and will be influenced by the greater inconvenience and cost of topical versus oral therapy.

IMMUNOMODULATORS

Azathioprine and 6-mercaptopurine

The topic of the use of azathioprine (AZA) and 6-mercaptopurine (6-MP) in the treatment of patients with UC and CD has been reviewed (Present, 1989). AZA and 6-MP are used in the treatment of patients with CD, used either alone or in combination with GS. However, the use of these immunomodulators remains controversial (Lennard-Jones, 1981; Singleton, 1981; Korelitz and Present, 1981). In an attempt to ascertain whether AZA or 6-MP is effective in preventing disease relapse in patients with UC in remission, Hawthorne *et al.* (1992) conducted a 1-year placebo-controlled double-blind trial of withdrawal of AZA in 79 patients who had been taking AZA for the previous 6 months, and who had been in clinical remission for a period of 2 months or more. A relapse rate of 36% was found in the AZA group, whereas a 59% relapse rate was seen in the placebo group. This suggests that AZA maintenance treatment in patients with UC is beneficial if patients have achieved remission while taking this drug. In a retrospective study in 81 UC patients unresponsive to standard treatment, with data collected over 18 years, it was possible to withdraw steroids in 48% of patients, or to reduce them in 13%, when patients were continued on 6-MP, 50 mg/day (Adler and Korelitz, 1991). This suggests that AZA may represent useful maintenance therapy in selected patients with UC, but it is not clear why AZA rather than SASP or mesalazine would be used.

In a retrospective study of patients with resistant and steroid-dependent CD, the addition of AZA 1.5–2 mg/kg per day may be useful (Present, 1989), as also is 6-MP 50–70 mg/day (Perrault *et al.*, 1991). In another retrospective study with a mean follow-up of 1.6 years, data were obtained in 78 patients with extensive, refractory, complicated, or steroid-dependent CD, mainly with ileocolonic involvement (O'Brien *et al.*, 1991). AZA (mean dosage, 1 mg/kg per day) and 6-MP controlled disease activity in 73%, demonstrated a corticosteroid-sparing effect in 76%, and reduced fistulization in 63%. These results took some time to appear, usually being evident after 3–4 months of therapy. About 10% of the patients withdrew because of adverse effects.

Lemann *et al.* (1990) retrospectively analysed the results obtained in 126 patients with CD who had been followed up to 15 years while on AZA (three were actually on 6-MP); 109 had active CD at the beginning of the study, 63 were steroid-dependent, and 23 were steroid-resistant. After 1 year of treatment with AZA 2 mg/kg per day, 64% were in remission, including 81% of those who had been in the steroid-dependent group. In patients with quiescent CD at the start of the follow-up and treated with AZA, only 15% had a relapse after 1 year.

Other retrospective and uncontrolled studies have also supported the use of immunosuppressive agents in patients with refractory UC or CD (Steinhart *et al.*, 1990; Lobo *et al.*, 1990). For example, Verhave *et al.* (1990) used 2 mg/kg per day of AZA in nine adolescents with UC and in 12 with CD who had relapsed during GS therapy, had severe side-effects due to GS, or who had disease resistant to GS treatment. A full response was seen in six of nine UC and six of 12 CD patients.

Several controlled trials of patients with chronic active CD in whom therapy with SASP or GS had failed have indicated that AZA/6-MP may be beneficial to achieve remission (Willoughby *et al.*, 1971; Rosenberg *et al.*, 1975; O'Donoghue *et al.*, 1978). Other trials that included only a few patients with active CD do not report an advantage of AZA compared with placebo (Rhodes *et al.*, 1971; Klein *et al.*, 1974). Recently, O'Brien *et al.* (1991), showed control of refractory disease, decreasing fistulization, and steroid 'sparing' in the majority of AZA-treated patients.

AZA may be a useful supplement to the use of GS: Ewe *et al.* (1993) reported on the effects of AZA (2.5 mg/kg per day) plus prednisolone versus prednisolone alone in 42 patients with active CD. Clinical activity was assessed by three different activity indices: the CDAI (Best *et al.*, 1979), the Dutch or VHAI Index (van Hees *et al.*, 1980), and a severity–activity index (based on the data of the ECCDS [Malchow *et al.*, 1984]). All 42 patients received prednisolone, 60 mg/day tapering to a maintenance dosage of 10 mg/day over 7 weeks. In addition, half of the patients took AZA, 2.5 mg/kg body weight per day. After 16 weeks of treatment, 76% of patients on AZA

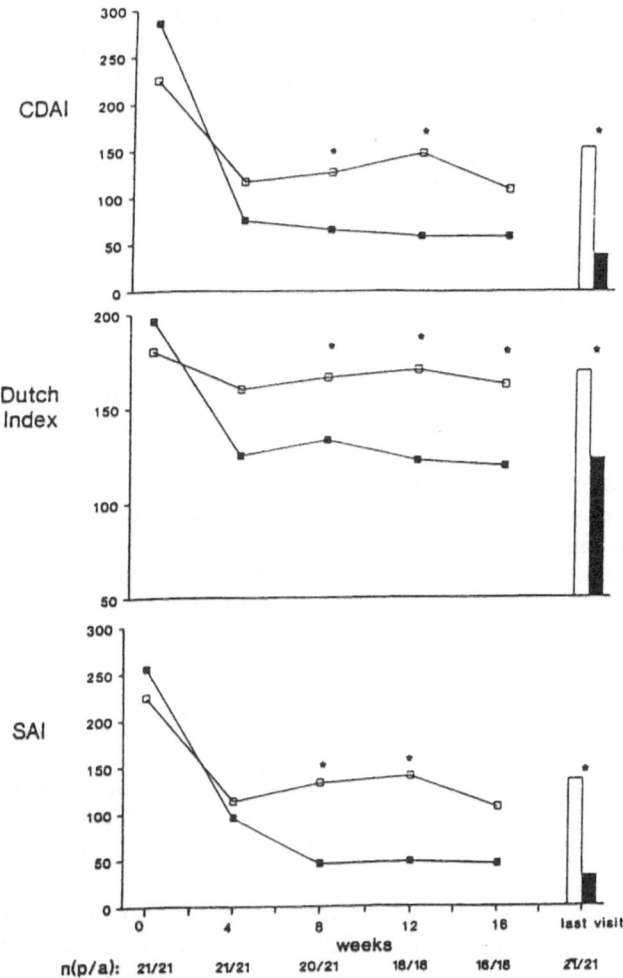

Fig. 11 Median of activity indices month by month in the AZA (■) and placebo-treated (□) groups; n = no. of patients. Last visit, median of activity indices (regular term or insufficient treatment) for CDAI, Dutch index, and SAI. $p < 0.05$ (Ewe *et al.*, 1993)

plus prednisolone therapy, but only 38% of patients on prednisolone therapy, were in remission, with a CDAI < 150. Two of the three activity indices showed that the combination of AZA plus prednisolone was superior to prednisolone alone (Fig. 11). The localization of CD did not substantially influence the proportions of treatment success or failure between the groups, with one possible exception: all six patients with Crohn's colitis responded to the combined treatment, as opposed to only two of five patients who received prednisolone alone ($p = 0.061$). In the AZA-treated group it was possible to taper the prednisolone dose according to the defined schedule in 57% of patients, whereas regular tapering of prednisolone in CD patients achieving remission on a placebo occurred in only 24%. Thus, the addition of AZA to prednisolone in patients with active CD had several advantages over treatment with prednisolone alone: remission was achieved more safely, more frequently, more quickly, and with a lower total dose of prednisolone. Serious side-effects were not recorded, and no patients on AZA had any evidence of bone marrow depression. Therefore, a recommendation of overlapping GS therapy during the first months of treatment with AZA/6-MP can be derived from these observations.

Although the response to AZA in the NCCDS was better than the response to placebo, the difference did not reach conventional levels of statistical significance (Summers et al., 1979). However, the NCCDS study has been criticized because of the withdrawal of GS therapy in many patients just before the beginning of the trial (Lennard-Jones, 1981; Korelitz and Present, 1981; Present et al., 1980). This concern was obviated in the study by Ewe et al. (1993); 20 of the 42 patients had been on GS therapy 4 weeks before randomization. A further point with regard to previous studies with AZA is the time before onset of benefit: a mean time of 3.1 months is needed for a clinical response (Present et al., 1980), with 20% of patients requiring more than 4 months to respond to 6-MP. Other investigators have shown that the median time interval for patients with CD refractory to conventional treatment to respond to AZA is 3 months (O'Brien et al., 1991). Four studies have now shown the steroid-'sparing' effect of AZA (Ewe et al., 1993; Rosenberg et al., 1975; Present et al., 1980; O'Brien et al., 1991). Indeed, a recent meta-analysis of eight randomized, double-blind, placebo-controllled trials in active or quiescent CD has demonstrated that 74% of patients respond, but usually after 16 weeks or longer (Pearson et al., 1994). Steroids may be reduced to 5 mg or less per day in 56% of patients treated with AZA, but in only 18% of steroid-treated patients not receiving AZA. In these studies the odds ratio was 9.3 for AZA use in active disease, 1.7 in quiescent disease, and 10.25 in patients with fistulae.

These recently reconfirmed positive effects of AZA have to be seen in relation to its potential adverse effects. The most hazardous factor is bone marrow depression, with white blood cell (WBC) counts below $2500/mm^3$ being reported in 2% of patients during more than 20 years of experience with 6-MP (Present et al., 1989). Bone marrow toxicity of AZA was higher in the short-term treatment phase of the NCCDS (Singleton et al., 1979). Two patients had to be withdrawn from this trial because of leukopenia, and 15% of patients on AZA had total WBC counts of $< 4000/mm^3$, requiring AZA dose reduction. Connell et al. (1992) reported two deaths among 714 patients with IBD who were treated with AZA; both deaths were related to bone marrow aplasia. Furthermore, leukopenia was unpredictable and occurred at any time between 0, 5 and 132 months of treatment (Connell et al., 1992, 1993). Other potentially serious AZA-associated complications include pancreatitis (Sturdevant et al., 1979). Theoretically, there may be genetic damage to the fetus with AZA (Present et al., 1989). Nonetheless, it has been suggested that a pregnancy in a patient with IBD on AZA can be safely continued in those who initially conceived while being treated with this immunosuppressant (Alstead et al., 1990). Many clinicians will remain cautious of continuing AZA during pregnancy, despite this favorable suggestion.

Cyclosporin

Sandborn and Tremaine (1992) discuss the utility of cyclosporin A (CyA) in patients with UC and CD. An initial report of the use of CyA in UC was not strongly encouraging (Baker and Jewell, 1989). On the other hand, Hanauer et al. (1990) gave 4 mg/kg per day of CyA i.v. to 15 patients with severe UC not responding to i.v. hydrocortisone 300 mg/day; 73% of these steroid-resistant patients showed clinical improvement within 5–8 days. CyA was then continued orally (6–8 mg/kg per day) and, at the end of 6 months, six of 11 patients were off steroids and a further three had greatly reduced their daily GS dose. To avoid surgery in non-responding UC patients, CyA 4 mg/kg per day i.v. was given in an uncontrolled study, with 70% of non-responding UC patients being able to progressively reduce their GS dosages (Lichtiger and Present, 1990). In a randomized, double-blind controlled trial in which CyA (4 mg/kg body weight per day) or placebo was administered by continuous i.v. infusion to 20 patients with severe UC whose condition had not improved after at least 7 days of i.v. corticosteroid therapy, 82% treated with CyA improved, as compared with those who received placebo (Lichter et al., 1994).

CyA, 5–7 mg/kg per day i.v. was used in a 3-month placebo-controlled trial in patients with active CD; after only 2 weeks there was 'a significant improvement in active CD without a dramatic change in CDAI' (Brynskov et al., 1989). A progressive decrease in CyA dose was associated with an increased relapse rate when these patients were seen in follow-up (Brynskov et al., 1991). This is similar to what happened when lower dosages (2 mg/kg per day) were used to prevent the onset of nephrotoxicity (Lobo et al., 1991). Two recently reported uncontrolled preliminary reports have suggested a possible role for i.v. CyA in patients with severely active CD (Gramlich and Barley, 1994; Leddin et al., 1994).

In a controlled trial of oral CyA performed for treatment of active CD (Brynskov et al., 1992), 71 patients with active CD of the terminal ileum, colon or both were randomly assigned to either oral placebo or CyA 5–7.5 mg/kg per day for 3 months. After 3 moths, 59% of the CyA group responded, compared with 32% in the placebo-treated group. The response to CyA was rapid, usually within 2 weeks. This is in marked contrast to the relatively slow response to AZA. Thus, oral or i.v. CyA may have a role in the management of some patients with active CD.

CyA has also been used for the treatment of fistulous CD that has not responded to GS, metronidazole or to antimetabolites; 76% (28 of 38 patients) had fistula closure initially, with 49% (17 of 35) remaining closed in long-term follow-up.

In a carefully performed Canadian placebo-controlled clinical trial, CyA (4.8 mg/kg) was shown to be ineffective for maintenance of remission in CD, as judged by the value of the CDAI or by QOL measures (Feagan et al.,

1994a); in fact, more patients worsened on CyA, as compared with placebo.

Sandborn et al. (1992) examined colonic tissue concentrations of CyA in two children with severe UC. Colonic tissue concentrations of CyA were higher in one patient responding to treatment, compared with the patient who did not respond. This suggests that varying tissue levels of CyA may be one of the factors explaining the variable response to this drug. This raises the possibility that the administered oral dose of CyA may not be adequate in some patients for them to achieve the desired clinical response (Bryskov et al., 1992).

There have been four uncontrolled studies evaluating the use of CyA enemas for refractory proctosigmoiditis (Brynskov et al., 1989; Ranzi et al., 1989; Sandborn et al., 1999). For example, 21 of 36 patients (58%) responded to initial therapy, with 13 of 36 patients (36%) remaining in remission after therapy was discontinued (Sandborn et al., 1993). Thus, there may be some role for the use of CyA enemas in patients with refractory distal colitis.

Methotrexate

Methotrexate has been proposed for use in patients with so-called refractory CD or UC: in an open study a weekly dose of 25 mg intramuscularly provided a favorable response (Kozarek et al., 1989). A further study showed the benefit of methotrexate in the treatment of CD patients refractory to AZA or 6-MP (Kozarek et al., 1991). A Canadian double-blind study of metotrexate in patients with acute CD is completed, and suggests that the addition of methotrexate to prednisone is superior to prednisone alone in patients with refractory active CD (Feagan et al., 1994b). The role of methotrexate as maintenance therapy in CD is under study.

Immunoglobulin and K76

Intravenous immunoglobulin therapy has been used for active, extensive and medically refractory idiopathic UC or CD (Levine et al., 1992): 12 young people with active UC not responding to SASP and/or GS received i.v. immunoglobulin 2 g/day during the induction phase, followed by 200–500 mg/kg every 2 weeks for 12 weeks. Six of the 12 UC patients were 1–17 years of age. Six of the 12 patients completed 12 or more weeks of therapy, and five of these six enjoyed an improvement in colitis activity and had a significant reduction in their prednisone dose.

K76, a monocarboxylic acid derivative of a culture supernatant of a fungus (*Stachybotrys complementi*), is a complement inhibitor which has been used in 21 patients with UC not responding to SASP or to GS (Kitano et al., 1992): 40% showed improvement with addition of K76.

Other immunomodulators

Fusidic acid is an antibiotic with T cell-specific immunosupressive effects. Eight patients with chronically active and medically resistant CD were treated for 8 weeks, with five improving (Langholz *et al.*, 1992).

An interleukin-1 receptor antagonist compound has been shown to be useful in a rabbit immune colitis model (Cominelli *et al.*, 1992). Open trials with chimeric monoclonal anti-CD_4 antibody have suggested efficacy in a small number of patients with CD or UC (Duesch *et al.*, 1992).

An open trial of T cell apheresis demonstrated remission achieved in 64 of 72 patients with chronically active CD (Holdstock *et al.*, 1979); remission was long-lasting. In contrast, in a later controlled trial, T cell apheresis allowed the doses of GS to be tapered, but relapse rates did not change (Bicks and Groshart, 1989).

ENTERAL AND PARENTERAL NUTRITION

Nutritional deficiencies are common in patients with IBD, especially those with CD. Replacement of established deficiencies is important, and management of the 'at-risk' patient is an important consideration. Nutritional therapy has been suggested to have a primary rather than an adjunctive role in the management of patients with IBD (O'Morain, 1990). This topic has been carefully reviewed (Seidman, 1993). A full discussion of this topic is beyond the scope of this presentation. Sitzmann *et al.* (1990) retrospectively reported the course of 22 patients with severe UC and 16 with Crohn's colitis, treated with GS plus total parenteral nutrition (TPN). Seventeen of the UC patients required colectomy, whereas 15 of the 16 patients with CD entered remission. Thus, TPN may have a role in the primary management of patients with CD, and not in those with UC. Home TPN for patients with short-bowel syndrome improves the CD patient's nutritional status and quality of life, and decreases the need for hospitalization or for surgery (Zinberg *et al.*, 1990). It has been recommended to use TPN only for patients with severe illness, either with obstruction or with the short-bowel syndrome (Sitzmann *et al.*, 1990; Galandiuk *et al.*, 1990).

Enteral nutrition with an elemental diet is as effective as TPN in the treatment of IBD (Caravo *et al.*, 1991). A number of studies have suggested the benefit of enteral nutrition for the patient with CD. For example, Teahon *et al.* (1990) assessed retrospectively the short- and long-term outcomes of 113 patients with CD who were treated primarily with an elemental diet. A remission was obtained in 85% of patients after 4 weeks, and surprisingly with follow-up of at least 5 years after use of elemental diet, the annual relapse rate was less than 10%. Giaffer *et al.* (1990) treated 30 patients with active CD with either an elemental diet or with a polymeric supplement containing intact protein. After 10 days, 12 of 16 patients (75%) on the elemental diet improved, compared with five of 14 (36%) on the polymeric diet.

It is controversial whether enteral nutrition can modify the long-term course of CD (Rigaud *et al.*, 1991; Giaffer *et al.*, 1990). In a large and well-designed multicenter study enrolling 107 patients with active CD randomized to receive only enteral nutrition with a liquid oligopeptide diet, or 6-methylprednisolone 48 mg/day plus SASP 3 g/day, after 6 weeks a higher

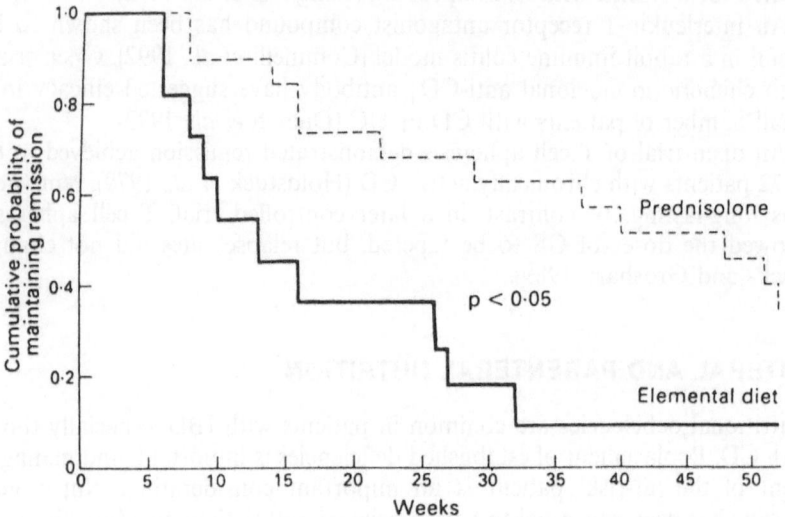

Fig. 12 Cumulative probability of maintaining remission during 1 year follow-up after treatment with prednisolone or elemental diet (Gorand *et al.*, 1993)

proportion of patients treated with these two drugs were in remission (41 of 52, 79%), as compared with those treated with enteral nutrition (29 of 55, 53%) (Lochs *et al.*, 1991). In contrast, in 42 patients with active CD treated with prednisolone or Vivonex Ten for 4 weeks, elemental diet was as effective in the short term as prednisolone in newly and previously diagnosed CD patients, and the benefit of this elemental diet was independent of the patient's nutritional status (Gorard *et al.*, 1993). The subsequent relapse after elemental diet-induced remission, however, is greater than after treatment with GS (Fig. 12).

Enteral nutrition can restore the increased intestinal permeability in CD to normal (Teahon *et al.*, 1991). The significance of this observation is unknown.

Are there specific nutrients ('gut fuels', such as short-chain fatty acids or glutamate) which might be beneficial when added to the diet or to enteral supplements? Butyrate is the major energy-yielding substrate for colonocytes, and sodium butyrate in the form of enemas 100 mmol/l has been used in a single-blind randomized crossover study in 10 patients with distal UC unresponsive to standard therapy (Scheppach *et al.*, 1992). Compared with placebo enemas, sodium butyrate enemas were effective. Senagore *et al.* (1992) compared short-chain fatty acid enemas (sodium acetate 60 mmol/l, sodium butyrate 40 mmol/l, and sodium propionate 30 mmol/l), versus hydrocortisone enemas (100 mg/60 ml) or mesalamine enemas (4 g/60 ml b.i.d.) in patients with nonspecific proctosigmoiditis; there was no difference in response rates. This suggests that short-chain fatty acid enemas may be useful treatment for some patients with distal UC. These are not yet in a commercially available form, but they may prove to be cheaper than 5-ASA-

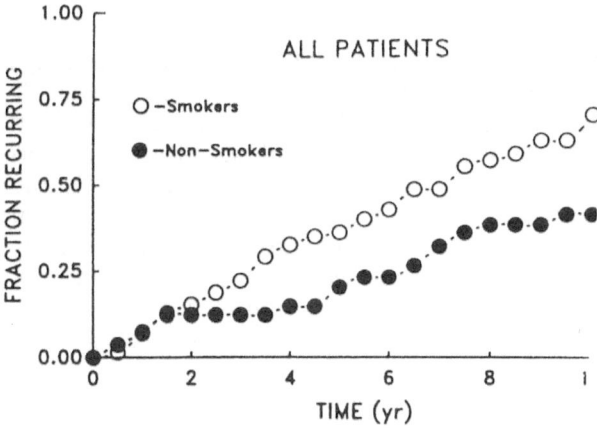

Fig. 13 Five- and 10-year cumulative recurrence rates in CD for smokers (36%, 70%) compared with nonsmokers (29%, 41%) ($p = 0.007$). Difference between the two groups at 5 years was 16% (CI_{95} 2.4–29.6); at 10 years the difference was 39% (CI_{95} 14–54%) (Sutherland *et al.*, 1990)

or GS-containing preparations. One pragmatic drawback for the widespread use of butyrate enemas is their foul odour! (Sutherland *et al.*, 1990).

LIFESTYLE MODIFICATION

Smoking may worsen the clinical course of patients with CD (Fig. 13) yet, curiously, smoking patients with UC may worsen when they give up their habit (Sutherland *et al.*, 1990). Nicotine chewing gum does not benefit the clinical course of patients with UC (Lashner *et al.*, 1990). To date, no controlled clinical trial has specifically stratified for smoking before patients were randomized; outcome results with budesonide appear to be similar in smokers versus non-smokers (Rutgeerts *et al.*, 1993; Greenberg *et al.*, 1993). There is anecdotal evidence from controlled trials in UC for clinical improvement with transdermal nicotine ('The Patch') (Scrivusta *et al.*, 1991).

Inhibition of cyclooxygenase by the use of nonsteroidal anti-inflammatory drugs (NSAID) is associated with colitis flaring in some patients, and there is clear evidence for the existence of NSAID-induced colitis in adults (Gibson *et al.*, 1992). Exacerbation of colitis by NSAID in rats is not related to elevated leukotriene B_4 levels, but is due instead to inhibition of cyclooxygenase products. Peripheral and axial arthralgias are common in patients with IBD, and these symptoms are treated with the management of the associated IBD, physiotherapy and the judicious use of acetaminophen.

The use of oral contraceptive agents may be a risk factor for the development of IBD, even after correcting for the adverse effect of smoking (Sutherland *et al.*, unpublished observations, 1994).

OTHER AGENTS

The use of lidocaine (Bjorck *et al.*, 1991) or bismuth subsalicylate enemas appears to be of some promise, as assessed in open studies (Ryder *et al.*, 1990). Clearly, these need to be validated in controlled clinical trials. There has been limited experience reported with sucralfate in patients with IBD (Wright *et al.*, 1992). Verapamil inhibits the release of LTB_4 from the rectal mucosa of patients with active UC (Gertner *et al.*, 1992); its clinical efficacy is unknown. An organic arsenical (Acetarsol®) has been found to be at least as effective as suppositories of prednisolone-21-phosphate (Connell *et al.*, 1965). A controlled clinical trial has been launched using TNFα. Interferon has been examined in open studies, and controlled clinical trials are soon to be initiated.

Hydroxychloroquine (Plaquenil®) (400 mg/day) has been used in a placebo-controlled trial, with no beneficial results noted (Mayer *et al.*, 1992). This contrasted with the early positive suggestion from an open trial in refractory UC (Mayer and Sachar, 1988).

A SOCIAL CONSCIENCE: WHAT IS THE COST?

There is a major impact of CD and UC in terms of the impaired quality of life of the sufferer, hospitalization and loss of income, and difficulty obtaining life insurance coverage, even though the mortality rate of UC and CD is not different now from that of an otherwise healthy community (Beck *et al.*, 1994). This pain and suffering is difficult to quantitate on a strictly dollar basis. Careful cost analyses of the medical therapy of IBD have not yet been formally completed, but the use of SASP-maintenance therapy in patients with UC results in a fall in the expected annual rate of relapse from approximately 80% to 20%. In CD, the annual risk of recurrence falls from approximately 50% to 25% with the use of mesalamine. When viewing strictly the cost of medications, there is considerable variation in the monthly expenditures for SASP tablets, enemas or suppositories of SASP, mesalamines, or GS (Table 1).

While GS is relatively inexpensive, the potential adverse effects go against its use for first-time or initial therapy. While SASP is as effective as the newer 5-ASA compounds, and is somewhat cheaper, there is concern for the much higher prevalence of adverse effects. This therefore provides the rational basis for the suggestion to begin all newly diagnosed patients with mild/moderately active CD or UC on one of the cost-effective formulations of mesalanine, in doses of at least 3 g/day (see Fig. 10). If 8 weeks of therapy is ineffective to achieve a remission, then it will be necessary to add prednisone in a dose of approximately 40 mg/day. If after a further 8 weeks the patient continues to be unwell, then the addition of i.v./p.o. CyA or AZA needs to be contemplated, and judicious timing of surgery considered.

Table 1 Publically quoted cost of one month supply of medications used to treat patients with active or remitted ulcerative colitis and Crohn's disease

	Representative dose		Cost ($/month)
1. Anti-inflammatories			
Sulfasalazine	4 g/day	8 x 30	$ 54.38
Mesalamine tablets			
Dipentum®	2[a]		$ 134.14
Asacol®	2[a]		$ 87.06
Mesasal®	2[a]		$ 76.79
Salofalk®	2[a]		$ 74.36
Pentasa®	2[a]		$ 80.66
Enemas – Salofalk®	1 per day	4 boxes	$ 192.81
Suppositories – Salofalk®	250 mg/day		$ 32.93
2. Antibiotics			
Metronidazole	1000[a]		$ 11.33 generic
Clofazimine			not available
3. Glucocorticosteroid tablets			
Deltasone	20[a]		$ 7.84
Enemas – Betnesol®	1 g h	1 box 7 enm	$ 16.09 5 boxes $48.00
Cortifoam 1 g h	1 g h	20 g	$ 85.75
4. Immunomodulators			
Azathioprine (6-MP)	150 mg/day		$ 92.45
Cyclosporine	600[a]		$1090.09
Methotrexate	25[a]		$ 181.32 generic
5. Nutrition[b]			
Parenteral	As needed		$ 250/day not stocked
Ensure	2/day		$ 1.98/can or
			$ 21.88/case
Boost	2/day		$ 1.68/can or $9.98 for 6
6. Antidiarrheal agents			
Lomotil®	20 mg/day	8 x 30	$ 120.88
Imodium®	16 mg/day	8 x 30	$ 156.60
Codeine	60 mg/day	2 x 30	$ 14.73
Questran®	8 g/day	Questran powder 378 g size $40.79 (21-day supply)	

[a]The dose of those medications may vary from patient to patient, and at different times. The doses shown here are representative. The costs represent a mean of two values quoted from a telephone survey conducted in Edmonton, in March 1994.

[b]The cost of these preparations varies widely. For example, the cost of TPN depends on whether the direct or the direct plus indirect costs are included. The figure of $250/day for TPN is considered to be a conservative estimate. There are numerous appropriate nutritional supplements which may benefit patients with IBD, and these range widely in price.

Acknowledgements

The author wishes to thank Drs R. McLeod, F. Martin, L. Sutherland and N. Williams for asking me to participate in the discussion of newer therapies in patients with inflammatory bowel disease, and to submit this manuscript for critical peer review. Permission from Dr L. Sutherland, to use Figs 5–8, is acknowledged with gratitude. The secretarial and word-processing assistance of Trudi Schmidt and Marlene Hoffmann is gratefully acknowledged.

I would also like to thank Mrs Peggy Kirdeikis for performing the telephone survey of the cost of medications used in Table 1.

Dedication

This work is dedicated to the memory of Grace and Arthur Lewis.

References

Adler DJ, Korelitz BI. The therapeutic efficacy of 6-mercaptopurine in refractory ulcerative colitis. Am J Gastroenterol. 1990;85:717–22.

Afdhal NH, Long A, Lennon J, Crowe J, O'Donaghue DP. Controlled trial of antimyobacterial therapy in Crohn's disease. Dig Dis Sci. 1991;36:449–53.

Alstead EM, Ritchie JK, Lennard-Jones JE, Farthing MUG, Lark ML. Safety of azathioprine in pregnancy in inflammatory bowel disease. Gastroenterology. 1990a;99:730–6.

Alstead EM, Ritchie JK, Lennard-Jones JE, Farthing MJG, Clark ML. Safety of azathioprine in pregnancy in inflammatory bowel disease. Gastroenterology. 1990b;99:443–6.

Angus P, Snook JA, Reid M, Jewell DP. Oral fluticasone propionate in active distal ulcerative colitis. Gut. 1992;33:711–14.

Arora S, Katkov WN, Cooley J et al. A double-blind, randomized, placebo-controlled trial of methotrexate in Crohn's disease. Immunol Microbiol Inflam Disorders, 1992;A591.

Aslan A, Triadafilopoulos GL. Fish oil fatty acid supplementation in active ulcerative colitis: a double blind placebo-controlled, crossover study. Am J Gastroenterol. 1992;87:432–7.

Azad Khan AK, Piris J, Truelove SC. An experiment to determine the active therapeutic moiety of sulfasalazine. Lancet. 1977;2:892–5.

Baker K, Jewell DP. Cyclosporin for the treatment of severe inflammatory bowel disease. Aliment Pharmacol Ther. 1989;3:143–9.

Bello C, Goldstein F, Thornton JJ. Alternate day prednisone treatment and treatment maintenance in Crohn's disease. Am J Gastroenterol. 1991;86:460–6.

Best WR, Becktel JM, Singleton JW, Kern FJ Jr. Development of a Crohn's disease activity index: National Cooperative Crohn's Disease Study. Gastroenterology. 1976;70:439–4.

Best WR, Becktel JM, Singleton JW. Rederived values of the eight coefficients of the Crohn's disease activity index (CDAI). Gastroenterology. 1979;77:843–6.

Bianchi Porro G, Campieri M, Bianchi P et al. Comparison of budesonide and methylprednisolone in the treatment of ulcerative colitis. Ital J Gastroenterol. 1991;23:640.

Bicks RO, Groshart KD. The current status of T-lymphocyte apheresis of Crohn's disease. J Clin Gastroenterol. 1989;11:136–8.

Biddle WL, Miner PB Jr. Long-term use of mesalamine enemas to induce remission in ulcerative colitis. Gastroenterology. 1990;99:113–18.

Bjorck S, Dahlstrom A, Ahlman H. Topical treatment with lidocaine in patients with ulcerative colitis. Gastroenterology. 1991;100:A198.

Bondesen S and the Danish 5-ASA Group. Mesalazine (Pentasa) as prophylaxis in Crohn's disease. A multicenter, controlled trial. Scand J Gastroenterol. 1991;26(Suppl.183):68.

Brignola C, Campieri M, Bassocchi G, Farrugia P, Tagnone A, Lanfranchi GA. A laboratory index for predicting relapse in asymptomatic patients with Crohn's disease. Gastroenterology. 1986;91:1490–4.

Brignola C, Campieri M, Farrugia P et al. The possible utility of steroids in the prevention of relapses of Crohn's disease in remission: a preliminary study. J Clin Gastroenterol. 1988;10:631–4.

Brignola C, Iannone P, Pasquali S et al. Placebo-controlled trial of oral 5-ASA in relapse prevention of Crohn's disease. Dig Dis Sci. 1992;37(1):29–32.

Brynskov J, Freund L, Rasmussen SN et al. A placebo-controlled, double-blind, randomized trial of cyclosporine therapy in active chronic Crohn's disease. N Engl J Med. 1989a;321:845–50.

Brynskov J, Freund L, Ostergaard Thomsen O, Anderson CB, Norby Rasmussen S, Binder V.

Treatment of refractory ulcerative colitis with cyclosporine enemas. Lancet. 1989;1:721–722.

Brynskov J, Freund L, Rasmussen SN et al. Final report on a placebo-controlled, double-blind, randomized, multicenter trial of cyclosporin treatment in active chronic Crohn's disease. Scand J Gastroenterol. 1991;26:689–95.

Brynskov J, Freund L, Campanini MC, Kampmann JP. Cyclosporin pharmacokinetics after intravenous and oral administration in patients with Crohn's disease. Scand J Gastroenterol. 1992;27:961–7.

Burke DA, Axon ATR, Clayden SA et al. The efficacy of tobramycin in the treatment of ulcerative colitis. Aliment Pharmacol Ther. 1990;4:123–9.

Campieri M, Lanfranchi GA, Bazzocchi G, Brignola C, Sarti F. Treatment of ulcerative colitis with high-dose 5-aminosalicylic acid enemas. Lancet. 1981;2:270–1.

Campieri M, De Franchis R, Porro GB, Ranzi T, Brunetti G, Barbara L. Mesalamine (5-aminosalicylic acid) suppositories in the treatment of ulcerative proctitis or distal proctosigmoiditis: a randomized controlled trial. Scand J Gastroenterol. 1990a;25:663–8.

Campieri M, Gionchetti P, Belluzzi A et al. Role of rectal formulations: enemas. Scand J Gastroenterol. 1990b;25(Suppl.172):63–5.

Campieri M, Gionchetti P, Belluzzi A et al. Topical treatment with 5-aminosalicylic acid in distal ulcerative colitis by using a new suppository preparation: a double-blind placebo controlled trial. Int J Colorectal Dis. 1990c;5:79–81.

Campieri M, Bianchi P, Bianchi Porro G et al. Therapeutic evaluation of mesalamine foam (Asacol) versus mesalamine enema in the treatment of distal ulcerative colitis. Gastroenterology. 1991a;100:A200.

Campieri M, Gionchetti P, Belluzzi A et al. Optimum dosage of 5-aminosalicylic acid as rectal enemas in patients with active ulcerative colitis. Gut. 1991b;32:929–31.

Canadian Inflammatory Bowel Disease Study Group. Oral budesonide in active Crohn's disease: interim report of a placebo controlled randomized trial. Immunol Microbiol Inflam Disorders. 1993;A675.

Canadian Inflammatory Bowel Disease Study Group. Budesonide 9 or 15 mg rapidly improves quality of life (qol) in active Crohn's disease. J Irvin Gut (In press).

Caprilli R, Andreoli A, Capurso L et al and the Gruppo Italiano Per Lo Studio Del Colon E Del Retto (Gisc). Oral mesalazine (5-aminosalicylic acid; Asacol) for the prevention of post-operative recurrence of Crohn's disease. Aliment Pharmacol Ther. 1994;8:35–43.

Caravo M, Camilo ME, Pinto Correia J. Nutritional support in Crohn's disease: which route? Am J Gastroenterol. 1991;86:317–21.

Christensen LA, Fallingborg J, Abildgaard K et al. Topical and systemic availability of 5-aminosalicylate: comparisons of 3 controlled release preparations in man. Aliment Pharmacol Ther. 1990;4:523–33.

Collawn C, Rubin P, Perez N et al. Phase II study of the safety and efficacy of a 5-lipoxygenase inhibitor in patients with ulcerative colitis. Am J Gastroenterol. 1992;87:342–6.

Cominelli F, Nast CCC, Duchini A, Lee M. Recombinant interleukin-1 receptor antagonist blocks the proinflammatory activity of endogenous interleukin-1 in rabbit immune colitis. Gastroenterology. 1992;103:65–71.

Connell AM, Lennard-Jones JE, Misiewicz JJ, Baron JH, Avery-Jones FA. Comparison of acetarsol and prednisolone-21-phosphate suppositories in the treatment of idiopathic proctitis. Lancet. 1965;1:238–9.

Connell WR, Kamm MA, Lennard-Jones JE, Ritchie JD. Bone marrow toxicity from azathioprine in inflammatory bowel disease: experience from 1963 patient years of therapy. Gut. 1992;33(Suppl.1):S10(abstr.).

Connell WR, Kamm MA, Ritchie JK, Lennard-Jones JE. Bone marrow toxicity caused by azathioprine in inflammatory bowel disease: 27 years of experience. Gut. 1993;34:1081–5.

Courtney MG, Nunes DP, Bergin CF et al. Randomised comparison of olsalazine and mesalamine in prevention of relapses in ulcerative colitis. Lancet. 1992;339:1279–81.

D'Arienzo A, Panarese A, Darmiento FP et al. 5-Aminosalicylic acid suppositories in the maintenance of remission in idiopathic proctitis or proctosigmoiditis: a double-blind placebo-controlled clinical trial. Am J Gastroenterol. 1990;85:1079–82.

Danielsson A, Hellers G, Lyrenas E et al. A controlled randomized trial of budesonide versus prednisolone retention enemas in active distal ulcerative colitis. Scand J Gastroenterol. 1987;22:987–92.

Danielsson A, Lofberg R, Persson T et al. A steroid enema, budesonide, lacking systemic effects for the treatment of distal ulcerative colitis or proctitis. Scand J Gastroenterol. 1992;27:9–12.

Danielsson A, Edsbacker S, Lofberg R et al. Pharmacokinetics of budesonide enema in patients with distal ulcerative colitis of proctitis. Aliment Pharmacol Ther. 1993;7:401–7.

Danish 5-ASa Group. Topical 5-aminosalicylic acid versus prednisolone in ulcerative proctosigmoiditis: a randomized double-blind multicenter trial. Dig Dis Sci. 1987;2:598–602.

Danish Budesonide Study Group. Budesonide enema in distal ulcerative colitis: a randomized dose-response trial with prednisolone enema as positive control. Scand J Gastroenterol. 1991;26:1225–30.

Deusch K, Reiter C, Mauthe B et al. Chimeric monoclonal anti-CD4 antibody therapy proves effective for treating inflammatory bowel disease. Gastroenterology. 1992;102:A615.

De Vos M, Verdievel H, Schoonjans R, Praet M, Bogaert M, Barbier F. Concentrations of 5-ASA and Ac-5-ASA in human ileocolonic biopsy homogenates after oral 5-ASA preparations. Gut. 1992;33:1338–42.

Dew MJ, Hughes P, Harris AD et al. Maintenance of remission in ulcerative colitis with oral preparation of 5-aminosalicylic acid. Br Med J. 1982;285:1012.

Dew MJ, Harris AD, Evans N et al. Maintenance of remission in ulcerative colitis with 5-aminosalicylic acid in high doses by mouth. Br Med J. 1983;287:23.

Dissanayake AS, Truelove SC. A controlled therapeutic trial of long-term maintenance treatment of UC with sulfasalazine. Gut. 1973;14:923.

Ewe K, Press AG, Singe CC et al. Azathioprine combined with prednisolone or monotherapy with prednisolone in active Crohn's disease. Gastroenterology. 1993;105:367–72.

Ewe K, Herfarth C, Malchow H, Jesdinsky HJ. Postoperative recurrence of Crohn's disease in relation to radicality of operation and sulfasalazine prophylaxis: a multicenter trial. Digestion. 1989;42:224–32.

Feagan BE, McDonald JWD, Rochon J et al. Low-dose cyclosporine for the treatment of Crohn's disease. N Engl J Med. 1994a;330:1846–51.

Feagan BG, Rochon J, Fedorak RN et al. Methotrexate for the treatment of Crohn's disease. In press, 1994b.

Feurle GE, Theuer D, Volasco S et al. Olsalazine versus placebo in the treatment of mild to moderate ulcerative colitis: A randomized double-blind trial. Gut. 1989;30:1354.

Fiorentini MT, Fracchia M, Galatola G, Barlotta A, Delapierre M. Acute pancreatitis during oral 5-aminosalicylic therapy. Dig Dis Sci. 1990;35:1180–2.

Fischer SH, Levine DS, Haggett RC. Immunoglobulin therapy for active and extensive idiopathic ulcerative colitis and Crohn's colitis. Gastroenterology. 1990;98:A170.

Florent C, Cortot A, Quandale P et al. Placebo-controlled trial of Claversal® in the prevention of early endoscopic relapse after 'curative' resection for Crohn's disease. Gastroenterology. 1992;102:A623.

Gaginella TS, Walsh RE. Sulfasalazine: multiplicity of action. Dig Dis Sci. 1992;37:801–12.

Galandiuk S, Oneill M, McDonald P, Fazio VW, Steigerr E. A century of home parenteral nutrition for Crohn's disease. Am J Surg. 1990;159:540–5.

Gendre JP, Mary JY, Florent C et al and the Groupe D'Etude Therapeutique Des Affections Inflammatories Digestives. Oral mesalamine (Pentasa) as maintenance treatment in Crohn's disease: a multicenter placebo-controlled study. Gastroenterology. 1993;104:435–9.

Gendre JP, Mary JY, Florent C et al. Does pentasa prevent relapses in quiescent Crohn's disease? A multicenter placebo-controlled trial (161 patients). Gastroenterology. 1990;98:A171.

Gertner DJ, Rampton DS, Stevens TRJ, Lennard-Jones JE. Verapamil inhibits in-vitro leukotriene B_4 release by rectal mucosa in active ulcerative colitis. Aliment Pharmacol Ther. 1992;6:163–8.

Giaffer MH, Cann P, Holdsworth CD. Long-term effects of elemental and exclusion diets for Crohn's disease. Aliment Pharmacol Ther. 1991;5:115–25.

Giaffer MH, Holdsworth CD, Lennard-Jones JE. Improved maintenance of remission in ulcerative colitis by balsalazide 4 g/day compared with 2 g/d. Aliment Pharmacol Ther. 1992;6:479–85.

Giaffer MH, North G, Holdsworth CD. Controlled trial of polymeric versus elemental diet in treatment of active Crohn's disease. Lancet. 1990;335:816–19.

Gibson GR, Whitacre EB, Ricotti CA. Colitis induced by nonsteroidal anti-inflammatory drugs:

report of four cases and review of the literature. Arch Intern Med. 1992;152:625–32.

Ginsberg AL, David ND, Nochomovitz LE. Placebo-controlled, double-blind trial of oral 4-aminosalicylic acid in ulcerative colitis. Gastroenterology. 1990;98:A172.

Gorard DA, Hunt JB, Payne-James JJ et al. Initial response and subsequent course of Crohn's disease treated with elemental diet or prednisolone. Gut. 1993;34:1198–202.

Gramlich LM, Barley RJ. Intravenous (IV) cyclosporine in refractory Crohn's disease for remission induction. Trends in Inflammatory Bowel Disease Therapy, Victoria, 6–9 April, Poster 15, 1994.

Green JRB, Swan CHJ, Rowlinson A et al. Short report: Comparison of two doses of balsalazide in maintaining ulcerative colitis in remission over 12 months. Aliment Pharmacol Ther. 1992;6:647–52.

Greenfield SM, Punchard NA, Teare JP, Thompson RPH. Review article: The mode of action of the aminosalicylates in inflammatory bowel disease. Aliment Pharmacol Ther. 1993;7:369–83.

Habal FM, Hui G, Greenberg GR. Oral 5-aminosalicylic acid for inflammatory bowel disease in pregnancy: Safety and clinical course. Gastroenterology. 1993;105:1057–60.

Halpern Z, Sold O, Baratz M, Konikoff F, Halak A, Gilat T. A controlled trial of beclomethasone versus betamethasone enemas in distal ulcerative colitis. J Clin Gastroenterol. 1991;13:38–41.

Hanauer S, Schwartz J, Roufail W et al. Dose-ranging study of oral mesalamine capsule (Pentasa) for active ulcerative colitis. Gastroenterology. 1986;96:A85 (abstr.).

Hanauer SB, Krawitt EL, Ropbinson et al. Long-term management of Crohn's disease with mesalamine capsules (Pentasa®). Am J Gastroenterol. 1988;88:1343.

Hanauer S, Beschcars L, Wilkinson C et al. Induction of remission in a dose-ranging study of oral mesalamine capsules. Gastroenterology. 1990;98:A174.

Hanauer SB. Sulfasalazine vs. steroids in Crohn's disease: David vs Goliath [editorial]? Gastroenterology. 1991;101:1130–1.

Hanauer ST, Krawitt EL, Robinson M, Rick GG, Safdi MA and the Pentasa® Crohn's Disease Compassionalt Use Study Group. Long-term management of Crohn's disease with mesalamine capsules (Pentasa®). Am J Gastroenterol. 1993;88:1343.

Hawthorne AB, Daneshmend TJ, Hawkey CJ et al. Treatment of ulcerative colitis with fish oil supplementation: A prospective 12 month randomized controlled trial. Gut. 1992a;33:922–8.

Hawthorne AB, Logan RFA, Hawkey CJ et al. Randomized controlled trial of azathioprine withdrawal in ulcerative colitis. Brit Med J. 1992b;305:20–2.

Hemphill DI, Greenberg GR, Steinhart AH. Sulfasalazine and mesalazine for maintenance therapy of Crohn's disease: a meta-analysis. Clin Inv Med. 1993;16:B46.

Hetzel DJ, Shearman DJ, Labrooy J et al. Olsalazine in the treatment of active ulcerative colitis. A placebo-controlled trial and assessment of drug deposition. J Gastroenterol Hepatol. 1986;1:257.

Holdstock GE, Fischer JA, Kembilin LT, Leohrig T. Plasmapheresis in Crohn's disease. Digestion. 1979;19:197–201.

International Mesalamine study Group. Coated oral 5-aminosalicylic acid versus placebo in maintaining remission of inactive Crohn's disease. Aliment Pharmacol Ther. 1990;4:55–64.

Ireland A, Mason CH, Jewell DP. Controlled trial comparing olsalazine and sulfasalazine for the maintenance treatment of ulcerative colitis. Gut. 1988;29:835–7.

Irvine EJ, Marshall JK. A meta-analysis of topical ASAs for distal ulcerative colitis (UC). Trends in Inflammatory Bowel Disease Therapy, Victoria, 6–9 April, Post 21, 1994.

Jarnerot G, Rolny P, Sandber-Gertzen H. Intensive intravenous treatment of ulcerative colitis. Gastroenterology. 1985;89:1005–13.

Jarnerot G, Lennard-Jones J, Bianchi-Porro G, Brynskov J, Campieri M, Present D. Medical treatment of refractory distal ulcerative colitis. Gastroenterol Int. 1991;4:93–8.

Jewell DP, Caprilli R, Mortensen N, Nicholls RJ, Wright JP. Indications and timing of surgery for severe ulcerative colitis. Gastroenterol Int. 1991;4:161–4.

Katz J. Treatment of Crohn's disease with 5-ASA. Am J Gastroenterol. 1993;88:1315–17.

Killerich S, Ladefoged K, Rannem T, Ranlov PJ. The Danish Olsalazine Study Group: Prophylactic effects of olsalazine v sulfasalazine during 12 months maintenance treatment of ulcerative colitis. Gut. 1992;33:252–5.

Kirsner JB, Shorter RG. Preface. In: Kirsner JB, Shorter RG, editors. Inflammatory bowel disease. Philadelphia: Lea & Febiger, 1975.

Kitano A, Matsumoto T, Nakamura S et al. New treatment of ulcerative colitis with K-76. Dis Colon Rectum. 1992;35:560-7.

Klein M, Binder HJ, Mitchell M, Aaronson R, Spiro H. Treatment of Crohn's disease with azathioprine: a controlled evaluation. Gastroenterology. 1974;66:916-22.

Korelitz BI, Present BH. Shortcomings of the national Crohn's disease study: the exclusion of azathioprine without adequate trial. Gastroenterology. 1981;80:193-200.

Kozarek RA, Patterson DJ, Gelfand MD, Botoman VA, Ball TJ, Wilske RR. Methotrexate induces clinical and histological remission in patients with refractory inflammatory bowel disease. Ann Intern Med. 1989;110:353-6.

Kozarek RA, Patterson DJ, Botoman VA, Ball TJ, Gelfand MD. Methotrexate (MTX) use in inflammatory bowel disease (IBD) patients who have failed azathioprine (AZ) or 6-mercaptupurine (6-MP). Gastroenterology. 1991;100:A222.

Kulerich S, Ladefoged K, Rannem T, Ranlov PJ, The Danish Olsalazine Study Group: Prophylactic effects of olsalazine v sulfasalazine during 12 months maintenance treatment of ulcerative colitis. Gut. 1992;33:252-5.

Kusunoki M, Moelein G, Shoji Y et al. Steroid complications in patients with ulcerative colitis. Dis Colon Rectum. 1992;35:1003-9.

Lamers C, Meijer J, Engels L et al. Comparative study of the topically acting glucocorticosteroid budesonide and 5-aminosalicylic acid enema therapy of proctitis and proctosigmoiditis. Am J Gastroenterol. 1991;100:A223.

Langholz E, Brynskov J, Bendtzen K, Vilien M, Binder V. Treatment of Crohn's disease with fusidic acid: an antibiotic with immunosuppressive properties similar to cyclosporin. Aliment Pharmacol Ther. 1992;6:495-502.

Lashner BA, Hanauer SB, Silverstein MD. Testine nicotine gum for ulcerative colitis patients. Experience with single patient trials. Dig Dis Sci. 1990;35:827-32.

Laursen LS, Stokolm M, Bukhave K, Rask-Madsen J, Lauritsen K. Disposition of 5-aminosalicylic acid by olsalazine and three mesalamine preparations in patients with ulcerative colitis: comparison of intraluminal colonic concentrations, serum values, and urinary excretion. Gut. 1990;31:1271-6.

Lechin F, van der Kijs B, Insavsti CL et al. Treatment of ulcerative colitis with clonidine. J Clin Pharmacol. 1985;25:19-26.

Leddin DJ, VeldLuyzenNanZanten S, Sidorow JJ, Stewart J, Tripathi D, Williams CN. Colectomy following treatment of Crohn's colitis with cyclosporine A (CyA). Trends in Inflammatory Bowel Disease Therapy, Victoria, 6-9 April, Poster 33, 1994.

Lemann M, Bonhomme P, Bitoun A, Messing B, Modigliani R, Rambaud JC. Treatment of Crohn's disease with azathioprine or 6-mercaptopurine: retrospective study in 126 patients [in French]. Gastroenterol Clin Biol. 1990;14:548-54.

Lennard-Jones JE. Azathioprine and 6-mercaptopurine have a role in the treatment of Crohn's disease. Dig Dis Sci. 1981;26:364-8.

Levine DS, Fischer SH, Christie DI, Haggitt RC, Ochs HD. Intravenous immunoglobulin therapy for active, extensive, and medically refractory idiopathic ulcerative or Crohn's colitis. Am J Gastroenterol. 1992;87:91-100.

Lichtenstein JE. Inflammatory conditions of the stomach and duodenum. Radiol Clin N Am. 1993;31:1315-33.

Lichter S, Present DH, Kornbluth A et al. Cyclosporine in severe ulcerative colitis refractory to steroid therapy. N Engl J Med. 1994;330:1841-5.

Lichtiger S, Present DH. Cyclosporine in treatment of severe active ulcerative colitis. Lancet. 1990;336:16-19.

Linn FV, Peppercorn MA. Drug therapy for inflammatory bowel disease: Part I. Am J Surg. 1992;164:85-9.

Lobo AJ, Foster PN, Burke DA, Johnston D, Axon ATR. The role of azathioprine in the management of ulcerative colitis. Dis Colon Rectum. 1990;33:374-7.

Lobo AJ, Juby LD, Rothwell J, Poole TW, Axon ATR. Long-term treatment of Crohn's disease with cyclosporine: the effect of a very low dose on maintenance of remission. J Clin Gastroenterol. 1991;13:42-5.

Lochs H, Steinhardt HJ, Klaus-Wentz B et al. Comparison of enteral nutrition and drug treatment in active Crohn's disease. Gastroenterology. 1991;101:881-8.

Löfberg R, Ostergaard-Thomsen O, Langholtz E et al. Budesonide versus prednisolone enema in active distal ulcerative colitis. A comparative eight week study. Gut. 1993;34(Suppl.):41.

Löfberg R, Rutgeerts P, Malchow H et al. Budesonide CIR for maintenance of remission in ileocecal Crohn's disease. A European multicenter placebo controlled trial for 12 months. Gastroenterology. 1994;106:A722.

Malchow H, Ewe K, Brandes JW et al. European Cooperative Crohn's Disease Study (ECCDS); results of drug treatment. Gastroenterology. 1984;86:249–66.

Mantzaris G, Hatzis A, Kontogiannis P, Triadaphyllou G. Intravenous tobramycin and metronidazole as an adjunct to corticosteroids in acute, severe ulcerative colitis.

Martin F, Sutherland L, Beck IT et al. Oral 5-ASA versus prednisone in short term treatment of Crohn's disease: a multicenter controlled trial. Can J Gastroenterol. 1990;4:452–7.

Mayer L, Schar DB, Present DH et al. Randomized double-blind placebo-controlled trial of hydroxychloroquine (Plaquenil) in the treatment of ulcerative colitis. Gastroenterology. 1992;102:A661.

Mayer L, Sachar DB. Efficacy of chloroquine in the treatment of inflammatory bowel disease. Gastroenterology. 1988;984:A293.

McIntyre PB, Rodrigues CA, Lennard-Jones JE et al. Balsalazide in the maintenance treatment of patients with ulcerative colitis, a double-blind comparison with sulfasalazine. Aliment Pharmacol Ther. 1988;2:237–43.

McLeod RS, Wolff BG, Steinhart H et al. Decreased recurrence following surgery for Crohn's disease (CD) using Salofalk 5-ASA tablets 3 gm/day. Trends in Inflammatory Bowel Disease Therapy, Victoria, 6–9 April 1994.

Mehta RP. Acute intestinal nephritis due to 5-aminosalicylic acid. Can Med Assoc J. 1990;143:1031–2.

Messori A, Brignola C, Trallori G et al. Effectiveness of 5-aminosalicylic acid (5-ASA) for maintaining remission in patients with Crohn's disease: a meta-analysis. Am J Gastroenterol. 1994;89:692–8.

Meyers S, Sachar DB, Present DH et al. Olsalazine sodium in the treatment of ulcerative colitis among patients intolerant of sulfasalazine. A prospective, randomised, placebo-controlled, double-blind, dose-ranging clinical trial. Gastroenterology. 1987;934:1255.

Miglioli M, Barbara L, Di Febo G et al. Topical administration of 5-aminosalicylic acid: a therapeutic proposal for the treatment of pouchitis (letter). N Engl J Med. 1989;320:257.

Miglioli M, Bianchi Porro G, Brunetti G, Sturniolo GC. Oral delayed-release mesalamine in the treatment of mild ulcerative colitis: a dose ranging study. Eur J Gastroenterol Hepatol. 1990a;2:2299.

Miglioli M, Porro GB, Brunetti G, Sturniolo GC. Oral delayed-release mesalamine in the treatment of mild ulcerative colitis: a dose ranging study. Eur J Gastroenterol Hepatol. 1990b;2:229.

Mihida YR, Jewell DP. Slow-release 5-aminosalicylic acid (Pentasa®) for the treatment of active Crohn's disease. Digestion. 1990;45:88–92.

Miner P, Schwartz J, Aora S et al. Maintenance of remission in ulcerative colitis patients with controlled-release mesalamine capsules (Pentasa®). Gastroenterology. 1992;102:A266.

Modigliani R, Mary JY, Simon JF et al. Clinical, biological, and endoscopic picture of attacks of Crohn's disease: evolution on prednisolone. Gastroenterology. 1990;98:811–18.

Mulder CJJ, Tytgat GNJ, Weterman IT et al. Double-blind comparison of slow-release 5-aminosalicylate and sulfasalazine in remission maintenance in ulcerative colitis. Gastroenterology. 1988;95:1449–53.

Nakshabendi IM, Duncan A, Russell RI. Is Asacol as effective as sulfasalazine in maintaining remission of Crohn's disease and ulcerative colitis? Postgrad Med J. 1992;68:189–91.

O'Brien JJ, Bayless TM, Bayless JA. Use of azathioprine of 6-mercaptopurine in the treatment of Crohn's disease. Gastroenterology. 1991;101:39–46.

O'Donoghue DP, Dawson AM, Powell-Tuck J, Brown RL, Lennard-Jones JE. Double-blind withdrawal trial of azathioprine as maintenance treatment for Crohn's disease. Lancet. 1978;2:955–7.

O'Morain CA. Does nutritional therapy in inflammatory bowel disease have a primary or an adjunctive role? Scand J Gastroenterol. 1990;25(Suppl.172):29–34.

Oliason G, Sjodhal R, Tagesson C. Glucocorticoid treatment in ileal Crohn's disease: relief of symptoms but not of endoscopically viewed inflammation. Gut. 1990;31:325–8.

Pearson DC, May GR, Fick GH, Sutherland LR. Azathioprine and 6-mercaptopurine in Crohn's disease: a meta-analysis. Trends in Inflammatory Bowel Disease Therapy, Victoria, 6–9 April, Post 8, 1994.

Perrault H, Greseth JLM, Tremaine WJ. 6-Mercaptopurine therapy in selected cases of corticosteroid-dependent Crohn's disease. Mayo Clin Proc. 1991;66:480–4.

Prantera C, Pallone F, Brunetti G, Cottone M, Miglioli M, The Italian IBD Study Group: Oral 5-aminosalicylic acid (Asacol) in the maintenance treatment of Crohn's disease. Gastroenterology. 1992;103:363–8.

Present DH. 6-Mercaptopurine and other immunosuppressive agents in the treatment of Crohn's disease and ulcerative colitis. Gastroenterol Clin N Am. 1989;18:57–71.

Present DH, Korelitz BI, Wisch N, Glass GL, Sachar DB, Pasternack BS. Treatment of Crohn's disease with 6-mercaptopurine. A long-term, randomized, double-blind study. N Engl J Med. 1980;302:981–7.

Present DH, Meltzer SJ, Krumholz MP, Wolke A, Korelitz BI. 6-Mercaptopurine in the management of inflammatory bowel disease: short- and long-term toxicity. Ann Intern Med. 1989;111:641–9.

Ranzi T, Campanini MC, Velio P, Quarto Di Palo F, Bianchi P. Treatment of chronic proctosigmoiditis with cyclosporin enemas. Lancet. 1989;2:97.

Rasmussen SN, Bondesen S, Hvidberg EF et al. Amino-salicylic acid in a slow-release preparation: bioavailability, plasma level and excretion in humans. Gastroenterology. 1982;83:1062–71.

Rasmussen SN, Lauritsen K, Tage-Jensen U et al. 5-aminosalicylic in the treatment of Crohn's disease. A 16-week double-blind, placebo-controlled, multicenter study with Pentasa®. Scand J Gastroenterol. 1987;22:877.

Record CO, Macrae K. Mesalamine versus olsalazine for prophylaxis of ulcerative colitis relapse. Lancet. 1992;340:1468.

Rhodes J, Bainton D, Beck P, Campbell H. Controlled trial of azathioprine in Crohn's disease. Lancet. 1971;2:1273–6.

Rigaud D, Cosnes J, Le Quintrec Y, Renne E, Gendre JP, Mignon M. Controlled trial comparing two types of enteral nutrition in treatment of active Crohn's disease: elemental polymeric diet. Gut. 1991;32:1492–7.

Rijk MCM, Van Hogezand RA, Van Schaik A, Van Tongeren JHM. Disposition of 5-aminosalicylic acid from 5-aminosalicylic acid-delivering drugs during accelerated intestinal transit in healthy volunteers. Scand J Gastroenterol. 1989;24:1179–85.

Rijk MCM, Van Hogezand RA, Van Lier HJJ et al. Sulfasalazine and prednisone compared with sulfasalazine for treating active Crohn's disease: a double-blind, randomized, multicenter trial. Ann Intern Med. 1991a;114:445–50.

Rijk MCM, Tongeren JHM. The relapse preventing effect and safety of sulfasalazine and olsalazine in patients with ulcerative colitis in remission. Gastroenterology. 1991b;100:A243.

Rijk MCM, Van Lier HJJ, Van Tongeren JHM. Relapse preventing effect and safety of sulfasalazine and olsalazine in patients with ulcerative colitis in remission: a prospective, double-blind, randomized multicenter study. Am J Gastroenterol. 1992;87:438–42.

Riley SA, Turnberg LA. Sulfasalazine and the aminosalicylates in the treatment of inflammatory bowel disease. Q J Med. 1990;278:551–62.

Riley SA, Mani V, Goodman MJ, Herd ME, Dutt S, Turnberg LA. Comparison of delayed-release 5-aminosalicylic acid (mesalamine) and sulfasalazine as maintenance treatment for patients with ulcerative colitis. Gastroenterology. 1988a;94:1383–8.

Riley SA, Mani V, Goodman MJ, Herd ME, Dutt S, Turnberg LA. Comparison of delayed-release 5-aminosalicylic acid (mesalamine) and sulfasalazine as maintenance treatment for patients with ulcerative colitis. Gastroenterology. 1988b;94:1449.

Riley SA, Tavares IA, Bishai PM, Bennet A, Mani V. Mesalamine release from coated tablets: effect of dietary fibre. Br J Clin Pharmacol. 1991;32:248–50.

Robinson M, Gilrick G, Balart L et al. Olsalazine in the treatment of mild to moderate ulcerative colitis. Gastroenterology. 1988;94:A381.

Rosenberg JL, Levin B, Wall AJ, Kirsner JB. A controlled trial of azathioprine in Crohn's disease. Am J Dig Dis. 1975;20:721–6.

Rosenberg W, Ireland A, Jewell D. High-dose methylprednisolone in the treatment of active ulcerative colitis. J Clin Gastroenterol. 1990;12:40–1.

Rutgeerts P. Comparative efficacy of coated, oral 5-aminosalicylic acid (Claversal®) and sulfasalazine for maintaining remission of ulcerative colitis. Aliment Pharmacol Ther. 1989;3:183.

Rutgeerts P, Geboes K, Vantrappen G, Beyls J, Kerremans R, Hiele M. Predictability of the postoperative course of Crohn's disease. Gastroenterology. 1990;99:956–63.

Rutgeerts P, Geboes K, Vantrappen G et al. Rifabutin and ethambutol do not help recurrent Crohn's disease in the neoterminal ileum. J Clin Gastroenterol. 1992;15:24–8.

Rutgeerts P, Lofberg R, Malchow H et al. Budesonide versus prednisolone for the treatment of active ileocecal Crohn's disease: a European multicenter trial. Gastroenterology. 1993;104A:772.

Ryder SD, Walker RJ, Jones H, Rhodes JM. Rectal bismuth subsalicylate as therapy for ulcerative colitis. Aliment Pharmacol Ther. 1990;4:333–8.

Salomon P, Kornbluth AA, Janowitz HD. Treatment of ulcerative colitis with fish oil n-3-omega-fatty acid: an open trial. J Clin Gastroenterol. 1990;12:157–61.

Salomon P, Kornbluth A, Aisennberg J et al. How effective are current drugs for Crohn's disease? J Clin Gastroenterol. 1992;14:211.

Sandberg-Gertzen H, Jarnerot G, Kraaz W. Azodisal sodium in the treatment of ulcerative colitis: a study of tolerance and relapse-prevention properties. Gastroenterology. 1986;90:1024–30.

Sandborn WJ, Tremaine WJ. Cyclosporine treatment of inflammatory bowel disease. Mayo Clin Proc. 1992;67:981–90.

Sandborn WJ, Strong RM, Forland SC, Chase RL, Cutler RE. Cyclosporin pharmacokinetics and colon tissue concentration after oral administration of retention enema in man. Gastroenterology. 1990;98:A202.

Sandborn WJ, Goldman DH, Lawson GM, Perrault J. Measurement of colonic tissue cyclosporine concentration in children with severe ulcerative colitis. J Pediatr Gastroenterol Nutr. 1992;15:125–9.

Sandborn WJ, Tremaine WJ, Schroeder KW et al. Cyclosporine enemas for treatment-resistant, mildly to moderately active, left-sided ulcerative colitis. Am J Gastroenterol. 1993;88:640–5.

Sandberg-Gertzen H, Jarnerot G, Kraaz W. Azodisal sodium in the treatment of ulcerative colitis. A study of tolerance and relapse-preventing properties. Gastroenterology. 1986;90:1024.

Scheppach W, Sommer H, Kirchner T et al. Effect of butyrate enemas on the colonic mucosa in distal ulcerative colitis. Gastroenterology. 1992;103:51–6.

Schreiber S, Howaldt S, Reinecker HC et al. Maintenance treatment of Crohn's disease: comparative study of 4-aminosalicylic acid and 5-aminosalicylic acid (Claversal®) slow release tablets. Gastroenterology. 1992;102:A692.

Schroeder KW, Tremaine WJ, Ilstrup DM. Coated oral 5-aminosalicylic acid therapy for mildly to moderately active ulcerative colitis: a randomized study. N Engl J Med. 1986;217:1625–9.

Schroeder KW, Tremaine WJ, Ilstrup DM. Coated oral 5-aminosalicylic acid therapy for mildly to moderately active ulcerative colitis: a randomized study. N Engl J Med. 1987;317:1625–9.

Scrivusta BD, Russell MAN, Masterson JG. Transdermal nicotine in ulcerative colitis. 1991;100:A252.

Selby WS, Barr GD, Ireland A et al. Olsalazine in active ulcerative colitis. Br Med J. 1985;291:1373.

Senagore AJ, Mackeigan JM, Scheider M, Ebrom S. Short-chain fatty acid enemas: a cost effective alternative in the treatment of nonspecific proctosigmoiditis. Dis Colon Rectum. 1992;35:923–7.

Singleton JW. Azathioprine has a very limited role in the treatment of Crohn's disease. Dig Dis Sci. 1982;26:368–71.

Singleton JW, Law DH, Kelley MI, Mekhjian HS, Sturdevant RAL. National Cooperative Crohn's Disease Study: adverse reactions to study drugs. Gastroenterology. 1979;77:870–82.

Singleton JW, Hanauer SB, Gitnick GL et al and the Pentasa Crohn's Study Group. Mesalamine capsules for the treatment of active Crohn's disease: results of a 16-week trial. Gastroenterology. 1993;104:1293–300.

Sitzmann JV, Converse RL Jr, Bayless TM. Favourable response to parenteral nutrition and medical therapy in Crohn's colitis. Gastroenterology. 1990;99:1647–52.

Sninsky CA, Cort DH, Shanahan F et al. Oral mesalamine (Asacol) for mildly to moderately active ulcerative colitis: a multicenter study. Ann Intern Med. 1991;115:350–5.

Steinhart AH, Baker JP, Brezezinski A, Prokipchuc EJ. Azathioprine therapy in chronic ulcerative colitis. J Clin Gastroenterol. 1990;12:271–5.

Stenson WF, Lauritsen K, Laursen LS et al. A clinical trial of Zileuton, a specific inhibitor of 5-lipoxygenase, in ulcerative colitis. Gastroenterology. 1991;100:A253.

Stenson WF, Cort D, Rodgers J et al. Dietary supplementation with fish oil in ulcerative colitis. Ann Intern Med. 1992;115:609–14.

Sturdevant RAL, Singleton JW, Deren JJ, Law DH, McCleery JL. Azathioprine-related pancreatitis in patients with Crohn's disease. Gastroenterology. 1979;77:883–86.

Summers WRW, Switz DM, Sessions JT et al. National Cooperative Crohn's Disease Study: results of drug treatment. Gastroenterology. 1979;77:847–69.

Sutherland LR. 5-Aminosalicylates for prevention of recurrence in patients with Crohn's disease: time for a reappraisal [editorial]? J Clin Gastroenterol. 1991;13:5–7.

Sutherland LR, Godet PG. Pharmacologic treatment of inflammatory bowel disease. Can Ther. 1994 (In press).

Sutherland LR, Ramcharan S, Bryant H, Fick G. Effect of cigarette smoking on recurrence of Crohn's disease. Gastroenterology. 1990a;98:1123–8.

Sutherland LR, Robinson M, Onstad G et al. A double-blind, placebo-controlled multicentre study of the efficacy and safety of 5-aminosalicylic acid (5-ASA) tablets in the treatment of ulcerative colitis. Falk Symposium Foundation, Freiburg, Germany, 1990b, p. 45.

Sutherland L, Singleton J, Session J et al. Double-blind, placebo-controlled trial of metronidazole in Crohn's disease. Gut. 1991;32:1071–75.

Sutherland LR, May GR, Schaeffer EA. Sulfasalazine revisited: a metaanalysis of 5-aminosalicylic acid in the treatment of ulcerative colitis. Ann Intern Med. 1993;118:540.

Teahon K, Bjarnason I, Pearson M, Levi AJ. Ten years' experience with an elemental diet in the management of Crohn's disease. Gut. 1990;31:1133–7.

Teahon K, Smethurst P, Pearson M, Levi AJ, Bjarnason I. The effect of elemental diet on intestinal permeability and inflammation in Crohn's disease. Gastroenterology. 1991;101:84–9.

Thomson ABR. Review article: new developments in the use of 5-aminosalicylic acid in patients with inflammatory bowel disease. Aliment Pharmacol Ther. 1991;5:449–70.

Thomson ABR, International Mesalazine Study Group. Coated oral 5-aminosalicylic acid versus placebo in maintaining remission in inactive Crohn's disease. Aliment Pharmacol Ther. 1990;4:55.

Tremaine WJ. Maintenance of remission in Crohn's disease: is 5-aminosalicylic acid the answer? Gastroenterology. 1992;103:694–704.

Tripathi RC, Kirschner BS, Kipp M et al. Corticosteroid treatment for inflammatory bowel disease in pediatric patients increases intraocular pressure. Gastroenterology. 1992a;102:1957–61.

Truelove SC, Jewell DP. Intensive intravenous regimen for severe attacks of ulcerative colitis. Lancet. 1974a;1:1067–70.

Truelove SC, Jewell DPL. Intravenous regimen for severe attacks of ulcerative colitis. Lancet. 1974b;1:1086–8.

Tytgat GNJ, Van Deventer SJH. Pouchitis. Int J Colon Dis. 1988;3:226–8.

Ursing B, Alm T, Barany F et al. A comparative study of metronidazole and sulfasalazine for active Crohn's disease: the cooperative Crohn's disease study in Sweden. II. Result. Gastroenterology. 1982;83:550–62.

Van Hees PAM, van Elteren PH, van Lier HJJ, van Tongeren JHM. An index of inflammatory activity in patients with Crohn's disease. Gut. 1980;21:279–86.

Van Hees PAM, Lier HJJ, Van Elteren PH et al. Effect of sulfasalazine in patients with active Crohn's disease: a controlled double-blind study. Gut. 1981;22:404.

Vantrappen G, Rutgeerts P. Recurrence of Crohn's disease in the neoterminal ileum after ileal resection and ileocolonic anastomosis. Verk K Acad Geneeskd Bldg. 1990;52:373–82.

Verhave M, Winter HS, Grand RJ. Azathioprine in the treatment of children with inflammatory bowel disease. J Pediatr. 1990;117:809–14.

Williams CN. Role of rectal formulations: suppositories. Scand J Gastroenterol. 1990;25(Suppl.172):60–2.

Willoughby JMT, Kumar PJ, Beckett J, Dawson AM. Controlled trial of azathioprine in Crohn's disease. Lancet. 1971;2:944–7.

Winter T, Dalton HR, Merrett MN, Campbell A, Jewell DP. Cyclosporin A retention enemas in refractory distal ulcerative colitis: an open trial. Gastroenterology. 1992;102:A947.

Wolf JL. Cipoflaxacin may be useful in Crohn's disease. Gastroenterology. 1990;98:A212.

Wright JP. Factors influencing first relapse in patients with Crohn's disease. J Clin Gastroenterol. 1992;15:12–16.

Wright JP, Boniface UA, Warner L. Sucralfate enemas in the treatment of ulcerative proctitis. Gastroenterology. 1992;102:A714.

Zaytoun AM, Cobden I, Al Mardini H, Record CO. Morphometric studies in rectal biopsy specimens from patients with ulcerative colitis: effect of oral 5-amino salicylic acid and rectal prednisolone treatment. Gut. 1991;32:183–7.

Zinberg J, Molinas S, Das KM. Double-blind placebo-controlled study of olsalazine in the treatment of ulcerative colitis. Am J Gastroenterol. 1990;85:562–6.

42
Therapy of IBD in 1994: a surgeon's perspective

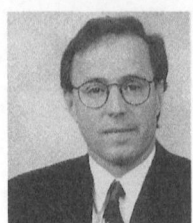

Z. COHEN

INTRODUCTION

The options of surgical therapy for ulcerative colitis patients include total proctocolectomy and Brooke ileostomy, total proctocolectomy and the continent ileostomy, subtotal colectomy and ileorectal anastomosis, as well as the pelvic pouch procedure. A stoma is required for the first two mentioned procedures, and no stoma is required for subtotal colectomy and ileorectal anastomosis and the pelvic pouch procedure. In our experience, as well as others, there are very few candidates that are now acceptable for a colectomy and ileorectal anastomosis alone. All of the above procedures achieve continence except for the conventional ileostomy, but the reoperation rates for all of the procedures vary from 25–50% with the continent ileostomy to ~10–12% following the pelvic pouch procedure. With all types of surgeries there may be failures of therapy. As will be discussed below, the morbidity following a pelvic pouch procedure is considerable, and must be weighed against doing this procedure versus a total proctocolectomy and Brooke ileostomy. However, it must be stated that surgery is curative for ulcerative colitis, and 'avoidance of colectomy' should not be the major outcome measure when one is assessing a patient for either medical or surgery therapy. The disease is completely removed with any form of total proctocolectomy and in most cases with the pelvic pouch procedure, although recently the transitional zone as well as 1–2 cm of anal mucosa may be left behind using a stapled technique for the pelvic pouch procedure. There have been no cancers reported in any of the pouches made for either the continent ileostomy or the pelvic pouch procedure. However, there have been two reported cases of cancer originating in the rectal cuff of patients who have had an incomplete mucosectomy where the indication for surgery was dysplasia[1].

Surgical options for patients with ulcerative colitis must therefore be presented in light of the psychological and psychosocial problems that may occur with patients undergoing a total proctocolectomy and Brooke ileostomy versus the technical difficulties, surgical complications and functional outcome of patients undergoing the pelvic pouch procedure.

In our own experience, as well as in others, since the mid-1970s the procedures of choice for patients with ulcerative colitis have shifted from total proctocolectomy and Brooke ileostomy to the continent ileostomy initially, and since the early 1980s almost exclusively to the pelvic pouch procedure. There are very few patients who are considered suitable candidates for the continent ileostomy, and again only a limited number of patients who wish to choose a total proctocolectomy and a Brooke ileostomy. Colectomy and ileorectal anastomosis in ulcerative colitis has become a rare procedure in our experience.

CONTROVERSIES RELATED TO THE PELVIC POUCH PROCEDURE

The pelvic pouch procedure has become the operation of choice in our own institution for patients undergoing surgery for ulcerative colitis. However, there remain areas of controversy. These include pouch configuration, anal sphincter pressure changes, the original diagnosis and pouchitis. Although there have been numerous studies with the 'J', 'S', 'H', 'K' and 'W' pouches, I believe that the pouch configuration in and of itself is not of much significance. The important fact is to have the ability to create more than one type of pouch, in case one has to change the pouch configuration in order to achieve more length to do a tension-free ileoanal anastomosis. It is well known that the resting anal pressure decreases following pelvic pouch surgery, and never really returns to be perfectly normal, although this does not seem to influence the functional results to a great extent. The original diagnosis is also important in that patients undergoing pelvic pouch surgery for ulcerative colitis have a poorer outcome in general than those undergoing the same surgery for familial polyposis. Pouchitis is a clinical syndrome which manifests itself usually with fatigue, anemia, changes in stool consistency and frequency, and often an endoscopic appearance of acute or chronic inflammation. Only in our own series has there been an association with stenosis at the outlet[2]. As far as age is concerned it is well described that patients over the age of 50 have a poorer result than those under the age of 50[3].

Quality-of-life assessments are, in and of themselves, quite difficult. However, in an attempt to delineate whether or not the pelvic pouch patients have a better outcome than those undergoing a Kock pouch or a conventional ileostomy, a study was undertaken using 36 patients having had a pelvic pouch, 28 with a Kock pouch and 30 with a conventional ileostomy[4]. These patients were chosen at random, but all had had their surgery at least 1 year previously and were in a stable condition. Using both the time trade-off technique and the direct questioning of objectives as methodological tools to assess quality of life, there were no significant differences in the patients undergoing the various procedures. However, what was evident was that all had an extremely good quality of life whichever surgical option was chosen.

Whether or not a mucosectomy and sutured anastomoses or a stapled anastomosis should be performed is still somewhat controversial, and if mucosa is left behind, what is the actual cancer risk? Another controversial area relates to whether or not a single versus a staged procedure should be performed, and whether an ileostomy should be performed in conjunction with the pelvic pouch procedure.

In most instances the stapled anastomosis does leave behind not only the transitional zone, but 1–2 cm of anal mucosa. Lofberg et al.[6] reported a case showing dysplasia and DNA aneuploidy in a pelvic pouch. This is the only reported case of dysplasia in either a pelvic pouch or a Kock pouch, and there have been no reports of cancer developing. Stern et al.[1] reported cancer in an ileoanal reservoir, but the cancer itself originated in the rectal mucosa that had been incompletely excised. This occurred in a patient who had a long rectal cuff where the indication for surgery was dysplasia. Thus if there is severe dysplasia in the anorectal area preoperatively, options to the pelvic pouch procedure should be considered. In addition, if severe extra-intestinal manifestations of ulcerative colitis exist, then a total mucosectomy and not a stapled anastomosis should be performed. There has been one other case report of cancer in a rectal cuff. However, it should be stressed that, with more recent techniques, (leaving no rectal cuff but only the residual anal mucosa) this problem should be minimized. In addition, there are very few cases of anal canal cancer developing in patients who have ulcerative colitis. Therefore, it is felt by ourselves, as well as most institutions, that a stapled anastomosis, leaving 1–2 cm of residual anorectal mucosa, is a safe and appropriate procedure.

We have also recently compared the outcome of patients who have had a hand-sewn ileoanal anastomosis to those who had a stapled ileoanal anastomosis with or without a defunctioning ileostomy[7]. Our patients were divided into three groups – group 1 were patients with a hand-sewn anastomosis and a defunctioning ileostomy, group 2 were those patients with a stapled ileoanal anastomosis and a defunctioning ileostomy, and group 3 were those patients with a stapled ileoanal anastomosis without a defunctioning ileostomy. The outcome measures were leak rate, surgical complications, reoperation rate and functional outcome. Factors analyzed for their effect on the leak rate included age, sex, steroid usage, weight, intraoperative difficulty, anastomotic staple technique, severity of disease at the distal margin and whether or not the patient had a previous subtotal colectomy.

The early surgical complications showed that the leak rate in group 1 patients was 12%, in group 2 patients it was 7% and in group 3 patients it was 18%. In group 3 patients, 13 out of 71 patients had a leak at the ileoanal anastomosis. However, only one of these required a reoperation in the form of a defunctioning ileostomy. The remainder were treated with intravenous antibiotics, drainage of the pouch with a rectal tube, and total parenteral nutrition if necessary. With this treatment regimen 11 of the 13 patients healed their leak and were fully continent. Their functional outcome was no different from those who did not have a leak.

Of the 22 patients who had a true single-stage procedure, seven or 32% of the patients developed a leak. In those patients who had a previous subtotal colectomy only 12% developed a leak. Other factors that influenced the leak rate were the amount of steroids utilized by patients preoperatively – those who were less than 40 years of age who had a 13% leak rate as opposed to those who were greater than 40 years of age who had a 35% leak rate and, in our own experience, males who had a 23% leak rate versus females who had an 11% leak rate.

It is therefore our experience, and our recommendation, that a true single-stage procedure should not be performed because of the high leak rate, but that a pelvic pouch procedure can be performed without a defunctioning ileostomy in patients who have already had a previous subtotal colectomy.

STRICTUREPLASTY IN THE MANAGEMENT OF CROHN'S DISEASE

The management of Crohn's disease has evolved since the mid-1930s from radical excision of bowel and lymph nodes to minimal surgical procedures including strictureplasty for obstructive disease. This is justified by the fact that Crohn's disease is a panintestinal disease which appears focally and cannot be cured. Our objective therefore should be to alleviate symptomatology. Surgery must be safe and provide minimal mortality and long-term survival, but it is not absolutely necessary to remove all diseased tissue, as not all of the diseased tissue will cause symptoms. It is also well known that stenosis can be overcome by either Heineke–Mikulicz or Finney-type strictureplasties. Our recent results following strictureplasty in patients from 1985 to 1993 revealed that we have performed a total of 143 strictureplasties in 37 patients, 25 of whom were males. The follow-up has been a mean of 50.2 months with a range of 2–92 months. Indications for strictureplasty in all have been obstruction. In one case a patient with duodenal obstruction underwent strictureplasty. The other sites of strictureplasty included the jejunum (85 strictureplasties), the ileum (54 strictureplasties), and the site of the previous ileocolonic anastomosis (3 strictureplasties).

In long-term follow-up of these 37 patients, 20 have not been rehospitalized or reoperated upon. Three have been rehospitalized but not reoperated upon, and 14 have been rehospitalized and reoperated upon. Of the 14 who have undergone reoperation, resection of the strictureplasty was carried out in nine, restrictureplasty in three, a new strictureplasty was carried out in six of the patients, and resection alone in eight. The indication in all of these patients for reoperation was obstruction and progression of their Crohn's disease. Variables that possibly affected the reoperation rate were compared. None of the following achieved statistical significance including the type of procedure – whether the strictureplasty was performed alone or with a resection, the type of strictureplasty, whether or not the patient had undergone previous surgery, the number of strictureplasties performed and the site of the disease. However, it must be stated that of 11 patients who underwent strictureplasty alone, only two have required reoperation (18%), whereas in those who have undergone strictureplasty and resection, 12 of 26 (46%) have required reoperation. The patients requiring strictureplasty alone may represent a subset of patients who have a specific type of disease which allows for a longer recurrence-free interval.

One can conclude, however, that strictureplasty is a safe procedure, as we have only had one leak and one fistula in our entire series. It is effective, at least in the short term, in overcoming obstruction. Active disease may become quiescent, although the natural history of the disease is usually progressive. Only those patients who have multiple obstructions and are at risk for developing a short bowel syndrome should have this procedure performed.

ASSESSMENT OF TRIALS USING METHOTREXATE AND CYCLOSPORINE

As mentioned previously, 'avoidance of colectomy', stated in many manuscripts, is a poor outcome measure of medical treatment, particularly when one can cure ulcerative colitis with a surgical procedure. What appears to be lacking in a number of assessments in both medical and surgical treatments is the quality of life produced with these interventions. It is therefore very important to assess the quality of life with validated instruments such as the time trade-off technique, direct questioning of objectives or the Inflammatory Bowel Disease Questionnaire, which has recently been described[8]. It is somewhat disheartening for a surgeon to read the medical literature when statements such as 'the goal of the acute phase of therapy is simply to avoid colectomy'[9] and 'Methotrexate studied by Kozarek's group has already proven to be efficacious in refractory inflammatory bowel disease'[9]. These statements were made in a recent paper by Simon Lichtiger[9]. Other statements such as 'the much-awaited controlled study from Brynskov showed effectiveness in 59% of those patients studied with moderate Crohn's disease'[10] and a report by C. N. Williams et al. stated that 'colectomy could be avoided in the majority of patients treated with cyclosporine for severe Crohn's colitis'[11].

In assessing the results of therapy of patients with Crohn's disease treated with methotrexate, Kozarek et al. in 1989 reported on a nonrandomized open-label preliminary 12-week trial in 21 patients who had refractory IBD[12]. Seventeen of these patients were on steroids. Twenty-five milligrams of methotrexate was used intramuscularly weekly for 12 weeks, and the patients were then switched to an oral form of the drug. These patients were followed clinically and objectively using a modified CDAI with an index score of 0–15 and a clinical activity index for ulcerative colitis of 0–15. The results showed that 11 of 14 Crohn's disease patients had their CDAI fall from 13.3 to 5.4, and five of seven ulcerative colitis patients had their clinical activity index fall from 13.3 to 6.3. Although these results were encouraging, there was no determination of the dose required, the route of administration or the length of treatment. The following year, the quotation by Lichtiger stated that treatment with methotrexate in this setting was efficacious[9]. However, in the follow-up paper by Kozarek's group in 1992[13], where the follow-up was for a 4-year period in 86 patients, 50% of the patients had already had a colectomy, and only 12 of 30 remained on methotrexate as well as steroids in the ulcerative colitis group. In the Crohn's disease group the follow-up was on 69 patients, and 51% remained on methotrexate plus prednisone. In the study there was no real assessment of the quality of life, and the conclusion was that a significant number of patients with severe IBD did become refractory to methotrexate. Although their early results might have been encouraging, the later follow-up showed a refractoriness to the drug as well as the potential for long-term side-effects if this drug were used. One must also consider the ethical dilemma of treating ulcerative colitis patients with long-term immunosuppressive drugs when one considers that ulcerative colitis is a potentially curable disease when treated surgically.

Arora et al.[14] reported on a double-blind placebo-controlled trial of methotrexate in Crohn's disease, and although there were fewer flare-ups of the disease on methotrexate, the side-effects were very significant and the compliance was poor, with only 31% of the patients on methotrexate completing a 52-week course of the drug.

As far as the use of cyclosporine in ulcerative colitis is concerned, Lichtiger et al. reported in 1990 on 24 patients who underwent both an acute and chronic phase of cyclosporine therapy[9]. Nineteen of 24 patients were considered acute responders and 13 of 19 patients were considered chronic responders. Overall the follow-up was short, and only 13 of 24 succeeded. These patients were followed using a modified clinical activity index with a score of > 12 determining severe disease, a score of ≤ 6 being success in the acute phase, or at least a 50% reduction in their score also being success in the acute phase. A score of ≤ 4 was required to represent a successful outcome in the chronic phase of their study. Once again, no quality-of-life assessments were undertaken in this study. The disease severity assessment was weighted with the following outcome measures: diarrhea, nocturnal diarrhea, blood in the stool, fecal incontinence, abdominal pain and cramping, general well-being, abdominal tenderness and antidiarrheals.

In the acute phase of this study whereby a score of ≤ 6, or a 50% reduction in the severity of the clinical index, indicated success, one could use examples which show that patients who have seven to nine bowel movements per day with some blood in the stool, abdominal cramping and localized tenderness, could have a score of 6. As far as a surgeon is concerned, localized tenderness can be a very serious problem, and one must question whether a patient with a clinical activity of 6 manifesting the symptoms mentioned above should be considered a success. In addition, a patient who feels poorly having five or six bowel movements per day could also have a score of 6. In the chronic phase, where success was related to a score of ≤ 4, a patient who had only an average general well-being with localized tenderness could also have a score of 4. In addition, a patient with severe or rebound tenderness with three or four bowel movements per day could have a score of 4. Of interest is the fact that six of the first 15 patients entered into the chronic phase actually had a clinical activity score of greater than 6 (average 7–9).

In a follow-up study reported in 1993 using i.v. cyclosporine 4 mg/kg per day, and switching to oral cyclosporine 8 mg/kg per day when a successful outcome was achieved, nine of 11 patients were successful in the acute phase on i.v. cyclosporine, and none of the nine on placebo were considered successful until some of these latter patients were crossed over to receive i.v. cyclosporine[15]. There appeared to be an advantage for the acute-phase therapy of i.v. cyclosporine in ulcerative colitis. What are the potential long-term side-effects using cyclosporine, and what might be the refractoriness of the disease to cyclosporine? What is the potential for malignancy if one were to maintain a patient on cyclosporine and steroids? These are very important questions to ask before suggesting cyclosporine use for these patients.

As far as cyclosporine use in Crohn's disease is concerned, Brynskov's study did show that 59% of patients on cyclosporine over a 3-month period did improve, but so did 32% of the placebo patients[10]. In addition, 36% of the patients relapsed after stopping the cyclosporine treatment, and this again brings up the question of how to treat the patient in the long term. The Canadian Crohn's Relapse Prevention Trial showed no improvement in the Crohn's patients treated with cyclosporine, and no improvement in the CDAI, or in the quality of life or percentage of steroids used[16]. In the low-activity stratum the placebo group did better than the cyclosporine-treated group. In the study reported by the Williams group[11], 'avoidance of colectomy' again was used as an outcome measure. Twenty-one percent had early colectomy. Another 21% came to colectomy an average of 73 weeks after initiation of therapy, and 21% of patients had surgery in the form of strictureplasty or small-bowel resection, but did not have their colons removed. Therefore, in assessing this study, only 27% of patients did not come to surgery. Of importance in this study was that there were three deaths: two were related to sepsis and one to a cerebrovascular accident. All of these deaths could be attributed to the use of cyclosporine. Although the conclusion from the study was that colectomy could be avoided in the majority of patients treated with cyclosporine for severe colitis, a surgical viewpoint would look upon this with extreme skepticism, and ask at what price is this avoidance of colectomy or surgery?

TOXICITY OF MEDICATIONS AND SURGERY

In addition to looking strictly at outcome measures one must consider the potential toxic effects of medical treatment and the potential morbidity incurred with surgery. The mainstay of therapy for patients with Crohn's disease and a number of patients with ulcerative colitis is steroids. However, the list of side-effects when using long-term corticosteroids is significant. These include moon facies in 47% of patients, acne in 30%, infection in 27%, striae in 23%, depression in 20%, hypertension in 13%, osteopenia in 30%, osteonecrosis in 4%, psychosis in 2% and growth retardation as well as pancreatitis and diabetes in a number of patients.

Cyclosporine also has a great potential for producing side-effects. In reviewing the literature on the use of cyclosporine in IBD, the following represent the major toxic effects as well as the percentages. Nephrotoxicity 7.5–10%, paraesthesias 36–45%, hypertension 20%, headache 5%, seizures and other neurological events 9–12%, hypertrichosis 25%, gastrointestinal distress 10%, gingival hypertrophy 5% and other miscellaneous causes[17]. In addition, one must stress once again that the use of cyclosporine and steroids in combination may in fact produce malignancy which heretofore has not been reported.

Methotrexate toxicity includes pneumonitis, gastrointestinal distress and biochemical liver abnormalities[14]. Although medical therapy is associated with very significant toxic effects, one must also consider the implications of ileostomies and pelvic pouch surgery in patients undergoing these procedures for ulcerative colitis. The sepsis, leak, abscess and fistula rate following the pelvic pouch procedure ranges from 8% to 15%. Although not specific for the operation, intestinal obstruction occurs in 10–20% of cases, pouchitis in 10–30% of cases, sexual dysfunction in both males and females in 5–10% of patients, strictures in 5%, loop ileostomy complications in 25% of patients and pouch excision in 5–8%[18,19].

Therefore, in summary, both medical and surgical therapies have their own resultant toxicity and morbidity, and this must be taken into consideration when managing these patients.

It is important to think of an IBD patient undergoing a combined multidisciplinary approach from both the physician and the surgeon. It is no longer acceptable for one or the other group to treat these patients in isolation, with their own biases. To that end it is my own viewpoint that both medical and surgical and/or combined trials of various medications or surgery should be undertaken. Importantly, before utilizing long-term immunosuppressive agents, one must consider the quality of life produced while being on medical agents versus surgical therapy.

For ulcerative colitis, therefore, it is my strong belief that long-term management of ulcerative colitis with potent immunosuppressives is potentially dangerous in a surgically curable disease. The results of surgery are certainly not perfect, but the quality of life will be improved with whatever surgical procedure is undertaken. 'Avoidance of colectomy' is a poor indicator of the results without factoring in quality-of-life measurements, and the perception of surgery or a stoma is far worse than reality for the patients.

In Crohn's disease, both medical and surgical therapies do have a role. Methotrexate and cyclosporine do not appear at the moment to be the long-term answer for these patients. As far as strictureplasty is concerned, although it is effective in overcoming obstructive episodes, it does not appear to change the natural history of the disease in the long term.

Management of patients with IBD can be extremely challenging and difficult. Patients, however, must be well aware of all of the options of therapy – both medical and surgical – and must be involved in the decision-making process. Gastroenterologists and surgeons must come together in their thinking about IBD patients, and continue to undertake trials of both medical and surgical therapies in order to determine the best management for any individual patient.

References

1. Stern H, Walfisch S, Mullen B, McLeod RS, Cohen Z. Cancer in an ileo-anal reservoir – a new late complication. Gut. 1990;3:473–5.
2. Fleshman JW, Cohen Z, McLeod RS, Stern H, Blair J. The ileal reservoir and ileo-anal anastomosis procedure – factors affecting technical and functional outcome. Dis Colon Rectum. 1989;31:10–16.
3. McIntyre TB, Pemberton J, Wolff B, Beart R, Dozois R. Comparing functional results one year and ten years after ileal pouch anal anastomosis for chronic ulcerative colitis. Dis Colon Rectum. 1994;37:303–7.
4. McLeod RS, Churchill N, Lock A, Vandenburg H, Cohen Z. Assessment of quality of life of patients with ulcerative colitis preoperatively and postoperatively. Gastroenterology. 1991;101:1307–13.
5. Cohen Z. Ileo-anal pouches – is mucosectomy necessary? Can J Gastroenterol. 1993;7:1–3.
6. Lofberg R, Liljeqvust L, Lindquist K, Veress B, Reinholt GP, Tribukait B. Dysplasia and DNA aneuploidy in a pelvic pouch. Dis Colon Rectum. 1991;34:280–4.
7. Cohen Z, Steven W, O'Connor B, Stern H, McLeod RS. Continuing evolution of the pelvic pouch procedure. Surgery. 1992;216:506–12.
8. Archambault A, Feagan B, Fedorak R et al. The Canadian Crohn's Disease Relapse Prevention Trial (CCRPT). Gastroenterology. 1992;102:A591.
9. Lichtiger S. Cyclosporine therapy in inflammatory bowel disease – open-label experience. Mount Sinai J Med. 1990;57:315–19.
10. Lichtiger S, Present DH. Preliminary report: cyclosporine in treatment of severe active ulcerative colitis. Lancet. 1990;336:16–19.
11. Leddin DJ, Vanzanten V, Sidorov JJ, Stewart J, Tripathi D, Williams CD. Colectomy following treatment of Crohn's colitis with cyclosporin. Post presentation. Trends in Inflammatory Bowel Disease Therapy. Victoria, British Columbia, April 1994.
12. Kozarek RA, Patterson DJ, Gelfand MD, Botoman VA, Ball TJ, Wilske KR. Methotrexate induces clinical and histologic remission in patients with refractory inflammatory bowel disease. Ann Intern Med. 1989;110:353–6.
13. Kozarek RA, Patterson DJ, Gelfand MD, Ball TJ, Botomon VA. Long-term use of methotrexate in inflammatory bowel disease: severe disease 3, Drug Therapy 2. Seventh inning stretch. Gastroenterology. 1992;102:A648(abstr.).
14. Arora S, Katkov WN, Cooley J et al. A double blind, randomized, placebo-controlled trial of methotrexate in Crohn's disease. Gastroenterology. 1993;102:A647.
15. Lichtiger S, Present DH, Kornbluth A, Hanauer S. Cyclosporin A in the treatment of severe, refractory ulcerative colitis: a double blinded placebo controlled trial. Gastroenterology. 1993;102(4):A732.
16. Archambault A, Feagan B, Fedorak R et al. The Canadian Crohn's Relapse Prevention Trial. Gastroenterology. 1992;4:A591.
17. Corman E, Reinus JF. Cyclosporine use in steroid-resistant Crohn's disease – grasping at new straws? Am J Gastroenterol. 1990;85:758–9.
18. Pemberton JH, Kelly KA, Beart RW, Dozois R, Wolff B, Ilstrup DM. Ileal pouch anal anastomosis for chronic ulcerative colitis – long term results. Ann Surg. 1987;206:504–13.
19. Salemans JM, Nagengast M, Lubbers EJ, Kuijpers JH. Postoperative and long-term results of ileal pouch anal anastomosis for ulcerative colitis in familial polyposis. Dig Dis Sci. 1992;37:1882–9.

Index